Curcumin in Health and Disease

Curcumin in Health and Disease

Special Issue Editor
Beatrice E. Bachmeier

MDPI • Basel • Beijing • Wuhan • Barcelona • Belgrade

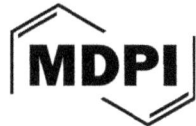

Special Issue Editor
Beatrice E. Bachmeier
Competence Center for Complementary
Medicine and Naturopathy,
Technical University
Germany

Editorial Office
MDPI
St. Alban-Anlage 66
4052 Basel, Switzerland

This is a reprint of articles from the Special Issue published online in the open access journal *International Journal of Molecular Sciences* (ISSN 1422-0067) from 2018 to 2019 (available at: https://www.mdpi.com/journal/ijms/special_issues/curcumin_health)

For citation purposes, cite each article independently as indicated on the article page online and as indicated below:

LastName, A.A.; LastName, B.B.; LastName, C.C. Article Title. *Journal Name* **Year**, *Article Number*, Page Range.

ISBN 978-3-03921-449-5 (Pbk)
ISBN 978-3-03921-450-1 (PDF)

Cover image courtesy of Beatrice E. Bachmeier.

© 2019 by the authors. Articles in this book are Open Access and distributed under the Creative Commons Attribution (CC BY) license, which allows users to download, copy and build upon published articles, as long as the author and publisher are properly credited, which ensures maximum dissemination and a wider impact of our publications.

The book as a whole is distributed by MDPI under the terms and conditions of the Creative Commons license CC BY-NC-ND.

Contents

About the Special Issue Editor vii

Beatrice E. Bachmeier and Dieter Melchart
Therapeutic Effects of Curcumin—From Traditional Past to Present and Future Clinical Applications
Reprinted from: *Int. J. Mol. Sci.* **2019**, *20*, 3757, doi:10.3390/ijms20153757 1

Ella Willenbacher, Shah Zeb Khan, Sara Cecilia Altuna Mujica, Dario Trapani, Sadaqat Hussain, Dominik Wolf, Wolfgang Willenbacher, Gilbert Spizzo and Andreas Seeber
Curcumin: New Insights into an Ancient Ingredient against Cancer
Reprinted from: *Int. J. Mol. Sci.* **2019**, *20*, 1808, doi:10.3390/ijms20081808 6

Panchanan Maiti, Jason Scott, Dipanwita Sengupta, Abeer Al-Gharaibeh and Gary L. Dunbar
Curcumin and Solid Lipid Curcumin Particles Induce Autophagy, but Inhibit Mitophagy and the PI3K-Akt/mTOR Pathway in Cultured Glioblastoma Cells
Reprinted from: *Int. J. Mol. Sci.* **2019**, *20*, 399, doi:10.3390/ijms20020399 19

Jochen Rutz, Sebastian Maxeiner, Eva Juengel, August Bernd, Stefan Kippenberger, Nadja Zöller, Felix K.-H. Chun and Roman A. Blaheta
Growth and Proliferation of Renal Cell Carcinoma Cells Is Blocked by Low Curcumin Concentrations Combined with Visible Light Irradiation
Reprinted from: *Int. J. Mol. Sci.* **2019**, *20*, 1464, doi:10.3390/ijms20061464 39

Vesselina Laubach, Roland Kaufmann, August Bernd, Stefan Kippenberger and Nadja Zöller
Extrinsic or Intrinsic Apoptosis by Curcumin and Light: Still a Mystery
Reprinted from: *Int. J. Mol. Sci.* **2019**, *20*, 905, doi:10.3390/ijms20040905 56

Mhd Anas Tomeh, Roja Hadianamrei and Xiubo Zhao
A Review of Curcumin and Its Derivatives as Anticancer Agents
Reprinted from: *Int. J. Mol. Sci.* **2019**, *20*, 1033, doi:10.3390/ijms20051033 69

Renata Novak Kujundžić, Višnja Stepanić, Lidija Milković, Ana Čipak Gašparović, Marko Tomljanović and Koraljka Gall Trošelj
Curcumin and its Potential for Systemic Targeting of Inflamm-Aging and Metabolic Reprogramming in Cancer
Reprinted from: *Int. J. Mol. Sci.* **2019**, *20*, 1180, doi:10.3390/ijms20051180 95

Anna Bielak-Zmijewska, Wioleta Grabowska, Agata Ciolko, Agnieszka Bojko, Grażyna Mosieniak, Łukasz Bijoch and Ewa Sikora
The Role of Curcumin in the Modulation of Ageing
Reprinted from: *Int. J. Mol. Sci.* **2019**, *20*, 1239, doi:10.3390/ijms20051239 119

Slawomir Kwiecien, Marcin Magierowski, Jolanta Majka, Agata Ptak-Belowska, Dagmara Wojcik, Zbigniew Sliwowski, Katarzyna Magierowska and Tomasz Brzozowski
Curcumin: A Potent Protectant against Esophageal and Gastric Disorders
Reprinted from: *Int. J. Mol. Sci.* **2019**, *20*, 1477, doi:10.3390/ijms20061477 141

Kathryn Burge, Aarthi Gunasekaran, Jeffrey Eckert and Hala Chaaban
Curcumin and Intestinal Inflammatory Diseases: Molecular Mechanisms of Protection
Reprinted from: *Int. J. Mol. Sci.* **2019**, *20*, 1912, doi:10.3390/ijms20081912 155

Martina Barchitta, Andrea Maugeri, Giuliana Favara, Roberta Magnano San Lio, Giuseppe Evola, Antonella Agodi and Guido Basile
Nutrition and Wound Healing: An Overview Focusing on the Beneficial Effects of Curcumin
Reprinted from: *Int. J. Mol. Sci.* **2019**, *20*, 1119, doi:10.3390/ijms20051119 . . . . **191**

Ryszard Pluta, Marzena Ułamek-Kozioł and Stanisław J. Czuczwar
Neuroprotective and Neurological/Cognitive Enhancement Effects of Curcumin after Brain Ischemia Injury with Alzheimer's Disease Phenotype
Reprinted from: *Int. J. Mol. Sci.* **2018**, *19*, 4002, doi:10.3390/ijms19124002 . . . . **205**

Nelson Ferreira, Maria João Saraiva and Maria Rosário Almeida
Uncovering the Neuroprotective Mechanisms of Curcumin on Transthyretin Amyloidosis
Reprinted from: *Int. J. Mol. Sci.* **2019**, *20*, 1287, doi:10.3390/ijms20061287 . . . . **221**

Lidia Czernicka, Agnieszka Grzegorczyk, Zbigniew Marzec, Beata Antosiewicz, Anna Malm and Wirginia Kukula-Koch
Antimicrobial Potential of Single Metabolites of Curcuma longa Assessed in the Total Extract by Thin-Layer Chromatography-Based Bioautography and Image Analysis
Reprinted from: *Int. J. Mol. Sci.* **2019**, *20*, 898, doi:10.3390/ijms20040898 . . . . **234**

Zwe-Ling Kong, Hsiang-Ping Kuo, Athira Johnson, Li-Cyuan Wu and Ke Liang B. Chang
Curcumin-Loaded Mesoporous Silica Nanoparticles Markedly Enhanced Cytotoxicity in Hepatocellular Carcinoma Cells
Reprinted from: *Int. J. Mol. Sci.* **2019**, *20*, 2918, doi:10.3390/ijms20122918 . . . . **246**

About the Special Issue Editor

Beatrice E. Bachmeier has a Master's degree in chemistry from the University of Regensburg, Germany and a PhD degree from the Medical Faculty of the Ludwig-Maximilians-University (LMU), Munich, Germany. After completing her PhD thesis, her continued preclinical research at the LMU led to her habilitation in the fields of oncology and molecular pathobiochemistry. Currently, she is Professor at the Medical Faculty of the LMU and Assistant Director of the Competence Center for Complementary Medicine and Naturopathy of the Technical University, Munich, Germany.

Her research interests are focused on the translation of experimental/preclinical research observations to clinical application with particular reference to the use of natural compounds in oncology. In this context, specific topics of her research encompass therapy resistance, molecular/diagnostic markers of efficacy, cellular pathways of natural compounds, and chemoprevention of cancer.

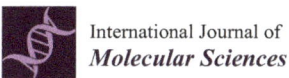

Editorial

Therapeutic Effects of Curcumin—From Traditional Past to Present and Future Clinical Applications

Beatrice E. Bachmeier [1,2,*] and Dieter Melchart [1,3]

1. Competence Center for Complementary Medicine and Naturopathy [CoCoNat], Technical University Munich, 80807 Munich, Germany
2. Institute of Laboratory Medicine, University Hospital, LMU Munich, 80807 Munich, Germany
3. Institute for Complementary and Integrative Medicine, University Hospital Zurich and University of Zurich, CH-8091 Zurich, Switzerland
* Correspondence: Beatrice.bachmeier@tum.de

Received: 18 July 2019; Accepted: 31 July 2019; Published: 1 August 2019

Abstract: The efficacy of the plant-derived polyphenol curcumin, in various aspects of health and wellbeing, is matter of public interest. An internet search of the term "Curcumin" displays about 12 million hits. Among the multitudinous information presented on partly doubtful websites, there are reports attracting the reader with promises ranging from eternal youth to cures for incurable diseases. Unfortunately, many of these reports are not based on scientific evidence, but they feed the desideratum of the reader for a "miracle cure". This circumstance makes it very difficult for researchers, who work in a scientifically sound and evidence-based manner on the therapeutic benefits (or side effects) of curcumin, to demarcate their results from sensational reports that circulate in the web and in other media. This is only one of many obstacles making it difficult to pave curcumin's way into clinical application; others are its nonpatentability and low economic usability. A further impediment comes from scientists who never worked with curcumin or any other natural plant-derived compound in their own labs. They have never tested these compounds in any scientific assay, neither in vitro nor in vivo; however, they claim, in a sometimes polemic manner, that everything that has so far been published on curcumin's molecular effects, is based on artefacts. The here presented Special Issue comprises a collection of five scientifically sound articles and nine reviews reporting on the therapeutic benefits and the molecular mechanisms of curcumin or of chemically modified curcumin in various diseases ranging from malignant tumors to chronic diseases, microbial infection, and even neurodegenerative diseases. The excellent results of the scientific projects that underlie the five original papers give reason to hope that curcumin will be part of novel treatment strategies in the near future—either as monotherapy or in combination with other drugs or therapeutic applications.

1. Curcumin's Therapeutic Potential and Novel Therapeutic Approaches

The natural polyphenol curcumin is derived from the plant *Curcuma longa* Linn, a member of the Zingiberaceae, naturally occurring throughout tropical and subtropical regions of the world. Curcumin has been used in Ayurveda and traditional Chinese medicine for thousands of years to treat inflammatory diseases and bacterial infections [1].

1.1. Neoplastic Diseases

Because of its anti-apoptotic and antiproliferative efficacy, its ability to interfere with several tumor progression associated signaling pathways, and to modulate tumor-associated miRNA expression, curcumin is regarded as antitumorigenic [2,3]. In addition, curcumin prevents formation of breast and prostate metastases in vivo [4–6]. The review by Willenbacher et al. in this issue summarizes some papers that have been published in the field of curcumin's antitumorigenic effects.

Curcumin is also potent against cancer types that are difficult to treat, like melanoma [7–9] or glioblastoma [10], as demonstrated by the work of Maiti et al. in this issue. They observed increased levels of autophagy and decreased levels of mitophagy markers, along with inhibition of the PI3K-Akt/mTOR pathway after treatment of glioblastoma cells with curcumin or solid lipid curcumin particles. Renal cell carcinoma is relatively rare, with rates of approximately 3% of all adult cancer patients; however, one-third of the patients have metastases at diagnosis and are resistant to most treatments like chemotherapy or radiation. In this context, complementary and alternative treatment strategies are highly desiderated by concerned patients. Blaheta and colleagues as well as Zöller and coworkers describe the very promising effects of a novel therapy combining the application of curcumin with visible light exposure. In detail, the combination therapy inhibits growth and proliferation of tumor cells and induces apoptosis.

In the context of curcumin's molecular modes of action, resulting in its antitumorigenic effects, it seems likely to draw some attention on its molecular structure. Tomeh and coworkers bring some light into this aspect by summarizing what is so far known on the correlation between molecular mechanisms, cellular pathways, and structural characteristics of curcumin and its derivatives.

1.2. Aging

The ability to modulate the transcription factor NFκB explains curcumin's anti-inflammatory effect [1,2,11–13]. Aging and age-related diseases also come along with chronic inflammation. The correlation between cancer and inflammation dates back to Virchow who suggested that "lymphoreticular" infiltrates reflect the origin of cancer at sites of chronic inflammation, and that there are striking similarities between ulcers, wound healing, and cancer [14]. The paper by Kujundži´ et al gives an overview on scientific data that would enable establishing connections and functional links between the specific of "inflamm-agin" and the cancer cell's metabolism, its proliferative potential, and curcumin's pleiotropic activity. In this context, Bielak-Zmijewska and coworkers also summarize scientific data on curcumin's ability to postpone progression of age-related diseases in which cellular senescence is directly involved. They furthermore point out that curcumin causes elongation of the lifespan of model organisms and alleviates aging symptoms. In addition, they discuss thoroughly curcumin's ability to modulate cellular senescence.

1.3. Inflammatory Disorders

Because of its scientifically evidenced characteristics to interfere with a variety of signal transduction pathways, transcription factors, and cellular processes, curcumin can potentially be applied in the treatment of many diseases (inflammatory disorders in particular). In this context, curcumin has been used to treat gastrointestinal diseases such as indigestion, flatulence diarrhea, and even gastric and duodenal ulcers [11,15,16]. Kwiecien and colleagues summarize in their review curcumin's protective effects against esophageal and gastric disorders. In addition, curcumin is potentially efficacious against intestinal inflammatory diseases. Burge and colleagues discuss the beneficial effects of curcumin on the microbiome, its antimicrobial properties, inhibition of TLR4/NFκB/AP-1 signal transduction, changes in cytokine profiles, and alterations to immune cell maturation and differentiation. The combination of all these molecular actions makes curcumin a promising candidate to treat intestinal inflammatory diseases like necrotizing enterocolitis, Crohn's disease, and ulcerative colitis.

Curcumin can also improve wound healing. Barchitta and coworkers point out that curcumin induces apoptosis of inflammatory cells during the early phase of wound healing and could accelerate the healing process by shortening the inflammatory phase. Moreover, curcumin might facilitate collagen synthesis, fibroblast migration, and differentiation.

1.4. Neurodegenerative Diseases

Lately, evidence has accumulated that curcumin has neuroprotective properties and is a candidate for the treatment of Alzheimer's disease. In their review, Pluta and colleagues focus on the role and mechanisms of curcumin in inhibiting ischemia/reperfusion brain injury and potential therapeutic strategies in the treatment of ischemic brain damage of the Alzheimer's disease phenotype. Comparably, Ferreira and colleagues also delineate neuroprotective characteristics by summarizing what is known about the role of curcumin on transthyretin amyloidosis. According to previous reports, curcumin modulates abnormal transthyretin (TTR) aggregation and inhibits its deposition in the tissue. The pleiotropic activities of curcumin provide multiple ways to tackle TTR pathophysiology, through direct interaction of curcumin with TTR, or indirect effects affecting signaling pathways associated with TTR amyloid fibril formation and clearance.

1.5. Infectious Diseases

The treatment of bacterial infections has become extremely challenging due to resistance against antibiotics available in the pharmaceutical market. Moreover, another important issue to be addressed is that common antibiotics evoke adverse events. In this context, phytotherapeutic approaches become popular for patients who are searching for alternatives to standard treatments. There are numerous reports that have already delineated not only the antibacterial but also the antiviral and antifungal activities of curcumin. [17]. In this Special Issue, Czernicka and coworkers focus on the antimicrobial potential of single components of the *Curcuma longa* crude extract against a variety of Gram-positive bacteria strains.

1.6. Remarks on Solubility and Bioavailability

Despite curcumin's therapeutic potential *in vitro* and *in vivo*, it has to be considered that the molecule is lipophilic and hardly soluble in water. Up to now it is not fully understood how curcumin reaches the target organ in order to exert its therapeutic effects and how it becomes metabolized in the human body. In order to overcome these pharmacological problems, several attempts have been undertaken to encapsulate curcumin into nanoparticles in order to ensure that curcumin is transported easily in the bloodstream. In the current issue, Kong and coworkers present their data on a novel formulation of curcumin-loaded mesoporous silica nanoparticles with higher antioxidant activity, antitumor activity, higher cytotoxicity, and stability as compared to the curcumin molecule itself. However, cytotoxicity of these nanoparticle carriers has to be explored in depth before we get too enthusiastic about this idea.

2. Conclusions

In recent years, curcumin's reputation regarding its therapeutic effects has been damaged. In molecular drug screening tests, and partly polemic publications, curcumin has been declared to belong to the PAINS (pan assay interference compounds) [18] and to yield confusing results because curcumin does not have one single drug target [19]. The authors of these disparagements gained their information from results generated in high-throughput screenings. However, high-throughput screenings are prone to technical artefacts and, therefore, are a deceptive tool because potential drug candidates could be missed. Additionally, the fact that curcumin, like many other natural compounds, has more than one drug target indicates its versatile applicability and its low risk to cause acquired therapy resistance [20–22].

A crucial state of mind is prerequisite for good quality of research and every reputable scientist questions not only the results of other fellow colleagues but also their own. It is our task and responsibility to provide good quality of research and, of course, it can happen that carelessly executed research projects and results are published—sometimes even in high ranked papers.

However, this holds true not only for curcumin but also for other bioactive compounds, no matter if they are plant-derived or if they have been developed and chemically synthesized in Pharma industry. While reasonable doubt is essential for scientifically sound results, it doesn't make sense to disparage everything that has so far been published on curcumin's therapeutic effects in treating chronic and neoplastic diseases and to declare that all results are artefacts. Instead, we should accept the challenge to distinguish between scientifically sound and false results; otherwise, we lose a promising candidate for complementary and alternative treatment strategies.

Additionally, we should not challenge treatment successes of Ayurveda or traditional Chinese medicine, where plant-derived compounds like curcumin have been applied efficaciously to treat inflammatory diseases and bacterial infections for thousands of years. To disclaim treatment success of traditional medicine would simply be ignorant.

Curcumin's detractors criticize that it has never been shown to be conclusively effective in a randomized, placebo-controlled clinical trial for any indication [19]. To this end it has to be considered that it is almost impossible to get financial support to conduct a clinical trial with a substance that cannot be patented and, therefore, is economically uninteresting. Another point is the study design—curcumin cannot be tested in randomized, placebo-controlled trials because, nowadays, clinical trials are performed in the form "study compound against standard therapy", otherwise the trial would not get a positive vote from the ethics committee. Therefore, the question is: against which compound should we test curcumin?

There is no doubt, that due to the comprehensive data from preclinical studies, together with first results from single patients or small cohorts, the next task on the list has to be to test Curcumin in well-designed clinical trials. However, the greatest challenge will be to find sponsors for clinical research on curcumin, as this promising plant-derived compound cannot be exploited economically.

Conflicts of Interest: The authors declare no conflict of interest.

References

1. Chainani-Wu, N. Safety and anti-inflammatory activity of curcumin: A component of tumeric [*Curcuma longa*]. *J. Altern. Complement. Med.* **2003**, *9*, 161–168. [CrossRef] [PubMed]
2. Bachmeier, B.E.; Killian, P.; Pfeffer, U.; Nerlich, A.G. Novel aspects for the application of Curcumin in chemoprevention of various cancers. *Front. Biosci.* **2010**, *2*, 697–717. [CrossRef]
3. Kronski, E.; Fiori, M.E.; Barbieri, O.; Astigiano, S.; Mirisola, V.; Killian, P.H.; Bruno, A.; Pagani, A.; Rovera, F.; Pfeffer, U.; et al. miR181b is induced by the chemopreventive polyphenol curcumin and inhibits breast cancer metastasis via down-regulation of the inflammatory cytokines CXCL1 and -2. *Mol. Oncol.* **2014**, *8*, 581–595. [CrossRef] [PubMed]
4. Bachmeier, B.E.; Killian, P.H.; Melchart, D. The Role of Curcumin in Prevention and Management of Metastatic Disease. *Int. J. Mol. Sci.* **2018**, *19*, 1716. [CrossRef] [PubMed]
5. Killian, P.H.; Kronski, E.; Michalik, K.M.; Barbieri, O.; Astigiano, S.; Sommerhoff, C.P.; Pfeffer, U.; Nerlich, A.G.; Bachmeier, B.E. Curcumin inhibits prostate cancer metastasis in vivo by targeting the inflammatory cytokines CXCL1 and -2. *Carcinogenesis* **2012**, *33*, 2507–2519. [CrossRef]
6. Bachmeier, B.; Nerlich, A.G.; Iancu, C.M.; Cilli, M.; Schleicher, E.; Vene, R.; Dell'Eva, R.; Jochum, M.; Albini, A.; Pfeffer, U. The chemopreventive polyphenol Curcumin prevents hematogenous breast cancer metastases in immunodeficient mice. *Cell. Physiol. Biochem.* **2007**, *19*, 137–152. [CrossRef] [PubMed]
7. Marin, Y.E.; Wall, B.A.; Wang, S.; Namkoong, J.; Martino, J.J.; Suh, J.; Lee, H.J.; Rabson, A.B.; Yang, C.S.; Chen, S.; et al. Curcumin downregulates the constitutive activity of NF-kappaB and induces apoptosis in novel mouse melanoma cells. *Melanoma Res.* **2007**, *17*, 274–283. [CrossRef]
8. Siwak, D.R.; Shishodia, S.; Aggarwal, B.B.; Kurzrock, R. Curcumin-induced antiproliferative and proapoptotic effects in melanoma cells are associated with suppression of IkappaB kinase and nuclear factor kappaB activity and are independent of the B-Raf/mitogen-activated/extracellular signal-regulated protein kinase pathway and the Akt pathway. *Cancer* **2005**, *104*, 879–890.
9. Bachmeier, B.E.; Iancu, C.M.; Killian, P.H.; Kronski, E.; Mirisola, V.; Angelini, G.; Jochum, M.; Nerlich, A.G.; Pfeffer, U. Overexpression of the ATP binding cassette gene ABCA1 determines resistance to Curcumin in M14 melanoma cells. *Mol. Cancer* **2009**, *8*, 129. [CrossRef]
10. Zhao, J.; Zhu, J.; Lv, X.; Xing, J.; Liu, S.; Chen, C.; Xu, Y. Curcumin potentiates the potent antitumor activity of ACNU against glioblastoma by suppressing the PI3K/AKT and NF-kappaB/COX-2 signaling pathways. *Onco Targets Ther.* **2017**, *10*, 5471–5482. [CrossRef]

11. Menon, V.P.; Sudheer, A.R. Antioxidant and anti-inflammatory properties of curcumin. *Adv. Exp. Med. Biol.* **2007**, *595*, 105–125. [PubMed]
12. Rahman, I.; Biswas, S.K.; Kirkham, P.A. Regulation of inflammation and redox signaling by dietary polyphenols. *Biochem. Pharmacol.* **2006**, *72*, 1439–1452. [CrossRef] [PubMed]
13. Jobin, C.; Bradham, C.A.; Russo, M.P.; Juma, B.; Narula, A.S.; Brenner, D.A.; Sartor, R.B. Curcumin blocks cytokine-mediated NF-kappa B activation and proinflammatory gene expression by inhibiting inhibitory factor I-kappa B kinase activity. *J. Immunol.* **1999**, *163*, 3474–3483. [PubMed]
14. Balkwill, F.; Mantovani, A. Inflammation and cancer: Back to Virchow? *Lancet* **2001**, *357*, 539–545. [CrossRef]
15. Goel, A.; Kunnumakkara, A.B.; Aggarwal, B.B. Curcumin as "Curecumin": From kitchen to clinic. *Biochem. Pharmacol.* **2008**, *75*, 787–809. [CrossRef]
16. Hatcher, H.; Planalp, R.; Cho, J.; Torti, F.M.; Torti, S.V. Curcumin: From ancient medicine to current clinical trials. *Cell. Mol. Life Sci.* **2008**, *65*, 1631–1652. [CrossRef] [PubMed]
17. Moghadamtousi, S.Z.; Kadir, H.A.; Hassandarvish, P.; Tajik, H.; Abubakar, S.; Zandi, K. A review on antibacterial, antiviral, and antifungal activity of curcumin. *BioMed Res. Int.* **2014**, *2014*, 186864.
18. Baell, J.; Walters, M.A. Chemistry: Chemical con artists foil drug discovery. *Nature* **2014**, *513*, 481–483. [CrossRef]
19. Nelson, K.M.; Dahlin, J.L.; Bisson, J.; Graham, J.; Pauli, G.F.; Walters, M.A. The Essential Medicinal Chemistry of Curcumin. *J. Med. Chem.* **2017**, *60*, 1620–1637. [CrossRef]
20. Heger, M. Drug screening: Don't discount all curcumin trial data. *Nature* **2017**, *543*, 40. [CrossRef]
21. Heger, M.; van Golen, R.F.; Broekgaarden, M.; Michel, M.C. The molecular basis for the pharmacokinetics and pharmacodynamics of curcumin and its metabolites in relation to cancer. *Pharmacol. Rev.* **2014**, *66*, 222–307. [CrossRef] [PubMed]
22. Lee, K.W.; Bode, A.M.; Dong, Z. Molecular targets of phytochemicals for cancer prevention. *Nat. Rev. Cancer* **2011**, *11*, 211–218. [CrossRef] [PubMed]

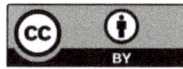

© 2019 by the authors. Licensee MDPI, Basel, Switzerland. This article is an open access article distributed under the terms and conditions of the Creative Commons Attribution (CC BY) license (http://creativecommons.org/licenses/by/4.0/).

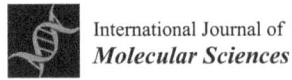

Review

Curcumin: New Insights into an Ancient Ingredient against Cancer

Ella Willenbacher [1], Shah Zeb Khan [2], Sara Cecilia Altuna Mujica [3], Dario Trapani [4], Sadaqat Hussain [5], Dominik Wolf [1], Wolfgang Willenbacher [1,6], Gilbert Spizzo [1,7] and Andreas Seeber [1,*]

1. Department of Internal Medicine V: Hematology and Oncology, Medical University of Innsbruck, Innsbruck 6020, Austria; ella.willenbacher@i-med.ac.at (E.W.); dominik.wolf@i-med.ac.at (D.W.); wolfgang.willenbacher@tirol-kliniken.at (W.W.); gilbert.spizzo@i-med.ac.at (G.S.)
2. Department of Clinical Oncology, BINOR Cancer Hospital, Bannu 28100, Pakistan; skhanizhere0@gmail.com
3. Department of Molecular Biology, Laboratorio Blau, Caracas 1071, Venezuela; altunamujica.md@gmail.com
4. Department of Oncology and Hematology, University of Milan, European Institute of Oncology, 20122 Milan, Italy; dario.trapani@ieo.it
5. Medical Oncology Department, KAMC NGHA, Riyadh 14413, Saudi Arabia; oncologysh@gmail.com
6. Oncotyrol, Center for Personalized Cancer Therapy, Innsbruck 6020, Austria
7. Oncologic Day Hospital, 39042 Bressanone, Italy
* Correspondence: andreas.seeber@tirol-kliniken.at; Tel.: 0043-50504-23001

Received: 14 March 2019; Accepted: 10 April 2019; Published: 12 April 2019

Abstract: Cancer patients frequently use complementary medicine. Curcumin (CUR) and its derivates (from the extract of *Curcuma longa* L.) represent some of the most frequently used ones, having a long history in traditional Asian medicine. CUR was demonstrated, both in vitro and in vivo, to have significant anti-inflammatory effects, thus potentially counteracting cancer-promoting inflammation, which is a hallmark of cancer. CUR modulate a plethora of signaling pathways in cancer cells, comprising the NF-κB (nuclear factor k-light-chain-enhancer of activated B cells), the JAK/STAT (Janus-Kinase/Signal Transducers and Activators of Transcription), and the TGF-β (transforming growth factor-β) pathways. Furthermore, CUR confers properties of electron receptors, which destabilize radical oxygen species (ROS), explaining its antioxidant and anti-apopototic effects. Although CUR has a low bioavailability, its role in advanced cancer treatment and supportive care was addressed in numerous clinical trials. After promising results in phase I–II trials, multiple phase III trials in different indications are currently under way to test for direct anti-cancer effects. In addition, CUR exerts beneficial effects on cancer treatment-related neurotoxcity, cardiotoxicity, nephrotoxicity, hemato-toxicity, and others. More efficient galenic formulations are tested to optimze CUR's usability in cancer treatment. This review should provide a comprehensive overview of basic science, and pre-clinical and clinical data on CUR in the field of oncology.

Keywords: curcumin; complementary medicine; cancer treatment; supportive care; antioxidants; anti-inflamation

---

1. Introduction

Cancer patients frequently use natural and herbal products during cancer treatment. A recent Italian review reported that half of all cancer patients use complementary and/or alternative medical (CAM) approaches [1]; however, the choice of CAM varies widely and may also depend on the cultural setting and availability of interventions and drugs.

Oncologic healthcare professionals should provide non-judgmental and evidence-based support to cancer patients and guarantee the safety of cancer treatment by adopting a clinical and research-based approach to complementary and alternative medicine. Numerous natural products or substances derived from plants or other life forms were evaluated in different medical conditions, especially in cancer.

Curcumin (CUR) and its derivates represent one of these products and are derived from the extract of *Curcuma longa* L. (turmeric rhizomes) [1,2]. Turmeric is a plant used for thousands of years in Asia, especially in the Vedic culture in India, where it is frequently used as a culinary spice or a dye and represents a component of traditional Chinese medicine and other medical cultures [3]. Curcuminoids include also demethoxycurcumin and bisdemethoxycurcumin, and most preparations that are available today are heterogenic biological mixtures of extracts of *Curcuma longa*. One must take into account that curcuminoids are of variable solubility [4], and the major problem when using curcuminoids is represented by its low bioavailability because of poor solubility [5]. Hence, high single doses of CUR are required to achieve detectable levels in serum of healthy volunteers [6]. Thus, different strategies were tested to overcome these limits, such as liposome-based formulations, and emulsion or microsphere preparations of CUR [7–9], all of which were developed with the ultimate goal of optimizing its bioavailability.

However, despite these unfavourable galenic properties, CUR displays several positive effects in vivo and in vitro. Due to its high concentration in the gastrointestinal tract for example, Shen et al. demonstrated a regulative effect of CUR with respect to microbial composition in the gastro-intestinal (GI) tract of C57BL/6 mice [10]. One of the most promising CUR effects, however, appears to be its anti-inflammatory potential. Tabrizi et al. summarized these effects by showing that CUR modulates inflammatory biomarkers such as IL-6 (Interleukin-6) and hs-CRP (high-sensitivity c-reactive protein) [11]. In line with these observations, a Cochrane analysis showed that CUR might be a safe and an effective therapy for maintenance of remission in quiescent ulcerative colitis [12].

Chronic inflammation is characterized as an emergent "hallmark of cancer" by driving malignant transformation on cancer progression [13]. Therefore, the capacity of the proven anti-inflammatory compound CUR to modulate signaling pathways in cancer cells was widely investigated. The most important of these are the NF-κB (nuclear factor k-light-chain-enhancer of activated B cells) pathway [14], the JAK/STAT (Janus-Kinase / Signal Transducers and Activators of Transcription) pathway [15], and the TGF-β axis [16]. All of these were demonstrated to be potentially modulated by CUR [14–16].

These pathways are particularly important in multiple neoplasia, and one of the most interesting aspects of recent research on CUR is the focus on cancer treatment and prophylaxis. Given the complexity of cancer medicine, natural products such as CUR might play a role in specific treatments, as well as in in supportive care. Thus, based on these observations, the present review aims to provide an overview on the most important aspects of CUR and cancer, focusing both on potential mechanisms of action, as well as results of clinical trials.

2. Effects of Curcumin on Tumor Cells, Metabolism, and Signaling Pathways

In addition to its anti-inflammatory properties, CUR was shown to exihibit antioxidant effects in cellular models both in vitro and in vivo. A molecular structure rich in phenol groups and biophysical characteristics allow CUR to interact with many different proteins at different stages, which may explain the diverse antitumor effects [17]. The regulation of enzymes and the activation and deactivation of growth pathways and programmed cell death make CUR a potential therapeutic agent for a broad spectrum of cancers, since the effects observed in cancer cell models could not be replicated in non-neoplastic cells. This fact may explain the low toxicity reported in interventional trials in humans [18].

It is still to be determined if the resulting putative anti-cancer effects derive from the products available after degradation, since CUR has a low oral bioavailability, undergoes first-pass metabolism, is hydrophobic, and consecutively does not reach high plasma levels [19]. Therefore, the synthesis of curcuminoid analogs may improve the bioavailability and effectiveness of CUR [20].

The presence of phenolic analogs in CUR confers properties of electron receptors, which destabilize radical oxygen species (ROS), explaining the observed antioxidant effects. There are multiple in vitro models demonstrating the avidity for electrons and an ROS scavenging activity [21]. CUR is, therefore, active in the repair mechanismns of DNA due to ultraviolet (UV) damage and stress, and it reduces ROS compounds that play a role in early carcinogenesis [22].

CUR further influences cytochrome P450 isoforms and has a direct effect on phase I and phase II metabolism, inhibiting the production of toxins that potentially act as carcinogens. This action on early cancer-initiating events may at least in part explain the protective potential of CUR with respect to malignant transformation and cancer progression [23].

In tumor cells, the interaction with ROS is considered as one of the main triggers of apoptosis. Syng-ai et al. [23] demonstrated that depletion of glutathione sensitized cells to CUR effects, and also downregulated the expression of Bcl-2 (B-cell lymphoma 2) in breast cancer and hepatoma cell cultures, which may be responsible for making them more vulnerable to apoptotic death. These effects were not observed in normal cells, which did not experience variation in superoxide generation.

The modulation of the inducible nitric oxide synthase gene expression derives lower concentrations of nitric oxide in macrophages, resulting in inhibition of carcinogenesis [24]. The effects of curcumin on GST (Glutathione-S-Transferase) metabolism, paired with the inhibition of immortalizing pathways and other enzymes that result in free ROS, contribute in the preliminary stages of cancer formation, and have direct involvement in the induction of apoptosis in tumor cells.

The interaction with other proteins has an anti-inflammatory effect. Pignanelli et al. [20] synthesized CUR analogs capable of efficiently killing triple-negative, inflammatory breast, p53-negative colorectal, and different blood cancer cell lines, by manipulating and increasing ROS species specifically in these cells, which translates to the induction of apoptosis. These analogs also proved to be more toxic and effective than natural CUR, with lower intracellular concentrations achieving the same effects.

CUR also has a direct effect on the synthesis of pro-inflammatory cytokines that perpetuate inflammation in favor of tumor growth. The inhibition of the COX2 (cyclooxygenase-2) and NF-κB genes derives an anti-inflammatory effect with a reduction in the synthesis of cytokines and pro-mitotic proteins, since genes regulated by NF-κB include cyclin-D1, Bcl-2, MMP-9 (matrix metalloproteinase-9), and several cytokines such as TNF-α (tumor necrosis factor-α) and many others [25]. In rat models of hemorrhagic resuscitation, Maheshwari et al. demonstrated that the exposure to CUR resulted in significant reduction of of pro-inflammatory cytokines such as IL-1α, IL-1β, IL-2, IL-6, and IL-10 to almost normal levels [26].

The antitumor effects of CUR revolve around the induction of apoptosis through the complex interaction of proteins in the STAT-3, HIF1/ROS (hypoxia inducible factor 1/reactive oxygen species), Wnt/β-catenin, and Sp-1 (specificity protein 1) pathways, as well as induction of the caspase pathways, mainly through the activation of caspase-3 and caspase-8, and endoplasmatic reticulum and mitochondrial stress [27]. The downregulation of the expression of anti-apoptotic genes such as Bcl-2 and Bcl-X makes cancer cells more vulnerable to apoptosis and, in cellular models with Bcl-2 overexpression, some analogs deactivate the Fas (CD95)-associated protein with death domain, resulting in programmed cell death [28]. CUR can also inhibit growth promoters and growth factors, such as EGFR (epithelial growth factor receptor) and cyclin D1 [28].

In prostate cancer cell and xenograft murine models, cyclohexanone curcumin analogs decreased invasion, migration, and ability to metastasize due to decreased matrix metalloproteinase production [29]. Other observations potentially explaining anti-metastatic properties include modulation of vascular endothelial growth factor (VEGF) synthesis, thus directly impacting angiogenesis [26]. Kunnumakkara et al. reported inhibition of VEGF production in orthotopic pancreatic and ovarian cancer cells implanted in mice [30].

A third path to cell death, autophagy, also known as type II cell death, is linked to CUR activity. The activation of the mTOR (mechanistic target of rapamycin) pathway seems to regulate autophagy in cancer cells through the complex mTORC1, and CUR deactivates this regulation by deactivation of the PI3K (Phosphoinositide 3-kinase)/Akt/mTOR pathway, extensively demonstrated in multiple cell culture models [31].

Another interaction with the mTOR pathway that leads to cell death is the inhibition of the aerobic glycolysis in anaerobic conditions (Warburg effect), which is promoted in cancer cells by the HIF1α pathway. Through the direct downregulation of pyruvate kinase M2 and modulation of mTOR, CUR decreases intracellular levels of HIF1α and glucose uptake, contributing to apoptosis [32].

The hepatocyte growth factor (HGF)/mesenchymal–epithelial transition factor (MET) axis is a further disregulated pathway in cancer which provokes tumor proliferation, as well as therapy escape [33]. As such, it is considered as a poor prognostic marker. In vitro data using different lung cancer cell lines showed that CUR inhibits HGF-induced migration and blocks the c-Met/Akt/mTOR signaling pathway. In a further mouse model, the authors illustrated that CUR induces an upregulation of epidermal markers (i.e., E-cadherin) and a downregulation of mesenchymal factors (i.e., vimentin). The authors concluded that these results suggest that CUR could inhibit epidermal-to-mesenchymal transition (EMT) by targeting the HFG/MET pathway [34].

CUR also demonstrates multiple effects on cancer stem cells, which remain dormant and unaffected by traditional chemotherapies and, therefore, enable tumor re-growth, leading to overt relapse after treatment. Varying doses and duration of administration of CUR on cancer stem cells using a wide array of cell cultures models (breast, colon, and lung cancer) showed antitumor activity, with a reduction in the formation of new spheres, activation of caspases, and other pro-apoptotic proteins, as well as downregulation of markers for stemness (CD133, CD44, ALDH1 [aldehyde dehydrogenasis]), increased availability, and activation of PARP (poly[ADP-ribose]-polymerase) inducing sensitivity to anti-cancer drugs like 5-fluoruracil and dasatinib in colon cancer cells, and cisplatinum in lung cancer cells [35]. Hedgehog signaling (HH) is a substantial pathway in cancer stem cells and in carcinogenesis. In the liver for example, HH signaling activation leads to the development of cirrhosis and liver cancer. The activation of this pathway correlates with a higly aggressive cancer by enhancing development of metatastasis and tumor growth [36]. HH signaling is essential to maintain the stemness in of cancer stem cells. In various two- and three-dimensional (2D and 3D) culture models, CUR decreased the activity of cancer stem cells by inhibiting tumor cell proliferation, downregulating cancer stem-cell markers (i.e., CD44 and Oct4 [octamer-binding transcription factor 4]), and inducing apoptosis [37–39]. Another research group showed in an in vitro experiment that CUR could not only inhibit proliferation and invasion by inhibiting the HH pathway, but could also induce expression of EMT-related markers [40].

There is evidence for the existence of synergistic effects with traditional anti-cancer therapies, due to the induction of apoptosis through the targeting of several pro-apoptotic and anti-proliferative pathways in different in vitro models. In an experimental model published by Zhang et al., the combination of CUR with cisplatinum in lung cancer xenograft murine models effectively demonstrated reduction of Sp-1 binding to CTR1 (copper uptake protein 1) promoters, increasing expression of CTR1 and Sp-1 and, thus, the uptake and sensitivity to cisplatinum in these cells [35]. Interestingly, antitumor effects were increased when both cisplatinum and CUR were combined and administered in increasing dosages, achieving significantly higher cell death and tumor regression rates compared to their application as monotherapy. Another possible synergistic interaction is with anti-EGFR therapy, targeting the EGFR/MAPK (mitogen-activated protein kinase) pathway known to stimulate cell proliferation [41]. Chen et al. [42] observed that simultaneous treatment with the anti-EGFR antibody cetuximab and CUR demonstrated suppression of the EGFR/MAPK pathway in oral cancer cells resistant to platinum.

Multiple observations of curcumin's anti-cancer effects were made in colon cancer xenograft models [43]. James and collegues demonstrated a direct effect on colon cancer stem cells derived from patients' metastatic tissue, noting a more dramatic decrease in formation of spheroids and expression of stemness biomarkers in cultures that received a combination of FOLFOX and CUR, suggesting there might be a synergistic effect, expressed also in longer DFS (disease-free survival) intervals of patients that received experimental therapy in this trial [44]. A summary of the interactions of CUR is listed in Table 1.

Table 1. Interactions between curcumin (CUR) and different pathways.

Pathway
Reduction of radical oxygen species (ROS)
Inhibiton of the production of toxins via cytochrome P450
Inhibition of COX2 and NF-κB
Reduction of proinflammatory cytokines (i.e., IL-1, IL-2)
Induction of caspase pathway (i.e. caspase-3)
Downregulation of anti-apoptotic genes (i.e., Bcl-2)
Inhibition of growth promoters (i.e., EGFR)
Decrease of MMP
Anti-metastatic properties (i.e., inhibition of VEGF)
Inhibition of PI3K/Akt/mTor pathway
Inhibtion of HIFα pathway
Downregulation of the HGF/MET pathway
Downregulation of stemness markers (i.e., CD133, CD44)
Inhibtion of the Hedghog signaling pathway

3. Clinical Data of Curcumin as a Therapeutical Anti-Cancer Compound

The first monotherapy assessment of pharmacokinetics and activity of CUR was reported in a phase I clinical trial assessing the safety of CUR in colorectal cancer patients, in a dose-finding design of an oral formulation [45]. No dose-limiting toxicities were observed in the 15 patients enrolled. Two patients (13%) exhibited stable disease by radiologic criteria after two months of treatment, receiving the treatment for a total of four months. One patient taking 450 mg of CUR daily and one patient allocated in the full dose group (3600 mg of CUR daily) developed significant diarrhea. However, the patient in the lower-dose cohort was able to optimize the management of this side effect with loperamide, while the patient taking the highest dose discontinued treatment, with rapid improvement of side effects. Accordingly, the authors defined a recommended phase II dose of 3600 mg daily as being suitable for further evaluations.

In a phase I dose-finding trial, CUR was analyzed in combination with docetaxel 100 mg/m^2 in 14 breast cancer patients [46]. Among eight patients evaluable for response, five (63%) showed a partial response. The maximal tolerated dose was established at 6000 mg daily for one week followed by two weeks off.

In a phase II clinical study conducted in patients with advanced pancreatic cancer, patients were enrolled to receive 8000 mg of CUR daily p.o. (per os) in combination with gemcitabine 1000 mg/m^2 intravenously weekly for three of four weeks [47]. CUR was split into two daily doses. Nearly one-third of the patients ($n = 5$) discontinued CUR due to toxicity and continued gemcitabine monotherapy. The principal adverse event causing the discontinuation of CUR was upper abdominal pain, presenting on average within two weeks from the beginning of the treatment, and not ameliorating with reduction of the CUR dose. Indeed, patients stopping CUR achieved a complete reversal of the symptoms, with no residual impairments. Time to progression was 2.5 months and overall survival was five months, consistent with the benefit achieved by gemcitabine in monotherapy of historical controls. In terms of disease control, five of 11 patients evaluable for response (45.5%) showed a clinical benefit, of which one (9.1%) had a partial response and four (36.4%) had a stable disease. The authors concluded that high-dose oral CUR in combination with chemotherapy is not an effective strategy, as the trial failed to demonstrate a safe feasibility of the combination regimen.

An additional phase II clinical trial conducted in patients with pretreated advanced pancreatic cancer ($n = 25$) received oral CUR 8000 mg daily as monotherapy until disease progression [1]. Of the patients evaluable for response ($n = 24$), two patients (8.3%) showed a clinical response. As expected, only low levels of CUR were detectable in plasma, i.e., 22–41 ng/mL at steady state. However, some pharmacodynamic assays along with the radiological tumor responses suggested a biologic activity at low bio-disponible plasma concentrations, with effects exerted on the expression of COX-2, NF-κB, and pSTAT3; no correlation of the cytokine change was demonstrated with either biologic activity or with clinical benefit [48].

The combination of CUR with tyrosine kinase inhibitors was investigated [49] in a cohort of patients receiving imatinib for CML (chronic myeloid leukemia) ($n = 50$), with or without turmeric powder (1500 mg daily). Patients who received CUR and imatinib together achieved a higher rate of clinical complete response compared to imatinib monotherapy. However, this finding was not statistically significant. Another imatinib combination was tested in a single patient with a pre-treated metastatic adenoid cystic parotid tumor, harbouring a c-KIT mutation [50]. The formulation used was intravenous CUR 225 mg/m^2 twice a week plus oral CUR 168 mg daily. The patient achieved a partial response still ongoing after 24 months of treatment.

As proof of concept, Capalbo et al. [51] provided a pivotal experience of a combination of CUR with monoclonal antibodies. The report described the case of an elderly platinum pre-treated cutaneous squamous cell carcinoma patient, receiving the EGFR monoclonal antibody blocker cetuximab combined with daily oral CUR phospholipid supplement (500 mg). Partial response was described, persistent for 11 months, with no evidence of tumor progression at the time of the last follow-up. The authors justified the decision to combine cetuximab with CUR as supposing to optimize the control of EGFR blocker-related skin adverse events based on a report ($n = 52$) by Wada et al. [52] and possibly potentiate the antineoplastic activity, overcoming the emergent resistance to EGFR blockers [53].

As a further attempt to optimize CUR bio-availability through drug delivery, liposomal CUR was tested in a phase I clinical trial in patients with advanced pre-treated solid tumors ($n = 32$) [54]. The liposomal formulation was administered intravenously as weekly infusion for eight weeks. Two patients experienced grade-3 anaemia and one patient experienced grade-3 hemolysis. One patient showed a clinical benefit, with a stable disease after four weeks.

The role of CUR was investigated in the prevention of cancer and treatment of pre-invasive tumors, reporting some preliminary results [55–57]. Oral and topic formulations were proposed, tailoring high-risk patients with CUR-based pharmacological interventions and tracking the reduction of pre-invasive lesions when exposed to CUR and related compounds. However, no definite role was defined in these settings, with discordant results in the clinical series, and results of ongoing trials are awaited.

The role of CUR in cancer treatment was addressed by numerous trials. Although apparently working at low plasma concentration, systemic bio-availability still represents an issue when dealing with CUR experiments in humans. Indeed, the optimization of CUR bio-availability through drug-delivery strategies provided more significant results, suggesting that in vitro and in vivo antitumoral activity can be replicated in the clinical setting by different pharmacological strategies. However, some of the results provided so far are no more than proof-of-concept studies, particularly for the combination with targeted agents, where only a few positive experiences are reported. Moreover, no phase III clinical trial provided results on the antitumor efficacy compared to the standard treatments, with efforts warranted in the definition of the disease most likely to benefit along with predictive biomarkers for better patient selection. For this, despite promising results and early signals of benefit, at present, no specific recommendation should be provided for CUR in the treatment of cancer, as data of safety are restricted to monotherapy and few combinations with selected agents, and data of activity are not mature enough. Eventually, the use of CUR to "adjuvate" the standard treatments should be discouraged unless new results will identify a precise setting of care as a pharmacological compound.

4. Role of Curcumin in Reducing Side Effects of Cytotoxic Drugs

Myelosuppresion is the most common side effect associated with chemotherapy. A murine model showed that, when CUR was administered after carboplatinum, it was able to reduce the length and depth of myelosuppression via reducing the DNA damage in the bone marrow [58].

One study found that use of CUR along with doxorubicin remarkably reduced the myocardial damage in albino rats [59]. The cardiac damage markers such as LDH (lactat dehydrogenasis) and CPK (creatininekinase) were also reduced, suggesting a protective role to anthracycline-induced cardiotoxicity. Another animal study on rats showed that cardiac damage due to doxorubicin was reduced due to CUR use [60]. CUR was shown to reduce the grade of lipid peroxidation and glutathione depletion—markers of oxidative stress. Furthermore, the levels of troponin, LDH, and a cardiac isoform of LDH decreased, along with an attenuation of pro-apoptotic signaling in myocardial cells, including pro-inflammatory mediators.

One experimental study on rats reported that CUR is effective in reducing weight loss and intestinal mucosal damage in 5-flurouracil use [61]. Importantly, no loss of the antineoplastic benefit of 5-flurouracil could be observed.

In a phase I study, a mucoadhesive formulation containing, among other compounds, CUR was tested as a mouth-washing solution for head and neck cancer patients. No genotoxic cellular damage was observed [62]. The formulation was shown to be clinically active with no apparent systemic adverse events.

The liver is the main site of metabolism of most chemotherapeutic drugs, and liver damage is a common toxicity of many cancer medicines. Cisplatinum damages the hepatocytes, resulting in the increase of serum ALT (alanine aminotransferasis) and AST (aspartate aminotransferasis). CUR pretreatment improved the hepatocyte damage due to cisplatinum in rats [63]. Another investigation showed that histopathologically confirmed methotrexate-induced liver damage in albino rats can be markedly reduced by post-methotrexate CUR administration [64].

Mitomycin-C is known for potentially causing severe toxicites to both kidney and bone marrow. An investigation was performed using a breast cancer xenograft model in which CUR was administered together with Mitomycin-C [65]. It showed that CUR decreased the kidney damage induced by Mitomycin-C, while at the same time sensitizing tumor cells to Mitomycin-C. Cisplatinum is broadly recognized to be able to provoke severe kidney injury causing acute kidney damage. When CUR was administered to the rats for three consecutive days concomitantly with cisplatinum, CUR showed a renal protective effect preserving kidney function by preventing mitochondrial bioenergetic alterations [66].

All the above evidence about CUR protective effects on chemotherapy-induced toxicities mostly are derived from animal experimental or in vitro studies. There is an unmet need to perform clinical trials in the future to confirm safety and efficacy of CUR in humans undergoing cancer therapy. As CUR is an unstable product with poor absorption and rapid systemic elimination, formulations with better bioavailability should be the focus in these these future investigations [67].

5. Perspective

Various preclinical studies highlighted the effects of CUR on NF-kB, STAT3, COX2, and CXCL-1 (chemokine [C-X-C motif] ligand 1) activity, leading to reduced inflammation and eventually also impacting tumor progression. Despite these promising in vitro and in vivo results, a clear clinical benefit could not be demonstrated in clinical trials. Thus, currently, a large amount of larger clinical studies are ongoing to investigate the effect of CUR in cancer patients in more detail.

At the moment, CUR is under evaluation against placebo in a phase II clinical trial (NCT02944578) in HIV (human immunodeficiency virus) -infected women with high-grade squamous intraepithelial lesions of the cervix. In another study, oral CUR is being tested for the treatment of cervical intraepithelial neoplasia (NCT02554344), assessing drug-induced tumor regression. CUR is also proposed as a chemo-preventive agent alternative to other anti-inflammatory drugs, as it inhibits COX activity and is, therefore, being tested in patients with familial adenomatous polyposis (FAP) (NCT00927485). For high-risk men under active surveillance for a biopsy-proven low-risk prostate cancer, a bioavailable formulation of CUR is expected to control disease and reduce the rates of clinically indicated interventions for prostate cancer, including the progression of locoregional disease or spread to distant sites requiring surgery or hormone therapy, respectively (NCT03769766). Similarly, the

NCT01975363 trial is assessing the role of daily oral CUR for obese women, as a risk-reducing strategy for high-risk patients defined by either genetic risk, namely harboring *BRCA* mutations, or clinically, when diagnosed with in situ ductal carcinoma.

In colorectal cancer, CUR showed its role in FAP and is now being tested actively in combination with conventional chemotherapy either to overcome resistance or to enhance the chemotherapeutic effects. In particular, an early study is testing CUR and a phospholipid mix with 5-floururacil, assessing the feasibility, safety, and effectiveness of the combination strategy (NCT02724202; NCT02439385). Moreover, a phase II clinical trial assessing the adjunctive benefit of CUR combined with paclitaxel for advanced breast cancer patients is ongoing (NCT03072992).

In breast cancer, whether for prevention in high-risk obese population or as an active role in reducing radiation-induced dermatitis or enhancing paclitaxel effects/reducing toxicities, CUR is making its way through ongoing trials in breast cancer.

Curcumin is also being studied for its protective effects in anthracycline-induced cardiotoxicity and chemotherapy-induced nephrotoxicity. It also reduces cisplatin resistance by inhibiting FEN-1 (Flap endonuclease 1) expression in animal models. Whether it is combined with tyrosine kinase inhibitors in lung cancer, with gemcitabine in pancreatic cancer, pre-cancerous lesions in cervical cancer, or its role in sarcoma, CUR is expected to show its promising effects.

NCT03211104 is a placebo-controlled, double-blind, randomized trial investigating whether CUR influences the course of prostate cancer patients treated with on/off hormonal deprivation therapy.

A larger phase III trial is investigating the risk-reducing potential of CUR in terms of recurrence-free survival for patients undergoing radical prostatectomy for an adenocarcinoma of the prostate (NCT02064673). In addition, another protocol is analyzing the role of CUR as a radio-sensitizing agent for prostate cancer patients, as assessed by tumor response.

Furthermore, the role of CUR associated with standard treatments for cancer is being evaluated for non-small-cell cancer patients, receiving tyrosine kinase inhibitors for advanced disease (NCT02321293). Table 2 summarizes the studies described in this section.

The role of CUR in cancer treatment was addressed by numerous trials. Although apparently working at low plasma concentration, systemic bio-availability still represents an issue when dealing with CUR experiments in humans. Indeed, the optimization of CUR bio-availability through drug-delivery strategies provided more significant results, suggesting that in vitro and in vivo antitumoral activity can be replicated in the clinical setting by different pharmacological strategies. However, some of the results provided so far are no more than proof-of-concept studies, particularly for the combination with targeted agents, where only a few positive experiences are reported. Moreover, no phase III clinical trial provided results on the antitumor efficacy compared to the standard treatments, with efforts warranted in the definition of the disease most likely to benefit along with predictive biomarkers for better patient selection. For this, despite promising results and early signals of benefit, at present, no specific recommendation should be provided for CUR in the treatment of cancer, as data of safety are restricted to monotherapy and few combinations with selected agents, and data of activity are not mature enough. Eventually, the use of CUR to "adjuvate" the standard treatments should be discouraged unless new results will identify a precise setting of care as a pharmacological compound.

Table 2. Currently ongoing clinical trials with curcumin.

NCT Number	Title	Cancer Type	Setting	Study Phase	Primary Objective
NCT02944578	Biomolecular Effects of Topical Curcumin in HSIL Cervical Neoplasia	Cervical pre-cancer lesions	Cancer prevention	2	Change in human papillomavirus (HPV)-related molecular target HPV E6/E7 messenger ribonucleic acid (mRNA) expression within HSIL lesions of the cervix
NCT02554344	Effect of Curcumin in Treatment of Squamous Cervical Intraepithelial Neoplasias (CINs)	Cervical pre-cancer lesions	Cancer prevention	1	Determine the safety and feasibility using curcumin in patients with CIN3 where toxicities will be graded according to the NCI Common Terminology Criteria for Adverse Events (CTCAE) Version 4.0.
NCT00927485	Use of Curcumin for Treatment of Intestinal Adenomas in Familial Adenomatous Polyposis (FAP)	Intestinal adenoma	Cancer prevention	na	To determine in a randomized, double-blinded, placebo-controlled study the tolerability and efficacy of curcumin to regress intestinal adenomas by measuring duodenal and colorectal/ileal polyp number, and polyp size in patients with FAP
NCT03769766	A Randomized, Double-Blind, Placebo-Controlled Trial of Curcumin to Prevent Progression of Biopsy Proven, Low-Risk Localized Prostate Cancer Patients Undergoing Active Surveillance	Prostate cancer	Cancer treatment/(neo)adjuvant treatment	3	The primary endpoint is the number of patients who have progressed at 2 years of follow-up defined as one of the following events: receipt of primary therapy for prostate cancer (e.g., prostatectomy, radiation, hormonal therapy) or pathologic progression (>4 cores involved, ≥50% of any core involved, or any Gleason score ≥7)
NCT01975363	Nanoemulsion Curcumin for Obesity, Inflammation, and Breast Cancer Prevention—A Pilot Trial	Breast cancer	Cancer prevention	na	To determine whether nanoemulsion curcumin modulates pro-inflammatory biomarkers in plasma and breast adipose tissue
NCT02724202	A Pilot, Feasibility Study of Curcumin in Combination with 5-FU for Patients With 5-FU-Resistant Metastatic Colon Cancer	Colorectal cancer	Metastatic treatment	1	Determine the safety using curcumin in patients with metastatic colon cancer; where toxicities will be graded according to the NCI Common Terminology Criteria for Adverse Events (CTCAE) Version 4.0 (time frame: 12 weeks)
NCT02439385	First-Line Avastin/FOLFIRI in Combination with Curcumin-Containing Supplement in Colorectal Cancer Patients with Unresectable Metastasis	Colorectal cancer	Metastatic treatment	2	Progression-free survival
NCT03072992	Study of Efficacy of Curcumin in Combination with Chemotherapy in Patients with Advanced Breast Cancer: Randomized, Double-Blind, Placebo-Controlled Clinical Trial	Advanced cancer	Metastatic treatment	2	Objective response rate (time frame: 4 weeks after the completion of the treatment)
NCT03211104	Comparison of Duration of Treatment Interruption with or without Curcumin During the Off Treatment Periods in Patients with Prostate Cancer Undergoing Intermittent Androgen Deprivation Therapy: A Randomized, Double-Blind, Placebo-Controlled Tria	Prostate cancer	Metastatic treatment	na	Duration of treatment interruption with or without curcumin (time frame: up to 42 months)
NCT02064673	Randomized Trial of Adjuvant Curcumin after Prostatectomy	Prostate cancer	Adjuvant treatment	3	Serum prostate-specific antigen (time frame: 3 years) Recurrence-free survival defined as a total serum prostate specific antigen of <0.2 ng/mL.
NCT02321293	A Phase I Open-Label Prospective Cohort Trial of Curcumin Plus Tyrosine Kinase Inhibitors for Epidermal Growth Factor Receptor (EGFR)-Mutant Advanced Non-Small-Cell Lung Cancer	Non-small-cell lung cancer	Metastatic setting	1	Feasibility and safety

6. Conclusions

The majority of studies analyzing CUR in cancer showed potentially beneficial effects on side effects and eventually also additive or even synsergistic effects on the efficacy of classical anti-cancer drugs. However, data from recent clinical trials are not sufficient to implement CUR as standard anti-cancer treatment. Large randomized trials are urgently needed to investigate the real effect of CUR in hemato-oncology. However, the efficacy of CUR as a complementary and/or alternative medical approach is promising. In addition, CUR causes no significant side effects and is cheap and easily available, even though its poor bioavailabity and fast metabolism remain major obstacles.

Funding: This research received no external funding.

Conflicts of Interest: The authors declare no conflict of interest.

References

1. Berretta, M.; Della Pepa, C.; Tralongo, P.; Fulvi, A.; Martellotta, F.; Lleshi, A.; Nasti, G.; Fisichella, R.; Romano, C.; De Divitiis, C.; et al. Use of Complementary and Alternative Medicine (CAM) in cancer patients: An Italian multicenter survey. *Oncotarget* **2017**, *8*, 24401–24414. [CrossRef]
2. Nelson, K.M.; Dahlin, J.L.; Bisson, J.; Graham, J.; Pauli, G.F.; Walters, M.A. The Essential Medicinal Chemistry of Curcumin. *J. Med. Chem.* **2017**, *60*, 1620–1637. [CrossRef] [PubMed]
3. Witkin, J.M.; Li, X. Curcumin, an active constiuent of the ancient medicinal herb *Curcuma longa* L.: Some uses and the establishment and biological basis of medical efficacy. *CNS Neurol. Disord. Targets* **2013**, *12*, 487–497. [CrossRef]
4. Payton, F.; Sandusky, P.; Alworth, W.L.J. NMR study of the solution structure of curcumin. *Nat. Prod.* **2007**, *70*, 143–146. [CrossRef] [PubMed]
5. Anand, P.; Kunnumakkara, A.B.; Newman, R.A.; Aggarwal, B.B. Bioavailability of curcumin: Problems and promises. *Mol. Pharm.* **2007**, *4*, 807–818.
6. Lao, C.D.; Ruffin, M.T., 4th; Normolle, D.; Heath, D.D.; Murray, S.I.; Bailey, J.M.; Boggs, M.E.; Crowell, J.; Rock, C.L.; Brenner, D.E. Dose escalation of a curcuminoid formulation. *BMC Complement. Altern. Med.* **2006**, *6*, 10. [CrossRef] [PubMed]
7. Feng, T.; Wei, Y.; Lee, R.J.; Zhao, L. Liposomal curcumin and its application in cancer. *Int. J. Nanomed.* **2017**, *12*, 6027–6044. [CrossRef]
8. Jyoti, K.; Bhatia, R.K.; Martis, E.; Coutinho, E.C.; Jain, U.K.; Chandra, R.; Madan, J. Soluble curcumin amalgamated chitosan microspheres augmented drug delivery and cytotoxicity in colon cancer cells: In vitro and in vivo study. *Colloids Surf. B Biointerfaces* **2016**, *148*, 674–683. [CrossRef] [PubMed]
9. Shinde, R.L.; Devarajan, P.V. Docosahexaenoic acid-mediated, targeted and sustained brain delivery of curcumin microemulsion. *Drug Deliv.* **2017**, *24*, 152–161. [CrossRef]
10. Shen, L.; Liu, L.; Ji, H.F. Regulative effects of curcumin spice administration on gut microbiota and its pharmacological implications. *Food Nutr. Res.* **2017**, *61*, 1361780. [CrossRef] [PubMed]
11. Tabrizi, R.; Vakili, S.; Akbari, M.; Mirhosseini, N.; Lankarani, K.B.; Rahimi, M.; Mobini, M.; Jafarnejad, S.; Vahedpoor, Z.; Asemi, Z. The effects of curcumin-containing supplements on biomarkers of inflammation and oxidative stress: A systematic review and meta-analysis of randomized controlled trials. *Phytother. Res.* **2018**, *33*, 253–262. [CrossRef]
12. Kumar, S.; Ahuja, V.; Sankar, M.J.; Kumar, A.; Moss, A.C. Curcumin for maintenance of remission in ulcerative colitis Cochrane. *Database Syst. Rev.* **2012**, *17*, CD008424.
13. Hanahn, D.; Weinberg, R.A. Hallmarks of cancer: The next generation. *Cell* **2011**, *144*, 646–6674. [CrossRef]
14. Marquardt, J.U.; Gomez-Quiroz, L.; Arreguin Camacho, L.O.; Pinna, F.; Lee, Y.H.; Kitade, M.; Domínguez, M.P.; Castven, D.; Breuhahn, K.; Conner, E.A.; et al. Curcumin effectively inhibits oncogenic NF-κB signaling and restrains stemness features in liver cancer. *J. Hepatol.* **2015**, *63*, 661–669. [CrossRef]
15. Rajasingh, J.; Raikwar, H.P.; Muthian, G.; Johnson, C.; Bright, J.J. Curcumin induces growth-arrest and apoptosis in association with the inhibition of constitutively active JAK-STAT pathway in T cell leukemia. *Biochem. Biophys. Res. Commun.* **2006**, *340*, 359–368. [CrossRef]

16. Thacker, P.; Karunagaran, D. Curcumin and emodin down-regulate TGF-β signaling pathway in human cervical cancer cells. *PLoS ONE* **2015**, *10*, e0120045. [CrossRef]
17. Matthew, C.; Fadus, A.; Lau, C.; Lynch, H.T. Curcumin: An age-old anti-inflammatory and anti-neoplastic agent. *J. Tradit. Complement. Med.* **2017**, *7*, 339–346.
18. Mahmood, K.; Zia, K.M.; Zuber, M.; Salman, M.; Anjum, M.N. Recent developments in curcumin and curcumin based polymericmaterials for biomedical applications: A review. *Int. J. Biol. Macromol.* **2015**, *81*, 877–890. [CrossRef]
19. Shen, L.; Ji, H.F. The pharmacology of curcumin: Is it the degradation products? *Trends Mol. Med.* **2012**, *18*, 138–144. [CrossRef]
20. Pignanelli, C.; Ma, D.; Noel, M.; Ropat, J.; Mansour, F.; Curran, C.; Pupulin, S.; Larocque, K.; Wu, J.; Liang, G. Selective Targeting of Cancer Cells by Oxidative Vulnerabilities with Novel Curcumin Analogs. *Nat. Sci. Rep.* **2017**, *7*, 1105. [CrossRef]
21. Leu, T.H.; Maa, M.C. The Molecular Mechanisms for the Antitumorigenic Effect of Curcumin. *Curr. Med. Chem. Anti-Cancer Agents* **2002**, *2*, 357–370.
22. Duvoix, A.; Blsius, R.; Delhalle, S.; Schnekenburger, M.; Morceau, F.; Henry, E.; Dicato, M.; Diederich, M. Chemopreventive and therapeutic effects of curcumin. *Cancer Lett.* **2005**, *223*, 181–190. [CrossRef]
23. Syng-ai, C.; Kumari, L.; Khar, A. Effect of curcumin on normal and tumor cells: Role of glutathione and bcl-2. *Mol. Cancer* **2004**, *3*, 1101–1108.
24. Sharma, R.A.; Gescher, A.J.; Steward, W.P. Curcumin: The story so far. *Eur. J. Cancer* **2005**, *41*, 1955–1968. [CrossRef]
25. Barati, N.; Momtazi-Borojeni, A.A.; Majeed, M.; Sahebkar, A. Potential therapeutic effects of curcumin in gastric cancer. *J. Cell Physiol.* **2018**, *234*, 2317–2328. [CrossRef]
26. Maheshwari, R.K.; Singh, A.K.; Gaddipati, J.; Srimal, R.C. Multiple biological activities of curcumin: A short review. *Life Sci.* **2006**, *78*, 2081–2087. [CrossRef]
27. Vallianou, N.G.; Evangelopoulos, A.; Schizas, N.; Kazazis, C. Potential Anticancer Properties and Mechanisms of Action of Curcumin. *Anticancer Res.* **2015**, *35*, 645–652.
28. Ravindran, J.; Prasad, S.; Aggarwal, B.B. Curcumin and Cancer Cells: How Many Ways Can Curry Kill Tumor Cells Selectively? *AAPS J.* **2009**, *11*, 495–510. [CrossRef]
29. Mapoung, S.; Suzuki, S.; Fuji, S.; Naiki-Ito, A.; Kato, H.; Yodkeeree, S.; Ovatlarnporn, C.; Takahashi, S.; Limtrakul Dejkriengkraikul, P. Cyclohexanone curcumin analogs inhibit the progression of castration-resistant prostate cancer in vitro and in vivo. *Cancer Sci.* **2018**. [CrossRef]
30. Kunnumakkara, A.B.; Bordoloi, D.; Harsha, C.; Banik, K.; Gupta, S.C.; Aggarwal, B.B. Curcumin mediates anticancer effects by modulating multiple cell signaling pathways. *Clin. Sci.* **2017**, *131*, 1781–1799. [CrossRef]
31. Shakeri, A.; Cicero, A.F.G.; Panahi, Y.; Mohajeri, M.; Sahebkar, A. Curcumin: A naturally occurring autophagy modulator. *J. Cell Physiol.* **2018**, *234*, 5643–5654. [CrossRef]
32. Siddiqui, F.A.; Prakasam, G.; Chattopadhyay, S.; Rehman, A.U.; Padder, R.A.; Ansari, M.A.; Irshad, R.; Mangalhara, K.; Bamezai, R.N.K.; Husain, M.; et al. Curcumin decreases Warburg effect in cancer cells by down-regulating pyruvate kinase M2 via mTOR-HIF1α inhibition. *Nat. Sci. Rep.* **2018**, *8*, 8323. [CrossRef]
33. Della Corte, C.M.; Fasano, M.; Papaccio, F.; Ciardiello, F.; Morgillo, F. Role of HGF-MET Signaling in Primary and Acquired Resistance to Targeted Therapies in Cancer. *Biomedicines* **2014**, *2*, 345–358. [CrossRef]
34. Jaio, D.; Wang, J.; Lu, W.; Tang, X.; Chen, J.; Mou, H.; Chen, Q.Y. Curcumin inhibited HGF-induced EMT and angiogenesis throuth regulating c-MET dependet PI3K/mTOR signaling pathways in lung cancer. *Mol. Ther. Oncolytics* **2016**, *3*, 16018.
35. Zhang, W.; Shi, H.; Chen, C.; Ren, K.; Xu, Y.; Liu, X.; He, L. Curcumin enhances cisplatin sensitivity of human NSCLC cell lines through influencing Cu-Sp1-CTR1 regulatory loop. *Phytomedicine* **2018**, *48*, 51–61. [CrossRef]
36. Della Corte, C.M.; Viscardi, G.; Papaccio, F.; Esposito, G.; Martini, G.; Ciardiello, D.; Martinelli, E.; Ciardiello, F.; Morgillo, F. Implication of the Hedgehog pathway in hepatocellularer carcinoma. *World J. Gastroenterol.* **2017**, *23*, 4330–4340. [CrossRef]
37. Li, X.; Wang, X.; Xie, C.; Zhu, J.; Meng, Y.; Chen, Y.; Li, Y.; Jiang, Y.; Yang, X.; Wang, S.; et al. Sonic hedgehog and Wnt/β-catenin pathwys mediate curcumin inhibition of breast cancer stem cells. *Anticancer Drugs* **2018**, *29*, 208–215.

38. Wang, D.; Kong, X.; Li, Y.; Qian, W.; Ma, J.; Wang, D.; Yu, D.; Zhong, C. Curcumin inhibits bladder cancer stem cells by suppressing Sonic Hedgehog pathway. *Biochem. Biophys. Res. Cummun.* **2017**, *493*, 521–527. [CrossRef]
39. Zhu, J.Y.; Yang, X.; Chen, Y.; Jiang, Y.; Wang, S.J.; Li, Y.; Wang, X.Q.; Meng, Y.; Zhu, M.M.; Ma, X.; et al. Curcumin Suppresses Lung Cancer Cells via Inhibiting Wnt/β-catenin and Sonic Hedgehog Pathways. *Phytother. Res.* **2017**, *31*, 680–688. [CrossRef]
40. Cao, L.; Xiao, X.; Lei, J.; Duan, W.; Ma, Q.; Li, W. Curcumin inhibits hypoxia-induced epithelial-mesenchymal transition in pancreatic cancer cell via suppression of the hedgehog signalling pathway. *Oncol. Rep.* **2016**, *35*, 3728–3734. [CrossRef]
41. Wilken, R.; Veena, M.S.; Wang, M.B.; Srivatsan, E.S. Curcumin: A review of anti-cancer properties and therapeutic activity in head and neck squamous cell carcinoma. *Mol. Cancer* **2011**, *10*, 12. [CrossRef]
42. Chen, C.; Chu, C.C.; Chiang, J.H.; Chiu, H.Y.; Yang, J.S.; Lee, C.Y.; Way, T.D.; Huang, H.J. Synergistic inhibitory effects of cetuximab and curcumin on human cisplatin-resistant oral cancer CAR cells through intrinsic apoptotic process. *Oncol. Lett.* **2018**, *16*, 6323–6330. [CrossRef]
43. Lu, W.D.; Qin, Y.; Yang, C.; Li, L.; Fu, Z.X. Effect of curcumin on human colon cancer multidrug resistance in vitro and in vivo. *Clinics* **2013**, *68*, 694–701. [CrossRef]
44. James, M.I.; Iwuji, C.; Irwing, G.; Karmokar, A.; Higgins, J.A.; Griffin-Teal, N.; Thomas, A.; Greaves, P.; Cai, H.; Patel, S.R.; et al. Curcumin inhibits cancer stem cell phenotypes in ex vivo models of colorectal liver metastases, and is clinically safe and tolerable in combination with FOLFOX chemotherapy. *Cancer Lett.* **2015**, *364*, 135–141. [CrossRef]
45. Sharma, R.A.; Euden, S.A.; Platton, S.L.; Cooke, D.N.; Shafayat, A.; Hewitt, H.R.; Marczylo, T.H.; Morgan, B.; Hemingway, D.; Plummer, S.M.; et al. Phase I Clinical Trial of Oral Curcumin. *Clin Cancer Res.* **2004**, *10*, 6847–6854. [CrossRef]
46. Bayet-Robert, M.; Kwiatkowski, F.; Leheurteur, M.; Gachon, F.; Planchat, E.; Abrial, C.; Mouret-Reynier, M.A.; Durando, X.; Barthomeuf, C.; Chollet, P. Phase I dose escalation trial of docetaxel plus curcumin in patients with advanced and metastatic breast cancer. *Cancer Biol.* **2010**, *9*, 8–14. [CrossRef]
47. Epelbaum, R.; Schaffer, M.; Vizel, B.; Badmaev, V.; Bar-Sela, G. Curcumin and gemcitabine in patients with advanced pancreatic cancer. *Nutr. Cancer* **2010**, *62*, 1137–1141. [CrossRef]
48. Dhillon, N.; Aggarwal, B.B.; Newman, R.A.; Wolff, R.A.; Kunnumakkara, A.B.; Abbruzzese, J.L.; Ng, C.S.; Badmaev, V.; Kurzrock, R. Phase II trial of curcumin in patients with advanced pancreatic cancer. *Clin. Cancer Res.* **2008**, *14*, 4491–4499. [CrossRef]
49. Ghalaut, V.S.; Sangwan, L.; Dahiya, K.; Ghalaut, P.S.; Dhankhar, R.; Saharan, R. Effect of imatinib therapy with and without turmeric powder on nitric oxide levels in chronic myeloid leukemia. *J. Oncol. Pharm. Pract.* **2012**, *18*, 186–190. [CrossRef]
50. Demiray, M.; Sahinbas, H.; Atahan, S.; Demiray, H.; Selcuk, D.; Yildirim, I.; Atayoglu, A.T. Successful treatment of c-kit-positive metastatic Adenoid Cystic Carcinoma (ACC) with a combination of curcumin plus imatinib: A case report. *Complement. Med.* **2016**, *27*, 108–113. [CrossRef]
51. Capalbo, C.; Belardinilli, F.; Filetti, M.; Capalbo, C.; Belardinilli, F.; Filetti, M.; et al. Effective treatment of a platinum-resistant cutaneous squamous cell carcinoma case by EGFR pathway inhibition. *Mol. Clin. Oncol.* **2018**, *9*, 30–34. [CrossRef]
52. Wada, K.; Lee, J.Y.; Hung, H.Y.; Shi, Q.; Lin, L.; Zhao, Y.; Goto, M.; Yang, P.C.; Kuo, S.C.; Chen, H.W.; et al. Novel curcumin analogs to overcome EGFR-TKI lung adenocarcinoma drug resistance and reduce EGFR-TKI-induced GI adverse effects. *Biorg. Med. Chem.* **2015**, *23*, 1507–1514. [CrossRef]
53. Li, S.; Liu, Z.; Zhu, F.; Fan, X.; Wu, X.; Zhao, H.; Jiang, L. Curcumin lowers erlotinib resistance in non-small cell lung carcinoma cells with mutated EGF receptor. *Oncol. Res.* **2013**, *21*, 137–144. [CrossRef]
54. Greil, R.; Greil-Ressler, S.; Weiss, L.; Schönlieb, C.; Magnes, T.; Radl, B.; Bolger, G.T.; Vcelar, B.; Sordillo, P.P. A phase 1 dose-escalation study on the safety, tolerability and activity of liposomal curcumin (Lipocurc™) in patients with locally advanced or metastatic cancer. *Cancer Chemother. Pharmacol.* **2018**, *82*, 695–706. [CrossRef]
55. Cruz-Correa, M.; Hylind, L.M.; Marrero, J.H.; Zahurak, M.L.; Murray-Stewart, T.; Casero, R.A., Jr.; Montgomery, E.A.; Iacobuzio-Donahue, C.; Brosens, L.A.; Offerhaus, G.J.; et al. Efficacy and Safety of Curcumin in Treatment of Intestinal Adenomas in Patients with Familial Adenomatous Polyposis. *Gastroenterology* **2018**, *155*, 668–673. [CrossRef]

56. Alfonso-Moreno, V.; López-Serrano, A.; Moreno-Osset, E. Chemoprevention of polyp recurrence with curcumin followed by silibinin in a case of multiple colorectal adenomas. *Rev. ESP Enferm. Dig.* **2017**, *109*, 875. [CrossRef]
57. Gattoc, L.; Frew, P.M.; Thomas, S.N.; Easley, K.A.; Ward, L.; Chow, H.S.; Ura, C.A.; Flowers, L. Phase I dose-escalation trial of intravaginal curcumin in women for cervical dysplasia. *Open Access J. Clin. Trials* **2017**, *9*, 1–10. [CrossRef]
58. Chen, X.; Wang, J.; Fu, Z.; Zhu, B.; Wang, J.; Guan, S.; Hua, Z. Curcumin activates DNA repair pathway in bone marrow to improve carboplatin-induced myelosuppression. *Sci. Rep.* **2017**, *7*, 17724. [CrossRef]
59. Swamy, A.; Gulliaya, S.; Thippeswamy, A.; Koti, B.; Manjula, D. Cardioprotective effect of curcumin against doxorubicin-induced myocardial toxicity in albino rats. *Indian J. Pharmacol.* **2012**, *44*, 73–77. [CrossRef]
60. Benzer, F.; Kandemir, F.M.; Ozkaraca, M.; Kucukler, S.; Caglayan, C. Curcumin ameliorates doxorubicin-induced cardiotoxicity by abrogation of inflammation, apoptosis, oxidative DNA damage, and protein oxidation in rats. *J. Biochem. Mol. Toxicol.* **2018**, *32*, e22030. [CrossRef]
61. Yao, Q.; Ye, X.; Wang, L.; Gu, J.; Fu, T.; Wang, Y.; Lai, Y.; Wang, Y.; Wang, X.; Jin, H.; et al. Protective effect of Curcumin on chemotherapy-induced intestinal dysfunction. *Int. J. Clin. Exp. Pathol.* **2013**, *6*, 2342–2349.
62. Santos Filho EXDArantes, D.A.C.; Oton Leite, A.F.; Batista, A.C.; Mendonça, E.F.; Marreto, R.N.; Naves, L.N.; Lima, E.M.; Valadares, M.C. Randomized clinical trial of a mucoadhesive formulation containing curcuminoids (Zingiberaceae) and Bidens pilosa Linn (Asteraceae) extract (FITOPROT) for prevention and treatment of oral mucositis—Phase I study. *Chem. Biol. Interact.* **2018**, *291*, 228–236. [CrossRef]
63. Palipoch, S.; Punsawad, C.; Koomhin, P.; Suwannalert, P. Hepatoprotective effect of curcumin and alpha-tocopherol against cisplatin-induced oxidative stress. *Tract. BMC Complement. Altern. Med.* **2014**, *14*, 111. [CrossRef]
64. Hemeida, R.A.; Mohafez, R.M. Curcumin Attenuates Methotraxate-Induced Hepatic Oxidative Damage in Rats. *J. Egypt Natl. Canc. Inst.* **2008**, *20*, 141–148.
65. Zhou, Q.-M.; Wang, X.-F.; Liu, X.-J.; Zhang, H.; Lu, Y.Y.; Huang, S.; Su, S.B. Curcumin improves MMC-based chemotherapy by simultaneously sensitising cancer cells to MMC and reducing MMC-associated side-effects. *Eur. J. Cancer* **2011**, *47*, 2240–2247. [CrossRef]
66. Ortega-Domínguez, B.; Aparicio-Trejo, O.E.; García-Arroyo, F.E.; León-Contreras, J.C.; Tapia, E.; Molina-Jijón, E.; Hernández-Pando, R.; Sánchez-Lozada, L.G.; Barrera-Oviedo, D.; Pedraza-Chaverri, J. Curcumin prevents cisplatin-induced renal alterations in mitochondrial bioenergetics and dynamic. *Food Chem. Toxicol.* **2017**, *107*, 373–385. [CrossRef]
67. Scarano, W.; Souza, P.D.; Stenzel, M.H. Dual-drug delivery of curcumin and platinum drugs in polymeric micelles enhance the synergistic effects: A double act for the treatment of multidrug-resistant cancers. *Biomater. Sci.* **2015**, *3*, 163–174. [CrossRef]

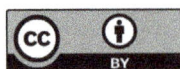 © 2019 by the authors. Licensee MDPI, Basel, Switzerland. This article is an open access article distributed under the terms and conditions of the Creative Commons Attribution (CC BY) license (http://creativecommons.org/licenses/by/4.0/).

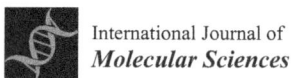

Article

Curcumin and Solid Lipid Curcumin Particles Induce Autophagy, but Inhibit Mitophagy and the PI3K-Akt/mTOR Pathway in Cultured Glioblastoma Cells

Panchanan Maiti [1,2,3,4,5,6,*], Jason Scott [5], Dipanwita Sengupta [4], Abeer Al-Gharaibeh [1,2] and Gary L. Dunbar [1,2,3,4,*]

1. Field Neurosciences Institute Laboratory for Restorative Neurology, Central Michigan University, Mt. Pleasant, MI 48859, USA; to.abeer@gmail.com
2. Program in Neuroscience, Central Michigan University, Mt. Pleasant, MI 48859, USA
3. Department of Psychology, Central Michigan University, Mt. Pleasant, MI 48859, USA
4. Field Neurosciences Institute, St. Mary's of Michigan, Saginaw, MI 48604, USA; Dipanwita.Sengupta@ascension.org
5. Department of Biology, Saginaw Valley State University, Saginaw, MI 48710, USA; jascott1@svsu.edu
6. Brain Research Laboratory, Saginaw Valley State University, Saginaw, MI 48710, USA
* Correspondence: maiti1p@cmich.edu (P.M.); dunba1g@cmich.edu (G.L.D.); Tel.: +1-9894973026 (P.M.); +1-9894973105 (G.L.D.)

Received: 20 November 2018; Accepted: 15 January 2019; Published: 18 January 2019

Abstract: Autophagy and the (PI3K-Akt/mTOR) signaling pathway play significant roles in glioblastoma multiforme (GBM) cell death and survival. Curcumin (Cur) has been reported to prevent several cancers, including GBM. However, the poor solubility and limited bioavailability of natural Cur limits its application in preventing GBM growth. Previously, we have shown the greater apoptotic and anti-carcinogenic effects of solid lipid Cur particles (SLCP) than natural Cur in cultured GBM cells. Here, we compared the autophagic responses on cultured U-87MG, GL261, F98, C6-glioma, and N2a cells after treatment with Cur or SLCP (25 µM for 24 h). Different autophagy, mitophagy, and chaperone-mediated autophagy (CMA) markers, along with the PI3K-AKkt/mTOR signaling pathway, and the number of autophagy vacuoles were investigated after treatment with Cur and or SLCP. We observed increased levels of autophagy and decreased levels of mitophagy markers, along with inhibition of the PI3K-Akt/mTOR pathway after treatments with Cur or SLCP. Cell survival markers were downregulated, and cell death markers were upregulated after these treatments. We found greater effects in the case of SCLP-treated cells in comparison to Cur. Given that fewer effects were observed on C-6 glioma and N2a cells. Our results suggest that SLCP could be a safe and effective means of therapeutically modulating autophagy in GBM cells.

Keywords: glioblastoma multiforme; autophagy; mitophagy; curcumin; chaperone-mediated autophagy; Akt/mTOR signaling; transmission electron microscopy

---

1. Introduction

According to the World Health Organization (WHO), glioblastoma multiforme (GBM) is one of the deadliest and most aggressive brain cancers, affecting millions of people world-wide. Histopathological analysis revealed that brain tumors account for 85% to 90% of all primary Central nervous system (CNS) tumors, and about 70% to 80% are of glial cell origins. Whereas among all primary brain tumors only 15% are GBM [1]. Importantly, most GBM patients survive on average for only 15 to 20 months following initial diagnosis [2]. Despite current neurosurgical, radiotherapy, and chemotherapeutic advancement, the GBM growth and proliferation cannot be effectively controlled. The most potent chemotherapeutic drug use to treat GBM is temozolomide (Temodar, TMZ), but resistance to TMZ limits its effectiveness. Moreover, neuroinflammation also increases after treatment of TMZ, making the development of alternative therapies critically important. In this context, several investigators have studied the anti-cancer and anti-inflammatory effects of curcumin (Cur) in human malignancies, including those found in various tissues, such as breast, prostate, colon, liver, and brain [3,4].

Several anti-cancer drugs have been tested to prevent GBM cell growth and metastasis [4]. Many of these drugs kill GBM cells by inducing apoptosis, autophagic cell death, or necrosis, whereas dysregulation of these major pathways promotes cancer development [5]. Although apoptosis is the most common form of programmed cell death (PCD), autophagic cell death also has significant roles in tumorigenesis [5]. It includes macroautophagy, microautophagy, and chaperones-mediated autophagy (CMA), which are highly conserved cellular-debris disposal mechanisms by which cellular organelles, misfolded protein aggregates, and pathogens or toxins are degraded through fusion of the resulting autophagosomes with lysosomes [6–8]. The beneficial effects of autophagy have been observed with anti-cancer drugs after their treatments in GBM cells, which may either induce or bypass the apoptotic pathway, depending on cellular stress [9]. Several experimental results from animal studies and cell culture studies have demonstrated that induction of autophagy or type-II PCD can induce or inhibit type-I PCD or apoptosis [10], which suggests that they are inter-linked for cell death and survival [11]. In addition, cancer cell growth and proliferation are also controlled by the phosphatidylinositol 3-kinase (PI3K)/Akt/mammalian target of rapamycin (mTOR, also known as the mechanistic target of rapamycin and FK506-binding protein 12-rapamycin-associated protein 1) sensitive mTOR-complex (PI3K-Akt/mTOR) pathway, which has inhibitory roles on the autophagic pathway. The Akt/mTOR pathway plays significant roles in the regulation of autophagy, as well as cancer cell growth and proliferation; inhibition of this pathway has activatory roles in the autophagy pathway and inhibitory roles on cancer cell proliferation. Therefore, targeting autophagy by inhibiting PI3K-Akt/mTOR might be a potent strategy to inhibit GBM growth and proliferation [12].

Curcumin (Cur), is the most active natural polyphenol present in the turmeric root of the herb, *Curcuma longa* [13]. For a long time, it has been known to function as a potent inhibitor of tumor growth, proliferation, invasion, angiogenesis, and metastasis. Cur has been applied for several cancer therapies, including GBM [14]. It can attenuate cancer growth by increasing oxidative stress, disrupting PI3k-Akt/mTOR signaling and induction of apoptosis, but it requires higher amounts to be effective against cancer cells [15]. Unfortunately, poor solubility and instability in physiological fluids limits its therapeutic application for targeting GBM [16,17]. Although various lipidated and nanotechnological approaches of Cur formulations have been shown to increase its solubility and bio-availability [15], none of these produce optimal levels. Recently, solid lipid particles (SLPs), conjugated with Cur (SLCPs), have been characterized by our laboratory [15,18,19] and those of others to increase Cur solubility, stability, and bioavailability [20–25], when tested in an in vitro model of GBM, as well as animal models and clinical trials of Alzheimer's disease [26,27].

Previously, we have reported that SLCPs induce a greater number of apoptotic deaths than natural Cur in U-87MG [19]. In the present study, we have designed the experiments to compare the autophagy mechanism, including mitophagy and the PI3K-Akt/mTOR pathway (which is one of the modulators of the autophagy pathway) in vitro, using GBM cells derived from human (U-87MG), mouse (GL261), and rat (F98) origins, their respective rat glial tumor cells (C6-glioma), and mouse neuroblastoma cells (N2a cells) after treatment with Cur and/or SLCP. Our results suggest that SLCP induced autophagy markers greater than natural Cur, as well as the inhibition of mitophagy and the significant disruption of the PI3K-Akt/mTOR pathway in all three GBM cells, without significant effects on C6-glioma and N2a cells.

2. Results

In this study, we have compared the levels of autophagy, including mitophagy markers and the PI3k-Akt/mTOR signaling pathway in cultured GBM cells after treatment with SLCP and or Cur.

2.1. SLCP Induced Autophagy Greater than Natural Cur in Different GBM Cells

We have investigated different autophagy markers, such as Atg5, Atg7, Beclin-1, LC3A/B, and p62, from all three GBM cell lines (U-87MG, GL261, and F98), and from C6-glioma and N2a cells. We observed that the Atg5 level was significantly increased ($p < 0.05$) in U-87MG and F98 cells, but not in GL261 after treatment with Cur and or SLCP in comparison to vehicle-treated groups (Figure 1A,B). Similarly, we found a significant increase ($p < 0.01$) in levels of Atg7 after Cur and or SLCP treatment in U-87MG and GL261, but not in F98 cells, in comparison to the vehicle-treated group (Figure 2A,C). Furthermore, the Beclin-1 level was also significantly increased ($p < 0.05$) in all three GBM cells after treatment with Cur or SLCP in comparison to the vehicle group (Figure 1A,D). We also observed that the ratio of LC3A/B-II/LC3A/B-I was significantly increased by Cur and or SLCP treatment in all three GBM cells lines in comparison to vehicle-treated cells (Figure 1A,D). SLCP-treated cells had more changes in autophagic markers, overall, than did Cur-treated cells. Similar to the Western blot data, the immunofluorescence intensity of Atg5, Atg7, Beclin-1, and LC3A/B all tended to increase in U-87MG cells after treatment with Cur and or SLCP, in comparison to vehicle-treated cells (Figure 1G).

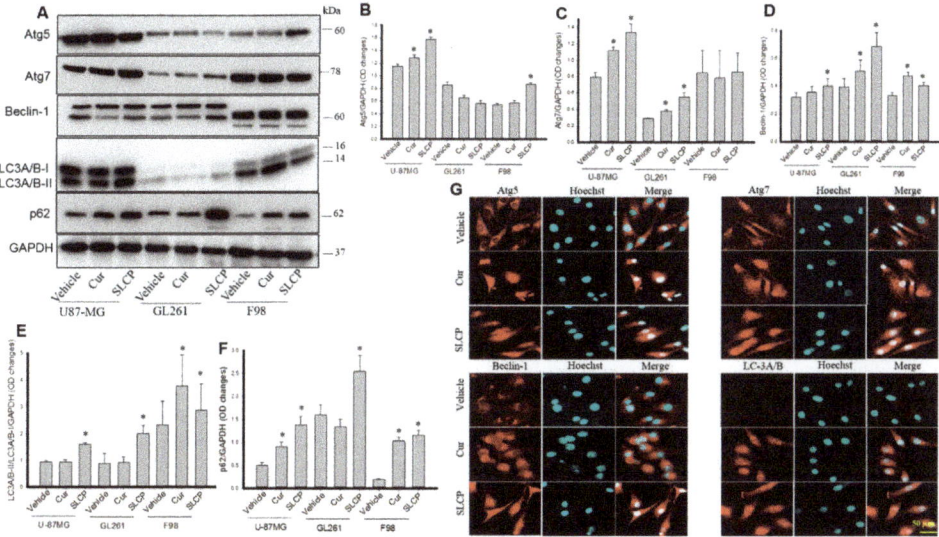

Figure 1. Changes of autophagy markers in GBM cells after treatment with Cur and or SLCP. (**A–F**): U-87MG, GL261, and F98 cells were treated with either Cur or SLCP (25 µM) for 24-h and then Western blots and immunocytochemistry (ICC) were performed. The Western blots data showed that there were significant increased levels of Atg5, Atg7, Beclin-1, LC3A/B, and p62 after treatment with SLCP and/or Cur. Values are represented as mean ± standard error of mean (SEM) from three independent observations. * $p < 0.05$ in comparison to the respective vehicle-treated group. (**G**): Immunocytochemisty (ICC) revealed apparent increases in ICC intensity of Atg5, Atg7, Beclin-1, and LC3/A/B in SLCP- and Cur-treated U-87MG cells in comparison to vehicle-treated cells. Scale bar indicates 50 µm and is applicable to all images.

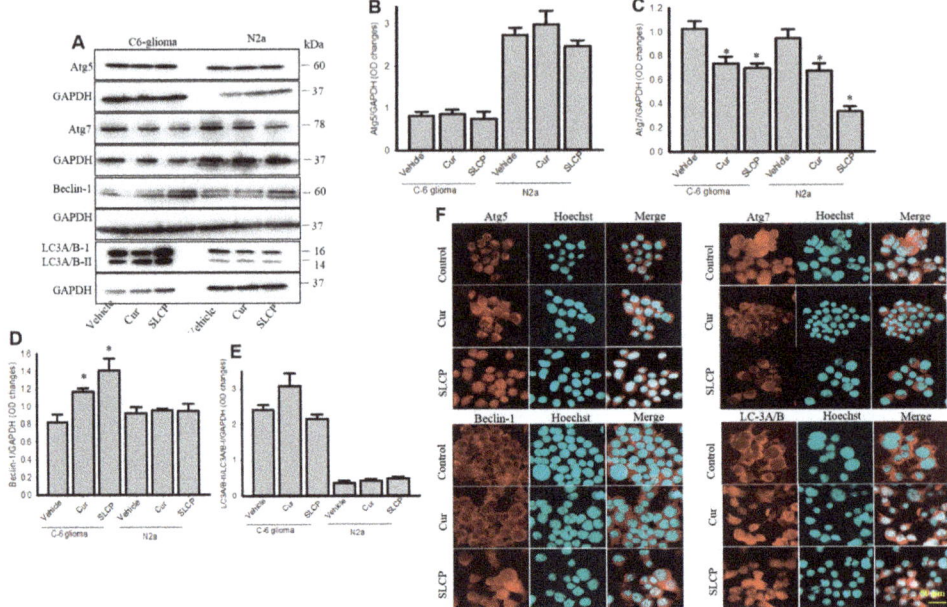

Figure 2. Changes of autophagy markers in C6-glioma and N2a cells after treatment with SLCP and Cur. C6-glima and N2a cells were treated with either Cur or SLCP (25 µM) for 24-h prior to performing Western blots and ICC. (**A–E**): The Western blots analyses revealed that there were no significant changes of autophagy markers following treatment, except Atg7 levels were significantly decreased in both cell lines (**C**) and Beclin-1 levels were increased in C6-glioma (**D**). Values are represented as mean ± SEM from three independent observations. * $p < 0.05$ in comparison to the respective vehicle-treated cells. (**F**): ICC of autophagy markers in N2a cells showed that there were no major changes of the immunofluorescent signal for these parameters. Scale bar indicates 50 µm and is applicable to all images.

2.2. Cur and or SLCP Treatment Has Little Influence on Autophagy Pathways in Rat Glial Tumor Cells (C6-Glioma) and Mouse Neuroblatsoma (N2a) Cells

We did not observe any significant changes of Atg5 (Figure 2A,B) and LC3A/B levels (Figure 2A,E) after treatment with Cur and or SLCP treatment. In addition, we observed very little differences of Atg7 levels in C6-glioma cells, and there was a decrease in N2a cells (Figure 2A,C) after Cur and or SLCP treatment. In contrast, Beclin-1 was increased in C6-glioma, but not in N2a cells (Figure 2A,D) after Cur and or SCLP treatment. The ICC of Atg5, Atg7, Beclin-1, and LC3A/B in U-87MG also showed comparable results, as shown in the Western blots after Cur and/or SLCP treatment (Figure 2F).

2.3. SLCP Inhibits Mitophagy Markers More than Cur in GBM Cells.

We also investigated the most important mitophagy markers, such as BNIP3L/NIX, FUNDC1, BNIP3, PINK-1, and HIF-1α, by Western blots. We observed that BNIP3L/NIX was significantly decreased in GL261 and F98 cells ($p < 0.05$) and there was a trend of reduction of this protein in U-87MG after treatment with Cur and SLCP, in comparison to the vehicle-treated group (Figure 3A,B). Similarly, the FUNDC1 level was also significantly decreased in SLCP-treated cells greater than the Cur treated and vehicle-treated group (Figure 3A,C). In addition, BNIP3, PINK-1, and HIF-1α levels were also significantly decreased ($p < 0.05$) in Cur and or SLCP-treated cells in comparison to the vehicle-treated group (Figure 3A,D,E). Whereas, we found a significant decrease of BNIP3L/NIX and

HIF-1α in C6-glioma and N2a cells after treatment with Cur and or SLCP (Figure 3F–I), whereas no significant changes were observed in the case of FUNDC1 protein in both the cell lines (Figure 3F,H).

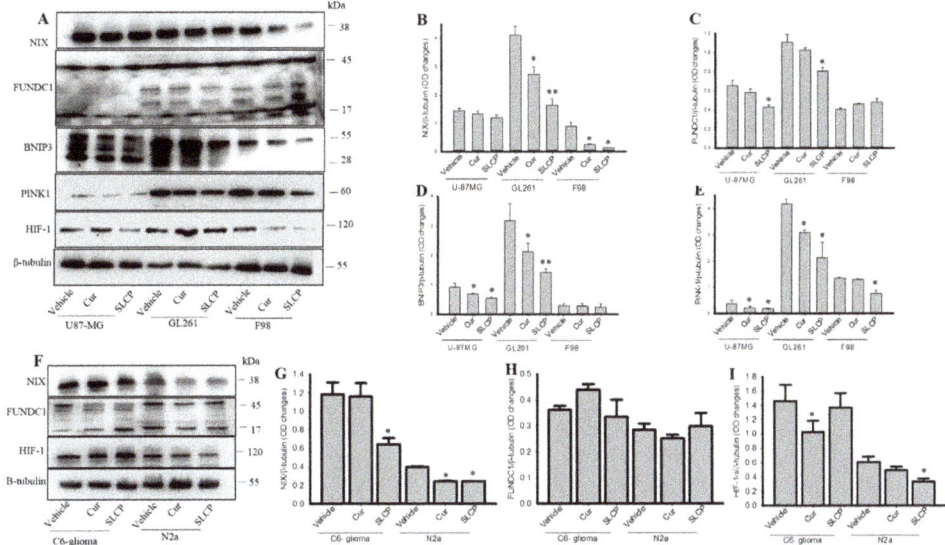

Figure 3. Mitophagy markers were down-regulated more in GBM cells by SLCP than by Cur. U-87MG, GL261, F98, C6-glioma, and N2a cells were treated with either Cur or SLCP (25 μM for 24-h) prior to Western blots analyses. The levels of BNIP3L/NIX, FUNDC1, BNIP3, PINK-1, and HIF-1α were significantly down-regulated ($p < 0.05$) after treatment of SLCP and or Cur in all three GBM cell lines (**A–E**), and SLCP showed greater decreases of these parameters than did Cur. Both NIX and HIF-1α were decreased in C6-glioma and N2a cells, but not FUNDC1 (**F–I**). Values are represented as mean ± SEM from three independent observations. * $p < 0.05$ and ** $p < 0.01$, in comparison to the respective vehicle-treated cells.

2.4. SLCP Inhibits PI3K-Akt/mTOR Pathway Activity in GBM Cells More than Cur does in GBM

We observed that PI3Kp85, phosphoPI3Kp85, total Akt, p-AKT, mTOR, and p-mTOR levels were significantly decreased in U-87MG, GL261, and F98 cell lines after treatment with Cur and or SLCP (Figure 4A–D). SLCP showed greater inhibition of the PI3k-Akt/mTOR pathway than Cur. Whereas in the case of C6-glioma and N2a cells, this pathway was mostly unaltered (Figure 4G–K).

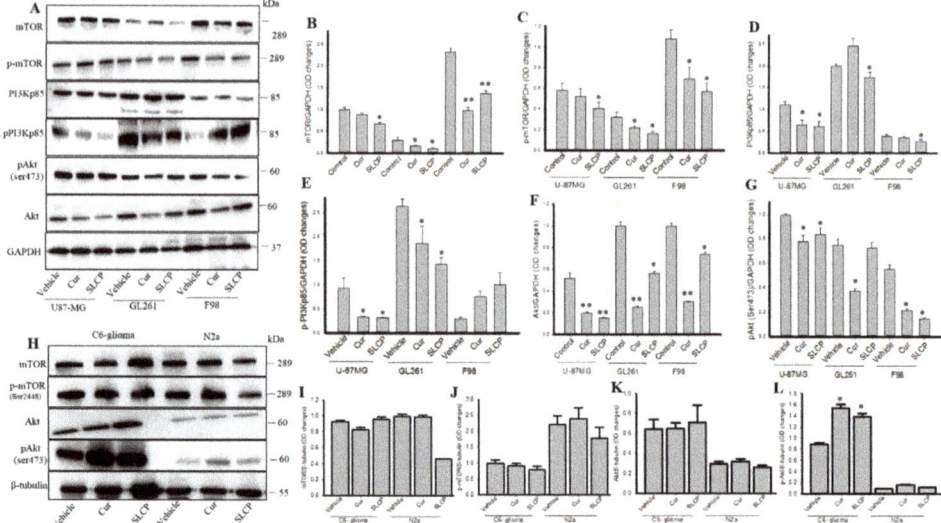

Figure 4. SLCP inhibited the PI3K-Akt/mTOR pathway greater than Cur in cultured GBM cells. U-87MG, GL261, F98, C6-glioma, and N2a cells were treated with either Cur or SLCP (25 μM for 24-h) prior to Western blots and ICC. (**A–G**): Western blots analyses revealed that PI3Kp85, pPI3Kp85, total Akt, p-Akt (Ser473), mTOR, and p-mTOR levels were significantly decreased in all three GBM cells after treatment with Cur and or SLCP, in comparison to the respective vehicle-treated cells. These parameters were unaltered in C6-glioma and or N2a cells (**H–L**), except that pAkt was significantly increased in C6-glioma after the treatment. Values are represented as mean ± SEM from three independent observations. * $p < 0.05$ and ** $p < 0.01$ in comparison to their respective vehicle-treated cells.

2.5. Cur and or SLCP Treatment Inhibited Chaperone-Mediated Autophagy (CMA) Markers in GBM Cells.

CMA markers, such as HSC70, were unaltered in all three GBM cell lines, but LAMP2A levels were significantly down-regulated after treatment with Cur and or SLCP (Figure 5A,D,E). In contrast, HSP70 was increased in all three cell lines after treatment with Cur and or SLCP (Figure 5A,B), and the HSP90 level was also diminished in U-87MG and GL261, but was increased in F98 cells treated with SLCP (Figure 5A,C).

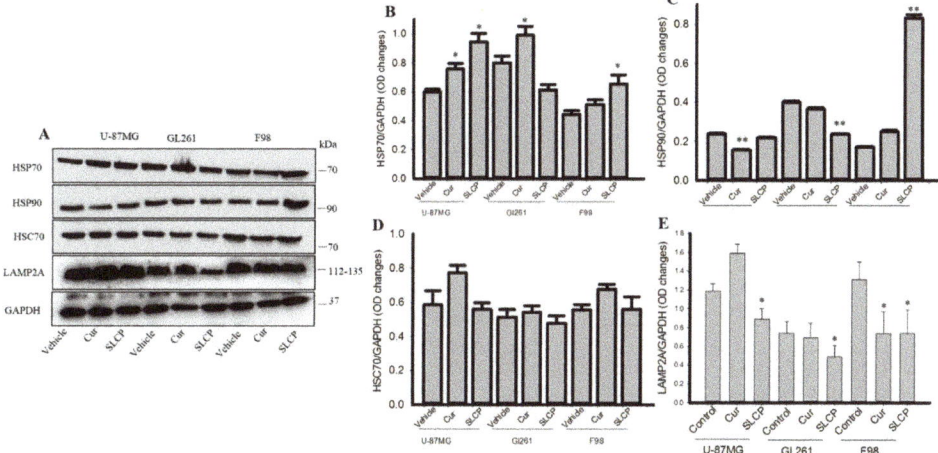

Figure 5. Chaperone-mediated autophagy markers were inhibited in GBM cells after SLCP or Cur treatment. U-87MG, GL261, F98, C6-glioma, and N2a cells were treated with either Cur or SLCP (25 µM for 24-h) prior to Western blots. HSC70 levels were unaltered by SLCP or Cur treatment, while LAMP2A levels were significantly decreased in all the GBM cell lines (**A,D,E**). There were significant increases in levels of HSP70 (**A,B**) and significant decreases in levels of HSP90 (**A,C**, but in F98 by SLCP) after treatment with Cur or SLCP treatments. The changes were more in the case of SLCP-treated cells in comparison to Cur-treated cells. Values are represented as mean ± SEM from two independent observations. * $p < 0.05$ and ** $p < 0.01$, in comparison to their respective vehicle-treated group.

2.6. Cell Survival and Cell Death Markers Were also Modulated by SLCP More than Cur in GBM Cells.

There was a significant increase ($p < 0.01$) in Bax and Cyt-c and caspase-3 levels in both Cur and SLCP-treated cells in comparison to vehicle-treated cells (Figure 6A–E). In contrast, there was a significant decrease of Bcl-2 in GL261 and F98 cells (Figure 6A,B). Unlike GBM cell lines, Bax and Bcl2 were unaltered in C6-glioma and N2a cells (Figure 6F,G), but Cas-3 (Figure 6F,J) levels were increased in C6-glioma, while being unaltered in N2a cells after Cur or SLCP treatment, in comparison to vehicle-treated cells.

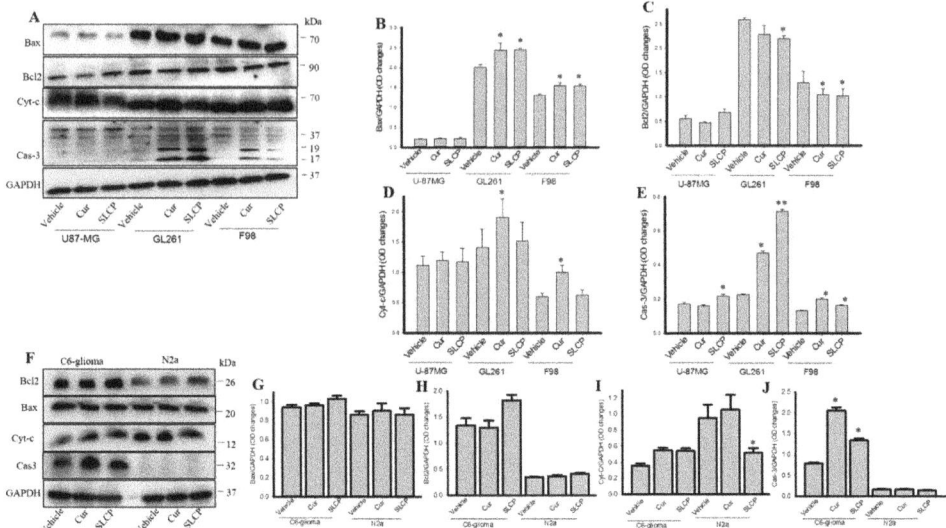

Figure 6. Cell death and cell survival markers in GBM cells. U-87MG, GL261, F98, C6-glioma, and N2a cells were treated with either Cur or SLCP (25 µM for 24-h) prior to Western blots analyses. Western blots analyses showed that SLCP and Cur treatments increased Bax, Cyt-c, and caspase-3 and decreased Bcl2 in all three GBM cell lines, in comparison to vehicle-treated cells (**A**–**E**). Cell survival and cell death markers were unaltered in the case of C6-glioma and N2a cells, except for Caspase-3, which was increased in C6-glioma after both of these treatments. Values are represented as mean ± SEM from two independent observations. * $p < 0.05$ and ** $p < 0.01$ in comparison to either in Cur-treated or to vehicle-treated cells.

2.7. SLCP Treatment Produced Greater Increases in the Number of Autophagy Vacuoles in U-87MG Cells than Did Cur Treatments

To investigate the degree of formation of autophagy vacuoles (AV) after Cur or SLCP-treatment, U-87MG cells were treated with SLCP and/or Cur for 24 h. TEM images indicated that there were significantly more autophagy vacuoles in SLCP-treated cells ($p < 0.01$) in comparison to Cur-treated cells (Cur: 61.00% and in SLCP: 163.84%) (Figure 7A,B). In addition, SLCP treatments increased membrane blebbing, cytoskeleton disorientation, and chromosomal condensation more in U-87MG cells than Cur-treated cells (Figure S1).

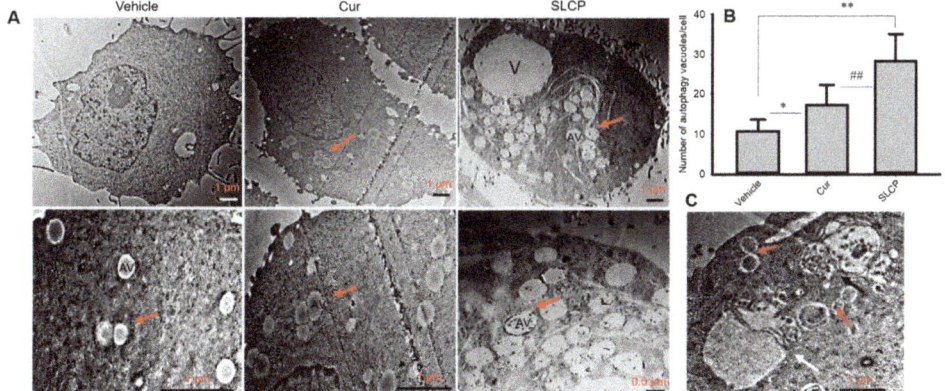

Figure 7. SLCP treatments resulted in more autophagy vacuole formations in U-87MG cells than did treatments with Cur. U-87MG cells were grown and treated with either Cur or SLCP (25 μM for 24-h). Cells were processed for TEM and images were taken with JEOL-TEM. (**A**): Representative TEM images showing that the numbers of autophagy vacuoles were significantly increased (**B**) in the case of SLCP-treated cells compared to Cur-treated cells. (**C**): Fusion of two autophagy vacuoles (red arrow), autophagolysosome complex (black arrow), and mitophagy (white arrow) after treatments with SLCP for 24 h. Scale bars indicate 1 μm. V-vacuole, AV-autophagy vacuoles, arrow indicates autophagy vacuoles. * $p < 0.05$ and ** $p < 0.01$ compared to vehicle group; ## $p < 0.01$ compared to Cur-treated cells.

3. Discussion

Accumulated experimental evidence supports the contention that the dysregulation of autophagy mechanisms significantly contributes to GBM cell death and survival [10]. In the present study, we compared the role of natural Cur or SLCP (a greater permeable solid lipid Cur formulation) on autophagy markers, including mitophagy and chaperone-mediated autophagy pathways in cultured GBM cells. We found a greater induction of autophagy markers, including an increased number of autophagy vacuoles, along with a significant decrease in the levels of mitophagy markers and inhibition of the PI3K-Akt/mTOR pathway by SLCP than by natural Cur in different GBM cell lines, without significantly affecting the rat glial tumor cells (C6-glioma) and mouse neuroblastoma (N2a) cells.

Given the present lack of effectiveness and the preponderance of side-effects when the current standard chemotherapies for GBM are used [28,29], many laboratories, including our own, have started investigating natural anti-cancer agents, such as Cur [2,30]. However, to avoid the poor solubility, rapid degradation, and limited bio-availability of natural Cur [17,23], we utilized more permeable solid lipid Cur particles (SLCP) [15,18,19]. Previously, we have demonstrated that SLCP has greater anti-cancer effects in U-87MG cells than does natural Cur [19]. However, its role in autophagy mechanisms in GBM cells remained unexplored. Given that Cur has been shown to induce autophagy, we hypothesized that using SLCP, with its higher solubility and greater membrane permeability, would have stronger modulatory effects on autophagy than natural Cur. Therefore, we investigated different autophagy markers in three different GBM cells (U-87MG, GL261, and F98) after treatment with Cur and or SLCP.

GBM cell metastasis can be prevented by induction of apoptosis [31]. However, cells can die by alternative pathways, such as autophagy. Interestingly, when autophagy is induced, either at earlier or later stages, it may lead to non-apoptotic cell death [32]. In addition, cells with a dysfunctional apoptotic pathway may undergo autophagic cell death [33]. Thus, the timing and magnitude of the cellular stresses seem to dictate whether autophagy or apoptosis will be activated. Moreover, autophagy preceded apoptosis, and this mechanism makes the cells more susceptible to death [10]. Given this, we sought to understand the mechanisms of autophagy, including mitochondrial autophagy (mitophagy) and CMA markers, in cultured GBM cells by comparing the treatment effects of SLCP with those of natural Cur.

To monitor the autophagy mechanism in GBM cells after treatment with Cur or SLCP, we investigated the Atg5, Atg7, Beclin-1 and LC3A/B, and p62. Atg5 and Atg7 are considered to be essential molecules for the induction of autophagy [34]. For example, defective Atg5 or Atg7 expression consequences decreased autophagic activity in animals [9]. In the present study, we observed an up-regulation of these two markers in all three GBM cells, (except Atg5 in U-87MG cells) (Figure 1) after treatment with Cur and or SLCP, suggesting the induction of autophagosome formation, which has been verified by transmission electron microscopic studies (Figure 7). Similarly, Beclin-1 is an important autophagosome initiation tumor suppressor protein, whose expression is reduced in many cancers. It interacts with Bcl-2 and can induce apoptosis by activating the function of mitochondrial permeability transition pore (MPTP) [35]. Overexpression of Beclin-1 in U-87MG cells enhances the capacity for cellular autophagy, whereas silencing of Beclin-1 decreases autophagic capacity [36]. We found an increase in beclin-1 levels after Cur and/or SLCP treatment, suggesting an enhancement of the autophagy pathway (Figure 1). Our findings are supported by Liang and colleagues, who also found that over-expression of Beclin-1 in U-87MG cells enhanced the capacity for cellular autophagy and induced apoptosis, whereas silencing of Beclin-1 decreased autophagic capacity [36].

LC3A/B is the key structural component of the autophagosome formation [37]. The amount of LC3-II reflects the number of autophagosomes and autophagy-related structures and a decrease of its level indicates an impairment of this process. Therefore, levels of LC3 are considered the most reliable marker to monitor autophagy. We observed an increase in the levels of LC3A/B-II after treatment with Cur or SLCP, indicating autophagosome formation was enhanced, which was supported by the recent in vitro work of Guo and colleagues [38]. Although the amount of LC3-II at a given time point does not necessarily estimate the autophagic activity, because inhibition of autophagosome degradation sometimes increases the amount of LC3-II, most cases reveal that increased amounts of LC3-II reflect the number of autophagosomes, thus increased levels of LC3A/B, suggesting that the autophagy mechanism was induced by these treatments (Figure 1). In addition, we also investigated the levels of sequestosome 1 (SQSTM1) or p62, which binds directly to LC3. Increased levels of LC3A/B-II and p62 indicate an increased accumulation of autophagosome formation, which is correlated with an increase in autophagic vacuoles (AV), as revealed by our TEM studies. Although increased levels of p62 inhibit autophagy mechanisms, and decreased levels can be observed when autophagy is induced, therefore, p62 levels may be used as a marker to study autophagic flux. We found that p62 levels were increased by Cur or SLCP treatment, which may be due to blocking of the fusion of autophagy vacuoles with lysosome or by the inhibition of a later maturation step of autophagosome degradation. The overall accumulated increase in AVs in cells by these treatments could induce autophagy-related cell death. Recently, Zanotto-Filho and colleagues showed that autophagy induction improves the efficacy of Cur and or TMZ combination therapy in animal models of glioblastomas, suggesting Cur is a potent autophagy inducer in GBM cells [39].

As GBM cells are resistant to apoptosis, the mammalian target for the rapamycin (mTOR) signaling pathway plays an important role [40]. In fact, the mTOR pathway has emerged as a major effector of cell growth and proliferation and is an attractive target for cancer therapy [41,42]. Indeed, mTOR and phosphorylated mTOR (p-mTOR, active form of mTOR) is a potent blocker of autophagy [43]. Thus, inhibiting the mTOR pathway could be a viable strategy to induce autophagy-related cell death to prevent GBM growth. These proteins are controlled by the cellular PI3K and Akt levels. Increases in PI3K activate Akt, which activates the mTOR pathway and induces tumorigenesis, whereas their inhibition prevents activation of this pathway [44]. We observed a significant decrease in levels of PI3Kp85, phosphorylated PI3Kp85, total Akt, p-Akt, mTOR, and p-mTOR after treatment with Cur and or SLCP, indicating PI3K-Akt/mTOR pathways were significantly affected by these treatments, which corresponds to recent findings of Yu and colleagues [45]. Decreased mTOR levels have been shown to induce autophagy [46]. Interestingly, we observed greater levels of PI3K-Akt/mTOR inhibition in SLCP-treated cells (Figure 4) than in Cur-treated cells, indicating greater induction of autophagy by SLCP than natural Cur, which was further supported by increased levels of autophagy markers and the number of AV (Figure 7). Recently, Guo and colleagues also reported that Cur may protect cells against oxidative stress-induced damage through induction of autophagy via inhibition of the Akt/mTOR pathway [38]. Similarly, using in vitro and in vivo models of GBM, Zhuang and colleagues also reported that Cur promotes differentiation of glioma-initiating cells by inducing autophagy [47]. Furthermore, Aoki and colleagues reported that Cur suppresses the growth of malignant gliomas in vitro and in vivo through induction of autophagy by inhibition of the Akt/mTOR/p70S6K pathway and activation of the ERK1/2 pathway [48]. The above observations were supported by the work of Zhao and colleagues, who reported that Cur potentiates the anti-tumor activities against GBM by suppressing the PI3K/AKT and NF-κB/COX-2 signaling pathways [14]. All these previous observations further supported and confirmed our findings.

In addition, we investigated the mitophagy markers. Mitophagy is a selective form of macroautophagy in which mitochondria are targeted for degradation in autophagolysosomes [49,50]. Although mitophagy is not a mechanism of autophagy, it is a special type of autophagy pathway, but it has beneficial effects, especially for the elimination of old and/or damaged mitochondria, thus maintaining the integrity of the mitochondrial pool. Inhibition of mitophagy has adverse effects on mitochondrial health and cell survival [49]. In addition, mitophagy also plays a key role in reducing mitochondrial mass [49]. We have investigated mitophagy markers, such as BNIP3L/NIX, FUNDC1, BNIP3, PINK-1, and HIF-1α (Figure 3). BNIP3L (Bcl2 and adenovirus E1B 19-kDa-interacting protein 3-like), also known as NIX, are the proteins which interact with Bcl2 and are involved in cell death and autophagy, suggesting that BNIP3L/NIX are implicated in the pathogenesis of cancer [51]. BNIP3L is required for interaction with Bcl2, the main anti-apoptotic protein present in mitochondria, whereas decreased levels of BNIP3L may inhibit interactions with Bcl2, thus indirectly inducing cell death [51]. Similarly, BNIP3 is another mitophagy marker, which has a similar role in mitophagy, like BNIP3L/NIX. We found a greater decrease in levels of both NIX and BNIP3 in the case of SLCP (Figure 3), which suggests that SLCP has greater capability to induce cell death. Moreover, in tumor cells, NIX and BNIP3 regulate mitophagy in response to hypoxia, and the deregulation of NIX and BNIP3 expression is associated with increased tumor growth [51]. One of the factors noted in most malignancies is the hypoxic environment, where hypoxia-inducing factor-1α (HIF-1α) levels increase. This factor is a positive regulator of NIX and BNIP3 expression. Therefore, reduction of HIF-1α may down-regulate NIX or BNIP3 levels. For example, knock-down of HIF-1α in glioma cells significantly impairs their migration in vitro, as well as their ability to invade into the brain parenchyma in vivo [52]. In addition, HIF-1α acts as an activator of angiogenic factors, such as placenta-like growth factor and platelet-derived growth factor. Therefore, decreased levels of HIF-1α may be one of the reasons for the down-regulation of NIX or BNIP3 levels, indicating a reduction of mitophagy and induction of cell death.

Like NIX and BNIP3, FUNDC1 is an adaptor molecule present at the outer membrane of mitochondria [53]. NIX, BNIP3, and FUNDC1 interact with Bcl-2 or Bcl-XL and modulate in binding with LC3 and recruit components of the autophagy machinery to the mitochondria. Therefore, inhibition of these adaptor proteins, along with decreased HIF-1α after treatment with Cur and or SLCP, indicates decreased mitophagy, which may lead to induction of cell death [49]. Greater inhibition of these proteins by SLCP treatment in comparison to Cur indicates SLCP is a stronger negative regulator on these proteins, which suggests that a greater amount of Cur is required to inhibit mitophagy, as well as induction of cell death. Given that mitophagy may also be regulated by PINK-1/Parkin, we investigated the levels of PINK-1 after treatment with Cur and or SLCP. We found a significant reduction of PINK-1 levels (Figure 3), suggesting Cur- and or SLCP-induced mitophagy is PINK-1 dependent. Other than PINK-1, mitophagy may also be regulated by the Parkin pathway, but the role of Parkin in the regulation of cell death is debated. Importantly, PINK1 shuttles between the cytosol and mitochondria in healthy cells. It plays a vital role in communicating the collapse of the mitochondrial membrane potential and it can stabilize on the outer membrane of depolarized mitochondria and recruit Parkin, which is initially inactive. In addition, PINK1 can phosphorylate Parkin on the ubiquitin-like (UBL) domain, resulting in an increase of its ubiquitin ligase activity and the formation of polyubiquitin chains on the surface of depolarized mitochondrial membranes, which could act as a Parkin activator by overcoming the autoinhibitory mechanism of Parkin. Therefore, we investigated the levels of PINK1 rather than Parkin.

In addition to macroautophagy and microautophagy, we also investigated the status of chaperone-mediated autophagy (CMA), which is a special type of autophagy for degradation of tiny proteins aggregates. It requires chaperones, such as heat shock cognate 70 (HSC70) and lysosome-associated membrane protein type 2A (LAMP-2A). Although HSC70 levels were unaltered, LAMP2A was significantly down regulated by Cur or SLCP, indicating CMA was also inhibited (Figure 5). In addition, we also checked whether the other chaperones, such as HSP70 and HSP90, were affected by Cur and or SLCP treatments in GBM cells. We observed that there was an upregulation of HSP70, whereas opposite effects were observed in the case of HSP90 in all these GBM cells (except F98 cells) after SLCP treatment. HSP90 become upregulated in cancer and the inhibition of HSP90 by Cur or SLCP suggested that Cur/SLCP acts as a HSP90-inhibitor [54].

Previously, we have confirmed that the SLCP induced greater cell death in U-87MG cells by using MTT, TUNEL, Annexin-V staining, and comet assays [19]. In support of our previous findings, we presently observed more membrane blebbing, actin or cytoarchitectural damage, and chromosomal condensation (Figure S1), as well as induction of cell-death related proteins and reduction of cell survival proteins (Figure 6) in the case of SLCP, when compared to Cur-treated cells. This finding indicates that a higher amount of Cur is required to damage the cells, which can be achieved more efficiently by SLCP treatments. Moreover, an increased number of autophagy vacuoles (Figure 7), chromosomal condensation, and membrane blebbing, as seen by TEM images (Figure S1), confirmed that SLCP can induce autophagy and cell death more efficiently than by using Cur (Figure 6). Extrapolating these results, we have assessed that Cur and SLCP have roles on autophagy mechanisms in cultured GBM cells, without affecting the rat glial tumor cell line (C6-glioma) or mouse neuroblastoma cell line (N2a cells). To this end, the C6-glioma and N2a cells that were treated with the same concentrations (25 µM) of Cur and/or SLCP consistently revealed the lowest levels of autophagy and cell death markers (Figures 2 and 6), which suggests that Cur and SLCP can specifically target its therapeutic effects on GBM cells (Type-IV glioma), rather than glial tumor or neuroblastoma cells. In addition, during cellular stress, pro-survival and pro-death processes are concomitantly activated, which depends on the degree of stress. Mild cellular stress causes damage to a few mitochondria, which are rapidly sequestered by autophagosomes, whereas severe stress induces mitochondrial damage and autophagy is unable to efficiently clear this. During these circumstances, mitochondria release pro-death proteins, such as cytochrome c, apoptosis inducing factor (AIF) and SMAC/Diablo, that can activate the cell death pathway. As treatment of Cur/SLCP induced cellular stress, therefore, it can induce mitochondrial damage and activate the cell death pathway. Overall, Cur or SLCP treatment induced cellular stress, which interfered in autophagy, mitophagy, and the cell death and survival pathway as observed in cultured GBM cells.

As autophagy determines cell death and survivability, therefore, the role of autophagy in GBM cell death and survivability after Cur and SLCP treatment needs to be critically analyzed. In fact, not only under disease conditions, but even under normal physiological conditions, the autophagy mechanism is active and can promote cell death or increase cell growth. For example, nutrient starvation, deprivation of supporting factors, or a hypoxic environment increases cell survivability [55,56]. Similarly, autophagy-dependent program cell death also occurs during mammalian embryogenesis [57] and in the case of apoptosis-resistant cells, such as in the absence of the pro-apoptotic proteins, Bax and Bak [58]. Moreover, many cellular environment autophagy cross-talks with the apoptotic machineries and directly inhibits apoptosis [59]. Therefore, the connections between autophagy and cell death are very complicated and controversial. In the case of cancer cells, autophagy may act as a tumor suppressor, as well as inducing tumor growth [60]. Some reports suggest that induction of autophagy can suppress tumor growth, whereas its prolonged activation may kill cancer cells with a high apoptotic threshold. In contrast, prolonged inhibition of autophagy may lead to cell survival instead of cell death. Most interestingly, the apoptotic pathways become mutated in human tumors, where autophagy plays alternative forms of PCD to prevent their growth. In our study, we found an induction of autophagy by Cur and or SLCP treatment, but whether autophagy was the mechanism by which GBM cells were dying (cell death by autophagy) or autophagy was present during cell death (cell death with autophagy) is an open question. As we know, when cell death is mediated by autophagy and if the cell death is prevented after inhibition of autophagy, then it is considered as "autophagic cell death". In our study, we did not investigate the cell death after inhibition of the autophagy mechanism, therefore, we were not sure whether it was a "autophagic cell death". However, the "autophagic cell death" is also characterized by the presence of abundant autophagosomes and lack of phagocytic activities, and we found many autophagosomes in U-87MG cells after treatment with Cur and or SLCP (Figure 7), which suggests that Cur and or SLCP may have partially induced cell death caused by autophagy, along with apoptotic death [19]. However, we prefer to describe this phenomenon as "cell death with autophagy" rather than an important effector mechanism of cell death because we do not have concrete evidence to confirm whether the cell death was caused by autophagy. Most importantly, Cur and/or SLCP treatment caused DNA damage [19], and disruption of the cytoskeleton (Figure S1), which induced autophagy and suppress tumor growth, suggesting that these treatments have a negative impact on GBM cell survivability. Therefore, further experiments are needed for a better understanding of the role of autophagy mechanisms on GBM cell death and survival after treatment with Cur and or SLCP in order to apply its beneficial role for GBM therapy.

4. Materials and Methods

4.1. Chemicals

Curcumin (Purity >65%; catalog no: C1386-50G (Sigma, St. Louis, MO, USA), propidium iodide (PI), and other accessory chemicals were procured from Sigma (St. Louis, MO, USA). Hoechst 33342 was purchased from ThermoFisher Scientific (Grand Island, NY, USA). Solid lipid particles containing Cur (SLCP or Longvida, which contains 26% pure Cur) were gifted from Verdure Sciences (Noblesville, IN, USA). The SLCP has been well characterized by us and others in collaboration with Verdure Sciences, including clinical studies in Alzheimer's disease [19,27]. The human origin GBM cell line (U-87MG; catalog no: HTB-14), rat GBM cells (F98, catalog no: ATCC® CRL2397™), mouse glioma (C6-glioma, catalog no: ATCC® CCL107™), and N2a (catalog no: ATCC® CCL-131™) cells were purchased from ATCC (Manassas, VA, USA), whereas the mouse GBM cell line (GL261) was procured from DCTD/DTP Tumor Repository at the National Cancer Institute. All the antibodies used in this study are documented in Table 1.

4.2. Cell Culture

U-87MG and N2a cells were grown with Eagle's Minimum Essential Medium (EMEM, GIBCO) containing 10% heat-inactivated fetal bovine serum (FBS), and penicillin/streptomycin (100 IU/mL penicillin and 100 µg streptomycin/mL). The Gl261 cells were cultured in Roswell Park Memorial Institute Medium-1640 (RPMI-1640), along with 10% FBS and pen/strep (100 IU/mL penicillin and 100 µg streptomycin/mL), and F98 cells were grown on Dulbeco's Modified Eagle's Medium (DMEM), along with 10% FBS and pen/strep, (100 IU/mL penicillin and 100 µg streptomycin/mL). The C6-glioma cells were grown in F12K media along with 2.5% FBS and 15% horse serum and 100 IU/mL penicillin and 100 µg streptomycin/mL. The cultures were maintained at 37 °C in a humidified atmosphere at 5% CO_2. Prior to the experiment, the cells were grown either in a 75 cm^2

culture flask, or on glass cover slips, with fresh media and antibiotics, but without growth factors, depending on the experimental setup.

Table 1. Sources of different antibodies used in this study.

Antibodies	Source	Type	Company	Catalog No.	Address
Atg5	Rabbit	Monoclonal	Cell signaling Technology	12994S	Danvers, MA, USA
Atg7	Rabbit	Monoclonal	Cell signaling Technology	8558S	Danvers, MA, USA
Beclin-1	Rabbit	Polyclonal	Cell signaling Technology	3738S	Danvers, MA, USA
LC3A/B	Rabbit	Polyclonal	Cell signaling Technology	4108S	Danvers, MA, USA
p62	Rabbit	Polyclonal	Cell signaling Technology	5114S	Danvers, MA, USA
mTOR	Rabbit	Polyclonal	Cell signaling Technology	2972S	Danvers, MA, USA
p-mTOR	Rabbit	Monoclonal	Cell signaling Technology	2971S	Danvers, MA, USA
PI3Kp85	Rabbit	Monoclonal	Cell signaling Technology	4292S	Danvers, MA, USA
BNIP3L/NIX	Rabbit	Monoclonal	Cell signaling Technology	12396S	Danvers, MA, USA
FUNDC1	Rabbit	Monoclonal	EMD Millipore	ABC506	Burlington, MA, USA
HIF-1α	Rabbit	Monoclonal	Cell signaling Technology	14179S	Danvers, MA, USA
PINK-1	Rabbit	Monoclonal	Cell signaling Technology	6946S	Danvers, MA, USA
Cyt-c	Rabbit	Monoclonal	Cell Signaling Technology	4272S	Danvers, MA, USA
Caspase-3	Rabbit	Monoclonal	Cell Signaling Technology	9661S	Danvers, MA, USA
Bax	Rabbit	Polyclonal	Cell signaling Technology	2772S	Danvers, MA, USA
Bcl-2	Mouse	Monoclonal	Santa Cruz Biotech	Sc-7382	Santa Cruz, CA, USA
Akt	Rabbit	Monoclonal	Cell signaling Technology	9272S	Danvers, MA, USA
pAkt (Ser473)	Rabbit	Monoclonal	Cell signaling Technology	4060S	Danvers, MA, USA
HSP70	Rabbit	Polyclonal	Cell signaling Technology	4872S	Danvers, MA, USA
HSP90	Rabbit	Polyclonal	Cell signaling Technology	4877S	Danvers, MA, USA
HSC70	Rabbit	Polyclonal	Cell signaling Technology	8444S	Danvers, MA, USA
LAMP2	Mouse	Polyclonal	Santa Cruz Biotech	sc-20004	Santa Cruz, CA, USA
GAPDH	Rabbit	Monoclonal	Cell signaling Technology	2118S	Danvers, MA, USA
β-tubulin	Rabbit	Monoclonal	Cell signaling Technology	2146S	Danvers, MA, USA

4.3. Curcumin and or SLCP Treatment

Cur was solubilized in pure methanol (100%), as described previously (28), and then diluted in the Hank's balanced salt solution (HBSS) to obtain its desired concentration before being added to the culture flask containing the cells. The final methanol concentration was ≤0.1% and the same amount of methanol was added to the vehicle-treated cell. The final Cur or SLCP concentration was 25 µM. This dose was selected on the basis of our dose dependent cell viability data (Figure S1) [34].

4.4. Immunocytochemistry and Confocal Imaging of Autophagy Markers.

Immunocytochemistry of Atg5, Atg7, Beclin-1, and LC3A/B were performed as described previously [24]. Briefly, U-87MG and N2a cells were grown (1 × 10^5/well) on a Petri-plate containing glass cover slips in EMEM with pen/strep (100 IU/mL penicillin and 100 µg streptomycin/mL) for 24 h and then treated with Cur and/or SLCP (25 µM) for another 24 h. Then, the cells were fixed with 4% paraformaldehyde after washing with cold PBS (0.1 mM, pH 7.4) and incubated with rabbit anti-Atg5, Atg7, Beclin-1, and LC3A/B monoclonal and polyclonal antibodies (1:200, see Table 1) overnight at 4 °C, followed by incubation with the respective secondary antibodies (1:500) tagged with Alexa-fluorophore 560 (Molecular Probes, OR) for 1 h at room temperature. Nuclei were stained with Hoechst 33342 (20 mM, ThermoFisher Scientific, Grand Island, NY, USA) for 5 min and visualized using a table top Fluoview confocal laser scanning microscope (FV1oi, Olympus) using appropriate filters for excitation and emission.

4.5. Transmission Electron Microscopy (TEM)

U-87MG cells were processed for TEM as described by Schrand and colleagues [61]. Briefly, U-87MG cells were grown in 60 mm Petri plate (~10^6 cells/mL) in EMEM with pen/strep (100 IU/mL penicillin and 100 µg streptomycin/mL) for 24 h. The next day, the cells were treated with Cur and or SLCP (25 µM) for 24 h. After treatment, the cells were thoroughly rinsed with fresh serum free media at room temperature (RT) for 3 times, 5 min each. Then, the cells were treated with 0.25% trypsin-EDTA solution for 1–2 min and the cell suspension was taken in a 15 mL conical tube and centrifuged for 5 min at 1000× g at room temperature. Supernatant was removed and 1 mL of fresh 2.5% glutaraldehyde/formaldehyde (dissolved in 0.1 mM PBS, pH 7.4) was added and kept for 2 h at RT. After fixation, the cells were thoroughly rinse with PBS, three times for 10 min each, and 1 mL of 1% osmium tetroxide (dissolved in PBS) was added and allowed for 1 h at RT. Then, the cell pellet was rinsed in PBS five times for 10 min each and then washed in double-distilled water (ddH$_2$O) two times for 10 min each. After centrifugation, the cell pellet was dehydrated through a graded series of ethanol concentrations (50%, 70%, 90%, and 100%) for 10 min each. The cells were treated with propylene oxide: ethanol mixture (1:1) for 30–45 min, then this mixture was replaced with 100% propylene oxide for 10 min, followed by a propylene oxide: resin (1:1) for 45 min before continuing in 100% resin overnight. The sample block was prepared with small plastic cubes at the flat face and cells reached the bottom of the capsule. For sectioning, stereomicroscope lenses were adjusted to the lowest magnification and the lighting was set to focus on the sample. A glass knife was inserted into the knife holder and positioned near the sample block face in the ultramicrotome. The block was trimmed manually by advancing the glass knife attached to the ultra-microtome while viewing the sample through the stereomicroscope lenses. An 80-nm thick section was made, and several sections were collected onto a TEM grid (300-mesh Cu, with support film such as formvar/carbon) and sections on grids were allowed to dry for a few minutes, then carefully placed in a grid storage box using fine-tipped tweezers. For staining, a piece of parafilm was placed in a glass petri dish, onto which a few drops of water or stain were added. Then, the grid was placed face down on a drop of ddH$_2$O for 1–2 min. Then, the grid was transferred face down onto a drop of 1% uranyl acetate and lead acetate (filtered through a 0.2-µm syringe filter) for 30 min, followed by the grid being dipped into a drop of double distilled H$_2$O to rinse. Then, the grids were blot dried using Whatman's filter paper and it was placed in a grid box for storage until imaging. At least 10 individual cells were imaged from each group and the number of autophagy vacuoles were counted from each of the cells manually.

4.6. Western Blot

To investigate different autophagy markers, Western blot was performed as described previously [19,24]. Briefly, after the stipulated period of each experiment, the media was removed and U-87MG, GL261, and F98 cells were washed with cold PBS, scrapped, collected in Eppendorf tubes, centrifuged, and pellets were lysed with cold radio-immunoprecipitation assay (RIPA) buffer, along with protease and phosphatase inhibitors. Total protein was measured from each of the samples by Pierce protein assay reagent. Equal amounts of protein, per lane, were loaded and electrophoresed on 10% Tris-glycine gel and transferred to PVDF membrane (Millipore, Bedford, MA). After probing with respective primary (1:1000; see Table 1) and secondary antibodies, the blots were developed with Immobilon^{TM} Western Chemiluminescent HRP-substrate (Millipore, Billeria, MA). The images were taken by a gel documentation system (Bio-Rad) with an automated exposure time. The relative optical density (OD) was measured using Image-J software (https://imagej.nih.gov/ij/). To ensure equal protein loading in each lane, the blots were probed with either β-tubulin or GAPDH.

4.7. Statistical Analysis

The data were expressed as mean ± SEM. Data were analyzed using one-way analysis of variance (ANOVA), followed by post-hoc Tukey HSD (honestly significant difference) test. Probability ≤0.05 was considered as statistically significant.

5. Conclusions

Overall, we demonstrated that Cur and or SLCP treatment induced autophagy and reduced mitophagy, probably through inhibition of the PI3K-Akt/mTOR signaling pathway in cultured GBM cells. In addition, cell death markers were induced, and cell survival markers were down-regulated by

Cur and or SLCP. Importantly, SLCP showed greater induction of autophagy and greater inhibition of mitophagy markers, along with greater disruption of the PI3K-Akt/mTOR signaling pathway than Cur. There were lowest treatment effects on autophagy and mitophagy in rat glial tumor cells and mouse neuroblastoma cells. Therefore, the data presented demonstrated that induction of autophagy and reduction of mitophagy by Cur and or SLCP treatment, suggesting that treatments with SLCP to prevent GBM cell growth and proliferation may have promising clinical utility.

Supplementary Materials: Supplementary materials can be found at http://www.mdpi.com/1422-0067/20/2/399/s1. Figure S1: SLCP induced greater changes of membrane, cytoskeleton, and nuclear morphology than Cur in U-87MG cells.

Author Contributions: Conceptualization, P.M.; methodology, P.M., J.S., A.A.-G., D.S.; validation, P.M.; formal analysis, P.M., investigation, P.M., J.S., A.A.-G., D.S.; resources, P.M., G.L.D., data curation, P.M.; writing, P.M., editing, P.M., G.L.D., visualization, P.M., J.S., A.A.-G., D.S., G.L.D.; supervision, P.M., and G.L.D.; project administration, P.M.; funding acquisition, G.L.D.

Funding: This work was supported by the Field Neurosciences Institute, St. Mary's of Michigan, and the John G. Kulhavi Professorship in Neurosciences at Central Michigan University.

Acknowledgments: We thank Verdure Sciences (Noblesville, IN) for donating the solid lipid curcumin particles for this study.

Conflicts of Interest: The authors declare no conflict of interest.

Abbreviations

GBM	Glioblastoma
SLCP	Solid lipid curcumin particles
Cur	Curcumin
Atg	Autophagy-related protein
Akt	Protein kinase B
PI3K	Phosphatidyl inositol-3 kinase
mTOR	Mechanistic target of rapamycin
HSP	Heat shock protein
TMZ	Temozolomide
PCD	Program cell death
ATP	Adenosine triphosphate
SLPs	Solid lipid particles
AD	Alzheimer's disease
PI	Propidium iodide
EMEM	Eagle's Minimum Essential Medium,
FBS	Fetal bovine serum
HBSS	Hank's balanced salt solution
DMEM	Dulbecco's Modified Eagle's Medium
FITC	Fluorescent isothiocyanate
DPBS	Dulbecco's phosphate buffer saline
ROS	Reactive oxygen species
BNIP3	Bcl-2/adenovirus E1B 19 kDa-interacting protein
Bax	Bcl$_2$-associated X protein
Bcl2	B-cell lymphoma 2
NF-kB	Nuclear factor kappa beta
ATCC	American type cell culture
SEM	Standard error of mean
PBS	Phosphate buffer saline
EDTA	Ethylene-di-amino-tetra-acetic-acid
RPM	Revolution per minute
mM	Millimolar

RIPA	Radio immunoprecipitation assay
SDS	Sodium dodecyl sulfate
BCA	Bicinchoninic acid assay
PVDF	Polyvinylidene fluoride
ANOVA	One-way analysis of variance
HSD	Honestly significant difference
μM	Micromolar
AU	Arbitrary unit
OD	Optical density
SDS-PAGE	Sodium dodecyl sulfate polyacrylamide gel electrophoresis
TBS	Tris buffer saline
CMA	Chaperone-mediated autophagy
HSC70	Heat shock cognate 70
LAMP-2A	Lysosome-associated membrane protein type 2A
G2/M	Gap2/mitosis
VEGF	Vascular endothelial growth factor

References

1. Davis, M.E. Glioblastoma: Overview of Disease and Treatment. *Clin. J. Oncol. Nurs.* **2016**, *20* (Suppl. 5), S2–S8. [CrossRef] [PubMed]
2. Sordillo, L.A.; Sordillo, P.P.; Helson, L. Curcumin for the Treatment of Glioblastoma. *Anticancer Res.* **2015**, *35*, 6373–6378. [PubMed]
3. Shanmugam, M.K.; Rane, G.; Kanchi, M.M.; Arfuso, F.; Chinnathambi, A.; Zayed, M.E.; Alharbi, S.A.; Tan, B.K.; Kumar, A.P.; Sethi, G. The multifaceted role of curcumin in cancer prevention and treatment. *Molecules* **2015**, *20*, 2728–2769. [CrossRef] [PubMed]
4. Abbruzzese, C.; Matteoni, S.; Signore, M.; Cardone, L.; Nath, K.; Glickson, J.D.; Paggi, M.G. Drug repurposing for the treatment of glioblastoma multiforme. *J. Exp. Clin. Cancer Res.* **2017**, *36*, 169. [CrossRef] [PubMed]
5. Shimizu, S.; Yoshida, T.; Tsujioka, M.; Arakawa, S. Autophagic cell death and cancer. *Int. J. Mol. Sci.* **2014**, *15*, 3145–3153. [CrossRef] [PubMed]
6. Mizushima, N.; Yoshimori, T.; Ohsumi, Y. The role of Atg proteins in autophagosome formation. *Annu. Rev. Cell Dev. Biol.* **2011**, *27*, 107–132. [CrossRef] [PubMed]
7. Mizushima, N.; Komatsu, M. Autophagy: Renovation of cells and tissues. *Cell* **2011**, *147*, 728–741. [CrossRef]
8. Yang, Z.; Klionsky, D.J. An overview of the molecular mechanism of autophagy. *Curr. Top. Microbiol. Immunol.* **2009**, *335*, 1–32.
9. Cuervo, A.M.; Bergamini, E.; Brunk, U.T.; Droge, W.; Ffrench, M.; Terman, A. Autophagy and aging: The importance of maintaining "clean" cells. *Autophagy* **2005**, *1*, 131–140. [CrossRef]
10. Boya, P.; Gonzalez-Polo, R.A.; Casares, N.; Perfettini, J.L.; Dessen, P.; Larochette, N.; Metivier, D.; Meley, D.; Souquere, S.; Yoshimori, T.; et al. Inhibition of macroautophagy triggers apoptosis. *Mol. Cell. Biol.* **2005**, *25*, 1025–1040. [CrossRef]
11. Song, X.; Lee, D.H.; Dilly, A.K.; Lee, Y.S.; Choudry, H.A.; Kwon, Y.T.; Bartlett, D.L.; Lee, Y.J. Crosstalk Between Apoptosis and Autophagy Is Regulated by the Arginylated BiP/Beclin-1/p62 Complex. *Mol. Cancer Res.* **2018**, *16*, 1077–1091. [CrossRef] [PubMed]
12. Amaravadi, R.K.; Lippincott-Schwartz, J.; Yin, X.M.; Weiss, W.A.; Takebe, N.; Timmer, W.; DiPaola, R.S.; Lotze, M.T.; White, E. Principles and current strategies for targeting autophagy for cancer treatment. *Clin. Cancer Res.* **2011**, *17*, 654–666. [CrossRef] [PubMed]
13. Prasad, S.; Aggarwal, B.B. Turmeric, the Golden Spice: From Traditional Medicine to Modern Medicine. In *Herbal Medicine: Biomolecular and Clinical Aspects*, 2nd ed.; Benzie, I.F.F., Wachtel-Galor, S., Eds.; CRC Press: Boca Raton, FL, USA, 2011.
14. Zhao, J.; Zhu, J.; Lv, X.; Xing, J.; Liu, S.; Chen, C.; Xu, Y. Curcumin potentiates the potent antitumor activity of ACNU against glioblastoma by suppressing the PI3K/AKT and NF-kappaB/COX-2 signaling pathways. *OncoTargets Ther.* **2017**, *10*, 5471–5482. [CrossRef] [PubMed]

15. Maiti, P.; Paladugu, L.; Dunbar, G.L. Solid lipid curcumin particles provide greater anti-amyloid, anti-inflammatory and neuroprotective effects than curcumin in the 5xFAD mouse model of Alzheimer's disease. *BMC Neurosci.* **2018**, *19*, 7. [CrossRef] [PubMed]
16. Anand, P.; Kunnumakkara, A.B.; Newman, R.A.; Aggarwal, B.B. Bioavailability of curcumin: Problems and promises. *Mol. Pharm.* **2007**, *4*, 807–818. [CrossRef] [PubMed]
17. Kumar, A.; Ahuja, A.; Ali, J.; Baboota, S. Conundrum and therapeutic potential of curcumin in drug delivery. *Crit. Rev. Ther. Drug Carrier Syst.* **2010**, *27*, 279–312. [CrossRef] [PubMed]
18. Maiti, P.; Hall, T.C.; Paladugu, L.; Kolli, N.; Learman, C.; Rossignol, J.; Dunbar, G.L. A comparative study of dietary curcumin, nanocurcumin, and other classical amyloid-binding dyes for labeling and imaging of amyloid plaques in brain tissue of 5x-familial Alzheimer's disease mice. *Histochem. Cell Biol.* **2016**, *146*, 609–625. [CrossRef] [PubMed]
19. Maiti, P.; Al-Gharaibeh, A.; Kolli, N.; Dunbar, G.L. Solid Lipid Curcumin Particles Induce More DNA Fragmentation and Cell Death in Cultured Human Glioblastoma Cells than Does Natural Curcumin. *Oxid. Med. Cell. Longev.* **2017**, *2017*, 9656719. [CrossRef] [PubMed]
20. Ma, Q.L.; Zuo, X.; Yang, F.; Ubeda, O.J.; Gant, D.J.; Alaverdyan, M.; Teng, E.; Hu, S.; Chen, P.P.; Maiti, P.; et al. Curcumin suppresses soluble tau dimers and corrects molecular chaperone, synaptic, and behavioral deficits in aged human tau transgenic mice. *J. Biol. Chem.* **2013**, *288*, 4056–4065. [CrossRef]
21. Frautschy, S.A.; Cole, G.M. Why pleiotropic interventions are needed for Alzheimer's disease. *Mol. Neurobiol.* **2010**, *41*, 392–409. [CrossRef]
22. Begum, A.N.; Jones, M.R.; Lim, G.P.; Morihara, T.; Kim, P.; Heath, D.D.; Rock, C.L.; Pruitt, M.A.; Yang, F.; Hudspeth, B.; et al. Curcumin structure-function, bioavailability, and efficacy in models of neuroinflammation and Alzheimer's disease. *J. Pharmacol. Exp. Ther.* **2008**, *326*, 196–208. [CrossRef] [PubMed]
23. Hu, S.; Maiti, P.; Ma, Q.; Zuo, X.; Jones, M.R.; Cole, G.M.; Frautschy, S.A. Clinical development of curcumin in neurodegenerative disease. *Expert Rev. Neurother.* **2015**, *15*, 629–637. [CrossRef] [PubMed]
24. Maiti, P.; Dunbar, G.L. Comparative Neuroprotective Effects of Dietary Curcumin and Solid Lipid Curcumin Particles in Cultured Mouse Neuroblastoma Cells after Exposure to Abeta42. *Int. J. Alzheimers Dis.* **2017**, *2017*, 4164872. [PubMed]
25. Maiti, P.; Manna, J.; Veleri, S.; Frautschy, S. Molecular chaperone dysfunction in neurodegenerative diseases and effects of curcumin. *Biomed. Res. Int.* **2014**, *2014*, 495091. [CrossRef] [PubMed]
26. Koronyo, Y.; Biggs, D.; Barron, E.; Boyer, D.S.; Pearlman, J.A.; Au, W.J.; Kile, S.J.; Blanco, A.; Fuchs, D.T.; Ashfaq, A.; et al. Retinal amyloid pathology and proof-of-concept imaging trial in Alzheimer's disease. *JCI Insight* **2017**, *2*, 93621. [CrossRef] [PubMed]
27. Koronyo, Y.; Salumbides, B.C.; Black, K.L.; Koronyo-Hamaoui, M. Alzheimer's disease in the retina: Imaging retinal abeta plaques for early diagnosis and therapy assessment. *Neurodegener. Dis.* **2012**, *10*, 285–293. [CrossRef] [PubMed]
28. Lata, S.; Molczyk, A. Side effects of temozolomide treatment in patient with glioblastoma multiforme—Case study. *Prz. Lek.* **2010**, *67*, 445–446.
29. Dinnes, J.; Cave, C.; Huang, S.; Milne, R. A rapid and systematic review of the effectiveness of temozolomide for the treatment of recurrent malignant glioma. *Br. J. Cancer* **2002**, *86*, 501–505. [CrossRef]
30. Rodriguez, G.A.; Shah, A.H.; Gersey, Z.C.; Shah, S.S.; Bregy, A.; Komotar, R.J.; Graham, R.M. Investigating the therapeutic role and molecular biology of curcumin as a treatment for glioblastoma. *Ther. Adv. Med. Oncol.* **2016**, *8*, 248–260. [CrossRef]
31. Fulda, S. Cell death-based treatment of glioblastoma. *Cell Death Dis.* **2018**, *9*, 121. [CrossRef]
32. Jawhari, S.; Ratinaud, M.H.; Verdier, M. Glioblastoma, hypoxia and autophagy: A survival-prone 'menage-a-trois'. *Cell Death Dis.* **2016**, *7*, e2434. [CrossRef] [PubMed]
33. Nikoletopoulou, V.; Markaki, M.; Palikaras, K.; Tavernarakis, N. Crosstalk between apoptosis, necrosis and autophagy. *Biochim. Biophys. Acta* **2013**, *1833*, 3448–3459. [CrossRef] [PubMed]
34. Arakawa, S.; Honda, S.; Yamaguchi, H.; Shimizu, S. Molecular mechanisms and physiological roles of Atg5/Atg7-independent alternative autophagy. *Proc. Jpn. Acad. Ser. B Phys. Biol. Sci.* **2017**, *93*, 378–385. [CrossRef] [PubMed]
35. Boutouja, F.; Brinkmeier, R.; Mastalski, T.; El Magraoui, F.; Platta, H.W. Regulation of the Tumor-Suppressor BECLIN 1 by Distinct Ubiquitination Cascades. *Int. J. Mol. Sci.* **2017**, *18*, 2541. [CrossRef] [PubMed]

36. Liang, X.H.; Jackson, S.; Seaman, M.; Brown, K.; Kempkes, B.; Hibshoosh, H.; Levine, B. Induction of autophagy and inhibition of tumorigenesis by beclin 1. *Nature* **1999**, *402*, 672–676. [CrossRef] [PubMed]
37. Koukourakis, M.I.; Kalamida, D.; Giatromanolaki, A.; Zois, C.E.; Sivridis, E.; Pouliliou, S.; Mitrakas, A.; Gatter, K.C.; Harris, A.L. Autophagosome Proteins LC3A, LC3B and LC3C Have Distinct Subcellular Distribution Kinetics and Expression in Cancer Cell Lines. *PLoS ONE* **2015**, *10*, e0137675. [CrossRef] [PubMed]
38. Guo, S.; Long, M.; Li, X.; Zhu, S.; Zhang, M.; Yang, Z. Curcumin activates autophagy and attenuates oxidative damage in EA. hy926 cells via the Akt/mTOR pathway. *Mol. Med. Rep.* **2016**, *13*, 2187–2193. [CrossRef]
39. Zanotto-Filho, A.; Braganhol, E.; Klafke, K.; Figueiró, F.; Terra, SR.; Paludo, F.J.; Morrone, M.; Bristot, I.J.; Battastini, A.M.; Forcelini, C.M.; et al. Autophagy inhibition improves the efficacy of curcumin/temozolomide combination therapy in glioblastomas. *Cancer Lett.* **2015**, *358*, 220–231. [CrossRef] [PubMed]
40. Duzgun, Z.; Eroglu, Z.; Biray Avci, C. Role of mTOR in glioblastoma. *Gene* **2016**, *575 Pt 1*, 187–190. [CrossRef]
41. Li, X.Y.; Zhang, L.Q.; Zhang, X.G.; Li, X.; Ren, Y.B.; Ma, X.Y.; Li, X.G.; Wang, L.X. Association between AKT/mTOR signalling pathway and malignancy grade of human gliomas. *J. Neurooncol.* **2011**, *103*, 453–458. [CrossRef]
42. Paquette, M.; El-Houjeiri, L.; Pause, A. mTOR Pathways in Cancer and Autophagy. *Cancers* **2018**, *10*, 18. [CrossRef] [PubMed]
43. Kim, Y.C.; Guan, K.L. mTOR: A pharmacologic target for autophagy regulation. *J. Clin. Investig.* **2015**, *125*, 25–32. [CrossRef] [PubMed]
44. Dobbin, Z.C.; Landen, C.N. The importance of the PI3K/AKT/MTOR pathway in the progression of ovarian cancer. *Int. J. Mol. Sci.* **2013**, *14*, 8213–8227. [CrossRef] [PubMed]
45. Yu, S.; Shen, G.; Khor, T.O.; Kim, J.H.; Kong, A.N. Curcumin inhibits Akt/mammalian target of rapamycin signaling through protein phosphatase-dependent mechanism. *Mol. Cancer Ther.* **2008**, *7*, 2609–2620. [CrossRef] [PubMed]
46. Kapuy, O.; Vinod, P.K.; Banhegyi, G. mTOR inhibition increases cell viability via autophagy induction during endoplasmic reticulum stress—An experimental and modeling study. *FEBS Open Bio* **2014**, *4*, 704–713. [CrossRef] [PubMed]
47. Zhuang, W.; Long, L.; Zheng, B.; Ji, W.; Yang, N.; Zhang, Q.; Liang, Z. Curcumin promotes differentiation of glioma-initiating cells by inducing autophagy. *Cancer Sci.* **2012**, *103*, 684–690. [CrossRef] [PubMed]
48. Aoki, H.; Takada, Y.; Kondo, S.; Sawaya, R.; Aggarwal, B.B.; Kondo, Y. Evidence that curcumin suppresses the growth of malignant gliomas in vitro and in vivo through induction of autophagy: Role of Akt and extracellular signal-regulated kinase signaling pathways. *Mol. Pharmacol.* **2007**, *72*, 29–39. [CrossRef]
49. Chourasia, A.H.; Boland, M.L.; Macleod, K.F. Mitophagy and cancer. *Cancer Metab.* **2015**, *3*, 4. [CrossRef]
50. Chourasia, A.H.; Tracy, K.; Frankenberger, C.; Boland, M.L.; Sharifi, M.N.; Drake, L.E.; Sachleben, J.R.; Asara, J.M.; Locasale, J.W.; Karczmar, G.S.; et al. Mitophagy defects arising from BNip3 loss promote mammary tumor progression to metastasis. *EMBO Rep.* **2015**, *16*, 1145–1163. [CrossRef]
51. Zhang, J.; Ney, P.A. Role of BNIP3 and NIX in cell death, autophagy, and mitophagy. *Cell Death Differ.* **2009**, *16*, 939–946. [CrossRef]
52. Mendez, O.; Zavadil, J.; Esencay, M.; Lukyanov, Y.; Santovasi, D.; Wang, S.C.; Newcomb, E.W.; Zagzag, D. Knock down of HIF-1alpha in glioma cells reduces migration in vitro and invasion in vivo and impairs their ability to form tumor spheres. *Mol. Cancer* **2010**, *9*, 133. [CrossRef] [PubMed]
53. Chen, M.; Chen, Z.; Wang, Y.; Tan, Z.; Zhu, C.; Li, Y.; Han, Z.; Chen, L.; Gao, R.; Liu, L.; et al. Mitophagy receptor FUNDC1 regulates mitochondrial dynamics and mitophagy. *Autophagy* **2016**, *12*, 689–702. [CrossRef] [PubMed]
54. Fan, Y.; Liu, Y.; Zhang, L.; Cai, F.; Zhu, L.; Xu, J. C0818, a novel curcumin derivative, interacts with Hsp90 and inhibits Hsp90 ATPase activity. *Acta Pharm. Sin. B* **2017**, *7*, 91–96. [CrossRef] [PubMed]
55. Klionsky, D.J.; Emr, S.D. Autophagy as a regulated pathway of cellular degradation. *Science* **2000**, *290*, 1717–1721. [CrossRef] [PubMed]
56. Reggiori, F.; Klionsky, D.J. Autophagy in the eukaryotic cell. *Eukaryot. Cell* **2002**, *1*, 11–21. [CrossRef] [PubMed]
57. Denton, D.; Nicolson, S.; Kumar, S. Cell death by autophagy: Facts and apparent artefacts. *Cell Death Differ.* **2012**, *19*, 87–95. [CrossRef] [PubMed]

58. Yonekawa, T.; Thorburn, A. Autophagy and cell death. *Essays Biochem.* **2013**, *55*, 105–117. [CrossRef] [PubMed]
59. El-Khattouti, A.; Selimovic, D.; Haikel, Y.; Hassan, M. Crosstalk between apoptosis and autophagy: Molecular mechanisms and therapeutic strategies in cancer. *J. Cell Death* **2013**, *6*, 37–55. [CrossRef]
60. Yang, Z.J.; Chee, C.E.; Huang, S.; Sinicrope, F.A. The role of autophagy in cancer: Therapeutic implications. *Mol. Cancer Ther.* **2011**, *10*, 1533–1541. [CrossRef]
61. Schrand, A.M.; Schlager, J.J.; Dai, L.; Hussain, S.M. Preparation of cells for assessing ultrastructural localization of nanoparticles with transmission electron microscopy. *Nat. Protoc.* **2010**, *5*, 744–757. [CrossRef]

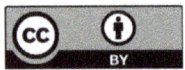

© 2019 by the authors. Licensee MDPI, Basel, Switzerland. This article is an open access article distributed under the terms and conditions of the Creative Commons Attribution (CC BY) license (http://creativecommons.org/licenses/by/4.0/).

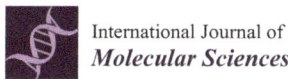

Article

Growth and Proliferation of Renal Cell Carcinoma Cells Is Blocked by Low Curcumin Concentrations Combined with Visible Light Irradiation

Jochen Rutz [1], Sebastian Maxeiner [1], Eva Juengel [1,2], August Bernd [3], Stefan Kippenberger [3], Nadja Zöller [3], Felix K.-H. Chun [1] and Roman A. Blaheta [1,*]

1. Department of Urology, Goethe-University, D-60590 Frankfurt am Main, Germany; Jochen.Rutz@kgu.de (J.R.); SebastianMaxeiner@gmx.de (S.M.); Eva.Juengel@unimedizin-mainz.de (E.J.); Felix.Chun@kgu.de (F.K.-H.C.)
2. Current address: Department of Urology and Pediatric Urology, University Medical Center Mainz, D-55131 Mainz, Germany
3. Department of Dermatology, Venereology, and Allergology, Goethe-University, D-60590 Frankfurt am Main, Germany; bernd@em.uni-frankfurt.de (A.B.); Kippenberger@em.uni-frankfurt.de (S.K.); nadjazoeller@netscape.net (N.Z.)
* Correspondence: blaheta@em.uni-frankfurt.de; Tel.: +49-69-6301-7109; Fax: +49-69-6301-7108

Received: 5 February 2019; Accepted: 21 March 2019; Published: 22 March 2019

Abstract: The anti-cancer properties of curcumin in vitro have been documented. However, its clinical use is limited due to rapid metabolization. Since irradiation of curcumin has been found to increase its anti-cancer effect on several tumor types, this investigation was designed to determine whether irradiation with visible light may enhance the anti-tumor effects of low-dosed curcumin on renal cell carcinoma (RCC) cell growth and proliferation. A498, Caki1, and KTCTL-26 cells were incubated with curcumin (0.1–0.4 µg/mL) and irradiated with 1.65 J/cm^2 visible light for 5 min. Controls were exposed to curcumin or light alone or remained untreated. Curcumin plus light, but not curcumin or light exposure alone altered growth, proliferation, and apoptosis of all three RCC tumor cell lines. Cells were arrested in the G0/G1 phase of the cell cycle. Phosphorylated (p) CDK1 and pCDK2, along with their counter-receptors Cyclin B and A decreased, whereas p27 increased. Akt-mTOR-signaling was suppressed, the pro-apoptotic protein Bcl-2 became elevated, and the anti-apoptotic protein Bax diminished. H3 acetylation was elevated when cells were treated with curcumin plus light, pointing to an epigenetic mechanism. The present findings substantiate the potential of combining low curcumin concentrations and light as a new therapeutic concept to increase the efficacy of curcumin in RCC.

Keywords: curcumin; renal cell cancer; tumor growth; tumor proliferation; cell cycling

1. Introduction

Cancer is the second most common cause of death in Europe. The incidence of renal cell carcinoma (RCC) is, compared to other cancer types, relatively rare, but both incidence and mortality are steadily increasing at a rate of approximately 2% to 3% per decade. Already, approximately 3% of all adult cancer patients suffer from malignant kidney tumors [1,2]. RCC is the most frequent form of kidney neoplasm, comprising about 90–95% of all renal melanomas [3]. Approximately one third of these patients have metastases at diagnosis, and 30–70% of patients with localized disease relapse within 5 years of surgery [4]. Since metastatic RCC (mRCC) is resistant to most treatments such as conventional chemotherapy or radiation, patients with mRCC can expect a 5 year survival rate of less than 10% [5]. The introduction of targeted agents including the tyrosine kinase inhibitors, sunitinib and sorafenib, and the mechanistic target of rapamycin (mTOR) inhibitors, temsirolimus and everolimus, have substantially improved patient outcome, but these drugs are not curative due to inevitable resistance development during therapy.

These unsatisfactory therapeutic options have opened patients' minds to complementary and alternative medicine (CAM) approaches to actively contribute to treatment, coupled with the hope of prolonging survival or even curing their disease. Up to 50% of cancer patients worldwide are applying CAM [6]. However, knowledge about the efficacy of a particular CAM is often limited due to the lack of evidence based studies. This holds true for the phytopharmacon curcumin, a yellow-orange pigment extracted from the rhizome of *Curcuma longa*, commonly known as tumeric. Apart from its use as a food additive and spice, anti-inflammatory and anti-oxidative qualities have been attributed to curcumin. It promotes the function of the immune system and acts as an antioxidant to capture free radicals, protecting living cells [7–9]. Recently, anti-tumorigenic effects in several in vitro and in vivo studies have shown that diverse biochemical processes and pathways triggering carcinogenesis are affected and modulated by curcumin [10]. Curcumin has been shown to inhibit cell proliferation, cell cycle progression, angiogenesis, and cell invasion as well as to induce apoptosis by altering the expression level of pro- and anti-apoptotic proteins [11]. Thus, curcumin is considered a promising possible future adjuvant in cancer management [12].

Low bioavailability, however, remains a serious problem with curcumin treatment. Due to poor water solubility, low absorption, and fast metabolization and clearance, a transfer to clinical use is hampered [13,14]. Human trials carried out so far have provided disappointing results [15–17].

Bernd et al. recently discovered that irradiation of tumor cells with visible light dramatically enhances the antitumor properties of curcumin [18]. Application of curcumin to tumor bearing nude mice followed by visible light exposure resulted in reduced tumor volumes, reduced proliferation rates, and the induction of apoptosis [19]. On the molecular level, inhibition of extracellular regulated kinases 1/2 and epidermal growth factor receptors along with DNA fragmentation and increased cleaved caspase-3 positive cells has been observed [20,21]. The present investigation was designed to determine the in vitro efficacy of curcumin combined with visible light exposure on RCC cell growth and proliferation.

2. Results

2.1. Cytotoxicity and Apoptosis

Curcumin (0.1–0.4 µg/mL) plus light (5500 lx) or curcumin alone did not impair the cell membrane integrity of all cell lines evaluated (Figure 1, representative for A498 cells), as indicated by lactate dehydrogenase (LDH) in the cell free supernatant.

Curcumin alone, up to 0.4 µg/mL, caused no increase of DNA fragments, as an indicator of apoptosis, in all three cell lines. When visible light was additionally applied, DNA fragments significantly increased in all three cell lines, even at 0.1 µg/mL curcumin (compared to the untreated control; Figure 2: representative for A498 cells, data not shown for Caki1 and KTCTL-26).

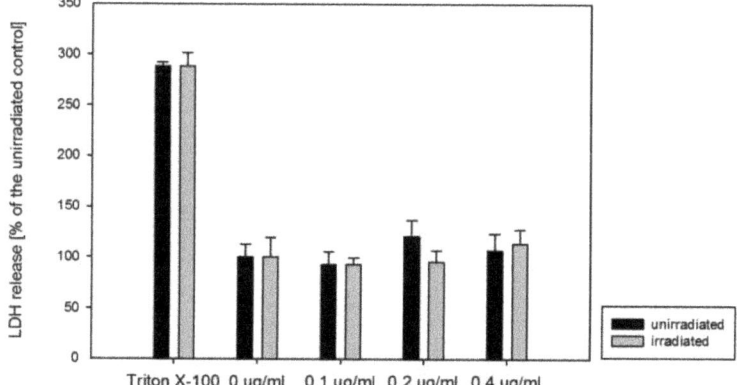

Figure 1. Lactate dehydrogenase (LDH) released from A498 renal cell carcinoma (RCC) cells incubated for 1 h with curcumin (0–0.4 µg/mL) and irradiated with 5500 lx visible light for 5 min (grey) or kept light protected (black). Twenty-four hours later, cell supernatants were prepared. Each column represents the mean ± S.D. of a representative experiment done in triplicate. Cells treated with 1% Triton X-100 served as a positive control.

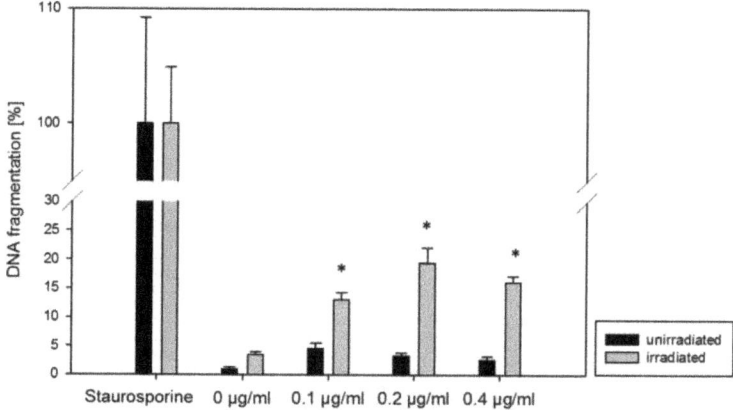

Figure 2. Histone-associated DNA fragments released from A498 RCC incubated for 1 h with curcumin (0–0.4 µg/mL) and irradiated with 5500 lx visible light for 5 min (grey) or kept light protected (black). Twenty-four hours later, cell supernatants were prepared. The positive control was incubated with 1 µM staurosporine (set to 100%). Each column represents the mean ± S.D. of a representative experiment done in triplicate. * indicates significant difference to cells with no curcumin (0 µg/mL).

2.2. Tumor Cell Proliferation

Treating the tumor cells with curcumin and subsequent irradiation evoked a significant dose-dependent decrease of the proliferative activity with maximum effects at 0.4 µg/mL (Figure 3). The most prominent effect was achieved in the KTCTL-26 cell line where the proliferation was decreased by 40% at a concentration of 0.1 µg/mL and up to 90% at a concentration of 0.4 µg/mL. Only the A498 cell line showed no significant proliferation decrease at the lowest concentration of 0.1 µg/mL. Application of visible light alone or curcumin alone led to no significant proliferation differences in any cell line.

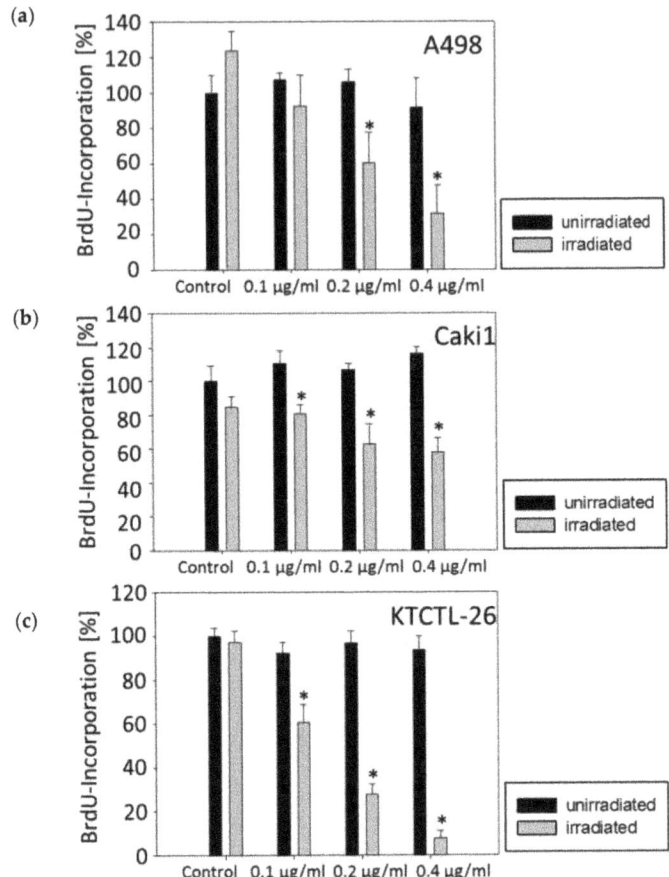

Figure 3. Cell proliferation in A498 (**a**), Caki1 (**b**), and KTCTL-26 (**c**) cells cultured with 0, 0.1, 0.2, and 0.4 µg/mL curcumin without (black bars) or with irradiation (grey bars). Irradiation was done with 5500 lx visible light for 5 min. Tumor cells were then subjected to the BrdU incorporation test following a further 24 h incubation in cell culture medium without curcumin. BrdU-incorporation is expressed as percentage of the untreated cells. Each experiment was done in triplicate and repeated five times. Data from one representative experiment are shown. * Indicates significant difference to controls.

2.3. Tumor Cell Growth

Curcumin applied at low doses of 0.1 or 0.2 µg/mL without irradiation caused no significant alteration in tumor cell number, compared to untreated controls (Figure 4). However, irradiation combined with 0.1 µg/mL (Caki1 and KTCTL-26) or 0.2 µg/mL curcumin (all cell lines) resulted in significantly decreased tumor cell number after 48 or 72 h.

The number of apoptotic A498 cells after 72 h was 21.25 ± 4.33% (0.1 µg/mL curcumin plus light) and 32.06 ± 5.68% (0.2 µg/mL curcumin plus light).

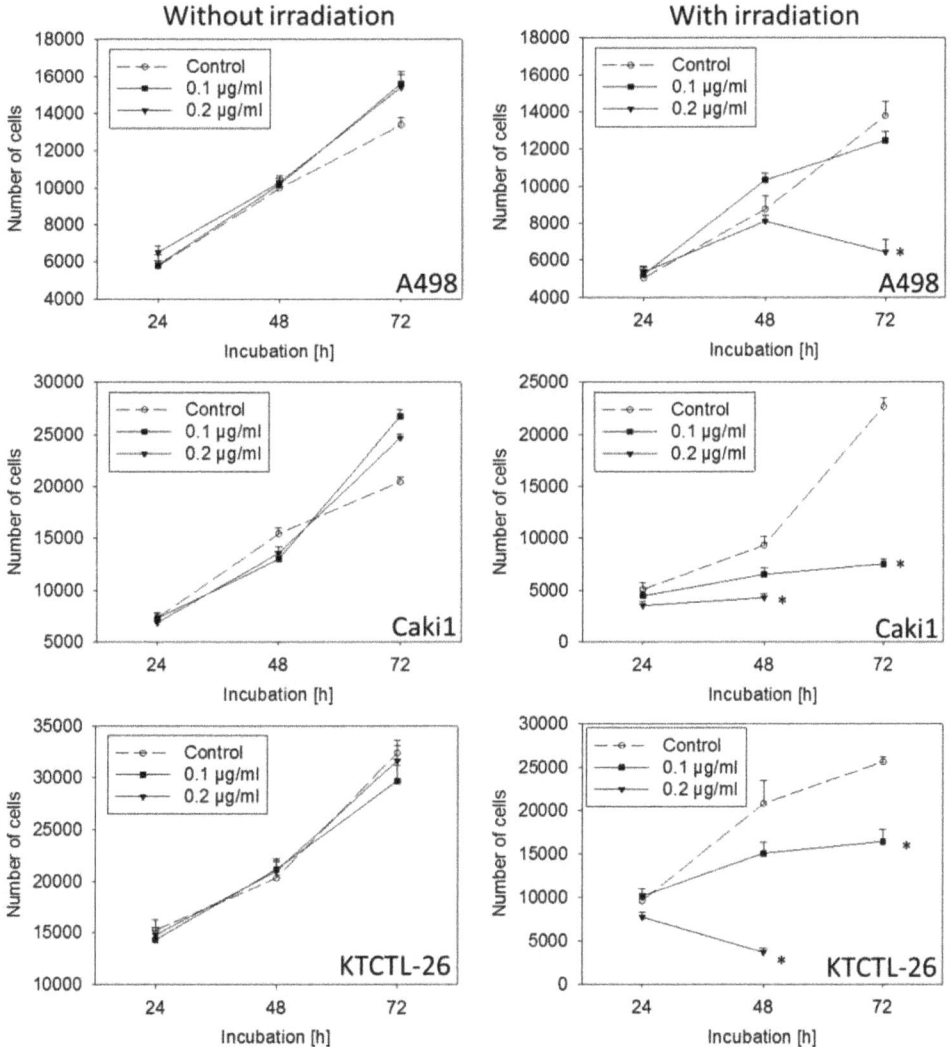

Figure 4. Growth of A498, Caki1, and KTCTL-26 renal cell cancer cells exposed to 0.1 or 0.2 μg/mL curcumin without or with irradiation. Irradiation was done with 5500 lx visible light for 5 min. Following light exposure, curcumin-containing medium was replaced by medium without curcumin. Tumor cell number was then evaluated after 24, 48, and 72 h. Controls remained untreated. Each experiment was done in triplicate and repeated six times. Data from one representative experiment are shown.* Indicates significant difference to controls.

2.4. Cell Cycle Progression

Low dosed curcumin combined with visible light induced a cell cycle arrest at the G0/G1-phase (Figure 5). G0/G1-phase arrest was accompanied by a decrease of cells in the S-phase (Caki1 and KTCTL-26) and/or G2/M-phase (A498 and KTCTL-26 cells). Treatment with curcumin or visible light alone did not significantly influence cell cycling.

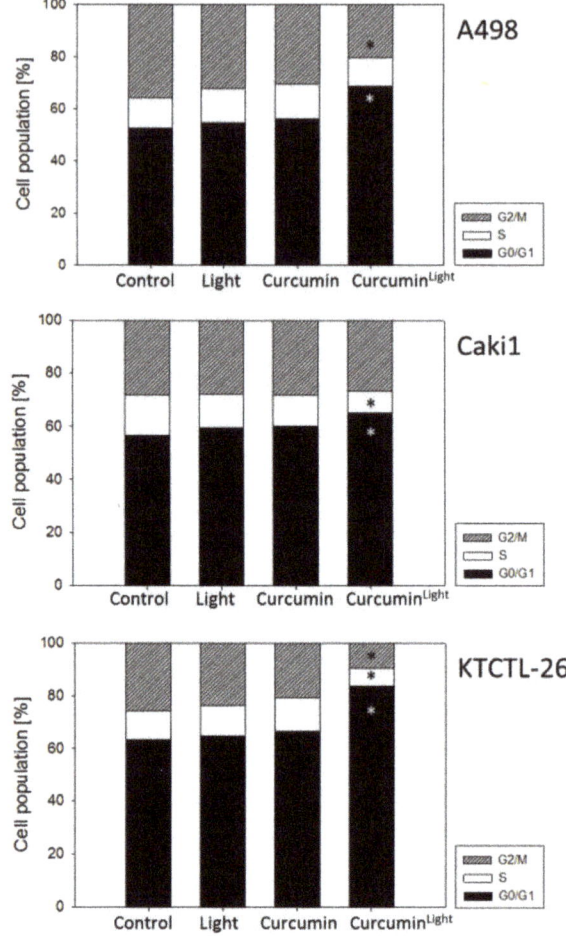

Figure 5. Cell cycle analysis of A498, Caki1, and KTCTL-26 cells treated with 0.2 µg/mL curcumin for 1 h, with or without irradiation (controls remained untreated). Analysis was done 24 h following curcumin exposure. The cell population is expressed as a percentage of the total cells analyzed. One representative experiment of three is shown. Mean $SD_{interassay}$ < 40%, mean $SD_{intraassay}$ < 10%. * Indicates significant difference to control.

The expression of cell cycle regulating proteins is depicted in Figure 6. Exposing the tumor cells to curcumin (0.2 µg/mL) or light did not induce significant changes of the protein expression level, compared to the untreated control cells. However, combining curcumin application with light irradiation, considerably diminished CDK1 and 2 (both total and phosphorylated), together with their respective binding partners Cyclin B and Cyclin A. CDK4 and Cyclin D1 were also reduced, although to a slighter extent, compared to CDK1/2 and Cyclin B/A. The tumor suppressor, p27, was down-regulated in Caki1 and KTCTL-26, whereas p19 was up-regulated in all cell lines analyzed. Bcl-2 decreased in all three cell lines, Bax was diminished in A498 and KTCTL-26, but enhanced in Caki1.

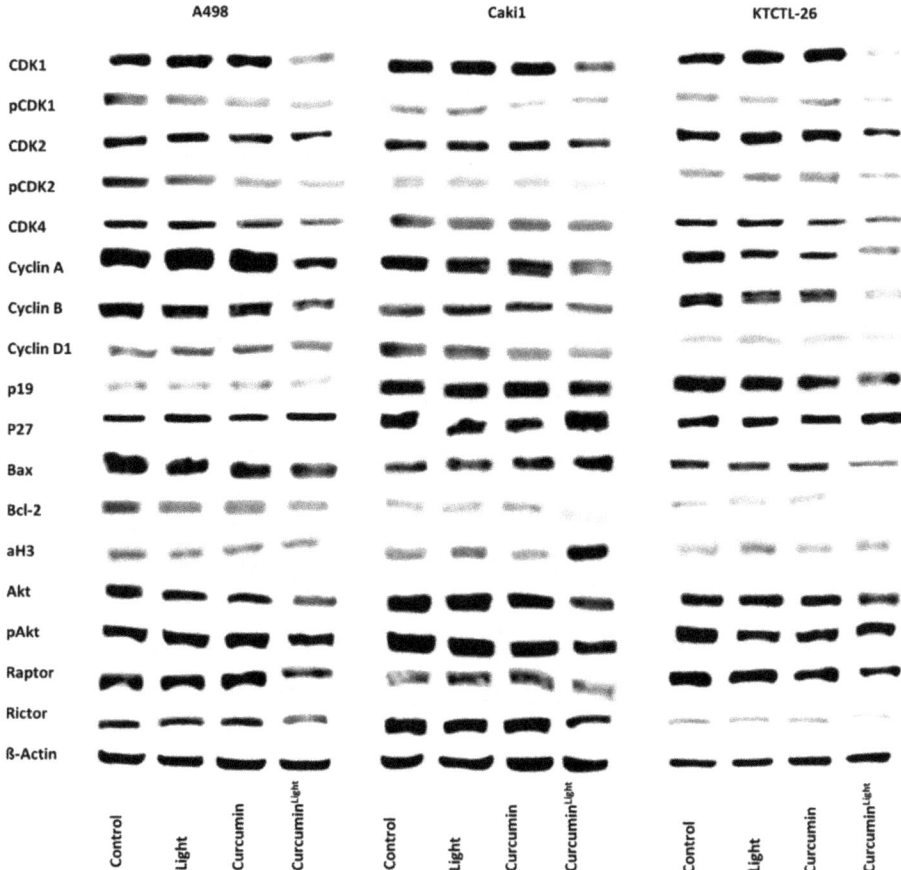

Figure 6. Influence of light, curcumin (0.2 µg/mL), and the combination of both (Curcumin[Light]) on the A498, Caki1, and KTCTL-26 cell cycle protein expression. The protein isolation was carried out 24 h after the respective treatment. β-Actin was used as an internal control. Each experiment was repeated three times. Data from one representative experiment are shown.

Akt and pAkt were reduced in the presence of curcumin plus light. The mTOR complexes Raptor and Rictor were also diminished by the treatment regimen in all cell lines, compared to controls.

The amount of deacetylated histones was not significantly influenced by light or curcumin alone compared to the untreated control in all three cell lines. However, 0.2 µg/mL curcumin in combination with visible light induced a significant overexpression of aH3 in Caki1 cells, pointing to an epigenetic mechanism. This finding was confirmed by the histone deacetylase (HDAC) expression assay pointing to a reduction of HDAC of about 25% (KTCTL-26), 35% (Caki1), and nearly 50% (A498) (Figure 7).

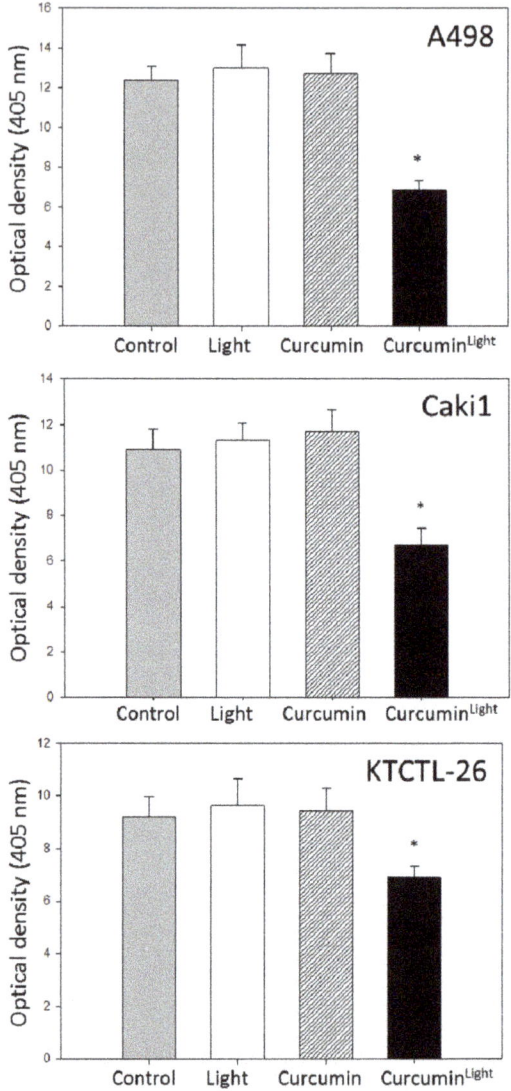

Figure 7. Histone deacetylation activity in A498, Caki1, and KTCTL-26 cell lines. Controls remained untreated (grey) after irradiation (white) or incubation with 0.2 µg/mL curcumin without (hatched) or with irradiation (black). Each experiment was done in triplicate and repeated five times. Data from one representative experiment are shown. * Indicates significant difference to control.

2.5. Knockdown Studies

Since curcumin strongly modified CDK1 and 2 as well as Cyclin A and B in all tumor cell lines, the physiologic relevance of these proteins was evaluated by siRNA knock-down. Down-regulation of CDK1 and Cyclin B or CDK2 and Cyclin A (Figure 8A) correlated with a significant growth blockade of A498, Caki1, and KTCTL-26 cells. Protein controls are shown in Figure 8B.

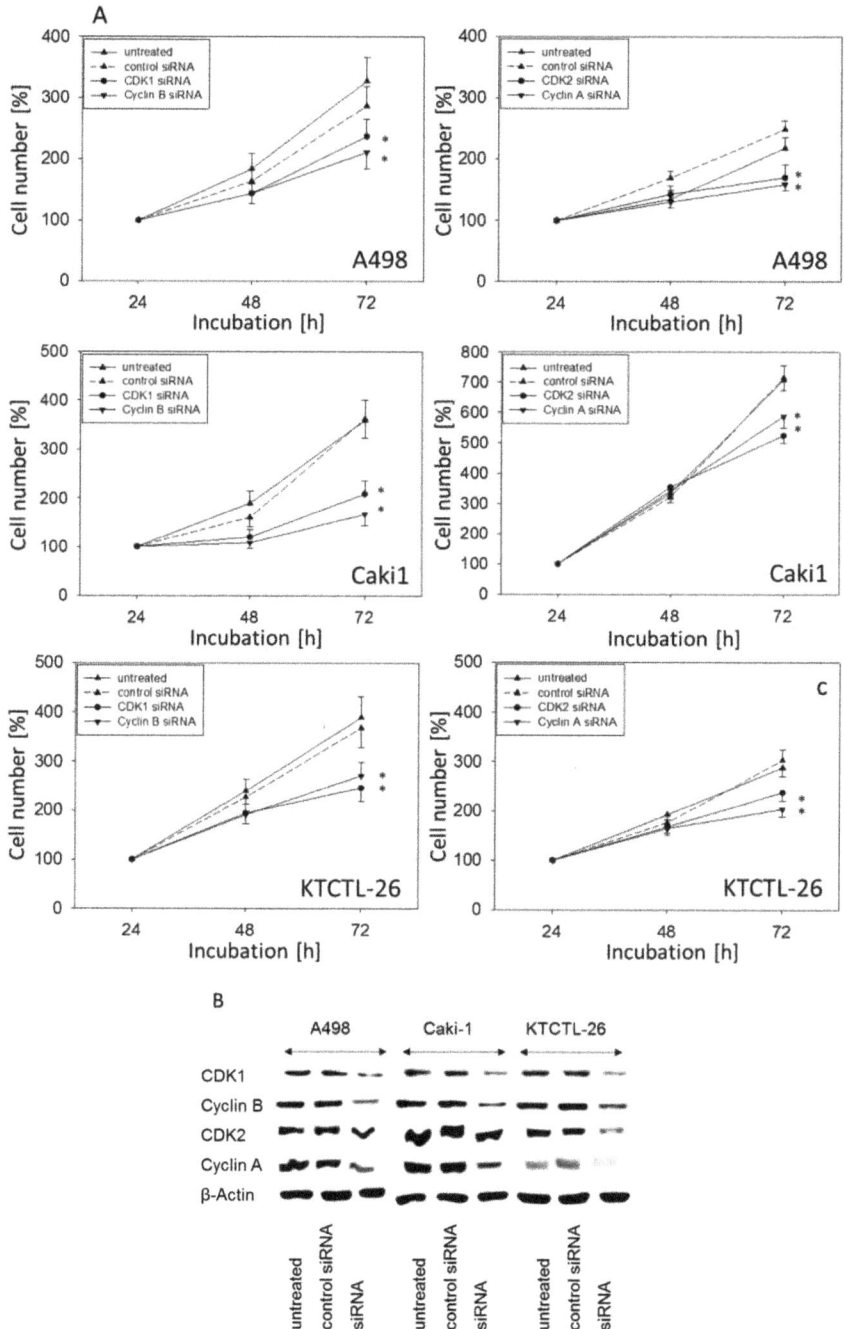

Figure 8. Influence of CDK1, Cyclin B, CDK2, and Cyclin A knock down on tumor cell growth. A498, Caki1, and KTCTL-26 cells were transfected with non-silencing control siRNA, CDK1, Cyclin B, CDK2, or Cyclin A siRNA (**A**). Cell number was set to 100% at 24 h. Knock down was controlled by Western blot (**B**). One representative from six experiments is shown. * indicates significant difference to controls.

3. Discussion

Light exposure greatly increased curcumin's anti-tumor properties. As low as 0.1 µg/mL (Caki1 and KTCTL-26) or 0.2 µg/mL curcumin (A498) significantly reduced tumor cell growth following irradiation, while 0.1 or 0.2 µg/mL curcumin alone or with light alone did not lead to growth-blocking effects in any of these cell lines. To achieve similar effects on RCC cell growth without irradiation, Caki1 cells required curcumin at a concentration of 2.9 µg/mL (8 µM) (data not shown). This coincides with data from others reporting an IC_{50} of 8 µM curcumin to block the growth of gastric cancer cell lines [22]. Even higher curcumin concentrations have been shown necessary to suppress proliferation of breast cancer (IC_{50}: 30–80 µM) [23], neuroblastoma (IC_{50}: 30 µM) [24], or bladder cancer cells (IC_{50}: 20 µM) [25].

The photodynamic effect is not restricted to RCC cells. A study, using skin keratinocytes, has shown that 0.2 µg/mL curcumin causes a significant proliferation inhibition when combined with visible light. This concentration was more than one magnitude lower than the lowest curcumin (without light) concentration providing pharmacological effects [21]. Curcumin plus light exposure has been shown to inhibit mitochondrial activity in nasopharyngeal carcinoma cell lines, whereas the same concentration without light did not [26].

Reduction of cell number was not caused by toxic effects as demonstrated by the LDH assay. However, Bcl-2 decreased in the RCC cell lines treated with 0.2 µg/mL curcumin–light, which may indicate apoptotic events. Indeed, the number of apoptotic cells evaluated after 72 h significantly increased when tumor cells were subjected to curcumin plus light. Dujic et al. have reported a strong increase of apoptotic nuclei in the keratinocyte cell line, HaCaT, 24 h after treatment with light and 1 µg/mL curcumin [21]. On the other hands, DNA fragments did not occur in a melanoma cell model until a curcumin concentration of 0.5 µg/mL was reached [27], and pilot studies on bladder cancer cells have demonstrated signs of early and late apoptosis at 0.4 but not at 0.1 µg/mL curcumin–light (data not shown). Sensitivity to curcumin in terms of apoptosis induction may thus depend on the tumor type.

The analysis of cell cycle progression revealed distinct modulations caused by curcumin. The number of cells in the S-phase (all cell lines) and the G2/M-phase (A498 and KTCTL-26) decreased, whereas the number of G0/G1-phase cells increased. A similar effect has also been observed on breast [23], prostate [28], and lung cancer cells [29]. However, the curcumin effect is not homogeneous. A G2/M-phase arrest has been ascribed to curcumin in a colon cancer [30], a thyroid carcinoma [31], and a colorectal cancer cell model [32].

Based on an investigation by Zhang et al., 10 µM curcumin blocked bladder cancer cells at the S-phase, whereas 15 µM led to a G2/M-phase arrest [25]. The mesothelioma cell line H-Meso-1 was blocked at G0/G1 in the presence of 12 µm curcumin, but stopped at G2/M with 25 µM curcumin [33]. Curcumin's mode of action, therefore, seems dose associated. Deng et al. recently reported dual effects on autophagy in RCC cells, closely depending on the curcumin concentration [34]. It seems reasonable to assume that the inhibition of RCC growth and proliferation by low-dosed curcumin–light observed in the present investigation is caused by a G0/G1 phase arrest.

Along with the G0/G1 block, the expression of CDK1 and CDK2 with their respective counterparts, Cyclin B and Cyclin A, as well as the Akt-mTOR signaling pathway, was significantly diminished in all cell lines in the presence of 0.2 µg/mL curcumin–light (but not in the presence of 0.2 µg/mL curcumin or light alone). Information about the influence of curcumin on the CDK-Cyclin-axis in RCC is sparse. Diminished expression of Cyclin B has been seen in the RCC cell line RCC-949 following curcumin exposure [35]. Treatment of glioma [36], lung [37], or pancreatic carcinoma cells [38] with curcumin has also been shown to cause a significant reduction of Cyclin B, along with CDK1, and Kuo et al. noted an additional decrease in the protein expression of Cyclin A in nasopharyngeal cancer cells [39]. In all these investigations, curcumin was applied at considerably higher concentrations than employed in the present investigation. In the RCC model from Zhang and colleagues, concentrations up to 100 µM were used [35]. The present data show clear evidence that light exposure to curcumin-treated

RCC cells strongly enhances the anti-tumor potency of this compound, whereby alteration of the CDK-Cyclin axis may be only one of several relevant mechanisms contributing to cell growth reduction by curcumin–light. The relevance of the respective CDKs and Cyclins is confirmed here, since protein knockdown significantly blocked tumor growth.

From a clinical viewpoint, loss of Akt and the mTOR-members, Rictor and Raptor, is of interest. The Akt/mTOR-pathway plays a crucial role in the pathogenesis of RCC, and various drugs targeting this signaling cascade have already been established and approved [40]. Unfortunately, neither the mTOR-inhibitors everolimus nor temsirolimus are able to permanently suppress Akt/mTOR. Rather, resistance develops under chronic therapy, leading to an increase in protein activity and relapse associated with tumor aggressiveness. Integrating curcumin into the oncotherapy might, therefore, optimize the current treatment concept. Combined curcumin and temsirolimus treatment has been shown to exert a synergistic effect on apoptosis in human RCC cells in vitro. The authors of that study concluded that pre-treatment or co-treatment of cells with curcumin might not only enhance the response to targeted drugs, but might also overcome drug resistance in human RCC [41].

The influence of curcumin on HDAC is difficult to interpret. There is little doubt that curcumin targets HDAC and that HDAC-suppression along with histone acetylation may contribute to the anti-cancer effects of curcumin [42]. Based on the present work, only Caki1 cells responded to curcumin–light in terms of elevated aH3, pointing to an epigenetic mechanism in this cell line. It is not clear why A498 and KTCTL-26 did not respond in the same manner. Marquardt et al. discovered that curcumin's influence on HDAC in liver cancer cells may depend on the extent of inhibition of NF-kB and downstream signaling [43]. Whether this may also hold true for bladder cancer cells remains to be seen.

The exact mechanism underlying the advantageous effect of light is not totally understood. Speculatively, light-dependent energy transfer during curcumin–protein interactions may enhance the influence of curcumin on protein function and cell regulation [18]. It has been postulated that both the photo-catalytic effect of curcumin and photo-activation are essential triggering factors [44]. A conceivable molecular mechanism of the photo-toxicity of curcumin might also be that curcumin photo-generates reduced forms of molecular oxygen [45]. Regardless of the exact mechanism, the present results demonstrate that combining curcumin with light irradiation could considerably enhance curcumin's anti-tumor potential.

Ongoing studies must now deal with the technical aspect of curcumin–light application in renal cancer. Introducing an optical fiber into RCC tumors of a mouse model with subsequent laser illumination of the vascular-acting photosensitizer WST11, either at a single wavelength (750 nm) or multispectrally (700 to 800 nm), induced necrosis in the RCC tissue, as evidenced by histological analysis. [46]. Baran et al. has suggested an interstitial optical fiber-based spectroscopy using sensitizers with high absorption at 780 nm or beyond to optimally treat RCC [47]. mTHPC (meso-tetra(hydroxyphenyl)chlorin), a photosensitizer that targets both vasculature and tissue, has been recommended by others, since its localization in RCC vasculature and tissue may produce a strong combined effect [48].

Based on pediatric epithelial liver tumor cell lines, evidence has been provided that irradiation with blue light (480 nm) amplifies the cytotoxic effects of low dosed curcumin. The authors concluded that combining low curcumin concentrations with light irradiation may compensate for low bioavailability and rapid degradation of curcumin in vivo [49]. From a technical viewpoint, irradiation of the tumor bed (including possible invisible micrometastases) with light after tumor resection could take place shortly after curcumin administration. Local laparoscopic light irradiation may be an optional treatment option [49]. Still, further investigation is required to explore whether curcumin specifically acts on the tumor cells or whether healthy tissues and cells may also be damaged by this compound.

Curcumin is not the only compound shown to have enhanced effects when combined with an energy source. Hypericin's anti-tumor effects have been shown to be enhanced when human

RCC cells are exposed to radiation or light in vitro, pointing to a clinical relevance of radiotherapy and intraoperative photodynamic therapy [50]. Ongoing studies must now deal with the technical feasibility of potentiating curcumin's anti-RCC activity with visible light. The next experimental step will, therefore, be to evaluate the effect of photodynamic therapy after curcumin administration in an RCC in vivo model.

4. Materials and Methods

4.1. Cell Culture

Renal carcinoma Caki1 and KTCTL-26 cell lines were purchased from LGC Promochem (Wesel, Germany). The A498 cells were derived from Cell Lines Service (Heidelberg, Germany). Caki1 and KTCTL-26 cells were chosen since both lines are derived from a clear cell renal cell carcinoma, which is the most common renal carcinoma tumor type. A498 served as the "classical" RCC cell line used as a model of ccRCC as well [51]. Both cell lines are von Hippel-Lindau (VHL) positive, whereas VHL function is disrupted in A498 cells. The tumor cells were grown and subcultured in RPMI 1640 medium supplemented with 10% fetal calf serum (FCS), 1% Glutamax (all Gibco/Invitrogen, Karlsruhe, Germany), 2% Hepes buffer, and 1% penicillin/streptomycin (both Sigma-Aldrich, München, Germany) at 37 °C in a humidified 5% CO_2 incubator. Subcultures from passages 5–30 were selected for experimental use.

4.2. Drug Treatment and Light Exposure

Curcumin was stored at -20 °C and was diluted in cell culture medium to a final concentration of 0.1–1 μg/mL (0.27–2.7 μM). Cells were treated for 1 h with curcumin and subsequently irradiated with visible light for 5 min (5500 lx, 10×40 W lamps, distance 45 cm, emission spectrum: 400–550 nm, cumulative dose 1.65 J/cm^2; Waldmann UV 801AL, Villingen-Schwenningen, Germany).

For irradiation, the cell culture medium was replaced by phenol red free PBS (Sigma-Aldrich). After irradiation PBS was replaced by cell culture medium containing no curcumin. Control cell cultures were exposed to visible light without curcumin, received curcumin without light exposure, or were treated with PBS alone. Tumor cells were then subjected to the assays listed below.

4.3. Cytotoxicity

Membrane integrity was quantified using a cytotoxicity detection kit (Roche Diagnostics, Penzberg, Germany) based on the release of lactate dehydrogenase (LDH) from damaged cells. Briefly, the cells were cultivated in 96-well plates (2×10^4 cells/0.33 cm^2) and treated with curcumin and light as aforementioned. The next day, cell-free supernatants were incubated with NAD$^+$, which is reduced by lactate dehydrogenase to NADH/H$^+$. Consecutively, NADH/H$^+$ reduces the yellow tetrazolium salt to a red-colored formazan salt. The amount of red color is proportional to the number of lysed cells. For quantification, the absorbance of the reaction product was measured at 490 nm using an ELISA reader.

4.4. Apoptosis

DNA fragmentation was chosen as an indicator of apoptosis. Quantification was performed with the Cell Death Detection ELISA (CDD; Roche, Mannheim, Germany) according to the manufacturer's instructions. In brief, cells were cultured in 96-well plates (2×10^4 cells/0.33 cm^2) and treated with curcumin and light as mentioned above. After 24 h, the cytosolic fraction was subjected to a sandwich enzyme-linked immunosorbent assay with the primary anti-histone antibody coated to the microtiter plate and the secondary anti-DNA antibody coupled to peroxidase. Optical density was measured at 530 nm by an ELISA reader.

Expression of Annexin V/propidium iodide (PI) was evaluated using the Annexin V-FITC Apoptosis Detection kit (BD Pharmingen, Heidelberg, Germany). Tumor cells were washed twice with

PBS-buffer, and then incubated with 5 μL of Annexin V-FITC and 5 μL of PI in the dark for 15 min at room temperature. Cells were analyzed on a FACScalibur (BD Biosciences, Heidelberg, Germany). The percentage of vital, necrotic, and apoptotic cells (early and late) in each quadrant was calculated using Cell-Quest software (BD Biosciences).

4.5. Measurement of Tumor Cell Growth and Proliferation

Cell growth was measured using the 3-(4,5-dimethylthiazol-2-yl)-2,5-diphenyltetrazolium bromide (MTT) dye reduction assay (Roche Diagnostics, Penzberg, Germany). Tumor cells (100 μL, 1×10^4 cells/mL) were plated into 96-well tissue culture plates. After 24, 48, and 72 h, MTT (0.5 mg/mL) was added for an additional 4 h. The reaction was stopped by lysing the cells in a buffer containing 10% SDS in 0.01 M HCl. After incubating the plates overnight at 37 °C and 5% CO_2, the absorbance at 570 nm was measured for each well using a microplate proliferation enzyme-linked immunosorbent assay (ELISA) reader. Each experiment was done in triplicate. After subtracting background absorbance, results were expressed as mean cell number.

Cell proliferation was measured using a BrdU cell proliferation ELISA kit (Calbiochem/Merck Biosciences, Darmstadt, Germany). Tumor cells, were seeded into 96-well tissue culture plates, incubated with 20 μL BrdU-labelling solution per well for 8 h, and fixed and detected using anti-BrdU mAb according to the manufacturer's instructions. Absorbance was measured at 450 nm after 24 h.

4.6. Cell Cycle Analysis

Cell cycle analysis was carried out with sub confluent tumor cells after 24 h cultivation with or without 0.2 μg/mL curcumin. Tumor cell populations were stained with propidium iodide, using a Cycle TEST PLUS DNA Reagent Kit (BD Biosciences, Heidelberg, Germany) and then subjected to flow cytometry with a FACScan flow cytometer (BD Biosciences). In total, 10,000 events were collected for each sample. Data acquisition was carried out using Cell-Quest software and cell cycle distribution was calculated using the ModFit software (BD Biosciences). The number of gated cells in the G1, G2/M, or S-phase is presented as %.

4.7. Histone Deacetylation

Histone deacetylation (HDAC) activity of renal cancer cells was quantified using the Color De Lys assay (Enzo Life sciences, Lörrach, Germany) according to the manufacturer's instructions. Cells were cultivated with curcumin and/or light as aforementioned. All substances were plated on a 96-well plate and the reaction was initiated by adding substrate and stopped by Color De Lys developer. Optical density was measured at a wavelength of 405 nm using an ELISA reader.

4.8. Western Blot Analysis

To investigate the level of the cell cycle regulating proteins in the three cell lines, tumor cell lysates were applied to a 7–12% polyacrylamide gel (depending on the proteins) and electrophoresed for 90 min at 100 V. The protein was then transferred to nitrocellulose membranes (1 h, 100 V). After blocking with nonfat dry milk for 1 h, the membranes were incubated overnight with monoclonal antibodies directed against the cell cycle proteins: CDK1/Cdc2 (IgG1, clone 1), pCDK1/Cdc2 (IgG1, clone 44/CDK1/Cdc2 (pY15)), CDK2 (IgG2a, clone 55), Cyclin A (IgG1, clone 25), Cyclin B (IgG1, clone 18), Cyclin D1 (IgG1, clone G124-36), p27 (IgG1, clone G173-524), CDK4 (IgG1, clone 97), p19 (IgG1, clone 52/p19 Skp1; all: BD Pharmingen), pCDK2 (Thr160 Cell Signaling). The mechanistic target of rapamycin (mTOR) pathway was investigated using the following monoclonal antibodies: Raptor (24C12 Cell Signaling), Rictor (D16H9; Cell Signaling), PKBα/Akt (IgG1 clone 55), anti phospho Akt (pAkt; IgG1, Ser472/Ser473, clone 104A282; both: BD Pharmingen). aH3 (Lys9), aH4 (Lys8; both Cell Signaling) and Bax (B-9:sc-7480), Bcl-2 (N-19:sc-492; both Santa Cruz). HRP-conjugated goat anti-mouse IgG and HRP-conjugated goat anti-rabbit IgG (both: 1:5.000; Upstate Biotechnology, Lake Placid, NY, USA) served as the secondary antibody. The membranes were briefly incubated with ECL detection reagent (ECL; Amersham/GE Healthcare, München, Germany) to visualize the proteins and then analyzed by the Fusion FX7 system (Peqlab, Erlangen, Germany). β-Actin (1:1.000; clone AC-15; Sigma-Aldrich, Taufenkirchen, Germany) served as the internal control.

4.9. Knockdown Studies of Cell Cycle Regulators

To determine whether CDK1, CDK2, Cyclin A, and Cyclin B impacted tumor cell growth in A498, Caki1, and KTCTL-26 cell lines, cells were transfected with the respective small interfering RNA (siRNA). Per batch, 3×10^5 cells/2.3 mL of medium were transfected with small interfering RNA (siRNA) directed against CDK1 (Hs_CDC2_10, gene ID: 983, target sequence: AAGGGGTTCCTAGTACTGCAA), CDK2 (gene ID: 1017, target sequence: AGGTGGTGGCGCTTAAGAAAA), Cyclin A (gene ID: 890, target sequence: GCCAGCTGTCAGGATAATAAA) or Cyclin B (Hs_CCNB1_6, gene ID: 891, target sequence: AATGTAGTCATGGTAAATCAA) (all from Qiagen, Hilden, Germany) or with an siRNA/transfection reagent (HiPerFect Transfection Reagent; Qiagen) at a ratio of 1:6. Non-treated cells and cells treated with 5 nM control siRNA (All stars negative control siRNA; Qiagen) served as controls. Subsequently, tumor cell growth was evaluated and Western blotting was done as indicated above.

4.10. Statistics

All experiments were performed three to six times. Statistical significance was calculated with the Wilcoxon–Mann-Whitney *U* test. Values are expressed as means ± S.D. Differences were considered statistically significant at a *p* value less than 0.05.

Author Contributions: Conceptualization, A.B. and R.A.B.; Investigation, J.R., S.M., S.K., and N.Z.; Methodology, E.J., S.K., and R.A.B.; Project administration, R.A.B.; Supervision, F.K.-H.C., A.B., and R.A.B.; Visualization, J.R., S.K., F.K.-H.C., and R.A.B.; Writing—original draft, J.R. and R.A.B.; Writing—review and editing, A.B., E.J., F.K.-H.C., and R.A.B.

Funding: This work was supported by the Brigitta & Norbert Muth Stiftung, Wiesbaden, Germany, the Alfons & Gertrud Kassel-Stiftung, Frankfurt, Germany, and the Friedrich-Spicker-Stiftung, Wuppertal, Germany.

Conflicts of Interest: The authors declare no conflict of interest.

References

1. Yu, S.S.; Quinn, D.I.; Dorff, T.B. Clinical use of cabozantinib in the treatment of advanced kidney cancer: efficacy, safety, and patient selection. *Onco Targets Ther.* **2016**, *9*, 5825–5837. [CrossRef] [PubMed]
2. Jayson, M.; Sanders, H. Increased incidence of serendipitously discovered renal cell carcinoma. *Urology* **1998**, *51*, 203–205. [CrossRef]
3. Gupta, K.; Miller, J.D.; Li, J.Z.; Russell, M.W.; Charbonneau, C. Epidemiologic and socioeconomic burden of metastatic renal cell carcinoma (mRCC): A literature review. *Cancer Treat. Rev.* **2008**, *34*, 193–205. [CrossRef] [PubMed]
4. Kroeger, N.; Choueiri, T.K.; Lee, J.-L.; Bjarnason, G.A.; Knox, J.J.; MacKenzie, M.J.; Wood, L.; Srinivas, S.; Vaishamayan, U.N.; Rha, S.-Y.; et al. Survival outcome and treatment response of patients with late relapse from renal cell carcinoma in the era of targeted therapy. *Eur. Urol.* **2014**, *65*, 1086–1092. [CrossRef]
5. Patil, S.; Manola, J.; Elson, P.; Negrier, S.; Escudier, B.; Eisen, T.; Atkins, M.; Bukowski, R.; Motzer, R.J. Improvement in overall survival of patients with advanced renal cell carcinoma: prognostic factor trend analysis from an international data set of clinical trials. *J. Urol.* **2012**, *188*, 2095–2100. [CrossRef]
6. Horneber, M.; Bueschel, G.; Dennert, G.; Less, D.; Ritter, E.; Zwahlen, M. How many cancer patients use complementary and alternative medicine: A systematic review and metaanalysis. *Integr. Cancer Ther.* **2012**, *11*, 187–203. [CrossRef] [PubMed]
7. Campbell, F.C.; Collett, G.P. Chemopreventive properties of curcumin. *Future Oncol.* **2005**, *1*, 405–414. [CrossRef] [PubMed]
8. Bose, S.; Panda, A.K.; Mukherjee, S.; Sa, G. Curcumin and tumor immune-editing: Resurrecting the immune system. *Cell Div.* **2015**, *10*, 6. [CrossRef]

9. Panda, A.K.; Chakraborty, D.; Sarkar, I.; Khan, T.; Sa, G. New insights into therapeutic activity and anticancer properties of curcumin. *J. Exp. Pharm.* **2017**, *9*, 31–45. [CrossRef]
10. Das, T.; Sa, G.; Saha, B.; Das, K. Multifocal signal modulation therapy of cancer: Ancient weapon, modern targets. *Mol. Cell. Biochem.* **2010**, *336*, 85–95. [CrossRef]
11. Sa, G.; Das, T. Anti cancer effects of curcumin: cycle of life and death. *Cell Div.* **2008**, *3*, 14. [CrossRef] [PubMed]
12. Núñez-Sánchez, M.A.; González-Sarrías, A.; Romo-Vaquero, M.; García-Villalba, R.; Selma, M.V.; Tomás-Barberán, F.A.; García-Conesa, M.-T.; Espín, J.C. Dietary phenolics against colorectal cancer—From promising preclinical results to poor translation into clinical trials: Pitfalls and future needs. *Mol. Nutr. Food Res.* **2015**, *59*, 1274–1291. [CrossRef]
13. Anand, P.; Kunnumakkara, A.B.; Newman, R.A.; Aggarwal, B.B. Bioavailability of curcumin: Problems and promises. *Mol. Pharm.* **2007**, *4*, 807–818. [CrossRef]
14. Burgos-Morón, E.; Calderón-Montaño, J.M.; Salvador, J.; Robles, A.; López-Lázaro, M. The dark side of curcumin. *Int. J. Cancer* **2010**, *126*, 1771–1775. [CrossRef] [PubMed]
15. Jalili-Nik, M.; Soltani, A.; Moussavi, S.; Ghayour-Mobarhan, M.; Ferns, G.A.; Hassanian, S.M.; Avan, A. Current status and future prospective of Curcumin as a potential therapeutic agent in the treatment of colorectal cancer. *J. of Cell. Physiol.* **2018**, *233*, 6337–6345. [CrossRef] [PubMed]
16. Hejazi, J.; Rastmanesh, R.; Taleban, F.-A.; Molana, S.-H.; Hejazi, E.; Ehtejab, G.; Hara, N. Effect of Curcumin Supplementation During Radiotherapy on Oxidative Status of Patients with Prostate Cancer: A Double Blinded, Randomized, Placebo-Controlled Study. *Nutr. Cancer* **2016**, *68*, 77–85. [CrossRef] [PubMed]
17. Mahammedi, H.; Planchat, E.; Pouget, M.; Durando, X.; Curé, H.; Guy, L.; Van-Praagh, I.; Savareux, L.; Atger, M.; Bayet-Robert, M.; et al. The New Combination Docetaxel, Prednisone and Curcumin in Patients with Castration-Resistant Prostate Cancer: A Pilot Phase II Study. *Oncol.* **2016**, *90*, 69–78. [CrossRef]
18. Bernd, A. Visible light and/or UVA offer a strong amplification of the anti-tumor effect of curcumin. *Phytochem. Rev.* **2014**, *13*, 183–189. [CrossRef]
19. Dujic, J.; Kippenberger, S.; Ramirez-Bosca, A.; Diaz-Alperi, J.; Bereiter-Hahn, J.; Kaufmann, R.; Bernd, A.; Hofmann, M. Curcumin in combination with visible light inhibits tumor growth in a xenograft tumor model. *Int. J. Cancer* **2009**, *124*, 1422–1428. [CrossRef]
20. Beyer, K.; Nikfarjam, F.; Butting, M.; Meissner, M.; König, A.; Ramirez Bosca, A.; Kaufmann, R.; Heidemann, D.; Bernd, A.; Kippenberger, S.; et al. Photodynamic Treatment of Oral Squamous Cell Carcinoma Cells with Low Curcumin Concentrations. *J. Cancer* **2017**, *8*, 1271–1283. [CrossRef]
21. Dujic, J.; Kippenberger, S.; Hoffmann, S.; Ramirez-Bosca, A.; Miquel, J.; Diaz-Alperi, J.; Bereiter-Hahn, J.; Kaufmann, R.; Bernd, A. Low concentrations of curcumin induce growth arrest and apoptosis in skin keratinocytes only in combination with UVA or visible light. *J. Invest. Dermatol.* **2007**, *127*, 1992–2000. [CrossRef] [PubMed]
22. Zheng, R.; Deng, Q.; Liu, Y.; Zhao, P. Curcumin Inhibits Gastric Carcinoma Cell Growth and Induces Apoptosis by Suppressing the Wnt/β-Catenin Signaling Pathway. *Med. Sci. Monit.* **2017**, *23*, 163–171. [CrossRef]
23. Moghtaderi, H.; Sepehri, H.; Delphi, L.; Attari, F. Gallic acid and curcumin induce cytotoxicity and apoptosis in human breast cancer cell MDA-MB-231. *BioImpacts* **2018**, *8*, 185–194. [CrossRef] [PubMed]
24. Namkaew, J.; Jaroonwitchawan, T.; Rujanapun, N.; Saelee, J.; Noisa, P. Combined effects of curcumin and doxorubicin on cell death and cell migration of SH-SY5Y human neuroblastoma cells. *In Vitro Cell. Dev. Biol. Anim.* **2018**, *54*, 629–639. [CrossRef] [PubMed]
25. Zhang, L.; Yang, G.; Zhang, R.; Dong, L.; Chen, H.; Bo, J.; Xue, W.; Huang, Y. Curcumin inhibits cell proliferation and motility via suppression of TROP2 in bladder cancer cells. *Int. J. Oncol.* **2018**, *53*, 515–526. [CrossRef]
26. Koon, H.; Leung, A.W.N.; Yue, K.K.M.; Mak, N.K. Photodynamic effect of curcumin on NPC/CNE2 cells. *J. Environ. Pathol. Toxicol. Oncol.* **2006**, *25*, 205–215. [CrossRef]
27. Buss, S.; Dobra, J.; Goerg, K.; Hoffmann, S.; Kippenberger, S.; Kaufmann, R.; Hofmann, M.; Bernd, A. Visible light is a better co-inducer of apoptosis for curcumin-treated human melanoma cells than UVA. *PloS ONE* **2013**, *8*, e79748. [CrossRef] [PubMed]

28. Sha, J.; Li, J.; Wang, W.; Pan, L.; Cheng, J.; Li, L.; Zhao, H.; Lin, W. Curcumin induces G0/G1 arrest and apoptosis in hormone independent prostate cancer DU-145 cells by down regulating Notch signaling. *Biomed. Pharmacother.* **2016**, *84*, 177–184. [CrossRef] [PubMed]
29. Lu, Y.; Wei, C.; Xi, Z. Curcumin suppresses proliferation and invasion in non-small cell lung cancer by modulation of MTA1-mediated Wnt/β-catenin pathway. *In Vitro Cell. Dev. Biol. Anim.* **2014**, *50*, 840–850. [CrossRef] [PubMed]
30. Liang, H.-H.; Huang, C.-Y.; Chou, C.-W.; Makondi, P.T.; Huang, M.-T.; Wei, P.-L.; Chang, Y.-J. Heat shock protein 27 influences the anti-cancer effect of curcumin in colon cancer cells through ROS production and autophagy activation. *Life Sci.* **2018**, *209*, 43–51. [CrossRef]
31. Schwertheim, S.; Wein, F.; Lennartz, K.; Worm, K.; Schmid, K.W.; Sheu-Grabellus, S.-Y. Curcumin induces G2/M arrest, apoptosis, NF-κB inhibition, and expression of differentiation genes in thyroid carcinoma cells. *J. Cancer Res. Clin. Oncol.* **2017**, *143*, 1143–1154. [CrossRef] [PubMed]
32. He, G.; Feng, C.; Vinothkumar, R.; Chen, W.; Dai, X.; Chen, X.; Ye, Q.; Qiu, C.; Zhou, H.; Wang, Y.; et al. Curcumin analog EF24 induces apoptosis via ROS-dependent mitochondrial dysfunction in human colorectal cancer cells. *Cancer Chemother. Pharm.* **2016**, *78*, 1151–1161. [CrossRef]
33. Masuelli, L.; Benvenuto, M.; Di Stefano, E.; Mattera, R.; Fantini, M.; de Feudis, G.; de Smaele, E.; Tresoldi, I.; Giganti, M.G.; Modesti, A.; et al. Curcumin blocks autophagy and activates apoptosis of malignant mesothelioma cell lines and increases the survival of mice intraperitoneally transplanted with a malignant mesothelioma cell line. *Oncotarget* **2017**, *8*, 34405–34422. [CrossRef]
34. Deng, Q.; Liang, L.; Liu, Q.; Duan, W.; Jiang, Y.; Zhang, L. Autophagy is a major mechanism for the dual effects of curcumin on renal cell carcinoma cells. *Eur. J. Pharm.* **2018**, *826*, 24–30. [CrossRef] [PubMed]
35. Zhang, H.; Xu, W.; Li, B.; Zhang, K.; Wu, Y.; Xu, H.; Wang, J.; Zhang, J.; Fan, R.; Wei, J. Curcumin Promotes Cell Cycle Arrest and Inhibits Survival of Human Renal Cancer Cells by Negative Modulation of the PI3K/AKT Signaling Pathway. *Cell Biochem. Biophys.* **2015**, *73*, 681–686. [CrossRef] [PubMed]
36. Cheng, C.; Jiao, J.-T.; Qian, Y.; Guo, X.-Y.; Huang, J.; Dai, M.-C.; Zhang, L.; Ding, X.-P.; Zong, D.; Shao, J.-F. Curcumin induces G2/M arrest and triggers apoptosis via FoxO1 signaling in U87 human glioma cells. *Mol. Med. Rep.* **2016**, *13*, 3763–3770. [CrossRef]
37. Chang, H.-B.; Chen, B.-H. Inhibition of lung cancer cells A549 and H460 by curcuminoid extracts and nanoemulsions prepared from Curcuma longa Linnaeus. *Int. J. Nanomed.* **2015**, *10*, 5059–5080.
38. Sahu, R.P.; Batra, S.; Srivastava, S.K. Activation of ATM/Chk1 by curcumin causes cell cycle arrest and apoptosis in human pancreatic cancer cells. *Br. J. Cancer* **2009**, *100*, 1425–1433. [CrossRef]
39. Kuo, C.-L.; Wu, S.-Y.; Ip, S.-W.; Wu, P.-P.; Yu, C.-S.; Yang, J.-S.; Chen, P.-Y.; Wu, S.-H.; Chung, J.-G. Apoptotic death in curcumin-treated NPC-TW 076 human nasopharyngeal carcinoma cells is mediated through the ROS, mitochondrial depolarization and caspase-3-dependent signaling responses. *Int. J. Oncol.* **2011**, *39*, 319–328.
40. Ciccarese, C.; Brunelli, M.; Montironi, R.; Fiorentino, M.; Iacovelli, R.; Heng, D.; Tortora, G.; Massari, F. The prospect of precision therapy for renal cell carcinoma. *Cancer Treat. Rev.* **2016**, *49*, 37–44. [CrossRef]
41. Xu, S.; Yang, Z.; Fan, Y.; Guan, B.; Jia, J.; Gao, Y.; Wang, K.; Wu, K.; Wang, X.; Zheng, P.; et al. Curcumin enhances temsirolimus-induced apoptosis in human renal carcinoma cells through upregulation of YAP/p53. *Oncol. Lett.* **2016**, *12*, 4999–5006. [CrossRef]
42. Soflaei, S.S.; Momtazi-Borojeni, A.A.; Majeed, M.; Derosa, G.; Maffioli, P.; Sahebkar, A. Curcumin: A Natural Pan-HDAC Inhibitor in Cancer. *Curr. Pharm. Des.* **2018**, *24*, 123–129. [CrossRef]
43. Marquardt, J.U.; Gomez-Quiroz, L.; Arreguin Camacho, L.O.; Pinna, F.; Lee, Y.-H.; Kitade, M.; Domínguez, M.P.; Castven, D.; Breuhahn, K.; Conner, E.A.; et al. Curcumin effectively inhibits oncogenic NF-κB signaling and restrains stemness features in liver cancer. *J. Hepatol.* **2015**, *63*, 661–669. [CrossRef]
44. Niu, T.; Tian, Y.; Cai, Q.; Ren, Q.; Wei, L. Red Light Combined with Blue Light Irradiation Regulates Proliferation and Apoptosis in Skin Keratinocytes in Combination with Low Concentrations of Curcumin. *PloS ONE* **2015**, *10*, e0138754. [CrossRef]
45. Bruzell, E.M.; Morisbak, E.; Tønnesen, H.H. Studies on curcumin and curcuminoids. XXIX. Photoinduced cytotoxicity of curcumin in selected aqueous preparations. *Photochem. Photobiol. Sci.* **2005**, *4*, 523–530. [CrossRef]

46. Neuschmelting, V.; Kim, K.; Malekzadeh-Najafabadi, J.; Jebiwott, S.; Prakash, J.; Scherz, A.; Coleman, J.A.; Kircher, M.F.; Ntziachristos, V. WST11 Vascular Targeted Photodynamic Therapy Effect Monitoring by Multispectral Optoacoustic Tomography (MSOT) in Mice. *Theranostics* **2018**, *8*, 723–734. [CrossRef]
47. Baran, T.M.; Wilson, J.D.; Mitra, S.; Yao, J.L.; Messing, E.M.; Waldman, D.L.; Foster, T.H. Optical property measurements establish the feasibility of photodynamic therapy as a minimally invasive intervention for tumors of the kidney. *J. Biomed. Opt.* **2012**, *17*, 98002-1. [CrossRef]
48. Kroeze, S.G.C.; Grimbergen, M.C.M.; Rehmann, H.; Bosch, J.L.H.R.; Jans, J.J.M. Photodynamic therapy as novel nephron sparing treatment option for small renal masses. *J. Urol.* **2012**, *187*, 289–295. [CrossRef]
49. Ellerkamp, V.; Bortel, N.; Schmid, E.; Kirchner, B.; Armeanu-Ebinger, S.; Fuchs, J. Photodynamic Therapy Potentiates the Effects of Curcumin on Pediatric Epithelial Liver Tumor Cells. *Anticancer Res.* **2016**, *36*, 3363–3372.
50. Wessels, J.T.; Busse, A.-C.; Rave-Fränk, M.; Zänker, S.; Hermann, R.; Grabbe, E.; Müller, G.-A. Photosensitizing and radiosensitizing effects of hypericin on human renal carcinoma cells in vitro. *Photochem. Photobiol.* **2008**, *84*, 228–235. [CrossRef]
51. Brodaczewska, K.K.; Szczylik, C.; Fiedorowicz, M.; Porta, C.; Czarnecka, A.M. Choosing the right cell line for renal cell cancer research. *Mol. Cancer* **2016**, *15*, 83. [CrossRef] [PubMed]

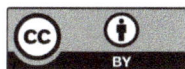

© 2019 by the authors. Licensee MDPI, Basel, Switzerland. This article is an open access article distributed under the terms and conditions of the Creative Commons Attribution (CC BY) license (http://creativecommons.org/licenses/by/4.0/).

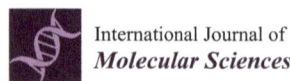

Communication

Extrinsic or Intrinsic Apoptosis by Curcumin and Light: Still a Mystery

Vesselina Laubach, Roland Kaufmann, August Bernd, Stefan Kippenberger and Nadja Zöller *

Department of Dermatology, Venereology and Allergology, Goethe University Frankfurt, 60590 Frankfurt, Germany; v.laubach@mail.de (V.L.); kaufmann@em.uni-frankfurt.de (R.K.); august.b@web.de (A.B.); Kippenberger@em.uni-frankfurt.de (S.K.)
* Correspondence: Nadja.Zoeller@kgu.de; Tel.: +49-69-6301-5090

Received: 24 January 2019; Accepted: 18 February 2019; Published: 19 February 2019

Abstract: Curcumin—a rhizomal phytochemical from the plant *Curcuma longa*—is well known to inhibit cell proliferation and to induce apoptosis in a broad range of cell lines. In previous studies we showed that combining low curcumin concentrations and subsequent ultraviolet A radiation (UVA) or VIS irradiation induced anti-proliferative and pro-apoptotic effects. There is still debate whether curcumin induces apoptosis via the extrinsic or the intrinsic pathway. To address this question, we investigated in three epithelial cell lines (HaCaT, A431, A549) whether the death receptors CD95, tumor necrosis factor (TNF)-receptor I and II are involved in apoptosis induced by light and curcumin. Cells were incubated with 0.25–0.5 µg/mL curcumin followed by irradiation with 1 J/cm^2 UVA. This treatment was combined with inhibitors specific for distinct membrane-bound death receptors. After 24 h apoptosis induction was monitored by quantitative determination of cytoplasmic histone-associated-DNA-fragments. Validation of our test system showed that apoptosis induced by CH11 and TNF-α could be completely inhibited by their respective antagonists. Interestingly, apoptosis induced by curcumin/light treatment was reversed by none of the herein examined death receptor antagonists. These results indicate a mechanism of action independent from classical death receptors speaking for intrinsic activation of apoptosis. It could be speculated that a shift in cellular redox balance might prompt the pro-apoptotic processes.

Keywords: curcumin; death receptor; apoptosis

1. Introduction

Phytochemicals have a crucial role in drug discovery and development [1,2]. Curcumin has been a part of traditional Asian medicine for thousands of years due to its extensive effects on cell physiology. It can be isolated from the rhizome of the ginger plant *Curcuma longa*. Curcumin is known for its anti-inflammatory, anti-oxidative, as well as its pro-apoptotic potential [3–7]. Taking into account the hardly existing toxicity of curcumin, it is predestined for the development of anti-tumorigenic therapeutic strategies. Targeting the low bioavailability of curcumin [8,9] strategies including encapsulation, inhibition of metabolic degradation and development of photodynamic therapies [6,10–20] have been developed. Reducing the proliferative potential of neoblastic cells as well as inducing pro-apoptotic effects is the mode of choice to target cancer cells [6,18]. These two criteria can be addressed by curcumin. Presently, there is debate whether curcumin induces apoptosis via the extrinsic or the intrinsic pathway. Treatment with high curcumin concentrations has been described to induce apoptosis depending on the cell type and tissue via the extrinsic as well as via the intrinsic pathway [21,22]. Characteristic of apoptosis induction via the extrinsic pathway is the binding of extracellular ligands to transmembrane death receptors, e.g., CD95 or tumor necrosis factor (TNF)-α receptors. Receptor clustering, binding with homologous trimeric ligands and recruitment of cytoplasmic adaptor proteins ultimately leads to auto-catalytic activation of pro-caspase-8 [23,24].

Caspase-8 thereafter cleaves and activates the effector caspases-3, -6, -7, leading to the substrate proteolysis, DNA fragmentation and cell death [24,25]. To evaluate whether curcumin in our experimental set up triggers apoptosis via the extrinsic pathway death receptor, specific antagonists were used.

2. Results

2.1. Death Receptor Specific Apoptosis Induction Was Cell Species Dependent

First of all, we determined to which death receptor agonist the herein investigated epidermal cell lines are susceptible. As shown in Figure 1, DNA fragmentation was induced in all three cell lines by a positive control (1 µg/mL staurosporine; black bars) which was set to 100%. Comparison of the DNA fragmentation of the respective untreated cultures (white bars) with CH11 treated cultures (striped bars), showed significantly higher DNA fragmentation in HaCaT and A431 cells. In contrast to the observed non-inducible DNA fragmentation in A549 by CH11, TNF-α (bricked bars) induced a clear increase of DNA fragmentation in comparison to the untreated control. Neither in HaCaT nor in A431 differed DNA fragmentation of the TNF-α treated cultures from the respective untreated cultures. Therefore, we further investigated CD95 related apoptosis induction in HaCaT and A431, and TNF-α related apoptosis induction in A549. Consecutively, we tested described death receptor antagonists to compensate for the pro-apoptotic stimuli. None of the used death receptor antagonists induced DNA fragmentation (Figure 2). In combination with the respective agonists all antagonists were able to reduce the pro-apoptotic impact of the agonists. In detail ZB4 completely neutralized the pro-apoptotic influence of CH11 in HaCaT (pointed bars) and A431 (striped bars; Figure 2a). The efficiency of the two investigated TNF-α antagonists varied in A549 (scaled bars; Figure 2b). Whereas anti-TNF-α RI completely neutralized the pro-apoptotic influence of TNF-α only a decreased but still significantly higher DNA fragmentation in comparison to the untreated control was observed after treatment with TNF-α and anti-TNF-α RII.

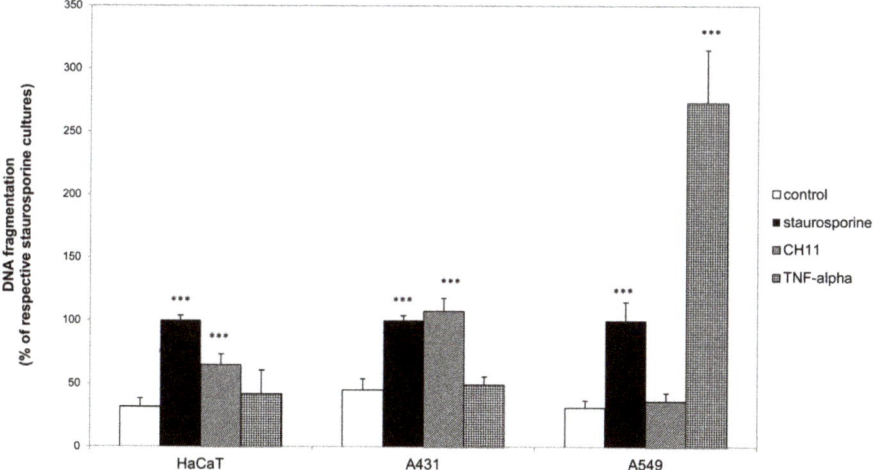

Figure 1. Death receptor agonist specific apoptosis induction. HaCaT, A431 and A549 cells were either left untreated (white bars) or were treated with 1 µg/mL staurosporine (black bars), with 1 µg/mL CH11 (striped bars) or 10 ng/mL tumor necrosis factor (TNF)-α (bricked bars). DNA fragmentation was evaluated after 24 h. The data displayed are representative of three experiments performed with comparable results. Average absorbance values (mean ± SD) from quintuplicate replicates per experimental condition were calculated. *** $p \leq 0.001$ versus the respective untreated control.

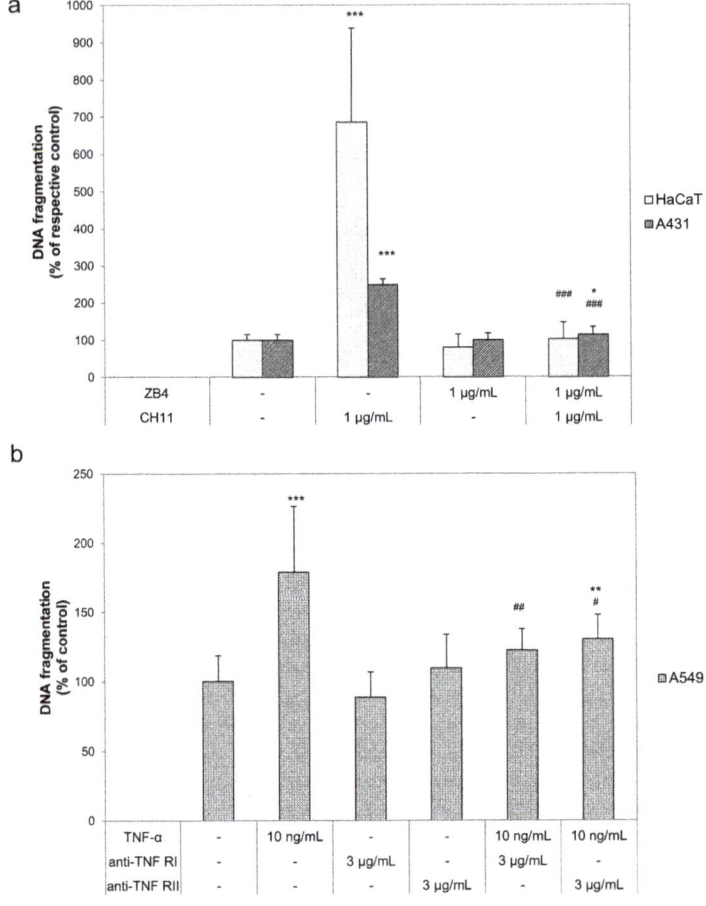

Figure 2. Death receptor specific antagonists reversed apoptosis induction. (**a**) HaCaT (pointed bars) and A431 (striped bars) cells were treated with 1 µg/mL CH11, 1 µg/mL ZB4 or their combination to investigate the CD95 receptor. (**b**) A549 (scaled bars) were treated with 10 ng/mL TNF-α, 3 µg/mL anti-TNF-α RI, 3 µg/mL anti-TNF-α RII or their combinations. DNA fragmentation was evaluated after 24 h. The data displayed are representative of three experiments performed with comparable results. Average absorbance values (mean ± SD) from quintuplicate replicates per experimental condition were calculated. * $p \leq 0.05$; ** $p \leq 0.01$; *** $p \leq 0.001$ versus the respective untreated control and # $p \leq 0.05$; ## $p \leq 0.01$; ### $p \leq 0.001$ versus the respective death receptor agonist.

2.2. Curcumin and Light Induced DNA Fragmentation Independent of the First Apoptosis Signal (FAS) Ligand and the TNF-α Receptors

After establishing the efficiency of the herein used death receptor antagonists their ability to influence DNA fragmentation in curcumin/light treated cultures was investigated. HaCaT and A431 cells were per-incubated with or without curcumin and ZB4 whereas A549 were pre-incubated with or without curcumin and anti-TNF-α RI or anti-TNF-α RII before irradiation with 1 J/cm^2 ultraviolet A radiation (UVA). Neither curcumin nor the antagonists under light-protected conditions induced DNA fragmentation (white bars; Figures 3 and 4). Likewise, the herein chosen UVA irradiation regimen did not induce significant DNA fragmentation in comparison to the light-protected controls. DNA fragmentation of cell cultures treated with curcumin and light (black bars; Figures 3 and 4) was significantly increased. DNA fragmentation of HaCaT after treatment with either 0.25 µg/mL or 0.5 µg/mL curcumin and UVA was 1600% higher in comparison to the light-protected control (Figure 3a). Blocking apoptosis via the first apoptosis signal (FAS) ligand by ZB4 did not change the amount of DNA fragmentation caused by the curcumin/light treatment. Comparable results were observed in A431 cells (Figure 3b). The combined treatment of curcumin and light induced a 300% higher DNA fragmentation than observed in the light-protected cultures. As observed in HaCaT cells, addition of ZB4 to A431 cells did not influence the curcumin/light induced DNA fragmentation. In A549 cells a curcumin concentration dependent increase of DNA fragmentation after irradiation was observed (Figure 4). Cultures that had been treated with 0.25 µg/mL curcumin and light showed a 500% higher DNA fragmentation compared to the light-protected control. Increasing the curcumin concentration to 0.5 µg/mL also increased the DNA fragmentation compared to the light-protected control to 800%. Independent of the applied curcumin concentration addition of anti-TNF-α RI and anti-TNF-α, RII was not able to significantly reduce the curcumin/light induced DNA fragmentation.

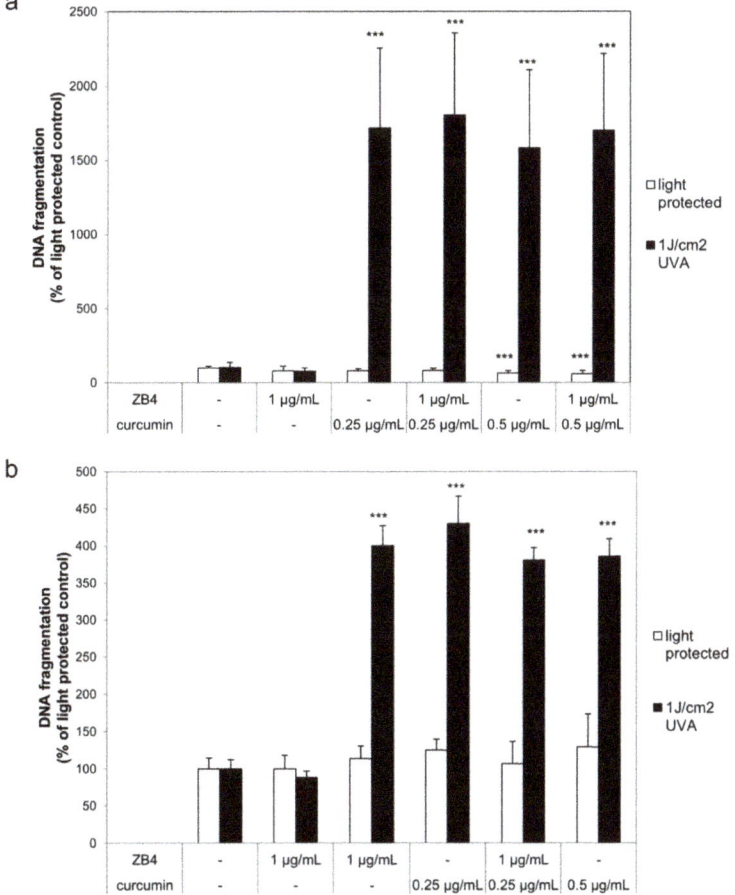

Figure 3. Curcumin does not induce apoptosis via CD95 HaCaT (**a**) and A431 (**b**) cells were pre-incubated with curcumin and ZB4. Thereafter the cells were irradiated with ultraviolet A radiation (UVA) followed by ZB4 exposure. DNA fragmentation was evaluated after 24 h. The applied ZB4 or curcumin concentrations had no effect on DNA fragmentation (white bars).

Combining curcumin with UVA (black bars) induced significant increase of DNA fragmentation. Addition of ZB4 did not reduce the curcumin/light induced DNA fragmentation. Data displayed are representative of four experiments performed with comparable results. Average absorbance values (mean ± SD) from quadruplicate replicates per experimental condition were calculated. *** $p \leq 0.001$ versus the respective untreated control.

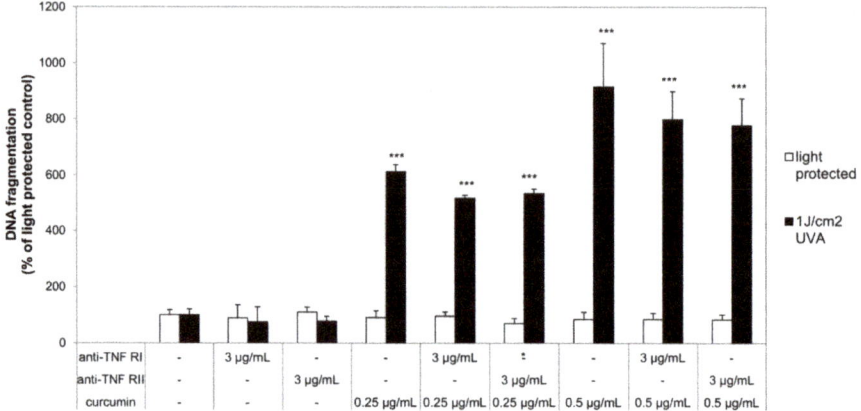

Figure 4. Curcumin does not induce apoptosis via TNF-α receptor I and II. A549 cells were pre-incubated with curcumin and anti-TNF-α RI or anti-TNF-α RII. Thereafter the cells were irradiated with UVA followed by anti-TNF-α RI or anti-TNF-α RII exposure. DNA fragmentation was evaluated after 24 h. The applied TNF-α receptor antagonists or curcumin concentrations had no effect on DNA fragmentation (white bars). Combining curcumin with UVA (black bars) induced a significant increase of DNA fragmentation. Neither anti-TNF-α RI nor anti-TNF-α RII reduced the curcumin/light induced DNA fragmentation. Data displayed are representative of four experiments performed with comparable results. Average absorbance values (mean ± SD) from quadruplicate replicates per experimental condition were calculated. * $p \leq 0.05$; *** $p \leq 0.001$ versus the respective untreated control.

2.3. Curcumin Increased the UVA Triggered H_2O_2 Generation

After establishing that curcumin in the herein described treatment regimen does not induce apoptosis through the classical death receptors, we were interested to monitor whether the combinatorial curcumin/light treatment induces a shift of the cellular redox balance. The H_2O_2 concentration was measured 1 h after the treatment. Irradiation with 1 J/cm^2 UVA induced a significant H_2O_2 generation increase of 1200% to 1400% in HaCaT and A431 cells (black bars, Figure 5). Under light-protected conditions (white bars) curcumin did not influence H_2O_2 generation in HaCaT cells (Figure 6a). Light treatment of A431 cells (Figure 6b) with curcumin induced an H_2O_2 increase of 7–11% in comparison to the respective controls. Comparing the UVA (black bars) induced H_2O_2 generation with the H_2O_2 generation of curcumin/light treated cultures revealed that in both cell species the H_2O_2 concentration was curcumin dependently increased. In HaCaT cultures treatment with 0.25 µg/mL curcumin induced a 15% higher H_2O_2 concentration, and treatment with 0.5 µg/mL curcumin a 29% higher H_2O_2 concentration than observed in the respective controls. Curcumin/light treatment of A431 cells showed a comparable influence on H_2O_2 generation. Treatment with 0.25 µg/mL curcumin induced a 20% increase whereas treatment with 0.5 µg/mL curcumin induced a 29% higher H_2O_2 concentration in comparison to the respective light-treated cultures.

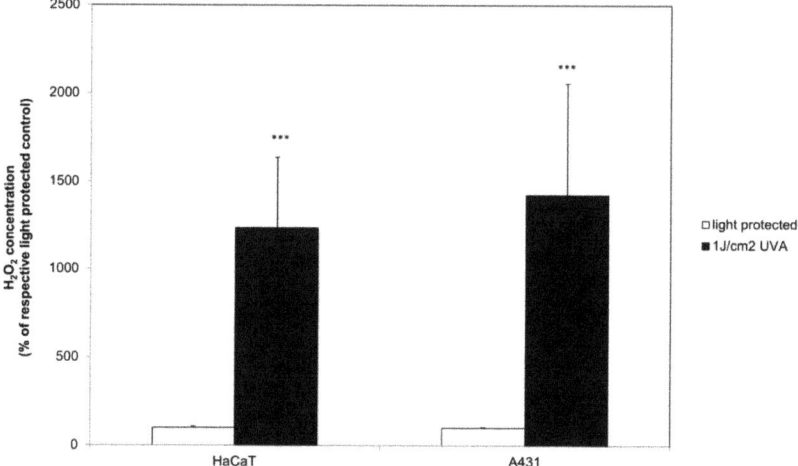

Figure 5. UVA induced H_2O_2 generation in HaCaT and A431. The data displayed are representative of four experiments performed with comparable results. Average luminescence values (mean ± SD) from triplicate replicates per experimental condition were calculated. *** $p \leq 0.001$ versus the respective light-protected control.

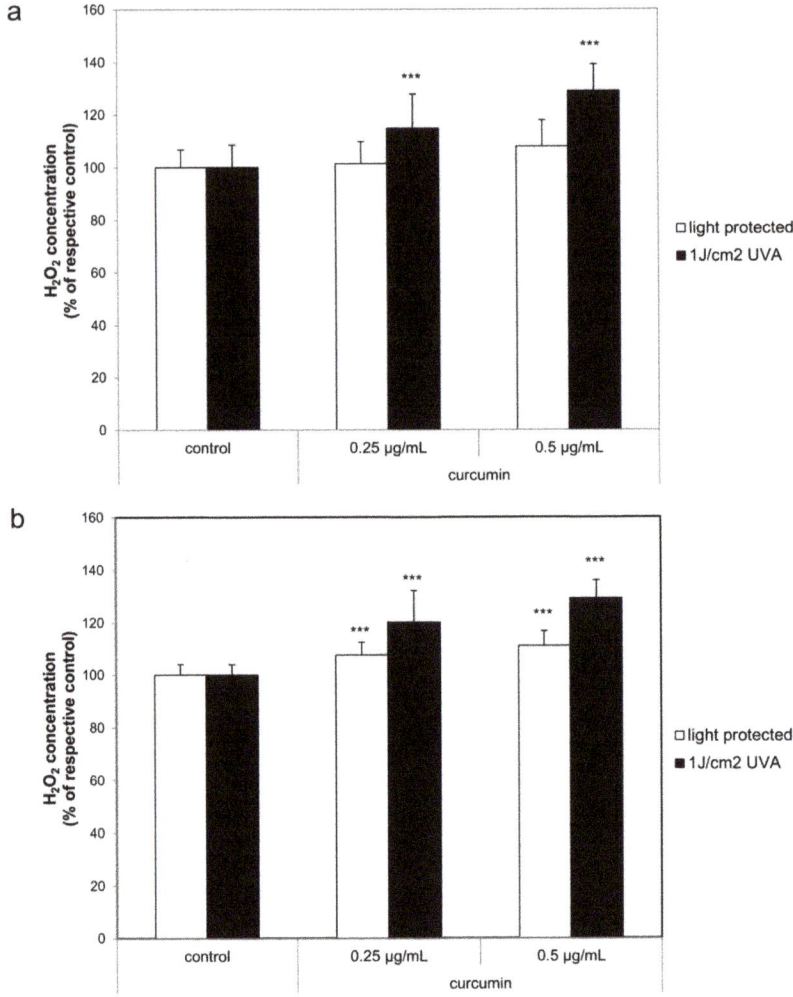

Figure 6. Curcumin enhanced the UVA triggered H_2O_2 generation in HaCaT (**a**) and A431 (**b**). The cells were pre-incubated with curcumin before irradiation with UVA. H_2O_2 generation was evaluated after 1 h. The data displayed are representative of four experiments performed with comparable results. Average luminescence values (mean ± SD) from triplicate replicates per experimental condition were calculated. *** $p \leq 0.001$ versus the respective control.

3. Discussion

Investigation of natural compounds that have been used for centuries in traditional medicine by scientific means has increased during the last decades. Curcumin is one of those phytochemicals with an anti-cancer potential showing a lower risk of inducing adverse events [26,27] than described for other cytostatic drugs. Curcumin influences an extensive spectrum of signaling pathways involved in cancer and inflammatory diseases [28–30]. Establishing a photodynamic treatment combining low curcumin concentrations and radiation with either UVA or VIS [6,16–18] was our approach to address the low bioavailability of curcumin [9]. As it is described that curcumin interacts, e.g., with the epidermal growth factor (EGF) receptor [31–33], we hypothesized that curcumin also directly interacts with different death receptors facilitating apoptosis via the extrinsic pathway. There are contradictory observations concerning the mode of apoptosis induction by curcumin. On the one hand, intrinsic apoptosis induction was observed in mamma carcinoma cells as well as in HL-60 and kidney carcinoma cells [21,34–37]. On the other hand, apoptosis induction via the CD95 receptor was observed, e.g., in melanoma cells while TNF-related apoptosis-inducing ligand (TRAIL) receptor triggered apoptosis was observed in ovarial and prostate carcinoma cells [22,38,39]. In this study we analyzed whether curcumin induced apoptosis in our treatment regimen via either the CD95 or the TNF-α receptor according to Schon et al. [40]. First, we showed that susceptibility to apoptosis inductors differed in the epithelial cell lines used. In particular, HaCaT and A431 seemed to be resistant to the applied TNF-α whereas A549 did not respond to FAS ligand specific apoptosis induction. Death receptor resistance can be acquired by cells through a broad variety of modulatory mechanisms [41,42]. We were furthermore interested whether curcumin might be able to overcome such resistances. The observed curcumin/irradiation dependent induction of DNA fragmentation was taken as a positive indicator of apoptosis [4,43,44]. Hence, DNA fragmentation was monitored to observe whether the herein investigated death receptor antagonists were able to reduce or inhibit the previously described pro-apoptotic influence of the combinatory treatment with low curcumin concentrations and light irradiation. In contrast to others that observed apoptosis induction by curcumin via the FAS ligand pathway [22,45,46], no FAS ligand-related apoptosis was measured in our experimental set up. The FAS ligand specific antagonist ZB4 failed to inhibit or reduce the pro-apoptotic influence of curcumin/light treatment in either of the investigated cell lines. Furthermore, inhibition of the TNF-α receptor I and II by specific antagonists in A549 cells did not change the curcumin/light triggered apoptosis. These observations indicate that in our experimental set up, a mechanism of apoptosis induction independent from classical death receptors is very likely. A possible alternative mode of action can be related to the observations of Kim et al. [47]. They showed that curcumin-related inhibition of EGF receptor phosphorylation and subsequent inhibition of the downstream kinases lead to activation of the effector caspase-3. It seems that curcumin triggers apoptosis in a cell specific manner by different pathways. This characteristic makes curcumin potentially useful to target a broad range of different tumor cells that are sensitive to different pro-apoptotic triggers. It is known that triggering apoptosis in cells that are non-responsive to death receptor agonists or chemotherapeutics is challenging [48]. Therefore, it is of great interest to identify or develop active agents that overcome such resistances [49–52]. The observations showing that curcumin in combination with UVA-boosted H_2O_2 generation indicated that a shift in the cellular redox balance might elicit the observed pro-apoptotic processes as also observed by others [53–58]. Future studies need to address this issue. Moreover, utilizing more complex systems, e.g., tissue cultured skin equivalents [59–61] and long-term analysis are advised to further analyze the potential of curcumin to overcome chemotherapeutic resistances.

4. Materials and Methods

4.1. Cell Culture and Identification of Death Receptor Agonist Susceptibility

The spontaneous immortalized human keratinocyte cell line HaCaT [62] (kindly provided by Prof. Norbert Fusenig (German Cancer Research Institute, Heidelberg, Germany)) and the human epidermoid carcinoma cell lines A431 (ATCC® CRL-1555™, American Culture Type Collection, Manassas, VA, USA) and A549 (ATCC® CCL-185™, American Culture Type Collection) were cultured in Dulbecco's Modified Eagle's Medium (D-MEM, Gibco, Karlsruhe, Germany) with GlutaMax supplemented with 10% (v/v) fetal calf serum (FCS, PAA, Cölbe, Germany) and 1% (v/v) penicillin/streptomycin solution (Gibco) in a 7.5% CO_2 atmosphere at 37 °C. The cells were either stimulated with 1 µg/mL staurosporine (Sigma-Aldrich, Traufkirchen, Germany) or with death receptor specific agonists: (anti-) Fas activating antibody (clone CH11, Merck Millipore, Darmstadt Germany) and TNF-α (R&D Systems, Wiesbaden-Nordenstadt, Germany). These death receptor agonists were combined with their respective antagonists: anti-Fas neutralizing antibody (clone ZB4, Merck Millipore) and anti-TNFα RI and anti-TNFα RII (both R&D Systems).

4.2. Irradiation Regimen

Curcumin (Sigma-Aldrich) was dissolved and applied as previously described [16,17]. Briefly, cells were incubated for 1 h in a medium containing 0.25–0.5 µg/mL curcumin, with or without the above mentioned death receptor antagonists. After replacement of the culture medium with PBS^{++} (Gibco) the cells were either kept light, and/or were irradiated with 1 J/cm^2 ultraviolet A (UVA, Waldmann, Villingen-Schwenningen, Germany). After irradiation PBS^{++} was replaced with culture medium with and without the above mentioned death receptor antagonists.

4.3. DNA Fragmentation

DNA fragmentation, the chosen apoptosis indicator, was quantified after 24 h. The adherent cells were lysed and DNA fragmentation was analyzed with the Cell Death Detection (CDD; Roche, Mannheim, Germany) enzyme-linked immunosorbent assay (ELISA), as described [16].

4.4. Monitoring of the Cellular Redox Balence

The generation of H_2O_2—monitored with the ROS-Glo™-H_2O_2 Assay (Promega, Mannheim, Germany) was chosen as the indicator for oxidative stress in relation to the herein described treatment regimen. Briefly, cells were pre-incubated for 1 h with PBS^{++} containing 0.25–0.5 µg/mL curcumin and were subsequently irradiated with 1 J/cm^2 UVA. After 1 h the assay was conducted as recommended by the manufacturer. The luminescence was recorded using a microplate luminometer (CentroPro LB962, Berthold Technologies, Bad Wildbach, Germany).

4.5. Presentation of Data and Statistical Analysis

All data are presented as mean values ± standard deviation. Statistical significance of the data was evaluated by the Wilcoxon-Mann-Whitney *U*-test (BiAS, version 11.06, epsilon-Verlag, Frankfurt, Germany). Each set of data was related to the referring untreated control (*) or the respective agonist (#). Differences were considered significant at *,# $p \leq 0.05$; **,## $p \leq 0.01$; ***,### $p \leq 0.001$.

Author Contributions: Conceptualization, S.K. and A.B.; methodology, V.L and N.Z.; validation, S.K., A.B. and N.Z.; formal analysis, V.L. and N.Z.; investigation, V.L.; resources, S.K. and A.B.; writing—original draft preparation, N.Z.; review and editing, N.Z.; visualization, N.Z.; supervision, S.K.; project administration, A.B. and R.K.; funding acquisition, A.B., S.K. and R.K.

Funding: This research received no external funding.

Conflicts of Interest: The authors declare no conflict of interest.

Abbreviations

TNF-α	tumor necrosis factor α
UVA	ultraviolet A
EGF	endothelial growth factor

References

1. Kadioglu, O.; Cao, J.; Saeed, M.E.; Greten, H.J.; Efferth, T. Targeting epidermal growth factor receptors and downstream signaling pathways in cancer by phytochemicals. *Target. Oncol.* **2015**, *10*, 337–353. [CrossRef] [PubMed]
2. Newman, D.J.; Cragg, G.M. Natural products as sources of new drugs over the last 25 years. *J. Nat. Prod.* **2007**, *70*, 461–477. [CrossRef]

3. Xu, Y.X.; Pindolia, K.R.; Janakiraman, N.; Noth, C.J.; Chapman, R.A.; Gautam, S.C. Curcumin, a compound with anti-inflammatory and anti-oxidant properties, down-regulates chemokine expression in bone marrow stromal cells. *Exp. Hematol.* **1997**, *25*, 413–422. [PubMed]
4. Zhu, L.; Han, M.B.; Gao, Y.; Wang, H.; Dai, L.; Wen, Y.; Na, L.X. Curcumin triggers apoptosis via upregulation of Bax/Bcl-2 ratio and caspase activation in SW872 human adipocytes. *Mol. Med. Rep.* **2015**, *12*, 1151–1156. [CrossRef] [PubMed]
5. Zhang, C.; Li, B.; Zhang, X.; Hazarika, P.; Aggarwal, B.B.; Duvic, M. Curcumin selectively induces apoptosis in cutaneous T-cell lymphoma cell lines and patients' PBMCs: Potential role for STAT-3 and NF-kappaB signaling. *J. Investig. Dermatol.* **2010**, *130*, 2110–2119. [CrossRef] [PubMed]
6. Dujic, J.; Kippenberger, S.; Ramirez-Bosca, A.; Diaz-Alperi, J.; Bereiter-Hahn, J.; Kaufmann, R.; Bernd, A.; Hofmann, M. Curcumin in combination with visible light inhibits tumor growth in a xenograft tumor model. *Int. J. Cancer* **2009**, *124*, 1422–1428. [CrossRef] [PubMed]
7. Calaf, G.M.; Ponce-Cusi, R.; Carrion, F. Curcumin and paclitaxel induce cell death in breast cancer cell lines. *Oncol. Rep.* **2018**, *40*, 2381–2388. [CrossRef] [PubMed]
8. Wang, Y.J.; Pan, M.H.; Cheng, A.L.; Lin, L.I.; Ho, Y.S.; Hsieh, C.Y.; Lin, J.K. Stability of curcumin in buffer solutions and characterization of its degradation products. *J. Pharm. Biomed. Anal.* **1997**, *15*, 1867–1876. [CrossRef]
9. Anand, P.; Kunnumakkara, A.B.; Newman, R.A.; Aggarwal, B.B. Bioavailability of curcumin: Problems and promises. *Mol. Pharm.* **2007**, *4*, 807–818. [CrossRef]
10. Schiborr, C.; Kocher, A.; Behnam, D.; Jandasek, J.; Toelstede, S.; Frank, J. The oral bioavailability of curcumin from micronized powder and liquid micelles is significantly increased in healthy humans and differs between sexes. *Mol. Nutrit. Food Res.* **2014**, *58*, 516–527. [CrossRef]
11. Hegge, A.B.; Bruzell, E.; Kristensen, S.; Tonnesen, H.H. Photoinactivation of Staphylococcus epidermidis biofilms and suspensions by the hydrophobic photosensitizer curcumin–effect of selected nanocarrier: Studies on curcumin and curcuminoides XLVII. *Eur. J. Pharm. Sci.* **2012**, *47*, 65–74. [CrossRef] [PubMed]
12. Wang, W.; Zhu, R.; Xie, Q.; Li, A.; Xiao, Y.; Li, K.; Liu, H.; Cui, D.; Chen, Y.; Wang, S. Enhanced bioavailability and efficiency of curcumin for the treatment of asthma by its formulation in solid lipid nanoparticles. *Int. J. Nanomed.* **2012**, *7*, 3667–3677. [CrossRef] [PubMed]
13. Yan, H.; Teh, C.; Sreejith, S.; Zhu, L.; Kwok, A.; Fang, W.; Ma, X.; Nguyen, K.T.; Korzh, V.; Zhao, Y. Functional mesoporous silica nanoparticles for photothermal-controlled drug delivery in vivo. *Angew. Chem. Int. Ed. Engl.* **2012**, *51*, 8373–8377. [CrossRef] [PubMed]
14. Shoba, G.; Joy, D.; Joseph, T.; Majeed, M.; Rajendran, R.; Srinivas, P.S. Influence of piperine on the pharmacokinetics of curcumin in animals and human volunteers. *Planta Med.* **1998**, *64*, 353–356. [CrossRef] [PubMed]
15. Singh, D.V.; Godbole, M.M.; Misra, K. A plausible explanation for enhanced bioavailability of P-gp substrates in presence of piperine: Simulation for next generation of P-gp inhibitors. *J. Mol. Model.* **2013**, *19*, 227–238. [CrossRef] [PubMed]
16. Buss, S.; Dobra, J.; Goerg, K.; Hoffmann, S.; Kippenberger, S.; Kaufmann, R.; Hofmann, M.; Bernd, A. Visible light is a better co-inducer of apoptosis for curcumin-treated human melanoma cells than UVA. *PLoS ONE* **2013**, *8*, e79748. [CrossRef] [PubMed]
17. Dujic, J.; Kippenberger, S.; Hoffmann, S.; Ramirez-Bosca, A.; Miquel, J.; Diaz-Alperi, J.; Bereiter-Hahn, J.; Kaufmann, R.; Bernd, A. Low concentrations of curcumin induce growth arrest and apoptosis in skin keratinocytes only in combination with UVA or visible light. *J. Investig. Dermatol.* **2007**, *127*, 1992–2000. [CrossRef]
18. Beyer, K.; Nikfarjam, F.; Butting, M.; Meissner, M.; König, A.; Ramirez Bosca, A.; Kaufmann, R.; Heidemann, D.; Bernd, A.; Kippenberger, S.; et al. Photodynamic Treatment of Oral Squamous Cell Carcinoma Cells with Low Curcumin Concentrations. *J. Cancer* **2017**, *8*, 1271–1283. [CrossRef]
19. Megalathan, A.; Kumarage, S.; Dilhari, A.; Weerasekera, M.M.; Samarasinghe, S.; Kottegoda, N. Natural curcuminoids encapsulated in layered double hydroxides: A novel antimicrobial nanohybrid. *Chem. Cent. J.* **2016**, *10*, 35. [CrossRef]
20. Park, K.; Lee, J.H. Photosensitizer effect of curcumin on UVB-irradiated HaCaT cells through activation of caspase pathways. *Oncol. Rep.* **2007**, *17*, 537–540. [CrossRef]

21. Kim, M.S.; Kang, H.J.; Moon, A. Inhibition of invasion and induction of apoptosis by curcumin in H-ras-transformed MCF10A human breast epithelial cells. *Arch. Pharm. Res.* **2001**, *24*, 349–354. [CrossRef] [PubMed]
22. Bush, J.A.; Cheung, K.J., Jr.; Li, G. Curcumin induces apoptosis in human melanoma cells through a Fas receptor/caspase-8 pathway independent of p53. *Exp. Cell Res.* **2001**, *271*, 305–314. [CrossRef] [PubMed]
23. Elmore, S. Apoptosis: A review of programmed cell death. *Toxicol. Pathol.* **2007**, *35*, 495–516. [CrossRef] [PubMed]
24. Hongmei, Z. Extrinsic and Intrinsic Apoptosis Signal Pathway Review. In *Apoptosis and Medicine*; Ntuli, T., Ed.; IntechOpen: London, UK, 2012; pp. 3–22.
25. Pfeffer, C.M.; Singh, A.T.K. Apoptosis: A Target for Anticancer Therapy. *Int. J. Mol. Sci.* **2018**, *19*, 448. [CrossRef] [PubMed]
26. Chainani-Wu, N. Safety and anti-inflammatory activity of curcumin: A component of tumeric (Curcuma longa). *J. Altern. Complement. Med.* **2003**, *9*, 161–168. [CrossRef] [PubMed]
27. Aggarwal, B.B.; Kumar, A.; Bharti, A.C. Anticancer potential of curcumin: Preclinical and clinical studies. *Anticancer Res.* **2003**, *23*, 363–398. [PubMed]
28. Goel, A.; Kunnumakkara, A.B.; Aggarwal, B.B. Curcumin as "Curecumin": From kitchen to clinic. *Biochem. Pharmacol.* **2008**, *75*, 787–809. [CrossRef] [PubMed]
29. Anand, P.; Sundaram, C.; Jhurani, S.; Kunnumakkara, A.B.; Aggarwal, B.B. Curcumin and cancer: An "old-age" disease with an "age-old" solution. *Cancer Lett.* **2008**, *267*, 133–164. [CrossRef] [PubMed]
30. Aggarwal, B.B.; Gupta, S.C.; Sung, B. Curcumin: An orally bioavailable blocker of TNF and other pro-inflammatory biomarkers. *Br. J. Pharmacol.* **2013**, *169*, 1672–1692. [CrossRef] [PubMed]
31. Squires, M.S.; Hudson, E.A.; Howells, L.; Sale, S.; Houghton, C.E.; Jones, J.L.; Fox, L.H.; Dickens, M.; Prigent, S.A.; Manson, M.M. Relevance of mitogen activated protein kinase (MAPK) and phosphotidylinositol-3-kinase/protein kinase B (PI3K/PKB) pathways to induction of apoptosis by curcumin in breast cells. *Biochem. Pharmacol.* **2003**, *65*, 361–376. [CrossRef]
32. Zhou, Y.; Zheng, S.; Lin, J.; Zhang, Q.J.; Chen, A. The interruption of the PDGF and EGF signaling pathways by curcumin stimulates gene expression of PPARgamma in rat activated hepatic stellate cell in vitro. *Lab. Investig.* **2007**, *87*, 488–498. [CrossRef] [PubMed]
33. Dorai, T.; Gehani, N.; Katz, A. Therapeutic potential of curcumin in human prostate cancer. II. Curcumin inhibits tyrosine kinase activity of epidermal growth factor receptor and depletes the protein. *Mol. Urol.* **2000**, *4*, 1–6. [PubMed]
34. Choudhuri, T.; Pal, S.; Agwarwal, M.L.; Das, T.; Sa, G. Curcumin induces apoptosis in human breast cancer cells through p53-dependent Bax induction. *FEBS Lett.* **2002**, *512*, 334–340. [CrossRef]
35. Choudhuri, T.; Pal, S.; Das, T.; Sa, G. Curcumin selectively induces apoptosis in deregulated cyclin D1-expressed cells at G2 phase of cell cycle in a p53-dependent manner. *J. Biol. Chem.* **2005**, *280*, 20059–20068. [CrossRef] [PubMed]
36. Bielak-Mijewska, A.; Piwocka, K.; Magalska, A.; Sikora, E. P-glycoprotein expression does not change the apoptotic pathway induced by curcumin in HL-60 cells. *Cancer Chemother. Pharmacol.* **2004**, *53*, 179–185. [CrossRef] [PubMed]
37. Woo, J.H.; Kim, Y.H.; Choi, Y.J.; Kim, D.G.; Lee, K.S.; Bae, J.H.; Min, D.S.; Chang, J.S.; Jeong, Y.J.; Lee, Y.H.; et al. Molecular mechanisms of curcumin-induced cytotoxicity: Induction of apoptosis through generation of reactive oxygen species, down-regulation of Bcl-XL and IAP, the release of cytochrome c and inhibition of Akt. *Carcinogenesis* **2003**, *24*, 1199–1208. [CrossRef] [PubMed]
38. Wahl, H.; Tan, L.; Griffith, K.; Choi, M.; Liu, J.R. Curcumin enhances Apo2L/TRAIL-induced apoptosis in chemoresistant ovarian cancer cells. *Gynecol. Oncol.* **2007**, *105*, 104–112. [CrossRef]
39. Deeb, D.; Jiang, H.; Gao, X.; Al-Holou, S.; Danyluk, A.L.; Dulchavsky, S.A.; Gautam, S.C. Curcumin [1,7-bis(4-hydroxy-3-methoxyphenyl)-1-6-heptadine-3,5-dione; C21H20O6] sensitizes human prostate cancer cells to tumor necrosis factor-related apoptosis-inducing ligand/Apo2L-induced apoptosis by suppressing nuclear factor-kappaB via inhibition of the prosurvival Akt signaling pathway. *J. Pharmacol. Exp. Ther.* **2007**, *321*, 616–625.
40. Schon, M.P.; Wienrich, B.G.; Drewniok, C.; Bong, A.B.; Eberle, J.; Geilen, C.C.; Gollnick, H.; Schon, M. Death receptor-independent apoptosis in malignant melanoma induced by the small-molecule immune response modifier imiquimod. *J. Investig. Dermatol.* **2004**, *122*, 1266–1276. [CrossRef]

41. Min, K.J.; Woo, S.M.; Shahriyar, S.A.; Kwon, T.K. Elucidation for modulation of death receptor (DR) 5 to strengthen apoptotic signals in cancer cells. *Arch. Pharm. Res.* **2019**, *42*, 88–100. [CrossRef]
42. Twomey, J.D.; Zhang, B. Circulating Tumor Cells Develop Resistance to TRAIL-Induced Apoptosis Through Autophagic Removal of Death Receptor 5: Evidence from an In Vitro Model. *Cancers* **2019**, *11*, 94. [CrossRef] [PubMed]
43. Chang, P.Y.; Peng, S.F.; Lee, C.Y.; Lu, C.C.; Tsai, S.C.; Shieh, T.M.; Wu, T.S.; Tu, M.G.; Chen, M.Y.; Yang, J.S. Curcumin-loaded nanoparticles induce apoptotic cell death through regulation of the function of MDR1 and reactive oxygen species in cisplatin-resistant CAR human oral cancer cells. *Int. J. Oncol.* **2013**, *43*, 1141–1150. [CrossRef] [PubMed]
44. Zhang, L.; Man, S.; Qiu, H.; Liu, Z.; Zhang, M.; Ma, L.; Gao, W. Curcumin-cyclodextrin complexes enhanced the anti-cancer effects of curcumin. *Environ. Toxicol. Pharmacol.* **2016**, *48*, 31–38. [CrossRef] [PubMed]
45. Wang, W.Z.; Li, L.; Liu, M.Y.; Jin, X.B.; Mao, J.W.; Pu, Q.H.; Meng, M.J.; Chen, X.G.; Zhu, J.Y. Curcumin induces FasL-related apoptosis through p38 activation in human hepatocellular carcinoma Huh7 cells. *Life Sci.* **2013**, *92*, 352–358. [CrossRef] [PubMed]
46. Lee, H.P.; Li, T.M.; Tsao, J.Y.; Fong, Y.C.; Tang, C.H. Curcumin induces cell apoptosis in human chondrosarcoma through extrinsic death receptor pathway. *Int. Immunopharmacol.* **2012**, *13*, 163–169. [CrossRef] [PubMed]
47. Kim, J.H.; Xu, C.; Keum, Y.S.; Reddy, B.; Conney, A.; Kong, A.N. Inhibition of EGFR signaling in human prostate cancer PC-3 cells by combination treatment with beta-phenylethyl isothiocyanate and curcumin. *Carcinogenesis* **2006**, *27*, 475–482. [CrossRef]
48. Chresta, C.M.; Arriola, E.L.; Hickman, J.A. Apoptosis and cancer chemotherapy. *Behring Inst. Mitt.* **1996**, 232–240.
49. Thulasiraman, P.; Garriga, G.; Danthuluri, V.; McAndrews, D.J.; Mohiuddin, I.Q. Activation of the CRABPII/RAR pathway by curcumin induces retinoic acid mediated apoptosis in retinoic acid resistant breast cancer cells. *Oncol. Rep.* **2017**, *37*, 2007–2015. [CrossRef]
50. Labbozzetta, M.; Notarbartolo, M.; Poma, P.; Maurici, A.; Inguglia, L.; Marchetti, P.; Rizzi, M.; Baruchello, R.; Simoni, D.; D'Alessandro, N. Curcumin as a possible lead compound against hormone-independent, multidrug-resistant breast cancer. *Ann. N. Y. Acad. Sci.* **2009**, *1155*, 278–283. [CrossRef]
51. Chatterjee, S.J.; Pandey, S. Chemo-resistant melanoma sensitized by tamoxifen to low dose curcumin treatment through induction of apoptosis and autophagy. *Cancer Biol. Ther.* **2011**, *11*, 216–228. [CrossRef]
52. Shankar, S.; Ganapathy, S.; Chen, Q.; Srivastava, R.K. Curcumin sensitizes TRAIL-resistant xenografts: Molecular mechanisms of apoptosis, metastasis and angiogenesis. *Mol. Cancer* **2008**, *7*, 16. [CrossRef] [PubMed]
53. Zhou, D.R.; Eid, R.; Boucher, E.; Miller, K.A.; Mandato, C.A.; Greenwood, M.T. Stress is an agonist for the induction of programmed cell death: A review. *Biochim. Biophys. Acta* **2019**. [CrossRef] [PubMed]
54. Jiang, S.; Zhu, R.; He, X.; Wang, J.; Wang, M.; Qian, Y.; Wang, S. Enhanced photocytotoxicity of curcumin delivered by solid lipid nanoparticles. *Int. J. Nanomed.* **2017**, *12*, 167–178. [CrossRef] [PubMed]
55. Moradi-Marjaneh, R.; Hassanian, S.M.; Rahmani, F.; Aghaee-Bakhtiari, S.H.; Avan, A.; Khazaei, M. Phytosomal curcumin elicits anti-tumor properties through suppression of angiogenesis, cell proliferation and induction of oxidative stress in colorectal cancer. *Curr. Pharm. Des.* **2019**. [CrossRef] [PubMed]
56. Jayakumar, S.; Patwardhan, R.S.; Pal, D.; Singh, B.; Sharma, D.; Kutala, V.K.; Sandur, S.K. Mitochondrial targeted curcumin exhibits anticancer effects through disruption of mitochondrial redox and modulation of TrxR2 activity. *Free Rad. Biol. Med.* **2017**, *113*, 530–538. [CrossRef] [PubMed]
57. Mortezaee, K.; Salehi, E.; Mirtavoos-Mahyari, H.; Motevaseli, E.; Najafi, M.; Farhood, B.; Rosengren, R.J.; Sahebkar, A. Mechanisms of apoptosis modulation by curcumin: Implications for cancer therapy. *J. Cell. Physiol.* **2019**. [CrossRef] [PubMed]
58. Gopal, P.K.; Paul, M.; Paul, S. Curcumin induces caspase mediated apoptosis in JURKAT cells by disrupting the redox balance. *Asian Pac. J. Cancer Prev.* **2014**, *15*, 93–100. [CrossRef] [PubMed]
59. Zöller, N.; Valesky, E.; Butting, M.; Hofmann, M.; Kippenberger, S.; Bereiter-Hahn, J.; Bernd, A.; Kaufmann, R. Clinical application of a tissue-cultured skin autograft: An alternative for the treatment of non-healing or slowly healing wounds? *Dermatology* **2014**, *229*, 190–198. [CrossRef] [PubMed]
60. Golinski, P.; Menke, H.; Hofmann, M.; Valesky, E.; Butting, M.; Kippenberger, S.; Bereiter-Hahn, J.; Bernd, A.; Kaufmann, R.; Zöller, N.N. Development and Characterization of an Engraftable Tissue-Cultured Skin

Autograft: Alternative Treatment for Severe Electrical Injuries. *Cells Tissues Organs* **2014**, *200*, 227–239. [CrossRef] [PubMed]
61. Zöller, N.N.; Kippenberger, S.; Thaci, D.; Mewes, K.; Spiegel, M.; Sattler, A.; Schultz, M.; Bereiter-Hahn, J.; Kaufmann, R.; Bernd, A. Evaluation of beneficial and adverse effects of glucocorticoids on a newly developed full-thickness skin model. *Toxicol. in Vitro* **2008**, *22*, 747–759. [CrossRef]
62. Boukamp, P.; Petrussevska, R.T.; Breitkreutz, D.; Hornung, J.; Markham, A.; Fusenig, N.E. Normal keratinization in a spontaneously immortalized aneuploid human keratinocyte cell line. *J. Cell Biol.* **1988**, *106*, 761–771. [CrossRef] [PubMed]

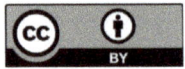

© 2019 by the authors. Licensee MDPI, Basel, Switzerland. This article is an open access article distributed under the terms and conditions of the Creative Commons Attribution (CC BY) license (http://creativecommons.org/licenses/by/4.0/).

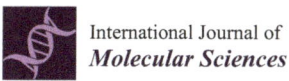

Review

A Review of Curcumin and Its Derivatives as Anticancer Agents

Mhd Anas Tomeh [1], Roja Hadianamrei [1] and Xiubo Zhao [1,2,*]

1. Department of Chemical and Biological Engineering, University of Sheffield, Sheffield S1 3JD, UK; matomeh1@sheffield.ac.uk (M.A.T.); rhadianamrei1@sheffield.ac.uk (R.H.)
2. School of Pharmaceutical Engineering and Life Science, Changzhou University, Changzhou 213164, China
* Correspondence: xiubo.zhao@sheffield.ac.uk; Tel.: +44-(0)-0114-222-8256

Received: 6 February 2019; Accepted: 21 February 2019; Published: 27 February 2019

Abstract: Cancer is the second leading cause of death in the world and one of the major public health problems. Despite the great advances in cancer therapy, the incidence and mortality rates of cancer remain high. Therefore, the quest for more efficient and less toxic cancer treatment strategies is still at the forefront of current research. Curcumin, the active ingredient of the *Curcuma longa* plant, has received great attention over the past two decades as an antioxidant, anti-inflammatory, and anticancer agent. In this review, a summary of the medicinal chemistry and pharmacology of curcumin and its derivatives in regard to anticancer activity, their main mechanisms of action, and cellular targets has been provided based on the literature data from the experimental and clinical evaluation of curcumin in cancer cell lines, animal models, and human subjects. In addition, the recent advances in the drug delivery systems for curcumin delivery to cancer cells have been highlighted.

Keywords: curcumin; anticancer; structure activity relationship; cellular pathway; mechanism of action; delivery system

1. Introduction

Cancer is the second most life-threatening disease and one of the main public health problems worldwide. In 2018, there were around 1.73 million new cases of cancer and more than 609,000 deaths in the United States alone [1]. Despite the tangible advances in cancer therapy, the reported incidence of the disease and the mortality have not declined in the past 30 years [2]. Understanding the molecular alterations that contribute to cancer development and progression is a key factor in cancer prevention and treatment. There are several common strategies for targeting specific cancer cells to inhibit tumor development, progression, and metastasis without causing severe side effects [3]. In addition to the chemically synthesized anticancer agents, several anticancer compounds with different modes of action have been extracted from plant sources, such as *Taxus brevifolia*, *Catharanthus roseus*, *Betula alba*, *Cephalotaxus* species, *Erythroxylum previllei*, *Curcuma longa*, and many others [4]. Among them, curcumin is the most important component of the rhizomes of *Curcuma longa* L. (turmeric) [5] and was extracted from turmeric plant in a pure crystalline form for the first time in 1870 [6]. Curcumin and its derivatives have received immense attention in the past two decades due to their biofunctional properties such as anti-tumor, antioxidant, and anti-inflammatory activities [7]. These properties are attributed to the key elements in the curcumin structure [8]. Therefore, a great deal of scientific work has shed light on the structure activity relationship (SAR) of curcumin in an attempt to improve its physiochemical and biological properties. Due to the importance of cancer as a leading cause of death and the ongoing quest for more efficient and less toxic anticancer agents, this review has mainly focused on the anticancer activity of curcumin. The applications of curcumin in other diseases are beyond the scope of this review and have been reviewed elsewhere [4,9].

The main mechanisms of action by which curcumin exhibits its unique anticancer activity include inducing apoptosis and inhibiting proliferation and invasion of tumors by suppressing a variety of cellular signaling pathways [10]. Several studies reported curcumin's antitumor activity on breast cancer, lung cancer, head and neck squamous cell carcinoma, prostate cancer, and brain tumors [11], showing its capability to target multiple cancer cell lines. In spite of all the above mentioned advantages, curcumin's applications are limited due to its low water solubility which results in poor oral bioavailability and also low chemical stability [7]. Another obstacle is the low cellular uptake of curcumin. Due to its hydrophobicity, the curcumin molecule tends to penetrate into the cell membrane and bind to the fatty acyl chains of membrane lipids through hydrogen binding and hydrophobic interactions, resulting in low availability of curcumin inside the cytoplasm [12,13]. To overcome these obstacles and improve the overall anticancer activity of curcumin, several structural modifications have been suggested to enhance selective toxicity towards specific cancer cells [14], increase bioavailability, or enhance stability [4,15]. Another approach is to use different delivery systems to improve curcumin's physiochemical properties and anticancer activity. This review focuses on the recent literature on the SAR of curcumin and its analogues and their anticancer activity in different cancer cell lines, animal models, and human clinical trials as well as different types of curcumin delivery systems that have been used for cancer therapy.

2. Structure Activity Relationship of Curcumin and Its Derivatives

Chemical structure modification does not only affect the receptor binding and pharmacological activity of a drug molecule but also alters its pharmacokinetics and physiochemical properties [4]. Determining the essential pharmacophores within a drug molecule requires a thorough study of its natural and synthetic analogues [11]. The chemical structure of curcumin is depicted in Figure 1A. As can be observed, it consists of two phenyl rings substituted with hydroxyl and methoxyl groups and connected via a seven carbon keto-enol linker (C7). While curcumin is naturally derived, its derivatives are generally produced by a chemical reaction between aryl-aldehydes and acetylacetone. This assembly method can yield multiple chemical analogues, such as compounds with alkyl substituents on the middle carbon of the linker (C7 moiety) [16,17]. A SAR study of curcumin derivatives demonstrates that the presence of a coplanar hydrogen donor group and a β-diketone moiety is essential for the antiandrogenic activity for the treatment of prostate cancer [17]. In addition, scanning 50 curcumin analogues showed that shortening the linker from seven carbon atoms (C7) to five carbon atoms (C5) improves the antiandrogenic activity [18]. As a result of introducing a methyl group at both C2 and C6 positions, a new curcumin derivative has been produced (Figure 1B). This derivative exhibited a steric hindrance effect toward metabolizing enzymes, such as alcohol dehydrogenase [14], and demonstrated significantly higher activity than curcumin in inhibiting endothelial cell proliferation and invasion both in vitro and in vivo [14]. Dimethylcurcumin or ASC-J9 (5-hydroxy-1, 7-bis (3, 4-dimethoxyphenyl)-1, 4, 6-heptatrien-3-one) is a newly developed curcumin analogue which enhances androgen receptor degradation and has been used for treatment of prostate cancer [19–21]. Moreover, it has also shown a significant antiproliferative effect against estrogen-dependent breast cancer cells [22]. Although methylation has enhanced the targetability and activity of the molecule, it has also increased its hydrophobicity massively compared to curcumin, which has limited its administrable dose in cancer therapy [23].

Furthermore, studies on the kinetic stability of synthetic curcumin derivatives have pointed out that glycosylation of the pharmacophore aromatic ring improves the compound's water solubility, which enhances its kinetic stability and leads to a better overall therapeutic response [24]. During phase I and phase II metabolism, the main routes of converting curcumin into a higher excretable form are oxidation, reduction, and conjugation (glucuronidation and sulfurylation). The conjugation reactions occur on the hydroxyl groups (4-OH) attached to the phenyl rings of curcumin. Thus, curcumin's kinetic stability can be enhanced by masking the 4-OH groups [25]. Another study has revealed a correlation between the hydrophobic property of the benzyl rings and androgen receptor affinity [26].

The benzyl rings are also crucial for inhibiting tumor growth, and adding hydrophobic substituents, such as CH_3 groups, on them (R1, R2, R3, R4 in Figure 1B) have been linked to the increased antitumor activity of curcumin derivatives [26,27]. O-methoxy substitution was found to be more effective in suppressing nuclear factor κ-light-chain-enhancer of activated B cells (NF-κB), but this modification has also affected the lipophilicity of curcumin [28]. A summary of the potential sites of modification on the curcumin molecule is illustrated in Figure 1B.

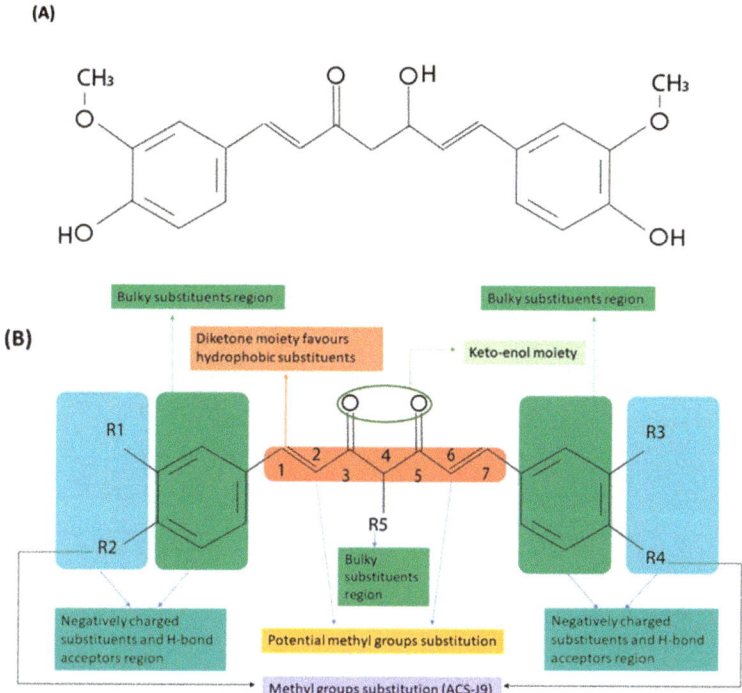

Figure 1. (A) Chemical structure of curcumin. (B) The main pharmacophores and potential substitution positions.

Some of the modified curcuminoids exhibit enhanced anticancer and anti-inflammatory activities compared to curcumin due to the low level of hydrogenation, high level of methoxylation, and unsaturation of the diketone moiety [29]. Ortho-methoxy substitution of the essential radical of curcuminoid alters the heptadiene moiety and the hydrogenation level [28]. A comparative study on curcumin and its derivatives revealed stronger antioxidant activity for several hydrogenated curcumin derivatives compared to the original curcumin compound [30]. For example, tetrahydrocurcumin (THC) exhibited higher antioxidant activity than dihydrocurcumin (DHC) and unmodified curcumin [31,32] (Table 1). Unlike curcumin, THC, which is a non-electrophilic derivative, failed to suppress the signal transducer and activator of transcription 3 (STAT3) signaling pathway and induce apoptosis. This suggests that the electrophilic nature of curcumin is essential for inhibiting the STAT3 signaling pathway during anticancer therapy [33]. Metallo-curcumin-conjugated DNA complexes have been constructed using $Cu^{2+}/Ni^{2+}/Zn^{2+}$ metal ions to improve curcumin solubility and enhance DNA-binding ability [34]. These complexes also showed a better antibacterial activity and significant toxicity to several prostate cancer cell lines [34] (Table 1).

In addition to anticancer and anti-inflammatory properties, curcuminoids exert antioxidant activity mainly through the chelating effect of the diketone moiety. The presence of metals such as

Cu^{2+}, Fe^{2+}, and Pb^{2+} boost the chelating power of curcumin derivatives [35]. The unsaturated diketone group in curcumin root is a Michael reaction acceptor, part of phase II enzyme inducers [4], which can be responsible for NF-κB suppression in cancer cells. However, an investigation on 72 different curcumin derivatives did not find a direct correlation between the inhibition of tumor growth through NF-κB and antioxidant activity [36]. O-methoxy substitution resulted in increased antioxidant activity of curcumin only when the methoxy group was not linked to the proton acceptor β-diketone moiety through conjugation [4]. The equilibrium between the keto and enol forms of curcumin relies on environmental factors such as pH. The keto form is dominant at acidic or neutral pH, while the enol form is more common in basic pH [37]. This unique property has been exploited in the discovery of new curcumin nanoassemblies with a buffering capacity that exhibit the "proton sponge effect" in endosomes and lysosomes [7].

Table 1. Changes to the pharmacological activity of curcumin derivatives compared to curcumin.

Curcumin Derivative	Chemical Modification	Activities	References
Dimethyl curcumin (ASC-J9)	Methyl groups substitution on R2 and R4	Enhanced activity toward prostate and breast cancer	[20–22,38]
Vanadium, gallium, and indium complexes	Metal complexation by the β-diketones	Enhanced cytotoxic activity	[39]
Tetrahydrocurcumin (THC)	Hydrogenated diketone moiety	Enhanced antioxidant activity but loss of DNA binding and STAT3 [a] inhibition properties	[31,33]
Modified aromatic rings curcumin compounds	Introduction of cyclohexane bridge	Improved mitochondrial membrane permeability during lymphoma therapy	[40]
Metallo-curcumin (Cu^{2+}/Ni^{2+}/Zn^{2+})	Metal complexation by the β-diketones	Enhanced water-solubility and improved DNA binding	[34]
Glycosylated curcumin derivative	Glycol groups substitution on the aromatic rings	Higher potency, aqueous solubility, and chelating properties	[41]
Cu^{2+} conjugate of synthetic curcumin analogues	Conjugation reaction on the keto-enol moiety	Stronger inhibition of TNF [b]-induced NF-κB [c] activation in leukemic KBM-5 cells	[42]
Cyclic curcumin derivatives	Boron trioxide-mediated aldol condensation	Enhanced cytostatic, antitumor, and antioxidant activity	[43]
Curcumin carbocyclic analogues	Introducing carboxyl group at the diketone moiety	Enhanced antioxidant activity and stronger inhibition of HIV [d] 1 protease	[44]
Hydrazinocurcumin	Replacing the diketone moiety with hydrazine derivative	Higher efficacy in inhibition of colon cancer progression via antagonism of Ca^{2+}/CaM [e] function	[45,46]
Semicarbazone	Introducing $NNHCONH_2$ at the keto-enol moiety	Enhanced antioxidant, antiradical, and antiproliferative activity	[47]

[a] STAT3: signal transducer and activator of transcription 3; [b] TNF: Tumor necrosis factor; [c] NF-κB: nuclear factor κ-light-chain-enhancer of activated B cells; [d] HIV: Human immunodeficiency virus; [e] Ca^{2+}/CaM: calcium/calmodulin.

Although curcumin has low water solubility and poor bioavailability, it enjoys a strong pharmacological effect in clinical applications [48]. A novel study attempted to explain this unique property of curcumin by testing the pharmacological effect of curcumin's metabolites resulting from physiological degradation. The parallel docking calculations of curcumin degradation products were found to be similar to those of curcumin because they share with the original compound the same binding pockets required for inhibiting several enzymes [48].

3. Different Types of Curcumin Delivery Systems Used in Cancer Therapy

Various delivery systems for curcumin have been formulated using different nanotechnologies in order to improve curcumin properties and targetability. For the rational design of the nanoformulations, several factors should be considered in order to enhance the efficacy and improve the cellular targeting of the anticancer agents. These factors include the nanoparticle size and shape, surface properties, and nanoparticle targeting ligands [49], as illustrated in Figure 2. A summary of the most commonly used curcumin delivery systems is introduced in this section.

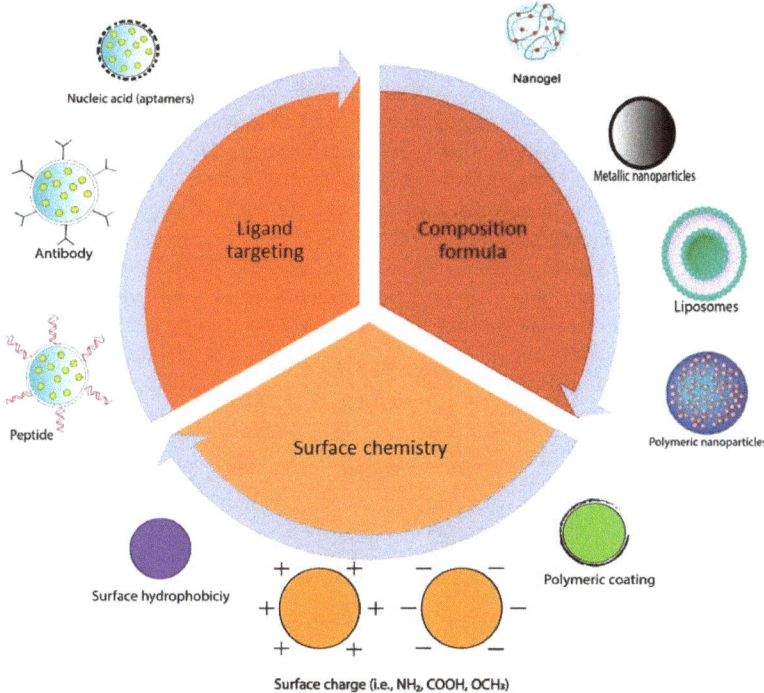

Figure 2. Examples of current nanoparticle design strategies used to improve targeting.

3.1. Polymeric Nanoparticles

Various polymers have been utilized to prepare nanoformulations for curcumin drug delivery to improve its biological activity [50]. The biocompatible and biodegradable polymers are preferred in the drug delivery systems due to lower risk of toxicity [51]. Therefore, biodegradable synthetic polymers such as PLGA (poly (D, L-lactic-co-glycolic acid) and natural polymers such as silk fibroin and chitosan have become widely used in drug delivery [52–54]. PLGA-curcumin nanoformulation was found to be as effective as curcumin at 15-fold lower concentration in inhibiting mRNAs for inflammatory cytokines (CXCR3 and CXCL10) and increasing anti-inflammatory cytokine interleukin-10 (IL-10) in the brain [55]. In vivo study in rats showed that the bioavailability of curcumin-PLGA nanospheres was increased nine-fold in comparison to unprocessed curcumin administrated with alkaloid compound piperine. However, curcumin/piperine coadministration enhanced curcumin activity by inhibiting hepatic and intestinal deactivation [56]. Another study compared the anticancer activity of curcumin-loaded PLGA nanoparticles (CUR-NPs) and curcumin-loaded PLGA nanoparticles conjugated to anti-P-glycoprotein (P-gp) (CUR-NPs-APgp). The latter formulation showed significantly more specific binding to cervical cancer cells KB-3-1 but lower entrapment efficiency compared to CUR-NPs [57]. Spherical PLGA nanospheres were also developed to encapsulate dimethyl curcumin (ASC-J9) and tested in breast cancer cells. The PLGA nanospheres were capable of releasing ASC-J9 intracellularly, leading to growth inhibition of estrogen-dependent MCF-7 cancer cells [22].

3.2. Liposomes

Nanoscale liposomes are emerging as one of the most useful drug delivery systems for anticancer agents. Recent advances in liposome formulations have resulted in improved treatment for drug-resistant tumors and reduced toxicity [58]. A liposome consists of a phospholipid bilayer shell and an aqueous core which makes it an ideal carrier for encapsulating both hydrophobic and hydrophilic compounds. Several liposome preparations have been utilized to encapsulate curcumin (Table 2). The liposomal lipid bilayer (such as egg yolk phosphatidyl choline (EYPC), dihexyl phosphate (DHP) and cholesterol) solubilizes curcumin. This preparation was found to stabilize loaded curcumin proportionally to its content [59]. Another work on liposomes tested coating liposomes with lipid–polymer conjugate N-dodecyl chitosan-N-[(2-hydroxy-3-trimethylamine) propyl] (HPTMA) chloride. Positively charged nanoliposomes for curcumin delivery have also been developed by incorporating polyethylene glycol (PEG) and cationic polyethyleneimine (PEI) into the formulation. Despite low encapsulation efficiency (45%), this formulation has demonstrated twenty-fold higher cytotoxic activity than unprocessed curcumin in various cell lines, including human HepG2 hepatocellular carcinoma, A549 lung carcinoma, HT29 colorectal carcinoma, and cervical carcinoma [60]. In liposomal gene delivery, an interesting work conducted by Fujita et al. [61] utilized curcumin to control siRNA release. By incorporating curcumin into the liposomal formula, siRNA release showed a bell-shaped pattern due to the dose-dependent increase in liposomal permeability induced by curcumin. Curcumin-loaded liposomes were also used to inhibit the production of IL-6 in macrophages. The liposomes were prepared by mixing curcumin solution with human serum albumin (HSA) solution and subsequently adding this mixture to a lipid mixture containing 1, 2-dipalmitoyl-sn-glycero-3-phosphocholine (DPPC), 1, 2-dipalmitoyl-sn-glycero-3-phospho-L-serine sodium salt (DPPS) and cholesterol. The designed system induced significant IL-6 suppression and reduction in the total number of macrophages [62] (Figure 3).

Table 2. Examples of recent curcumin delivery systems.

Nanoformulation	Particle Size	Application	Outcome	Reference
Curcumin-loaded liposomal PMSA [a] antibodies	100–150 nm	Human prostate cancer (LNCa, C4-2B)	Enhanced antiproliferative efficacy and targeting	[63]
Curcumin-loaded magnetic silk nanoparticles	100–350 nm	Human breast cancer (MDA-MB-231) cells	Enhanced cellular uptake and growth inhibition	[54]
Curcumin/MPEG [b]-PCL [c] micelles	27 ± 1.3 nm	Colon carcinoma (C-26) cells	Enhanced cancer growth inhibition	[64]
Curcumin nanoemulsion	<200 nm	Human ovarian adenocarcinoma cells (SKV3)	Increased cytotoxicity	[65]
Curcumin loaded liposomes coated with N-dodecyl chitosan-HPTMA [d] chloride	73 nm	Murine fibroblasts (NIH3T3) and murine melanoma (B16F10) cells	Specific toxicity in murine melanoma (but not in fibroblasts)	[66]
Curcumin-PLGA [e] nanoparticles	248 ± 1.6 nm	Erythroleukemia type 562 cells	Improved clinical management of leukemia	[65]
Curcumin loaded lipo-PEG [f]-PEI [g] complexes	269 nm	Melanoma (B16F10) and colon carcinoma (CT-26) cells	Increased cytotoxicity	[67]
Curcumin–chitosan nanoparticles	100–250 nm	Melanomas	Enhanced antitumor effect	[68]

Table 2. *Cont.*

Nanoformulation	Particle Size	Application	Outcome	Reference
ApoE [h] peptide-functionalized curcumin-loaded liposomes	132 nm	RBE4 cell monolayer	Increased accumulation in brain capillary endothelium	[69]
Curcumin-crosslinked polymeric Nanogels	10–200 nm	Breast and pancreatic cancers	Higher stability and enhanced antitumor effect	[70]
Curcumin-loaded chitin nanogels	70–80 nm	Human skin melanoma (A385) and human dermal fibroblasts (HDF)	Specific toxicity in skin melanoma (lower toxicity in HDF)	[70]
Curcumin-loaded lipid-core nanocapsules	196 ± 1.4 nm	Rat C6 and U251MG glioma cell lines	Decreased tumor size and prolonged survival	[71]
Liposome-encapsulated curcumin	Not reported	Head and neck squamous cell carcinoma (HNSCC) cell lines (CAL27 and UM-SCC1)	Cancer growth suppression both in vitro and in vivo	[72]

[a] PMSA: Prostate membrane specific antigen; [b] MPEG: Monomethoxy poly ethylene glycol; [c] PCL: Poly(ε-caprolactone); [d] HPTMA: N-[(2-hydroxy-3-trimethylamine) propyl; [e] PLGA: Polylactic-co-glycolic acid; [f] PEG: Poly ethylene glycol; [g] PEI: Polyethyleneimine; [h] ApoE: Apolipoprotein E.

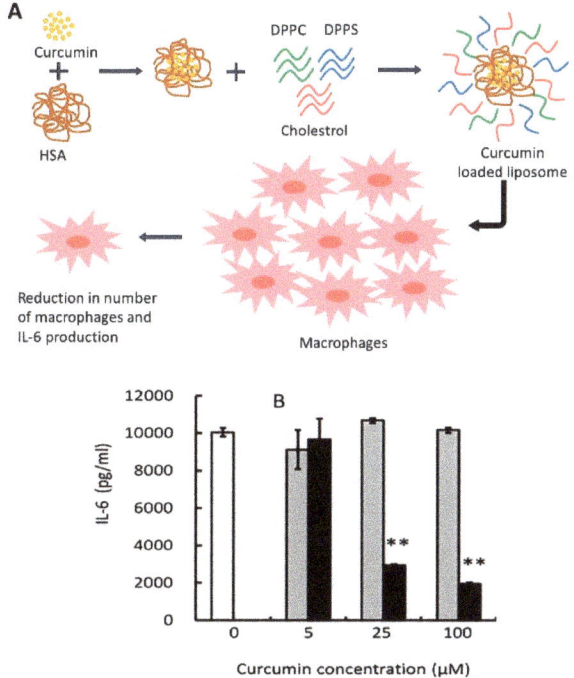

Figure 3. (**A**) Schematic representation of curcumin-loaded liposomes inducing a reduction in the number of macrophages [62]. HSA: human serum albumin; DPPC: 1, 2-dipalmitoyl-sn-glycero-3-phosphocholine; DPPS: 1, 2-dipalmitoyl-sn-glycero-3-phospho-L-serine. (**B**) curcumin-loaded liposomes inhibit production of IL-6; white, grey, and black columns represent control, unloaded liposomes, and curcumin-loaded liposomes respectively. Reprinted from Amano et al. [62].

3.3. Nanogels

Although hydrogels and nanogels have gained considerable attention in the past decade as a promising drug delivery system, only a few studies have investigated the curcumin-nanogel delivery in cancer therapy. There are several polymeric hydrogel nanoparticle systems that have been prepared recently using synthetic or natural polymers. Among the natural polymers, chitosan, chitin, and alginate are the most studied for the preparation of nanogels in drug delivery [73]. On the other hand, the most commonly used synthetic polymers are polyvinyl alcohol (PVA), polyethylene oxide (PEO), polyethyleneimine (PEI), polyvinyl pyrrolidone (PVP), and poly-N-isopropylacrylamide (PNIAA) [74]. One of the main advantages of natural hydrogels over synthetic ones when used in drug delivery is biodegradability and biocompatibility [70,74]. Additionally, nanogels possess unique features, including large surface area for drug entrapment and a porous structure for drug loading and release [70,75]. A curcumin-loaded chitin nanogel has been used as a transdermal system for the treatment of skin cancer [70] (Table 2) and has shown more specific toxicity towards human skin melanoma (A375) in comparison to human dermal fibroblast (HDF) cells without compromising the antitumor activity of curcumin [70]. In another study, a hybrid nanogel system consisting of alginate, chitosan, and pluronic polymers was prepared via the polycationic crosslinking method and tested on a HeLa cell line [76]. This delivery system demonstrated very high entrapment efficiency, and a significant difference in cell proliferation was observed between the cells treated with unprocessed curcumin and the cells treated with curcumin-loaded hybrid nanogel [76].

3.4. Peptide and Protein Formulations

As discussed earlier, hydrogels and polymeric materials have shown promising results in curcumin drug delivery. However, a few limitations have arisen in processing clinical applications, including toxicity of unreacted monomers, post-crosslinking shrinkage or fragility of the polymer gels, and rapid discharge of a large amount of the loaded drug during the initial burst release in drug carrier [77]. In an attempt to address these limitations, self-assembling peptide systems have been developed. Peptides provide several benefits when introduced to drug delivery systems, such as biocompatibility, desirable hydrophilicity, and mild processing conditions [78]. A recent study investigated the physical properties and therapeutic efficacy of a curcumin-loaded, self-assembling (MAX8) peptide (β-hairpin) hydrogel system. This newly developed system has combined multiple advantages such as enhanced delivery, curcumin stabilization, and controlled drug release by changing the MAX8 peptide concentration [79]. In another example, an amphiphilic polypeptide (β-casein) was able to self-assemble into micelles. Encapsulation of curcumin within the hydrophobic core of the β-casein micelles increased its aqueous solubility by 2500 times [80]. Human serum albumin (HSA) is one of the most commonly used proteins in nanoparticle preparation due to its excellent biocompatibility [81]. Curcumin-loaded HSA nanoparticles have been produced through the homogenization of aqueous HSA solution (to crosslink the HSA molecules) and curcumin dissolved in chloroform. This formulation improved the curcumin solubility by 300 times but only achieved 7.2% curcumin loading efficiency, which was likely due to entrapment of curcumin within the albumin hydrophobic cavity through hydrophobic interactions [82]. Recently, silk fibroin (SF) protein has attracted tremendous attention due to its excellent biocompatibility and multiple biomedical applications [83]. Since its approval by the FDA, several studies have investigated its potential applications in drug delivery [84]. Magnetic silk nanoparticles (MSPs) were used to deliver curcumin to MDA-MB-231 breast cancer cells. As illustrated in Figure 4, these particles were fabricated using the salting-out method to convert silk from its α-helix form to the β-sheet (the insoluble) form, thus providing a hydrophobic surface for curcumin loading. The designed nanoformulation managed to achieve a small particle size (100–350 nm), cell internalization, and the possibility for additional targeting using an external magnetic field on the target tissue [54].

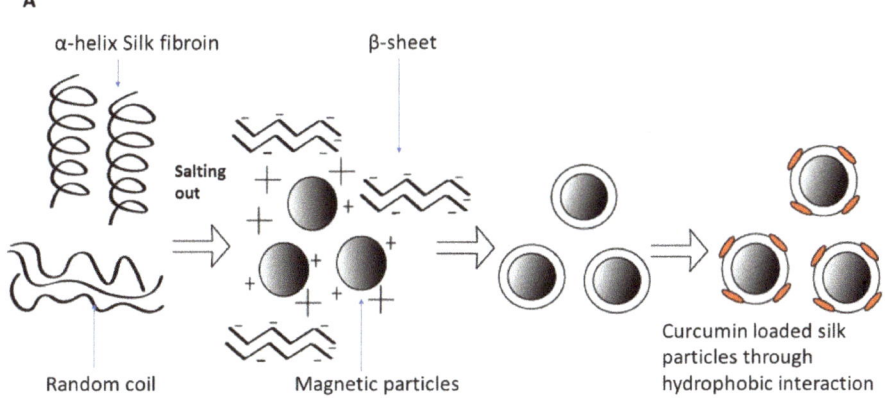
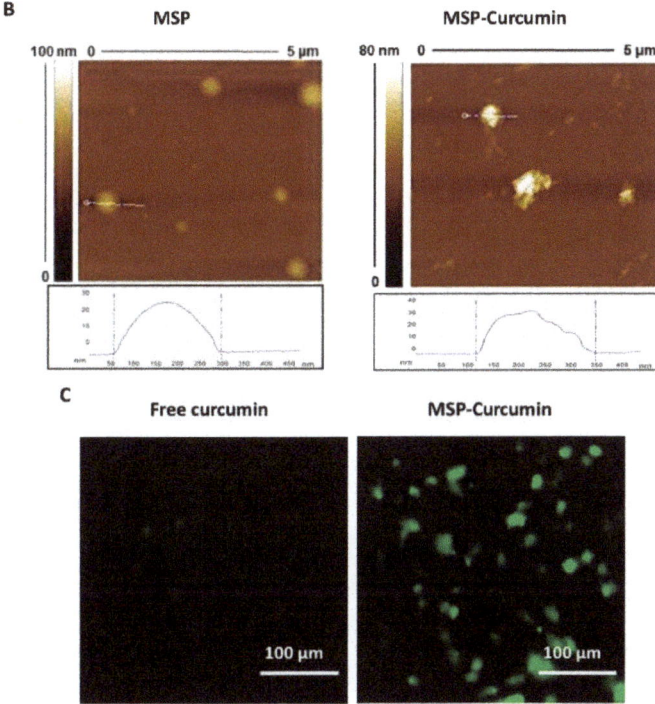

Figure 4. (**A**) Fabrication of magnetic silk particles (MSP) for curcumin delivery. (**B**) Atomic force microscopy (AFM) images of MSP before and after curcumin loading. (**C**) Representative microscopic images of MDA-MB-231 cells incubated with free curcumin and curcumin-loaded MSP showing a significant improvement of curcumin cellular uptake. Reprinted from Song et al. [54], copyright © 2017 ACS.

3.5. Cyclodextrin Complexes

Cyclodextrins are cyclic oligosaccharides which consist of a hydrophilic outer layer and a lipophilic core. In drug delivery, these complexes provide several beneficial properties, including enhanced solubility, increased bioavailability, and improved stability of the loaded drug. There are different types of cyclodextrins, such as natural (α, β, and γ), chemically modified, and polymerized cyclodextrins, that vary in water solubility and molecular weight [85]. There are also different cyclodextrin complexes, including inclusion complexes and self-assembled cyclodextrins (Figure 5A). Few studies have used cyclodextrins as carriers in curcumin delivery to enhance bioavailability, minimize degradation, and reduce nonselective toxicity [86]. A β-cyclodextrin–curcumin self-assembling preparation has shown higher uptake of curcumin by DU145 prostate cancer cells compared to unprocessed curcumin [86] As shown in Figure 5B, a significant increase in cellular uptake of cyclodextrin–curcumin (CD–CUR) inclusion complexes (CD5, CD10, CD20, and CD30) by cancer cells was observed compared to free curcumin. Another study found a complementary therapeutic effect of curcumin–cyclodextrin complexes in lung cancer. Administration of these complexes to mice with orthotopically implanted lung tumors resulted in improved bioavailability of curcumin and a significant reduction in tumor size [87].

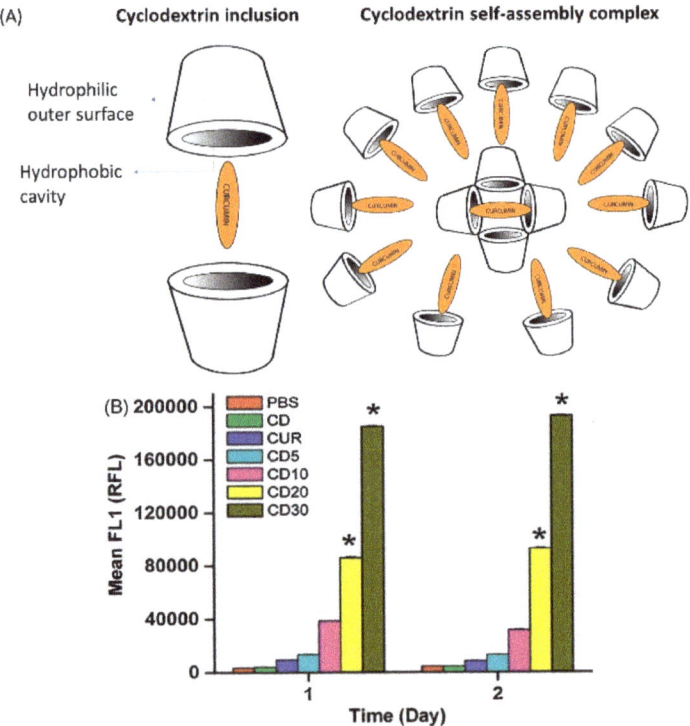

Figure 5. (**A**) Schematic structure of cyclodextrin–curcumin (CD–CUR) inclusion and self-assembled complexes (**B**) Fluorescence-activated cell sorting (FACS) analysis for cellular uptake of curcumin and different CD–CUR (CD5, CD10, CD20, and CD30) inclusion complexes treated in DU145 prostate cancer. * $p < 0.05$ represents significant difference from the curcumin uptake. Reprinted from Yallapu et al. [86] with permission from the copyright holder Elsevier.

4. Anticancer Activity of Curcumin

One of the main causes of cancer is the loss of balance between cell proliferation and cell death [88]. When the cells skip death due to the absence of the apoptotic signals, uncontrolled cell proliferation occurs, leading to different types of cancer [89]. The apoptotic signals are generated through two major pathways: the intrinsic pathway and the extrinsic pathway. The intrinsic pathway works through stimulating the mitochondrial membrane to inhibit expression of antiapoptotic proteins Bcl-2 and

Bcl-Xl [90]. Curcumin disturbs the balance in the mitochondrial membrane potential, leading to enhanced suppression of the Bcl-xL protein [91]. The extrinsic apoptotic pathway works through increasing the death receptors (DRs) on cells and triggering the tumor necrosis factor (TNF)-related apoptosis. Curcumin also contributes to this pathway by upregulating the expression of death receptors DR 4 and DR 5 [92–94]. In vitro studies showed a remarkable ability of curcumin and its derivatives to induce apoptosis in different cell lines by inhibiting or downregulating intracellular transcription factors. These factors include NF-κB, activator protein 1 (AP-1), cyclooxygenase II (COX-2), nitric oxide synthase, matrix metalloproteinase-9 (MMP-9), and STAT3 [33,73]. A recent work has found a new anticancer mechanism for curcumin by decreasing the glucose uptake and lactate production (Warburg effect) in cancer cells via downregulation of pyruvate kinase M2 (PKM2). The inhibition of PKM2 was achieved by suppressing the mammalian target of rapamycin-hypoxia-inducible factor 1α (TOR-HIF1α) [95]. Several studies have investigated the ability of curcumin and its derivatives to suppress multiple different carcinomas by interacting with different molecular targets (Figure 6).

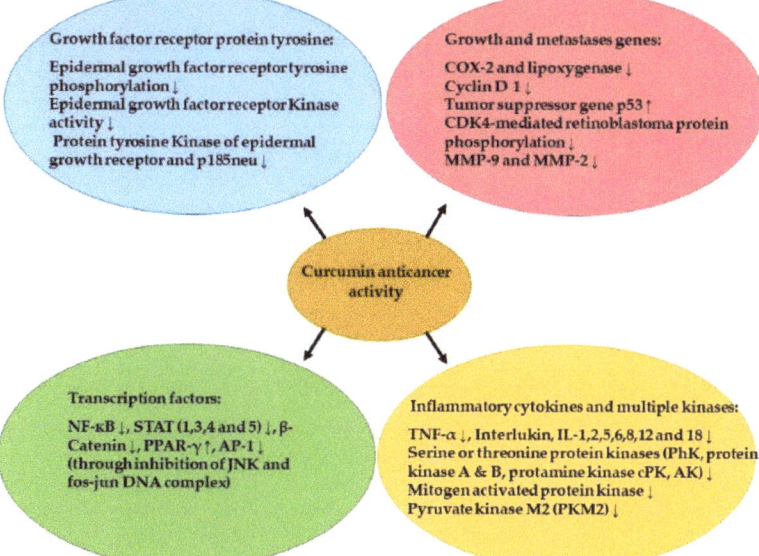

Figure 6. The main molecular targets of curcumin in cancer cells. ↑: Increase; ↓: Decrease; MMP: Matrix metalloproteinase; AP-1: Activation protein-1.

4.1. In Vitro and In Vivo Studies

Curcumin has shown very promising results in suppressing cancer cell growth and proliferation in several different types of cancer, such as prostate, colorectal, breast, pancreatic, brain, head, and neck cancers. What comes next is a summary of the anticancer activity of curcumin and its derivatives in different types of cancer based on the data from in vitro studies in different cancer cell lines and animal studies.

4.1.1. Prostate Cancer

A recent estimate reported by the American Cancer Society revealed that 2.9 million men have been diagnosed with prostate cancer (PCa) in the United States [20], making it the second leading cause of cancer death in men [96]. Curcumin has shown a strong ability to inhibit proliferation and induce apoptosis in prostate cancer both in vitro and in vivo [97] by interfering with a number of cellular pathways, including mitogen-activated protein kinase (MAPK), epidermal growth factor receptor

(EGFR), and nuclear factor κ (NFκB) [98,99]. A recent study has revealed the ability of curcumin to activate protein kinase D1 (PKD1), leading to attenuation of the oncogenic signaling by β-catenin and MAPK [100] and consequent inhibition of prostate cancer [100]. Moreover, PKD1 was found to be severely downregulated following progression from androgen-dependent to androgen-independent prostate cancer [100], and to affect the motility and invasion of prostate cancer via interaction with E-cadherin [101]. Therefore, it has been considered as a new therapeutic target for cancer in general and for prostate cancer in particular [102]. In addition to curcumin, some of its derivatives have also shown anticancer activity against prostate cancer. Metallo-curcumin conjugated DNA complexes exhibited significant toxicity to prostate cancer cells (PC3, 22Rv1, TRAMP-C1, LNCaP, and DU145) [34]. Dimethyl curcumin (ASC-J9) has also shown very good activity in enhancing androgen receptor degradation in androgen-dependent prostate cancer [20,38].

4.1.2. Colorectal Cancer

Colorectal cancer comes third behind prostate cancer and lung cancer as the most common form of malignant cancer [103]. Although patients diagnosed with colorectal carcinoma undertake surgical removal of the tumor tissue along with chemotherapy, more than half of the patients suffer from relapses [104]. Administration of curcumin was found to reduce M (1) G levels in the malignant colorectal cells without changing COX-2 protein levels [105]. In addition, curcumin treatment was able to downregulate miR-21 gene, which is overexpressed in colorectal cancer cells, by inhibiting AP-1 (activator protein) binding to miR-21 promoter [101]. Treating HCT 116 colorectal cancer cells with curcumin resulted in a cell cycle arrest in the G_2/M phase via miR-21 gene regulation and inhibited the tumor tissue growth [101]. However, an in vivo study in mice with colorectal cancer demonstrated an improved response to radiation therapy when combined with curcumin due to its ability to target nuclear factor (NF-κB) [106]. Another study has managed to enhance curcumin inhibition activity against colon cancer cells by combining it with ERRP, a pan-erb B inhibitor [107].

4.1.3. Head and Neck Squamous Cell Carcinoma

Head and neck squamous cell carcinoma (HNSCC) is the sixth most common form of cancer worldwide, with more than 30,000 diagnosed cases every year [108]. HNSCC generally arises in the oral cavity, paranasal cavities, larynx, and pharynx [10]. In vitro studies of curcumin in different head and neck cancer cell lines have proven its ability to inhibit cell growth due to its effects on a number of cellular pathways involved in cell proliferation, most notably NF-κB and STAT3, which are found to be overexpressed in several head and neck carcinomas [109,110]. Curcumin was shown to downregulate NF-κB and inhibit the interleukin-6 (IL-6)-mediated phosphorylation of STAT3, thus inhibiting the proliferation of the cancer cells [110,111].

4.1.4. Breast Cancer

Breast cancer has shown an alarming record as a leading cause of death in women [112]. Despite lumpectomy, radiation therapy, chemotherapy, and endocrine therapy, the recurrence rate of breast cancer has been reported to be still high based on a meta-analysis of 21 retrospective studies [113]. Therefore, there is still a need for more efficient therapeutic strategies. In a study on MCF-10A human mammary epithelial cells and MCF-7 breast cancer cells [114], a tangible drop in telomerase activity was observed as a result of treatment with curcumin in a concentration-dependent manner which was correlated to downregulation of hTERT by curcumin but not through the c-Myc mRNA pathway [114]. The effect of curcumin on cell-cycle regulatory proteins, matrix metalloproteinases (MMPs), and NF-κB was evaluated in MDA-MB-231 and BT-483 breast cancer cell lines [115]. In agreement with the previous studies on other breast cancer cell lines, this study also confirmed the ability of curcumin to downregulate NF-κB, leading to an antiproliferative effect [115,116]. However, a decrease in cyclic D1 in MDA-MB-231 cells and a decrease in CDK4 BT-483 were observed after treatment with curcumin [115]. Combining arabinogalactan and curcumin enhanced apoptosis induction by increasing

ROS levels, disturbing the mitochondrial membrane and decreasing glutathione in MDA-MB-231 cell line [117]. Moreover, curcumin led to the inhibition of breast tumor via overexpression of the *p53* gene and reduction of antigen ki-67 levels [117]. Another study on MDA-MB-231 cells has shown that curcumin also inhibits inflammatory cytokines CXCL1/2. Inhibiting CXCL1 and 2 by curcumin results in inhibiting the expression of a series of metastasis-promoting genes such as chemotactic receptor CXCR4 [118,119]. Dimethyl curcumin (ASC-J9) has also been reported to be effective against estrogen-dependent breast cancer via inhibiting several types of steroid receptors [22,120].

4.1.5. Brain Cancer and Glioblastoma

The incidence rate of central nervous system (CNS) tumors, including brain tumors, are predicted to increase by 6% in the UK between 2014 and 2035 [121]. Glioblastoma (GBM), which is the most common malignant brain cancer in humans, accounts for about 15% of all CNS tumors [122,123]. In the treatment of brain tumors and GBM, surgical intervention and radiation therapy are limited due to infiltration of cancer cells into the healthy brain, leading to damaging effects after treatment [124]. Therefore, alternative therapies using naturally derived compounds such as curcumin with less side effects than the conventional treatments are receiving more attention. Curcumin has multiple molecular targets (Figure 6), therefore, combating brain tumors may take different cellular pathways, including apoptosis, autophagy, angiogenesis, invasion, and metastasis [123]. Although penetrating the blood–brain barrier (BBB) is considered the rate-limiting step for many anticancer agents, curcumin was able to cross the BBB in high levels [125]. Moreover, an in vivo study using human glioma U-87 cells xenografted into athymic mice showed that curcumin is able to suppress glioma angiogenesis through inhibiting MMP-9 and downregulating endothelial cell markers (CD31 and CD105 mRNA) [125]. Curcumin was also able to induce G2/M cell cycle arrest by increasing protein kinase 1 (DAPK1) in U-251 malignant glioblastoma cells, which indicates that suppressing DAPK1 by curcumin does not only induce cell arrest but also inhibits STAT3 and NF-κB and activates caspase-3 [126].

4.2. Clinical Studies

In addition to the studies carried out in human cell cultures or in animal models, there have been several clinical studies carried out in human subjects to evaluate the efficacy and safety of treatment with curcumin in different types of cancer either alone or in combination with other chemotherapy agents. A summary of an excerpt of these clinical studies is provided in Table 3.

Table 3. Clinical studies of curcumin in the prevention/treatment of different types of cancer.

Type of Cancer	Type of Study	No of Patients	Dose of Curcumin	Endpoints	Results	References
BPH [a]	Pilot product evaluation study	61	1g/day for 24 weeks	Signs and symptoms, quality of life	Reduced signs and symptoms, improved quality of life	[127]
Breast	Phase I clinical trial	14	0.5–8 g/day for 7 days plus docetaxel	Maximal tolerated dose of curcumin, toxicity, safety, efficacy, levels of VEGF [b] and tumor markers	No cancer progression, partial response in some patients, low frequency of toxic effects, decreased levels of VEGF	[128]
CML [c]	Randomized controlled trial	50	5 g TID [d] for 6 weeks plus imatinib (400 mg BD [e])	Plasma nitric oxide levels	Reduced nitric oxide levels	[129]

Table 3. Cont.

Type of Cancer	Type of Study	No of Patients	Dose of Curcumin	Endpoints	Results	References
Colorectal	dose-escalation pilot study	15	40–200 mg/day for 29 days	Blood COX-2 [f] activity and PGE2 [g] levels	Dose-dependent decrease in PGE2 levels	[130]
	Phase I does-escalation trial	15	0.45–3.6 g/day for 4 months	Levels of curcumin and its metabolites in plasma urine, and feces; levels of PGE2 and glutathione S-transferase activity in blood	Dose-dependent decrease in PGE2 levels, low concentrations of curcumin and its metabolites in plasma and urine	[131]
	Phase I does-escalation trial	12	0.45 g, 1.8 g, 3.6 g per day for 7 days	Concentration of curcumin and its metabolites in plasma and colorectal tissue	Biologically active concentrations of curcumin in the colorectal tissue	[105]
	Phase I clinical trial	126	360 mg TID for 10–30 days	Serum levels of TNF-α [h], $p53$ expression in tumor tissue	Decreased serum levels of TNF-α, increased expression of $p53$ in colorectal tissue	[132]
	Phase II clinical trial	44	2 g/day and 4 g/day for 1 month	Concentration of PGE2 and 5-HETE [i] within ACF [j] and normal mucosa, total ACF number	Reduced number of ACF with dose of 4 g	[133]
	Pilot study	26	2.35 g/day for 14 days	Safety, tolerance, levels of curcumin in colonic mucosa	Safe and well tolerated, Prolonged biologically active levels of curcumin achieved in colon tissue	[134]
HNSCC [k]	Pilot study	21	1 g single dose	IκKβ [l] kinase activity, cytokine levels in saliva	Reduced IκKβ activity in the salivary cells	[135]
Intestinal Adenoma	Randomized controlled trial	44	1.5 g BID for 12 months	total number of polyps, mean polyp size, adverse effects	No significant clinical response, very few adverse effects	[136]
Pancreatic	Phase II clinical trial	25	8 g/day for 8 weeks	Tumor response, tumor markers, adverse effects	Poor oral bioavailability, biological response in only 2 patients, no toxicities	[137]
	Phase II clinical trial	17	8 g/day for 4 weeks	Time to tumor progression (TTP) and toxicity profile	TTP of 1–12 months (median 2 months), high frequency of side effects	[138]
	Phase I/II clinical trial	21	8 g/day for 14 days plus gemcitabine	patient compliance, toxicity, efficacy	Safe and well tolerated, median overall survival time of 161 days	[139]
	Phase I clinical trial	16	200–400 mg/day for 9 months	Safety, pharmacokinetics, NF-κB [m] activity, cytokine levels, efficacy and quality of life	Safe, highly bioavailable, no significant changes in NF-κB activity or cytokine levels, improved quality of life	[140]
Prostate	Randomized controlled trial	85	100 mg plus 40 mg soy isoflavones for 6 months	Serum PSA [n] levels	Decreased levels of PSA in patients with an initial PSA ≥ 10 μg/mL	[141]
	Randomized controlled trial	40	3 g/day for 3 months as a supplement to radiotherapy	biochemical and clinical progression-free survivals, alterations in the activity of antioxidant enzymes	Considerable antioxidant effect, decreased levels of PSA	[142]
Solid tumors	Randomized controlled trial	80	180 mg/day for 8 weeks	Changes in quality of life, serum levels of inflammatory mediators	Improved quality of life, reduced levels of inflammatory mediators	[143]

[a] BPH: benign prostatic hypertrophy; [b] VEGF: vascular endothelial growth factor; [c] CML: chronic myeloid leukemia; [d] TID: three times daily; [e] BD: Twice daily; [f] COX-2: cyclooxygenase-2; [g] PGE2: Prostaglandin E2; [h] TNF-α: tumor necrosis factor α; [i] 5-HETE: 5-hydroxyeicosatetraenoic acid; [j] ACF: aberrant crypt foci; [k] HNSCC: Head and neck squamous cell carcinoma; [l] IκKβ: IκB kinase β; [m] NF-κB: Nuclear factor κB; [n] PSA: prostate-specific antigen.

4.2.1. Colorectal Cancer

The pharmacology of curcumin in humans was studied in a dose-escalation study by Sharma et al. [131] on fifteen patients with histologically proven advanced adenocarcinoma of the colon or rectum refractory to standard chemotherapies. The patients received doses of curcumin between 0.45 and 3.6 g per day orally for up to four months. Subsequently, levels of curcumin and its metabolites in plasma, urine, and feces were measured. In addition, glutathione S-transferase (GST) activity, levels of oxidative DNA adduct (M_1G), and the extent of ex vivo induction of prostaglandin E2 (PGE2) in patient blood leukocytes were measured as biomarkers of curcumin activity. Intact curcumin and its glucuronide and sulfate conjugates were detected in plasma at a concentration of 10 nmol/L and also in urine. No dose-limiting toxicity was observed. No effect on basal PGE2 levels in leukocytes was observed after administration of curcumin at any of the doses, nor were there any changes in the lipopolysaccharide (LPS)-induced production of PGE2 at doses between 0.45 and 1.8 g per day. However, administration of 3.6 g curcumin per day led to 62% and 57% reductions in the inducible PGE2 levels in patient blood samples 1 h after administration on days 1 and 29, respectively, compared to the baseline levels. Total GST activity and M_1G levels in leukocytes showed considerable differences between patients, but no treatment-related effects were observed. Based on these results, they suggested a daily oral dose of 3.6 g of curcumin for a Phase II trial in cancers in sites outside the gastrointestinal tract which require systemic effects [131].

The pharmacological activity of curcumin in the colorectum was also studied by Garcea et al. [105] as measured by the levels of M_1G and COX-2 in 12 patients with colorectal carcinoma following oral administration of curcumin at doses of 450 mg, 1800 mg, or 3600 mg per day. Blood samples and biopsy samples of the normal and malignant colorectal tissue were taken from the patients at designated time points and analyzed for the levels of curcumin, curcumin metabolites (curcumin sulfate and curcumin glucuronide), M_1G, and COX-2. Higher concentrations of curcumin were observed in normal compared to malignant colorectal tissues of patients receiving 3.6 g/day of curcumin, with trace levels of curcumin in the peripheral blood circulation. Curcumin metabolites were also detected in the colorectum of these patients. On the other hand, baseline M_1G levels were 2.5-fold higher in malignant tissue as compared with normal tissue in the same group of patients, which were reduced significantly after the administration of curcumin. Nevertheless, the levels of COX-2 in malignant colorectal tissue were not reduced by curcumin. Based on these findings, they suggested that a daily dose of 3.6 g of curcumin can reach pharmacologically active concentrations in the colorectum with minimal distribution outside the gastrointestinal system [105].

The mechanism of anticancer activity of curcumin in colorectal cancer was investigated by a number of researchers. In 2001, Plummer et al. [130] conducted a dose-escalation pilot study of the effects of Curcuma extract (containing curcumin and desmethoxycurcumin) on the inhibition of COX-2 activity and consequently the levels of PGE2 in 15 patients with advanced colorectal cancer. The patients were divided into five groups receiving doses between 40 and 200 mg of curcuminoids once per day via the oral route for a minimum of 29 days. Comparison of the PGE2 levels in blood samples from patients showed a significant difference between patients in different groups and decreased levels of PGE2 with an increased dose of curcumin, which clearly indicates dose-dependent inhibition of COX-2 by curcumin [130].

This was further investigated by Carroll et al. [133] who carried out a nonrandomized, open-label clinical trial to assess the effects of oral curcumin in prevention of colorectal cancer. In the study, 44 smokers with eight or more aberrant crypt foci (ACF) on screening colonoscopy were included and were divided into two groups receiving either 2 g or 4 g of curcumin per day via the oral route for 30 days. The levels of PGE2 and 5-hydroxyeicosatetraenoic acid (5-HETE) within ACF were assessed, as well as the reduction in the number and/or proliferation of ACF (measured by rectal endoscopy and Ki-67 immunohistochemistry assay, respectively). ACF reduction was used as a measure of the cancer preventive efficacy of curcumin, assuming that reducing the concentrations of PGE2 and 5-HETE in the colorectal mucosa would result in reduced epithelial crypt proliferation and ACF formation.

No reduction in the levels of PGE2 or 5-HETE within ACF or normal mucosa was observed with any doses of curcumin, nor was there any reduction in the levels of Ki-67 in normal mucosa. By the same way, there were no changes in the number of ACF in the group treated with 2 g of curcumin. However, a significant reduction in the number of ACF was observed in the group treated with 4 g of curcumin, which was associated with a significant increase in the plasma levels of curcumin conjugates, indicating the effect of systematically delivered curcumin conjugates on the reduction of ACF number, rather than locally delivered curcumin [133].

He et al. [132] investigated the effects of curcumin on the expression of *p53* in the colorectum tissue and the serum levels of TNF-α in patients with colorectal cancer. A total of 126 patients diagnosed with colorectal cancer were randomly divided into two groups receiving either curcumin (360 mg three times per day per oral route) or placebo during the period ahead of surgery. Colorectal biopsy samples and blood samples were obtained from the patients before and after treatment and were analyzed for *p53* expression and serum TNF-α levels respectively. A significant reduction in the serum levels of TNF-α was observed in the patients treated with curcumin, whereas no such effect was observed in the placebo group. In the same way, the number of apoptotic cells was increased after treatment with curcumin compared to baseline values, whereas no significant change was observed in the placebo group. Moreover, treatment with curcumin increased the expression of *p53* and Bax and inhibited expression of Bcl-2 in the colorectal tissue [132].

More recently, the safety and efficacy of curcumin in familial adenomatous polyposis was evaluated in a double-blinded randomized trial by Cruz-Correa et al. [136]. In this study, 44 patients with familial adenomatous polyposis with at least five intestinal adenomatous polyps who had not undergone colectomy were included in this trial and were randomly allocated to two groups receiving either pure curcumin (3 g per day orally) or placebo for 12 months. The main outcome measures were the number and size of lower gastrointestinal tract polyps, which were assessed every four months for one year. At the end of the study, no significant difference was found in the mean number or mean size of polyps between the curcumin group and the placebo group. The adverse effects were very few, and not significantly different from the placebo group. These results show the low efficacy but high safety of oral curcumin at the administered dose in patients with familial adenomatous polyposis [136].

4.2.2. Pancreatic Cancer

The efficacy of curcumin in the treatment of pancreatic cancer was investigated in a nonrandomized, open-label, phase II clinical trial conducted by Dhillon et al. [137]. In this study, 25 patients with histologically confirmed pancreatic adenocarcinoma were treated with a combination of curcuminoids (curcumin, desmethoxycurcumin, and bisdesmethoxycurcumin), at a dose of 8 g per day for eight weeks. The patients did not receive any chemotherapy or radiotherapy from four weeks before commencing the trial and also during the trial. Tumor response (as per the classic Response Evaluation Criteria in Solid Tumors criteria), tumor markers, and serum cytokine levels were assessed after 8 weeks. In addition, the effect of orally administered curcumin on constitutive and tumor necrosis factor-α–induced binding expression of NF-κB, COX-2, and phosphorylated signal transducer and activator of transcription 3 (pSTAT3) in peripheral blood mononuclear cells pretherapy and on day 8 were determined, as well as curcumin pharmacokinetics.

Low steady-state levels of curcumin glucuronide and curcumin sulfate indicated poor oral bioavailability. As a result, only two patients showed a clinical biological response to curcumin therapy, and one other patient showed a brief tumor regression accompanied by a considerable increase in serum cytokine levels (IL-6, IL-8, IL-10, and IL-1 receptor antagonists). On the other hand, curcumin down-regulated the expression of NF-κB, COX-2, and pSTAT3 in peripheral blood mononuclear cells obtained from patients. No treatment-related toxic effects were reported in any patients [137].

In a more recent study by Epelbaum et al. [138], patients with either advanced local or metastatic pancreatic cancer were treated with a combination of curcumin (8 g/day per oral) and gemcitabine (1000 mg/m^2 IV once per week) for three out of four weeks of each chemotherapy cycle. The primary outcome was time to tumor progression and the main secondary outcome was toxicity profile. In the study, eight out of seventeen patients were noncompliant with curcumin due to abdominal pain, five of which discontinued treatment before two weeks and three received adjusted doses of curcumin for the rest of the study (4 g/day). One patient died during the first cycle due to cardiac problems not associated with curcumin. One patient developed grade II neutropenia and one patient grade I thrombocytopenia. The time to tumor progression was between one and twelve months (median two months), and the overall survival time was between one and 24 months (median 6). Based on these results, they concluded that the combination therapy with curcumin and gemcitabine in pancreatic cancer is feasible; however, the dose of curcumin should be less than 8 g/day [138].

4.2.3. Prostate Cancer

In a double-blinded, randomized, placebo-controlled trial by Hejazi et al. [142], the effect of curcumin on the oxidative status of patients with prostate cancer during radiotherapy was evaluated. In this study, 40 patients were included in the trial and were randomly assigned to receive either curcuminoids (curcumin, desmethoxycurcumin, and bisdesmethoxycurcumin, 3 g per day per oral route) or placebo prior to and during external-beam radiation therapy. The outcome measures for oxidative status were the plasma total antioxidant capacity (TAC), superoxide dismutase (SOD) activity, catalase activity, and glutathione peroxidase activity, three months after radiotherapy. In addition, the level of prostate specific antigen (PSA) was used as a measure of successful treatment.

A significant increase in TAC and a significant decrease in SOD activity was observed after radiotherapy compared to the baseline (pretreatment) values, suggesting an antioxidant effect of curcumin, whereas no significant changes were observed in catalase activity and glutathione peroxidase activity. The levels of PSA were significantly reduced compared to baseline levels in both groups, indicating successful treatment; nevertheless, there was no significant difference between the two groups, indicating that curcumin did not affect the efficacy of the radiotherapy [142].

The effect of a combination of curcumin and soy isoflavones on the expression of PSA in men with elevated levels of PSA (but neither prostate cancer nor prostatic intraepithelial neoplasia) was investigated in a randomized placebo-controlled double-blind study by Ide et al. [141]. A total of 85 patients were included in this study and were randomly assigned to receive either a supplement containing a combination of isoflavones and curcumin or placebo. Systematic prostate biopsy was performed on the patients before and six months after treatment, and the levels of PSA were determined. The curcumin/isoflavone treatment considerably decreased the levels of PSA in the patients with an initial PSA $\geq$ 10 µg/mL as compared to the placebo group who did not show such change, which they attributed to the synergistic antiandrogen effect of curcumin and isoflavones [141]. However, since there was no comparison between the effects of treatment with isoflavones alone and curcumin alone compared to combination therapy on the levels of PSA, it is hard to accept the authors' claim that the combination therapy has advantages over monotherapy as no such evidence is provided.

4.2.4. Breast Cancer

Bayet-Robert et al. [128] evaluated the feasibility and tolerability of a combination of curcumin and docetaxel in 14 patients with metastatic or locoregionally recurrent advanced breast cancer in an open-label phase I dose escalation clinical trial. The patients received an I.V. infusion of Docetaxel (100 mg/m^2) every three weeks for six chemotherapy cycles, and oral curcumin (starting from 500 mg/day and increased until a dose-limiting toxicity would occur) for seven consecutive days in each cycle (from five days before to two days after administration of docetaxel). The primary endpoint was the maximal tolerated dose of curcumin when administered in combination with a standard dose of docetaxel in the patients. Secondary outcomes were toxicity, safety, and clinical response to the combination therapy, as well as levels of CEA tumor marker and vascular endothelial growth factor (VEGF) as a positive endogenous modulator of angiogenesis.

The maximal tolerated dose of curcumin was found to be 8 g/day as in higher doses, dose-limiting toxicities (neutropenia, anemia, and severe diarrhea) were observed, leading to the discontinuation of the trial in two patients. Other toxicities (oral cavity mucositis, hand-foot syndrome, nail changes, dermal changes, conjunctivitis, and fatigue) were either not persistent or were treated easily so did not affect the continuation of the trial. However, due to noncompliance of a number of patients with the doses higher than 6 g/day, in the end, this dose was recommended as the maximal tolerated dose to be considered for phase II clinical trials. In terms of clinical and biological response (decrease in CEA tumor marker across the treatment and regression of nonmeasurable lesions), some degree of improvement was observed in most patients, with five patients showing a partial response to treatment and three patients having stable disease at least six weeks after the last cycle of treatment. No disease progression was observed in any of the patients. Moreover, curcumin/docetaxel combination significantly decreased the levels of VEGF after three cycles of treatment [128].

4.2.5. Head and Neck Cancer

Kim et al. [135] performed a pilot study in patients with head and neck squamous cell carcinoma (HNSCC) to determine the effect of curcumin on inhibiting IκB kinase β (IκKβ) activity and suppressing the proinflammatory cytokines. The patients were asked to chew curcumin tablets (2 mg), their saliva samples were collected before and after chewing the tablets, and the IκKβ activity was measured, as well as the levels of salivary cytokines interleukin (IL)-6 and IL-8. Curcumin resulted in a reduction in IκKβ activity in the salivary cells of HNSCC patients. There was a brief reduction in IL-8 expression in eight of 21 post-curcumin samples; however, this reduction was not statistically significant. On the other hand, there was a marked decrease in the expression of other cytokines, including IL-10, IFN-γ, IL-12p70, and IL-2 clustered together, and also granulocyte macrophage colony stimulating factor (GMCSF) and TNF-α clustered together. These results show the inhibitory effect of curcumin on IκKβ activity in the salivary cells of patients with HNSCC; therefore, they suggested considering IκKβ as a biomarker for detecting the effect of curcumin in head and neck cancer [135].

5. Conclusions and Future Perspectives

Curcumin, the active ingredient of the *Curcuma longa* extract, has been studied widely over the past few decades for its anti-inflammatory, antioxidant, anticancer, and antiandrogenic effects. Curcumin has shown considerable anticancer effects against several different types of cancer, including prostate cancer, breast cancer, colorectal cancer, pancreatic cancer, and head and neck cancer both in vitro and in vivo. Furthermore, its efficacy and safety in cancer patients either alone or in combination with other anticancer agents has been proven in several clinical studies with human subjects. Curcumin is believed to exert its anticancer activity via multiple mechanisms, interfering with different cellular pathways and inducing/inhibiting the production of various types of cytokines, enzymes or growth factors such as MAPK, EGF, NFκB, PKD1, COX-2, STAT3, TNF-α, and IκKβ. However, the anticancer application of curcumin has been limited mainly due to its low water solubility, which results in low cellular uptake and poor oral bioavailability, as well as low chemical stability. In order to overcome these limitations, different approaches have been made, such as structural modification and the use of drug delivery systems. The key pharmacophores contributing to the biological activity of curcumin are known to be the hydrogen donor group, the β-diketone moiety, the phenyl rings, and the substituent groups on them. Chemical modification of these moieties has led to curcumin derivatives with higher efficacy and/or enhanced water solubility or stability. In addition, various types of delivery systems have been developed for curcumin delivery to cancer cells or animal xenografts using a variety of natural or synthetic polymers, lipids, or proteins, some of which have improved the stability and/or cellular uptake of curcumin, thus giving rise to a stronger anticancer response.

In spite of the tremendous effort to improve the physicochemical and biological properties of curcumin, there are still several issues to be addressed in regard to its bioavailability, potency, and specificity for the target tissue. The medicinal chemistry approaches to improving the pharmacological properties of curcumin have not managed to increase its potency significantly, and the curcumin derivatives are not more potent than curcumin itself. Due to the low potency of curcumin and its derivatives, higher doses are required to see a therapeutic response, which increases the adverse effects and reduces the patient compliance. Another drawback of the structural modification is that it is difficult to achieve a balance between efficacy and solubility, and in most cases, one has been sacrificed in favor of the other. Most of the structural modifications that improve curcumin efficacy make the molecule more hydrophobic and reduce its solubility. Therefore, more work has to be done in this regard to overcome this problem. Although various types of drug delivery systems have been used to enhance the cellular uptake and efficacy of curcumin, most of these formulations have remained at the proof of concept level and have not been evaluated in clinical trials. There is a lack of clinical studies to evaluate the safety and efficacy of these curcumin delivery systems in humans before they can find their way to the pharmaceutical market. Moreover, most of the currently developed drug delivery systems for curcumin lack specificity for the target tissue. Hence, there is still much room for improvement in the curcumin delivery systems in terms of selectivity for specific tumor tissues. Tissue-specific curcumin delivery enhances the local drug concentrations in the site of action and therefore results in higher efficacy (with lower doses of curcumin) and less adverse effects.

Funding: This research was funded by EPSRC, grant numbers EP/N007174/1 and EP/N023579/1; The Royal Society, grant numbers RG160662 and IE150457; and Jiangsu specially appointed professors program. R.H. was funded by the University of Sheffield studentship.

Conflicts of Interest: The authors declare no conflict of interest.

References

1. Siegel, R.L.; Miller, K.D.; Jemal, A. Cancer statistics, 2018. *CA Cancer J. Clin.* **2018**, *68*, 7–30. [CrossRef] [PubMed]
2. Gupta, A.P.; Pandotra, P.; Sharma, R.; Kushwaha, M.; Gupta, S. Chapter 8—Marine Resource: A Promising Future for Anticancer Drugs. In *Studies in Natural Products Chemistry*; Elsevier: Amsterdam, The Netherlands, 2013; Volume 40, pp. 229–325.
3. Umar, A.; Dunn, B.K.; Greenwald, P. Future directions in cancer prevention. *Nat. Rev. Cancer* **2012**, *12*, 835. [CrossRef] [PubMed]
4. Gupta, A.P.; Khan, S.; Manzoor, M.M.; Yadav, A.K.; Sharma, G.; Anand, R.; Gupta, S. Chapter 10—Anticancer Curcumin: Natural Analogues and Structure-Activity Relationship. In *Studies in Natural Products Chemistry*; Atta ur, R., Ed.; Elsevier: Amsterdam, The Netherlands, 2017; Volume 54, pp. 355–401.
5. Alibeiki, F.; Jafari, N.; Karimi, M.; Peeri Dogaheh, H. Potent anti-cancer effects of less polar Curcumin analogues on gastric adenocarcinoma and esophageal squamous cell carcinoma cells. *Sci. Rep.* **2017**, *7*, 2559. [CrossRef] [PubMed]
6. Goel, A.; Kunnumakkara, A.B.; Aggarwal, B.B. Curcumin as "Curecumin": From kitchen to clinic. *Biochem. Pharm.* **2008**, *75*, 787–809. [CrossRef] [PubMed]
7. Nagahama, K.; Utsumi, T.; Kumano, T.; Maekawa, S.; Oyama, N.; Kawakami, J. Discovery of a new function of curcumin which enhances its anticancer therapeutic potency. *Sci. Rep.* **2016**, *6*, 30962. [CrossRef] [PubMed]
8. Aggarwal, B.B.; Deb, L.; Prasad, S. Curcumin differs from tetrahydrocurcumin for molecular targets, signaling pathways and cellular responses. *Molecules* **2014**, *20*, 185–205. [CrossRef] [PubMed]
9. Gera, M.; Sharma, N.; Ghosh, M.; Huynh, D.L.; Lee, S.J.; Min, T.; Kwon, T.; Jeong, D.K. Nanoformulations of curcumin: An emerging paradigm for improved remedial application. *Oncotarget* **2017**, *8*, 66680–66698. [CrossRef] [PubMed]
10. Kunnumakkara, A.B.; Bordoloi, D.; Padmavathi, G.; Monisha, J.; Roy, N.K.; Prasad, S.; Aggarwal, B.B. Curcumin, the golden nutraceutical: Multitargeting for multiple chronic diseases. *Br. J. Pharm.* **2017**, *174*, 1325–1348. [CrossRef] [PubMed]
11. Anand, P.; Sundaram, C.; Jhurani, S.; Kunnumakkara, A.B.; Aggarwal, B.B. Curcumin and cancer: An "old-age" disease with an "age-old" solution. *Cancer Lett.* **2008**, *267*, 133–164. [CrossRef] [PubMed]
12. Barry, J.; Fritz, M.; Brender, J.R.; Smith, P.E.; Lee, D.K.; Ramamoorthy, A. Determining the effects of lipophilic drugs on membrane structure by solid-state NMR spectroscopy: The case of the antioxidant curcumin. *J. Am. Chem. Soc.* **2009**, *131*, 4490–4498. [CrossRef] [PubMed]
13. Tsukamoto, M.; Kuroda, K.; Ramamoorthy, A.; Yasuhara, K. Modulation of raft domains in a lipid bilayer by boundary-active curcumin. *Chem. Commun.* **2014**, *50*, 3427–3430. [CrossRef] [PubMed]

14. Koo, H.-J.; Shin, S.; Choi, J.Y.; Lee, K.-H.; Kim, B.-T.; Choe, Y.S. Introduction of Methyl Groups at C2 and C6 Positions Enhances the Antiangiogenesis Activity of Curcumin. *Sci. Rep.* **2015**, *5*, 14205. [CrossRef] [PubMed]
15. Agrawal, A.K.; Gupta, C.M. Tuftsin-bearing liposomes in treatment of macrophage-based infections. *Adv. Drug Deliv. Rev.* **2000**, *41*, 135–146. [CrossRef]
16. Chen, W.-F.; Deng, S.-L.; Zhou, B.; Yang, L.; Liu, Z.-L. Curcumin and its analogues as potent inhibitors of low density lipoprotein oxidation: H-atom abstraction from the phenolic groups and possible involvement of the 4-hydroxy-3-methoxyphenyl groups. *Free Radic. Biol. Med.* **2006**, *40*, 526–535. [CrossRef] [PubMed]
17. Ohtsu, H.; Xiao, Z.; Ishida, J.; Nagai, M.; Wang, H.K.; Itokawa, H.; Su, C.Y.; Shih, C.; Chiang, T.; Chang, E.; et al. Antitumor agents. 217. Curcumin analogues as novel androgen receptor antagonists with potential as anti-prostate cancer agents. *J. Med. Chem.* **2002**, *45*, 5037–5042. [CrossRef] [PubMed]
18. Lin, L.; Shi, Q.; Su, C.Y.; Shih, C.C.; Lee, K.H. Antitumor agents 247. New 4-ethoxycarbonylethyl curcumin analogs as potential antiandrogenic agents. *Bioorg. Med. Chem.* **2006**, *14*, 2527–2534. [CrossRef] [PubMed]
19. Shi, Q.; Shih, C.C.; Lee, K.H. Novel Anti-Prostate Cancer Curcumin Analogues That Enhance Androgen Receptor Degradation Activity. *Anti-Cancer Agents Med. Chem.* **2009**, *9*, 904–912. [CrossRef]
20. Cheng, M.A.; Chou, F.-J.; Wang, K.; Yang, R.; Ding, J.; Zhang, Q.; Li, G.; Yeh, S.; Xu, D.; Chang, C. Androgen receptor (AR) degradation enhancer ASC-J9® in an FDA-approved formulated solution suppresses castration resistant prostate cancer cell growth. *Cancer Lett.* **2018**, *417*, 182–191. [CrossRef] [PubMed]
21. Lin, T.H.; Izumi, K.; Lee, S.O.; Lin, W.J.; Yeh, S.; Chang, C. Anti-androgen receptor ASC-J9 versus anti-androgens MDV3100 (Enzalutamide) or Casodex (Bicalutamide) leads to opposite effects on prostate cancer metastasis via differential modulation of macrophage infiltration and STAT3-CCL2 signaling. *Cell Death Dis.* **2013**, *4*, e764. [CrossRef] [PubMed]
22. Verderio, P.; Pandolfi, L.; Mazzucchelli, S.; Marinozzi, M.R.; Vanna, R.; Gramatica, F.; Corsi, F.; Colombo, M.; Morasso, C.; Prosperi, D. Antiproliferative Effect of ASC-J9 Delivered by PLGA Nanoparticles against Estrogen-Dependent Breast Cancer Cells. *Mol. Pharm.* **2014**, *11*, 2864–2875. [CrossRef] [PubMed]
23. Qiu, X.; Du, Y.; Lou, B.; Zuo, Y.; Shao, W.; Huo, Y.; Huang, J.; Yu, Y.; Zhou, B.; Du, J.; et al. Synthesis and identification of new 4-arylidene curcumin analogues as potential anticancer agents targeting nuclear factor-kappaB signaling pathway. *J. Med. Chem.* **2010**, *53*, 8260–8273. [CrossRef] [PubMed]
24. Ferrari, E.; Lazzari, S.; Marverti, G.; Pignedoli, F.; Spagnolo, F.; Saladini, M. Synthesis, cytotoxic and combined cDDP activity of new stable curcumin derivatives. *Bioorg. Med. Chem.* **2009**, *17*, 3043–3052. [CrossRef] [PubMed]
25. Cao, Y.K.; Li, H.J.; Song, Z.F.; Li, Y.; Huai, Q.Y. Synthesis and biological evaluation of novel curcuminoid derivatives. *Molecules* **2014**, *19*, 16349–16372. [CrossRef] [PubMed]
26. Xu, G.; Chu, Y.; Jiang, N.; Yang, J.; Li, F. The Three Dimensional Quantitative Structure Activity Relationships (3D-QSAR) and docking studies of curcumin derivatives as androgen receptor antagonists. *Int. J. Mol. Sci.* **2012**, *13*, 6138–6155. [CrossRef] [PubMed]
27. Yadav, B.; Taurin, S.; Rosengren, R.J.; Schumacher, M.; Diederich, M.; Somers-Edgar, T.J.; Larsen, L. Synthesis and cytotoxic potential of heterocyclic cyclohexanone analogues of curcumin. *Bioorg. Med. Chem.* **2010**, *18*, 6701–6707. [CrossRef] [PubMed]
28. Sandur, S.K.; Pandey, M.K.; Sung, B.; Ahn, K.S.; Murakami, A.; Sethi, G.; Limtrakul, P.; Badmaev, V.; Aggarwal, B.B. Curcumin, demethoxycurcumin, bisdemethoxycurcumin, tetrahydrocurcumin and turmerones differentially regulate anti-inflammatory and anti-proliferative responses through a ROS-independent mechanism. *Carcinogenesis* **2007**, *28*, 1765–1773. [CrossRef] [PubMed]
29. Sugiyama, Y.; Kawakishi, S.; Osawa, T. Involvement of the beta-diketone moiety in the antioxidative mechanism of tetrahydrocurcumin. *Biochem. Pharm.* **1996**, *52*, 519–525. [CrossRef]
30. Somparn, P.; Phisalaphong, C.; Nakornchai, S.; Unchern, S.; Morales, N.P. Comparative antioxidant activities of curcumin and its demethoxy and hydrogenated derivatives. *Biol. Pharm. Bull.* **2007**, *30*, 74–78. [CrossRef] [PubMed]
31. Anand, P.; Thomas, S.G.; Kunnumakkara, A.B.; Sundaram, C.; Harikumar, K.B.; Sung, B.; Tharakan, S.T.; Misra, K.; Priyadarsini, I.K.; Rajasekharan, K.N.; et al. Biological activities of curcumin and its analogues (Congeners) made by man and Mother Nature. *Biochem. Pharm.* **2008**, *76*, 1590–1611. [CrossRef] [PubMed]

32. Khopde, S.M.; Priyadarsini, K.I.; Guha, S.N.; Satav, J.G.; Venkatesan, P.; Rao, M.N. Inhibition of radiation-induced lipid peroxidation by tetrahydrocurcumin: Possible mechanisms by pulse radiolysis. *Biosci. Biotechnol. Biochem.* **2000**, *64*, 503–509. [CrossRef] [PubMed]
33. Hahn, Y.-I.; Kim, S.-J.; Choi, B.-Y.; Cho, K.-C.; Bandu, R.; Kim, K.P.; Kim, D.-H.; Kim, W.; Park, J.S.; Han, B.W.; et al. Curcumin interacts directly with the Cysteine 259 residue of STAT3 and induces apoptosis in H-Ras transformed human mammary epithelial cells. *Sci. Rep.* **2018**, *8*, 6409. [CrossRef] [PubMed]
34. Vellampatti, S.; Chandrasekaran, G.; Mitta, S.B.; Lakshmanan, V.-K.; Park, S.H. Metallo-Curcumin-Conjugated DNA Complexes Induces Preferential Prostate Cancer Cells Cytotoxicity and Pause Growth of Bacterial Cells. *Sci. Rep.* **2018**, *8*, 14929. [CrossRef] [PubMed]
35. Dairam, A.; Limson, J.L.; Watkins, G.M.; Antunes, E.; Daya, S. Curcuminoids, curcumin, and demethoxycurcumin reduce lead-induced memory deficits in male Wistar rats. *J. Agric. Food Chem.* **2007**, *55*, 1039–1044. [CrossRef] [PubMed]
36. Weber, W.M.; Hunsaker, L.A.; Roybal, C.N.; Bobrovnikova-Marjon, E.V.; Abcouwer, S.F.; Royer, R.E.; Deck, L.M.; Vander Jagt, D.L. Activation of NFκB is inhibited by curcumin and related enones. *Bioorg. Med. Chem.* **2006**, *14*, 2450–2461. [CrossRef] [PubMed]
37. Bernabe-Pineda, M.; Ramirez-Silva, M.T.; Romero-Romo, M.; Gonzalez-Vergara, E.; Rojas-Hernandez, A. Determination of acidity constants of curcumin in aqueous solution and apparent rate constant of its decomposition. *Spectrochim. Acta Part A Mol. Biomol. Spectrosc.* **2004**, *60*, 1091–1097. [CrossRef]
38. Soh, S.F.; Huang, C.K.; Lee, S.O.; Xu, D.; Yeh, S.; Li, J.; Yong, E.L.; Gong, Y.; Chang, C. Determination of androgen receptor degradation enhancer ASC-J9((R)) in mouse sera and organs with liquid chromatography tandem mass spectrometry. *J. Pharm. Biomed. Anal.* **2014**, *88*, 117–122. [CrossRef] [PubMed]
39. Mohammadi, K.; Thompson, K.H.; Patrick, B.O.; Storr, T.; Martins, C.; Polishchuk, E.; Yuen, V.G.; McNeill, J.H.; Orvig, C. Synthesis and characterization of dual function vanadyl, gallium and indium curcumin complexes for medicinal applications. *J. Inorg. Biochem.* **2005**, *99*, 2217–2225. [CrossRef] [PubMed]
40. Thompson, K.H.; Böhmerle, K.; Polishchuk, E.; Martins, C.; Toleikis, P.; Tse, J.; Yuen, V.; McNeill, J.H.; Orvig, C. Complementary inhibition of synoviocyte, smooth muscle cell or mouse lymphoma cell proliferation by a vanadyl curcumin complex compared to curcumin alone. *J. Inorg. Biochem.* **2004**, *98*, 2063–2070. [CrossRef] [PubMed]
41. Benassi, R.; Ferrari, E.; Grandi, R.; Lazzari, S.; Saladini, M. Synthesis and characterization of new beta-diketo derivatives with iron chelating ability. *J. Inorg. Biochem.* **2007**, *101*, 203–213. [CrossRef] [PubMed]
42. Zambre, A.P.; Kulkarni, V.M.; Padhye, S.; Sandur, S.K.; Aggarwal, B.B. Novel curcumin analogs targeting TNF-induced NF-kappaB activation and proliferation in human leukemic KBM-5 cells. *Bioorg. Med. Chem.* **2006**, *14*, 7196–7204. [CrossRef] [PubMed]
43. Youssef, D.; Nichols, C.E.; Cameron, T.S.; Balzarini, J.; De Clercq, E.; Jha, A. Design, synthesis, and cytostatic activity of novel cyclic curcumin analogues. *Bioorg. Med. Chem. Lett.* **2007**, *17*, 5624–5629. [CrossRef] [PubMed]
44. Bhullar, K.S.; Jha, A.; Youssef, D.; Rupasinghe, H.P. Curcumin and its carbocyclic analogs: Structure-activity in relation to antioxidant and selected biological properties. *Molecules* **2013**, *18*, 5389–5404. [CrossRef] [PubMed]
45. Shim, J.S.; Kim, D.H.; Jung, H.J.; Kim, J.H.; Lim, D.; Lee, S.K.; Kim, K.W.; Ahn, J.W.; Yoo, J.S.; Rho, J.R.; et al. Hydrazinocurcumin, a novel synthetic curcumin derivative, is a potent inhibitor of endothelial cell proliferation. *Bioorg. Med. Chem.* **2002**, *10*, 2987–2992. [CrossRef]
46. Shim, J.S.; Lee, J.; Park, H.-J.; Park, S.-J.; Kwon, H.J. A New Curcumin Derivative, HBC, Interferes with the Cell Cycle Progression of Colon Cancer Cells via Antagonization of the Ca2+/Calmodulin Function. *Chem. Biol.* **2004**, *11*, 1455–1463. [CrossRef] [PubMed]
47. Dutta, S.; Padhye, S.; Priyadarsini, K.I.; Newton, C. Antioxidant and antiproliferative activity of curcumin semicarbazone. *Bioorg. Med. Chem. Lett.* **2005**, *15*, 2738–2744. [CrossRef] [PubMed]
48. Shen, L.; Liu, C.-C.; An, C.-Y.; Ji, H.-F. How does curcumin work with poor bioavailability? Clues from experimental and theoretical studies. *Sci. Rep.* **2016**, *6*, 20872. [CrossRef] [PubMed]
49. Davis, M.E.; Chen, Z.G.; Shin, D.M. Nanoparticle therapeutics: An emerging treatment modality for cancer. *Nat. Rev. Drug Discov.* **2008**, *7*, 771–782. [CrossRef] [PubMed]
50. Sun, M.; Su, X.; Ding, B.; He, X.; Liu, X.; Yu, A.; Lou, H.; Zhai, G. Advances in nanotechnology-based delivery systems for curcumin. *Nanomedicine* **2012**, *7*, 1085–1100. [CrossRef] [PubMed]

51. Naksuriya, O.; Okonogi, S.; Schiffelers, R.M.; Hennink, W.E. Curcumin nanoformulations: A review of pharmaceutical properties and preclinical studies and clinical data related to cancer treatment. *Biomaterials* **2014**, *35*, 3365–3383. [CrossRef] [PubMed]
52. Danhier, F.; Ansorena, E.; Silva, J.M.; Coco, R.; Le Breton, A.; Préat, V. PLGA-based nanoparticles: An overview of biomedical applications. *J. Control. Release* **2012**, *161*, 505–522. [CrossRef] [PubMed]
53. Fredenberg, S.; Wahlgren, M.; Reslow, M.; Axelsson, A. The mechanisms of drug release in poly(lactic-co-glycolic acid)-based drug delivery systems—A review. *Int. J. Pharm.* **2011**, *415*, 34–52. [CrossRef] [PubMed]
54. Song, W.; Muthana, M.; Mukherjee, J.; Falconer, R.J.; Biggs, C.A.; Zhao, X. Magnetic-Silk Core–Shell Nanoparticles as Potential Carriers for Targeted Delivery of Curcumin into Human Breast Cancer Cells. *ACS Biomater. Sci. Eng.* **2017**, *3*, 1027–1038. [CrossRef]
55. Dende, C.; Meena, J.; Nagarajan, P.; Nagaraj, V.A.; Panda, A.K.; Padmanaban, G. Nanocurcumin is superior to native curcumin in preventing degenerative changes in Experimental Cerebral Malaria. *Sci. Rep.* **2017**, *7*, 10062. [CrossRef] [PubMed]
56. Shaikh, J.; Ankola, D.D.; Beniwal, V.; Singh, D.; Kumar, M.N.V.R. Nanoparticle encapsulation improves oral bioavailability of curcumin by at least 9-fold when compared to curcumin administered with piperine as absorption enhancer. *Eur. J. Pharm. Sci.* **2009**, *37*, 223–230. [CrossRef] [PubMed]
57. Punfa, W.; Yodkeeree, S.; Pitchakarn, P.; Ampasavate, C.; Limtrakul, P. Enhancement of cellular uptake and cytotoxicity of curcumin-loaded PLGA nanoparticles by conjugation with anti-P-glycoprotein in drug resistance cancer cells. *Acta Pharmacol. Sin.* **2012**, *33*, 823–831. [CrossRef] [PubMed]
58. Malam, Y.; Loizidou, M.; Seifalian, A.M. Liposomes and nanoparticles: Nanosized vehicles for drug delivery in cancer. *Trends Pharmacol. Sci.* **2009**, *30*, 592–599. [CrossRef] [PubMed]
59. Karewicz, A.; Bielska, D.; Gzyl-Malcher, B.; Kepczynski, M.; Lach, R.; Nowakowska, M. Interaction of curcumin with lipid monolayers and liposomal bilayers. *Colloids Surf. B Biointerfaces* **2011**, *88*, 231–239. [CrossRef] [PubMed]
60. Li, X.; Nan, K.; Li, L.; Zhang, Z.; Chen, H. In vivo evaluation of curcumin nanoformulation loaded methoxy poly(ethylene glycol)-graft-chitosan composite film for wound healing application. *Carbohydr. Polym.* **2012**, *88*, 84–90. [CrossRef]
61. Fujita, K.; Hiramatsu, Y.; Minematsu, H.; Somiya, M.; Kuroda, S.I.; Seno, M.; Hinuma, S. Release of siRNA from liposomes induced by curcumin. *J. Nanotechnol.* **2016**, *2016*. [CrossRef]
62. Amano, C.; Minematsu, H.; Fujita, K.; Iwashita, S.; Adachi, M.; Igarashi, K.; Hinuma, S. Nanoparticles Containing Curcumin Useful for Suppressing Macrophages In Vivo in Mice. *PLoS ONE* **2015**, *10*, e0137207. [CrossRef] [PubMed]
63. Thangapazham, R.L.; Puri, A.; Tele, S.; Blumenthal, R.; Maheshwari, R.K. Evaluation of a nanotechnology-based carrier for delivery of curcumin in prostate cancer cells. *Int. J. Oncol.* **2008**, *32*, 1119–1123. [CrossRef] [PubMed]
64. Gou, M.; Men, K.; Shi, H.; Xiang, M.; Zhang, J.; Song, J.; Long, J.; Wan, Y.; Luo, F.; Zhao, X.; et al. Curcumin-loaded biodegradable polymeric micelles for colon cancer therapy in vitro and in vivo. *Nanoscale* **2011**, *3*, 1558–1567. [CrossRef] [PubMed]
65. Ganta, S.; Amiji, M. Coadministration of Paclitaxel and curcumin in nanoemulsion formulations to overcome multidrug resistance in tumor cells. *Mol. Pharm.* **2009**, *6*, 928–939. [CrossRef] [PubMed]
66. Karewicz, A.; Bielska, D.; Loboda, A.; Gzyl-Malcher, B.; Bednar, J.; Jozkowicz, A.; Dulak, J.; Nowakowska, M. Curcumin-containing liposomes stabilized by thin layers of chitosan derivatives. *Colloids Surf. B Biointerfaces* **2013**, *109*, 307–316. [CrossRef] [PubMed]
67. Lin, Y.-L.; Liu, Y.-K.; Tsai, N.-M.; Hsieh, J.-H.; Chen, C.-H.; Lin, C.-M.; Liao, K.-W. A Lipo-PEG-PEI complex for encapsulating curcumin that enhances its antitumor effects on curcumin-sensitive and curcumin-resistance cells. *Nanomed. Nanotechnol. Biol. Med.* **2012**, *8*, 318–327. [CrossRef] [PubMed]
68. Li, X.; Chen, S.; Zhang, B.; Li, M.; Diao, K.; Zhang, Z.; Li, J.; Xu, Y.; Wang, X.; Chen, H. In situ injectable nano-composite hydrogel composed of curcumin, N,O-carboxymethyl chitosan and oxidized alginate for wound healing application. *Int. J. Pharm.* **2012**, *437*, 110–119. [CrossRef] [PubMed]
69. Re, F.; Cambianica, I.; Zona, C.; Sesana, S.; Gregori, M.; Rigolio, R.; La Ferla, B.; Nicotra, F.; Forloni, G.; Cagnotto, A.; et al. Functionalization of liposomes with ApoE-derived peptides at different density affects cellular uptake and drug transport across a blood-brain barrier model. *Nanomed. Nanotechnol. Biol. Med.* **2011**, *7*, 551–559. [CrossRef] [PubMed]

70. Mangalathillam, S.; Rejinold, N.S.; Nair, A.; Lakshmanan, V.K.; Nair, S.V.; Jayakumar, R. Curcumin loaded chitin nanogels for skin cancer treatment via the transdermal route. *Nanoscale* **2012**, *4*, 239–250. [CrossRef] [PubMed]
71. Zanotto-Filho, A.; Coradini, K.; Braganhol, E.; Schröder, R.; de Oliveira, C.M.; Simões-Pires, A.; Battastini, A.M.O.; Pohlmann, A.R.; Guterres, S.S.; Forcelini, C.M.; et al. Curcumin-loaded lipid-core nanocapsules as a strategy to improve pharmacological efficacy of curcumin in glioma treatment. *Eur. J. Pharm. Biopharm.* **2013**, *83*, 156–167. [CrossRef] [PubMed]
72. Wang, D.; Veena, M.S.; Stevenson, K.; Tang, C.; Ho, B.; Suh, J.D.; Duarte, V.M.; Faull, K.F.; Mehta, K.; Srivatsan, E.S.; et al. Liposome-encapsulated curcumin suppresses growth of head and neck squamous cell carcinoma in vitro and in xenografts through the inhibition of nuclear factor kappaB by an AKT-independent pathway. *Clin. Cancer Res.* **2008**, *14*, 6228–6236. [CrossRef] [PubMed]
73. Lee, W.-H.; Loo, C.-Y.; Young, P.M.; Traini, D.; Mason, R.S.; Rohanizadeh, R. Recent advances in curcumin nanoformulation for cancer therapy. *Expert Opin. Drug Deliv.* **2014**, *11*, 1183–1201. [CrossRef] [PubMed]
74. Hamidi, M.; Azadi, A.; Rafiei, P. Hydrogel nanoparticles in drug delivery. *Adv. Drug Deliv. Rev.* **2008**, *60*, 1638–1649. [CrossRef] [PubMed]
75. Stuart, M.A.C.; Huck, W.T.S.; Genzer, J.; Müller, M.; Ober, C.; Stamm, M.; Sukhorukov, G.B.; Szleifer, I.; Tsukruk, V.V.; Urban, M.; et al. Emerging applications of stimuli-responsive polymer materials. *Nat. Mater.* **2010**, *9*, 101. [CrossRef] [PubMed]
76. Das, R.K.; Kasoju, N.; Bora, U. Encapsulation of curcumin in alginate-chitosan-pluronic composite nanoparticles for delivery to cancer cells. *Nanomed. Nanotechnol. Biol. Med.* **2010**, *6*, 153–160. [CrossRef] [PubMed]
77. Hatefi, A.; Amsden, B. Biodegradable injectable in situ forming drug delivery systems. *J. Control. Release* **2002**, *80*, 9–28. [CrossRef]
78. Chung, H.J.; Park, T.G. Self-assembled and nanostructured hydrogels for drug delivery and tissue engineering. *Nano Today* **2009**, *4*, 429–437. [CrossRef]
79. Altunbas, A.; Lee, S.J.; Rajasekaran, S.A.; Schneider, J.P.; Pochan, D.J. Encapsulation of curcumin in self-assembling peptide hydrogels as injectable drug delivery vehicles. *Biomaterials* **2011**, *32*, 5906–5914. [CrossRef] [PubMed]
80. Esmaili, M.; Ghaffari, S.M.; Moosavi-Movahedi, Z.; Atri, M.S.; Sharifizadeh, A.; Farhadi, M.; Yousefi, R.; Chobert, J.-M.; Haertlé, T.; Moosavi-Movahedi, A.A. Beta casein-micelle as a nano vehicle for solubility enhancement of curcumin; food industry application. *LWT—Food Sci. Technol.* **2011**, *44*, 2166–2172. [CrossRef]
81. Lomis, N.; Westfall, S.; Farahdel, L.; Malhotra, M.; Shum-Tim, D.; Prakash, S. Human Serum Albumin Nanoparticles for Use in Cancer Drug Delivery: Process Optimization and In Vitro Characterization. *Nanomaterials* **2016**, *6*, 116. [CrossRef] [PubMed]
82. Kim, T.H.; Jiang, H.H.; Youn, Y.S.; Park, C.W.; Tak, K.K.; Lee, S.; Kim, H.; Jon, S.; Chen, X.; Lee, K.C. Preparation and characterization of water-soluble albumin-bound curcumin nanoparticles with improved antitumor activity. *Int. J. Pharm.* **2011**, *403*, 285–291. [CrossRef] [PubMed]
83. Dal Pra, I.; Freddi, G.; Minic, J.; Chiarini, A.; Armato, U. De novo engineering of reticular connective tissue in vivo by silk fibroin nonwoven materials. *Biomaterials* **2005**, *26*, 1987–1999. [CrossRef] [PubMed]
84. Vepari, C.; Kaplan, D.L. Silk as a Biomaterial. *Prog. Polym. Sci.* **2007**, *32*, 991–1007. [CrossRef] [PubMed]
85. Gidwani, B.; Vyas, A. A Comprehensive Review on Cyclodextrin-Based Carriers for Delivery of Chemotherapeutic Cytotoxic Anticancer Drugs. *BioMed Res. Int.* **2015**, *2015*, 198268. [CrossRef] [PubMed]
86. Yallapu, M.M.; Jaggi, M.; Chauhan, S.C. beta-Cyclodextrin-curcumin self-assembly enhances curcumin delivery in prostate cancer cells. *Colloids Surf. B Biointerfaces* **2010**, *79*, 113–125. [CrossRef] [PubMed]
87. Rocks, N.; Bekaert, S.; Coia, I.; Paulissen, G.; Gueders, M.; Evrard, B.; Van Heugen, J.C.; Chiap, P.; Foidart, J.M.; Noel, A.; et al. Curcumin–cyclodextrin complexes potentiate gemcitabine effects in an orthotopic mouse model of lung cancer. *Br. J. Cancer* **2012**, *107*, 1083. [CrossRef] [PubMed]
88. Wong, R.S.Y. Apoptosis in cancer: From pathogenesis to treatment. *J. Exp. Clin. Cancer Res.* **2011**, *30*, 87. [CrossRef] [PubMed]
89. Bauer, J.H.; Helfand, S.L. New tricks of an old molecule: Lifespan regulation by p53. *Aging Cell* **2006**, *5*, 437–440. [CrossRef] [PubMed]
90. Tuorkey, M.J. Curcumin a potent cancer preventive agent: Mechanisms of cancer cell killing. *Interv. Med. Appl. Sci.* **2014**, *6*, 139–146. [CrossRef] [PubMed]

91. Balasubramanian, S.; Eckert, R.L. Curcumin suppresses AP1 transcription factor-dependent differentiation and activates apoptosis in human epidermal keratinocytes. *J. Biol. Chem.* **2007**, *282*, 6707–6715. [CrossRef] [PubMed]
92. Moragoda, L.; Jaszewski, R.; Majumdar, A.P. Curcumin induced modulation of cell cycle and apoptosis in gastric and colon cancer cells. *Anticancer Res.* **2001**, *21*, 873–878. [PubMed]
93. Ashour, A.A.; Abdel-Aziz, A.A.; Mansour, A.M.; Alpay, S.N.; Huo, L.; Ozpolat, B. Targeting elongation factor-2 kinase (eEF-2K) induces apoptosis in human pancreatic cancer cells. *Apoptosis* **2014**, *19*, 241–258. [CrossRef] [PubMed]
94. Lee, H.P.; Li, T.M.; Tsao, J.Y.; Fong, Y.C.; Tang, C.H. Curcumin induces cell apoptosis in human chondrosarcoma through extrinsic death receptor pathway. *Int. Immunopharmacol.* **2012**, *13*, 163–169. [CrossRef] [PubMed]
95. Siddiqui, F.A.; Prakasam, G.; Chattopadhyay, S.; Rehman, A.U.; Padder, R.A.; Ansari, M.A.; Irshad, R.; Mangalhara, K.; Bamezai, R.N.K.; Husain, M.; et al. Curcumin decreases Warburg effect in cancer cells by down-regulating pyruvate kinase M2 via mTOR-HIF1α inhibition. *Sci. Rep.* **2018**, *8*, 8323. [CrossRef] [PubMed]
96. Ahmed, A.; Ali, S.; Sarkar, F.H. Advances in androgen receptor targeted therapy for prostate cancer. *J. Cell. Physiol.* **2014**, *229*, 271–276. [CrossRef] [PubMed]
97. Dorai, T.; Cao, Y.C.; Dorai, B.; Buttyan, R.; Katz, A.E. Therapeutic potential of curcumin in human prostate cancer. III. Curcumin inhibits proliferation, induces apoptosis, and inhibits angiogenesis of LNCaP prostate cancer cells in vivo. *Prostate* **2001**, *47*, 293–303. [CrossRef] [PubMed]
98. Mukhopadhyay, A.; Bueso-Ramos, C.; Chatterjee, D.; Pantazis, P.; Aggarwal, B.B. Curcumin downregulates cell survival mechanisms in human prostate cancer cell lines. *Oncogene* **2001**, *20*, 7597–7609. [CrossRef] [PubMed]
99. McCarty, M.F. Targeting multiple signaling pathways as a strategy for managing prostate cancer: Multifocal signal modulation therapy. *Integr. Cancer Ther.* **2004**, *3*, 349–380. [CrossRef] [PubMed]
100. Sundram, V.; Chauhan, S.C.; Jaggi, M. Emerging roles of protein kinase D1 in cancer. *Mol. Cancer Res.* **2011**, *9*, 985–996. [CrossRef] [PubMed]
101. Mudduluru, G.; George-William, J.N.; Muppala, S.; Asangani, I.A.; Kumarswamy, R.; Nelson, L.D.; Allgayer, H. Curcumin regulates miR-21 expression and inhibits invasion and metastasis in colorectal cancer. *Biosci. Rep.* **2011**, *31*, 185–197. [CrossRef] [PubMed]
102. LaValle, C.R.; George, K.M.; Sharlow, E.R.; Lazo, J.S.; Wipf, P.; Wang, Q.J. Protein kinase D as a potential new target for cancer therapy. *Biochim. Biophys. Acta* **2010**, *1806*, 183–192. [CrossRef] [PubMed]
103. Nautiyal, J.; Banerjee, S.; Kanwar, S.S.; Yu, Y.; Patel, B.B.; Sarkar, F.H.; Majumdar, A.P. Curcumin enhances dasatinib-induced inhibition of growth and transformation of colon cancer cells. *Int. J. Cancer* **2011**, *128*, 951–961. [CrossRef] [PubMed]
104. Carrato, A. Adjuvant treatment of colorectal cancer. *Gastrointest. Cancer Res.* **2008**, *2*, S42–S46. [PubMed]
105. Garcea, G.; Berry, D.P.; Jones, D.J.; Singh, R.; Dennison, A.R.; Farmer, P.B.; Sharma, R.A.; Steward, W.P.; Gescher, A.J. Consumption of the putative chemopreventive agent curcumin by cancer patients: Assessment of curcumin levels in the colorectum and their pharmacodynamic consequences. *Cancer Epidemiol. Prev. Biomark.* **2005**, *14*, 120–125.
106. Kunnumakkara, A.B.; Diagaradjane, P.; Guha, S.; Deorukhkar, A.; Shentu, S.; Aggarwal, B.B.; Krishnan, S. Curcumin sensitizes human colorectal cancer xenografts in nude mice to gamma-radiation by targeting nuclear factor-kappaB-regulated gene products. *Clin. Cancer Res.* **2008**, *14*, 2128–2136. [CrossRef] [PubMed]
107. Xu, H.; Yu, Y.; Marciniak, D.; Rishi, A.K.; Sarkar, F.H.; Kucuk, O.; Majumdar, A.P. Epidermal growth factor receptor (EGFR)-related protein inhibits multiple members of the EGFR family in colon and breast cancer cells. *Mol. Cancer Ther.* **2005**, *4*, 435–442. [CrossRef] [PubMed]
108. Vokes, E.E.; Weichselbaum, R.R.; Lippman, S.M.; Hong, W.K. Head and neck cancer. *N. Engl. J. Med.* **1993**, *328*, 184–194. [CrossRef] [PubMed]
109. Chun, K.S.; Keum, Y.S.; Han, S.S.; Song, Y.S.; Kim, S.H.; Surh, Y.J. Curcumin inhibits phorbol ester-induced expression of cyclooxygenase-2 in mouse skin through suppression of extracellular signal-regulated kinase activity and NF-kappaB activation. *Carcinogenesis* **2003**, *24*, 1515–1524. [CrossRef] [PubMed]

110. Chakravarti, N.; Myers, J.N.; Aggarwal, B.B. Targeting constitutive and interleukin-6-inducible signal transducers and activators of transcription 3 pathway in head and neck squamous cell carcinoma cells by curcumin (diferuloylmethane). *Int. J. Cancer* **2006**, *119*, 1268–1275. [CrossRef] [PubMed]
111. LoTempio, M.M.; Veena, M.S.; Steele, H.L.; Ramamurthy, B.; Ramalingam, T.S.; Cohen, A.N.; Chakrabarti, R.; Srivatsan, E.S.; Wang, M.B. Curcumin suppresses growth of head and neck squamous cell carcinoma. *Clin. Cancer Res.* **2005**, *11*, 6994–7002. [CrossRef] [PubMed]
112. Ananthakrishnan, P.; Balci, F.L.; Crowe, J.P. Optimizing surgical margins in breast conservation. *Int. J. Surg. Oncol.* **2012**, *2012*, 585670. [CrossRef] [PubMed]
113. Houssami, N.; Macaskill, P.; Marinovich, M.L.; Dixon, J.M.; Irwig, L.; Brennan, M.E.; Solin, L.J. Meta-analysis of the impact of surgical margins on local recurrence in women with early-stage invasive breast cancer treated with breast-conserving therapy. *Eur. J. Cancer* **2010**, *46*, 3219–3232. [CrossRef] [PubMed]
114. Ramachandran, C.; Fonseca, H.B.; Jhabvala, P.; Escalon, E.A.; Melnick, S.J. Curcumin inhibits telomerase activity through human telomerase reverse transcritpase in MCF-7 breast cancer cell line. *Cancer Lett.* **2002**, *184*, 1–6. [CrossRef]
115. Liu, Q.; Loo, W.T.Y.; Sze, S.C.W.; Tong, Y. Curcumin inhibits cell proliferation of MDA-MB-231 and BT-483 breast cancer cells mediated by down-regulation of NFκB, cyclinD and MMP-1 transcription. *Phytomedicine* **2009**, *16*, 916–922. [CrossRef] [PubMed]
116. Bachmeier, B.; Nerlich, A.G.; Iancu, C.M.; Cilli, M.; Schleicher, E.; Vene, R.; Dell'Eva, R.; Jochum, M.; Albini, A.; Pfeffer, U. The chemopreventive polyphenol Curcumin prevents hematogenous breast cancer metastases in immunodeficient mice. *Cell. Physiol. Biochem.* **2007**, *19*, 137–152. [CrossRef] [PubMed]
117. Moghtaderi, H.; Sepehri, H.; Attari, F. Combination of arabinogalactan and curcumin induces apoptosis in breast cancer cells in vitro and inhibits tumor growth via overexpression of p53 level in vivo. *Biomed. Pharmacother.* **2017**, *88*, 582–594. [CrossRef] [PubMed]
118. Müller, A.; Homey, B.; Soto, H.; Ge, N.; Catron, D.; Buchanan, M.E.; McClanahan, T.; Murphy, E.; Yuan, W.; Wagner, S.N.; et al. Involvement of chemokine receptors in breast cancer metastasis. *Nature* **2001**, *410*, 50. [CrossRef] [PubMed]
119. Bachmeier, B.E.; Mohrenz, I.V.; Mirisola, V.; Schleicher, E.; Romeo, F.; Hohneke, C.; Jochum, M.; Nerlich, A.G.; Pfeffer, U. Curcumin downregulates the inflammatory cytokines CXCL1 and -2 in breast cancer cells via NFkappaB. *Carcinogenesis* **2008**, *29*, 779–789. [CrossRef] [PubMed]
120. Yang, Z.; Chang, Y.J.; Yu, I.C.; Yeh, S.; Wu, C.C.; Miyamoto, H.; Merry, D.E.; Sobue, G.; Chen, L.M.; Chang, S.S.; et al. ASC-J9 ameliorates spinal and bulbar muscular atrophy phenotype via degradation of androgen receptor. *Nat. Med.* **2007**, *13*, 348–353. [CrossRef] [PubMed]
121. UK, C.R. Brain, Other CNS and Intracranial Tumours Statistics. 2019. Available online: https://www.cancerresearchuk.org/health-professional/cancer-statistics/statistics-by-cancer-type/brain-other-cns-and-intracranial-tumours#heading-Zero (accessed on 14 February 2019).
122. Grossman, S.A.; Batara, J.F. Current management of glioblastoma multiforme. *Semin. Oncol.* **2004**, *31*, 635–644. [CrossRef] [PubMed]
123. Klinger, N.V.; Mittal, S. Therapeutic potential of curcumin for the treatment of brain tumors. *Oxid. Med. Cell. Longev.* **2016**, *2016*. [CrossRef] [PubMed]
124. Chintala, S.K.; Tonn, J.C.; Rao, J.S. Matrix metalloproteinases and their biological function in human gliomas. *Int. J. Dev. Neurosci.* **1999**, *17*, 495–502. [CrossRef]
125. Perry, M.C.; Demeule, M.; Regina, A.; Moumdjian, R.; Beliveau, R. Curcumin inhibits tumor growth and angiogenesis in glioblastoma xenografts. *Mol. Nutr. Food Res.* **2010**, *54*, 1192–1201. [CrossRef] [PubMed]
126. Wu, B.; Yao, H.; Wang, S.; Xu, R. DAPK1 modulates a curcumin-induced G2/M arrest and apoptosis by regulating STAT3, NF-κB, and caspase-3 activation. *Biochem. Biophys. Res. Commun.* **2013**, *434*, 75–80. [CrossRef] [PubMed]
127. Ledda, A.; Belcaro, G.; Dugall, M.; Luzzi, R.; Scoccianti, M.; Togni, S.; Appendino, G.; Ciammaichella, G. Meriva(R), a lecithinized curcumin delivery system, in the control of benign prostatic hyperplasia: A pilot, product evaluation registry study. *Panminerva Med.* **2012**, *54*, 17–22. [PubMed]
128. Bayet-Robert, M.; Kwiatkowski, F.; Leheurteur, M.; Gachon, F.; Planchat, E.; Abrial, C.; Mouret-Reynier, M.A.; Durando, X.; Barthomeuf, C.; Chollet, P. Phase I dose escalation trial of docetaxel plus curcumin in patients with advanced and metastatic breast cancer. *Cancer Biol. Ther.* **2010**, *9*, 8–14. [CrossRef] [PubMed]

129. Ghalaut, V.S.; Sangwan, L.; Dahiya, K.; Ghalaut, P.S.; Dhankhar, R.; Saharan, R. Effect of imatinib therapy with and without turmeric powder on nitric oxide levels in chronic myeloid leukemia. *J. Oncol. Pharm. Pract.* **2012**, *18*, 186–190. [CrossRef] [PubMed]
130. Plummer, S.M.; Hill, K.A.; Festing, M.F.; Steward, W.P.; Gescher, A.J.; Sharma, R.A. Clinical development of leukocyte cyclooxygenase 2 activity as a systemic biomarker for cancer chemopreventive agents. *Cancer Epidemiol. Prev. Biomark.* **2001**, *10*, 1295–1299.
131. Sharma, R.A.; Euden, S.A.; Platton, S.L.; Cooke, D.N.; Shafayat, A.; Hewitt, H.R.; Marczylo, T.H.; Morgan, B.; Hemingway, D.; Plummer, S.M.; et al. Phase I clinical trial of oral curcumin: Biomarkers of systemic activity and compliance. *Clin. Cancer Res.* **2004**, *10*, 6847–6854. [CrossRef] [PubMed]
132. He, Z.Y.; Shi, C.B.; Wen, H.; Li, F.L.; Wang, B.L.; Wang, J. Upregulation of p53 expression in patients with colorectal cancer by administration of curcumin. *Cancer Investig.* **2011**, *29*, 208–213. [CrossRef] [PubMed]
133. Carroll, R.E.; Benya, R.V.; Turgeon, D.K.; Vareed, S.; Neuman, M.; Rodriguez, L.; Kakarala, M.; Carpenter, P.M.; McLaren, C.; Meyskens, F.L., Jr.; et al. Phase IIa clinical trial of curcumin for the prevention of colorectal neoplasia. *Cancer Prev. Res.* **2011**, *4*, 354–364. [CrossRef] [PubMed]
134. Irving, G.R.; Howells, L.M.; Sale, S.; Kralj-Hans, I.; Atkin, W.S.; Clark, S.K.; Britton, R.G.; Jones, D.J.; Scott, E.N.; Berry, D.P.; et al. Prolonged biologically active colonic tissue levels of curcumin achieved after oral administration–a clinical pilot study including assessment of patient acceptability. *Cancer Prev. Res.* **2013**, *6*, 119–128. [CrossRef] [PubMed]
135. Kim, S.G.; Veena, M.S.; Basak, S.K.; Han, E.; Tajima, T.; Gjertson, D.W.; Starr, J.; Eidelman, O.; Pollard, H.B.; Srivastava, M.; et al. Curcumin treatment suppresses IKKbeta kinase activity of salivary cells of patients with head and neck cancer: A pilot study. *Clin. Cancer Res.* **2011**, *17*, 5953–5961. [CrossRef] [PubMed]
136. Cruz-Correa, M.; Hylind, L.M.; Marrero, J.H.; Zahurak, M.L.; Murray-Stewart, T.; Casero, R.A., Jr.; Montgomery, E.A.; Iacobuzio-Donahue, C.; Brosens, L.A.; Offerhaus, G.J.; et al. Efficacy and Safety of Curcumin in Treatment of Intestinal Adenomas in Patients with Familial Adenomatous Polyposis. *Gastroenterology* **2018**, *155*, 668–673. [CrossRef] [PubMed]
137. Dhillon, N.; Aggarwal, B.B.; Newman, R.A.; Wolff, R.A.; Kunnumakkara, A.B.; Abbruzzese, J.L.; Ng, C.S.; Badmaev, V.; Kurzrock, R. Phase II trial of curcumin in patients with advanced pancreatic cancer. *Clin. Cancer Res.* **2008**, *14*, 4491–4499. [CrossRef] [PubMed]
138. Epelbaum, R.; Schaffer, M.; Vizel, B.; Badmaev, V.; Bar-Sela, G. Curcumin and gemcitabine in patients with advanced pancreatic cancer. *Nutr. Cancer* **2010**, *62*, 1137–1141. [CrossRef] [PubMed]
139. Kanai, M.; Yoshimura, K.; Asada, M.; Imaizumi, A.; Suzuki, C.; Matsumoto, S.; Nishimura, T.; Mori, Y.; Masui, T.; Kawaguchi, Y.; et al. A phase I/II study of gemcitabine-based chemotherapy plus curcumin for patients with gemcitabine-resistant pancreatic cancer. *Cancer Chemother. Pharmacol.* **2011**, *68*, 157–164. [CrossRef] [PubMed]
140. Kanai, M.; Otsuka, Y.; Otsuka, K.; Sato, M.; Nishimura, T.; Mori, Y.; Kawaguchi, M.; Hatano, E.; Kodama, Y.; Matsumoto, S.; et al. A phase I study investigating the safety and pharmacokinetics of highly bioavailable curcumin (Theracurmin) in cancer patients. *Cancer Chemother. Pharmacol.* **2013**, *71*, 1521–1530. [CrossRef] [PubMed]
141. Ide, H.; Tokiwa, S.; Sakamaki, K.; Nishio, K.; Isotani, S.; Muto, S.; Hama, T.; Masuda, H.; Horie, S. Combined inhibitory effects of soy isoflavones and curcumin on the production of prostate-specific antigen. *Prostate* **2010**, *70*, 1127–1133. [CrossRef] [PubMed]
142. Hejazi, J.; Rastmanesh, R.; Taleban, F.A.; Molana, S.H.; Hejazi, E.; Ehtejab, G.; Hara, N. Effect of Curcumin Supplementation During Radiotherapy on Oxidative Status of Patients with Prostate Cancer: A Double Blinded, Randomized, Placebo-Controlled Study. *Nutr. Cancer* **2016**, *68*, 77–85. [CrossRef] [PubMed]
143. Panahi, Y.; Saadat, A.; Beiraghdar, F.; Sahebkar, A. Adjuvant therapy with bioavailability-boosted curcuminoids suppresses systemic inflammation and improves quality of life in patients with solid tumors: A randomized double-blind placebo-controlled trial. *Phytother. Res.* **2014**, *28*, 1461–1467. [CrossRef] [PubMed]

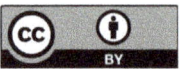 © 2019 by the authors. Licensee MDPI, Basel, Switzerland. This article is an open access article distributed under the terms and conditions of the Creative Commons Attribution (CC BY) license (http://creativecommons.org/licenses/by/4.0/).

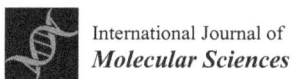

Review

Curcumin and its Potential for Systemic Targeting of Inflamm-Aging and Metabolic Reprogramming in Cancer

Renata Novak Kujundžić [1], Višnja Stepanić [1], Lidija Milković [2], Ana Čipak Gašparović [2], Marko Tomljanović [1] and Koraljka Gall Trošelj [1,*]

[1] Laboratory for Epigenomics, Ruđer Bošković Institute, Division of Molecular Medicine, 10 000 Zagreb, Croatia; rnovak@irb.hr (R.N.K.); stepanic@irb.hr (V.S.); Marko.Tomljanovic@irb.hr (M.T.)
[2] Laboratory for Oxidative Stress (LabOS), Ruđer Bošković Institute, Division of Molecular Medicine, 10 000 Zagreb, Croatia; Lidija.Milkovic@irb.hr (L.M.); Ana.Cipak.Gasparovic@irb.hr (A.Č.G.)
* Correspondence: troselj@irb.hr; Tel.: +385-1-4560-972

Received: 25 January 2019; Accepted: 5 March 2019; Published: 8 March 2019

Abstract: Pleiotropic effects of curcumin have been the subject of intensive research. The interest in this molecule for preventive medicine may further increase because of its potential to modulate inflamm-aging. Although direct data related to its effect on inflamm-aging does not exist, there is a strong possibility that its well-known anti-inflammatory properties may be relevant to this phenomenon. Curcumin's binding to various proteins, which was shown to be dependent on cellular oxidative status, is yet another feature for exploration in depth. Finally, the binding of curcumin to various metabolic enzymes is crucial to curcumin's interference with powerful metabolic machinery, and can also be crucial for metabolic reprogramming of cancer cells. This review offers a synthesis and functional links that may better explain older data, some observational, in light of the most recent findings on curcumin. Our focus is on its modes of action that have the potential to alleviate specific morbidities of the 21st century.

Keywords: curcumin; oxidative metabolites; inflamm-aging; cancer; metabolic reprogramming; direct protein binding; IL-17; STAT3; SHMT2

1. Introduction

During the past one and a half decades, we have been witnessing increased interest in natural compounds and their applications to everyday life. This fact should not be surprising, especially in the field of preventive medicine. Thanks to various interventions including, but not limited to, vaccination, high hygienic standards, avoidance of smoking and alcohol abuse, healthy diet, maintenance of body weight and exercising, human life span is extended. According to the World Health Organization (WHO), the average global life expectancy for those born in 2016 is 72.0 years (males 69.8 years; females 74.2 years), with a significant differential depending on the geographical region: African region (only) 61.2 years, versus European region 77.5 years [1]. The United Nations Department of Economic and Social Affairs (DESA) has forecasted that global life expectancy at birth, for both sexes combined, is going to rise to 76.9 years by years 2045–2050 [2].

However, an inevitable trade-off of extended lifespan is the increased incidence of various age-related diseases, of which cancer is certainly a very important one.

Chronic inflammation is common to aging and age-related diseases. The concept of a causal relationship between inflammation and cancer dates back to Rudolf Virchow who suggested, in his lectures in 1858, that the "lymphoreticular infiltrate" reflects the origin of cancer at sites of chronic inflammation. He pointed out that there are striking similarities between ulcers, wound healing, and cancer [3,4]. More than a century later, Harold F. Dvorak published an essay in the New England Journal of Medicine entitled "Tumors: Wounds that do not heal. Similarities between tumor stroma generation and wound-healing." He proposed that solid tumors act as parasites that promote a wound-healing response to acquire the stroma needed for their survival and growth [5]. Aging is often accompanied by an impaired healing response [6], accumulation of senescent cells, and chronic inflammation [7].

The link between aging and inflammation is very accurately coined in the term "inflamm-aging", which denotes the up-regulation of certain pro-inflammatory cytokines at older ages, and is associated with chronic diseases. This term was originally introduced in 2006 [8], to describe the imbalance between inflammatory and anti-inflammatory networks, which results in a low grade chronic, age-associated, pro-inflammatory status. Currently, deregulated cytokine production is appreciated as a very important consequence of the remodeling of the immune system in old age (recently reviewed) [9]. It has been recognized that, in older subjects, high levels of interleukins IL-6 and IL-1, tumor necrosis factor-alpha (TNF-α), and C-reactive protein (CRP) are associated with an increased risk of morbidity and mortality [10].

The rate of cancer incidence is increasing, especially in the Western world. According to GLOBOCAN 2018, there have been 18.1 million new reported cases of cancer in 2018 (9.5 million males and 8.6 million females). The same database predicted 9.6 million cancer deaths in 2018 (5.4 million males and 4.2 million females) [11]. For 2040, the International Agency for Research on Cancer predicted 29.5 million newly diagnosed cancer patients, and 16.4 million cancer deaths [12].

Early detection screenings represent a valid effort in fighting cancer. In the same setting, the era of biotechnology implemented in molecular medicine, enables an insightful understanding of the molecular mechanisms of action of natural compounds which have been used in traditional medicine for centuries. One such compound is curcumin, which possesses properties relevant to successful cancer chemoprevention. This is particularly important for the elder population.

2. Curcumin and Inflamm-aging

The natural source of curcumin is the rhizome of the medicinal plant, *Curcuma longa*, a perennial herb in the family *Zingiberaceae* [13]. The curcuminoid complex, found in the rhizome of turmeric (2.5–6%) contains: curcumin (CUR - diferuloylmethane, ~85%); demethoxycurcumin (DEM, ~15%); bis-demethoxycurcumin (bis-DEM, ~5%) and cyclocurcumin [14]. In the commercially available formulations, the major curcuminoid complexes are reported to be in a similar range: 77% of CUR; 17% of DEM; and 3% of bis-DEM) [15]. By 2022, the U.S. curcumin market is expected to approach 40 million dollars [16]. It is also recognized that over 52% of curcumin production will be used for pharmaceutical applications, in the U.S.

Well-known for its healing properties, curcumin has been extensively used in traditional Ayurveda, Unani and Siddha medicine for treating various diseases. An early mention of curcumin in modern medical literature was in 1937, appearing in the Lancet, one of the most prestigious clinical medical journals [17]. The article, describing curcumin applications to humans, was written by Albert Oppenheimer—then an assistant professor at the American University of Beirut, Lebanon, who applied curcumin orally (up to 800 mg daily) for the treatment of 67 patients suffering from various forms of subacute, recurrent, or chronic cholecystitis. The positive therapeutic response recorded then, was the basis for future interest in curcumin and its healing properties, especially its anti-inflammatory properties, which were among the first studied [18].

Is it reasonable to conclude that the anti-inflammatory property of curcumin may be used for alleviating inflamm-aging? If that is so, can it explain the beneficial effects of curcumin in various experimental models of diseases of elderly humans? We will present some older and some very recent data which we consider central in the context of this puzzle.

In 2009, Smith et al. published data showing that the total projected cancer incidence will increase in the U.S. by approximately 45%, in only 20 years, from 1.6 million (2010) to 2.3 million, in 2030 [19].

This prediction seems to be very accurate since, for 2019, 1,762,450 new cases and 606,880 cancer deaths were estimated to occur in the U.S. [20]. The Smith's study predicted something that was way ahead of the time when the article was published. A 67% increase in cancer incidence was anticipated for older adults [19]. Eight years later, in 2017, Nolen et al. have shown that cancer prevalence and cancer incidence increases until ages 85-89, after which the rates decrease until 100+ [21].

Inflammation has been recognized as a strong contributor to the acquisition of core hallmark cancer capabilities [22]. The most recent data convincingly show that the high level of pro-inflammatory cytokines (such as IL-6 and IL-8) may predict some crucial prognostic parameters in cancer patients [23,24]. In addition to an increased level of IL-6 and IL-8, colorectal cancer patients also have alterations in their serum amino-acid profile. Low levels of serum glutamine, histidine, alanine and high glycine levels were shown to be associated with advanced stage of cancer and with poor cancer-specific survival (N = 336; univariate analysis) [25].

There are also quite convincing data on neuroinflammation as a crucial process in the pathogenesis of the two the most common neurodegenerative diseases in the elder population: Alzheimer's disease (AD) and Parkinson's disease (PD) [26]. Based on numerous data, it has been proposed that both disorders are strongly related to inflamm-aging [27,28]. As recently reviewed, three shared strong mediators of inflammatory reaction are increased in patients suffering from these two disorders: IL-6, IL-1β and TNF-α [29].

These inflammatory molecules are integrative parts of the canonical activation of the NF-kappa B (nuclear factor kappa-light-chain-enhancer of activated B cells; NF-κB) signaling pathway. Generally, this pathway has been considered as protumorigenic, although there are several models showing its opposite action [30]. During the last few years, the interleukin 17 (IL-17) has become the focus of various types of research, including the research related to cancer, Alzheimer's and Parkinson's disease. There are several models in which the communication between NF-κB and IL-17 takes the place. The most recent data indicate that IL-17 can promote the proliferation and migration of glioma cells via PI3K/AKT1/NF-κB-p65 activation [31].

2.1. Inflamm-Aging, Interleukin-17 and Curcumin

Originally, in 2002, human colonic subepithelial myofibroblasts (SEMFs) were used as a model system for showing that SEMFs secrete IL-6, IL-8, and MCP-1 (Monocyte Chemoattractant Protein-1), in response to IL-17 [32]. The most recent data point out the critical role for IL-17-producing T lymphocytes in sporadic PD, in humans. In vitro, the midbrain neurons (MBNs) were shown to increasingly die consequentially to the upregulation of IL-17 receptor (IL-17R) and NF-κB activation [33]. The involvement of IL-17-producing T lymphocytes in the onset of Alzheimer's disease was also shown, in the animal model [34].

Although majority studies performed so far indicate the presence/an increase of IL-17 as a negative prognostic factor for cancer patients, the results are not entirely conclusive and depend on numerous factors. These include the type of the tumor, the types of genetic aberrations, which may significantly vary, and the host's immune response. Of importance, different cell types expressing IL-17 can play different roles, not only in the tumor microenvironment, but, it seems, may provide insight into the overall picture of the malignant tumor. In a cohort of 573 gastric cancer patients [35], high levels of IL-17+ neutrophils were shown in the tumorous tissue, where the high level of IL-17 induced the migration of neutrophils into gastric cancer, via cancer cell–derived CXC chemokines. These neutrophils were further shown to stimulate the proangiogenic activity of tumor cells, both in vitro and in vivo. The increase in IL-17-expressing cells in peripheral blood, particularly Th17, was associated with tumor progression in HNC (Head and Neck Carcinoma) patients (N = 120) [36].

While there are many data on curcumin and NF-κB, there are only a few of them in relation to curcumin and its effect on IL-17producing cells. In relation to HNC, it is quite interesting that the testing in 2015 of a novel microgranular curcumin formulation (15 patients and eight healthy volunteers) showed that curcumin strongly decreases the serum level of IL-17 at one hour post-ingestion; p = 0.0342 [37].

2.2. Breast Tissue Inflamm-Aging and Curcumin

There are many research papers discussing curcumin's action on sex-hormone related cancer (breast, ovary, prostate), in vitro. In breast cancer cells, the effects obtained depend not only on the status of estrogen and progesterone receptors (estrogen receptor; ER and progesterone receptor; PR), but also on the specific genetic/epigenetic cellular background. A 20 year old paper presented the strong inhibitory action of curcumin alone and in combination with isoflavonoids in both ER-positive human breast cancer cells (MCF-7 and T47D) and ER-negative MDA-MB-231 cells exposed to environmental estrogens (pesticide o,p'-DDT and the pollutants 4-nonylphenol and 4-octylphenol) [38]. The mechanism of curcumin's inhibitory effect on MCF-7 and MDA-MB-231 was explained four years later [39]. Curcumin exerts antiproliferative effects on MCF-7 cells through: (a) inhibiting the exogenous 17-β estradiol's stimulatory growth effect on these cells; (b) blocking the expression of downstream ER-responsive genes, pS2 and TGF-α, when applied in high concentrations. In MDA-MB-231 cells, this mechanism was absent. Instead, curcumin strongly decreased the level of MMP-2 (matrix metalloproteinase 2).

In this paper, we reinforce the fact that breast cancer has been recognized as a systemic disease [40]. There is strong experimental data showing that postmenopausal breast cancer in obese women also can be considered as „breast inflamm-aging" disease. At the outset of the pathophysiological process, subclinical, local breast inflammation, characterized by crown-like structures (CLS) consisting of dead adipocytes surrounded by macrophages, occurs in breast white adipose tissue [41]. This type of inflammation is paralleled by increased NF-κB binding activity joined with elevated levels of proinflammatory mediators and a key enzyme in the biosynthesis of estrogen in menopause, aromatase (estrogen synthase) [42]. Through aromatization of androgen precursors in adipose tissue (through tissue specific reactions), this enzyme makes a strong link between inflammation, obesity, and an increased risk for hormone receptor-positive breast cancer [43].

On the other hand, lipolysis, which is also increased in obesity, results in increased concentrations of free fatty acids [44]. Saturated fatty acids trigger the activation of NF-κB in macrophages resulting in increased production of proinflammatory mediators which additionally induce aromatase in preadipocytes [45]. Thus, there is a complete *circulus vitiosus*, associated with increased activity of NF-κB, which can be modified by curcumin.

As shown in vitro, curcumin can significantly suppress the inductive effects of stearic acid–treated macrophages, on aromatase mRNA and aromatase activity in preadipocytes, through suppression of NF-κB and Akt signaling pathways [46]. In the cited paper [46], a mixture of multiple polyphenols (Zyflamend; curcumin included), was given to animals kept on a high-fat-diet. As a result, the increased levels of aromatase mRNA and its activity in the mammary glands were partially suppressed. Although this data constitutes a solid basis for future research on chemoprevention in humans, there is one obvious problem. Measurement of the effect which occurs locally requires a biopsy. This significant obstacle is one, but not the only one, of the major reasons for serious gaps in this area of research [47].

There is no data, to the best of our knowledge showing the organ-specific, local effects and/or systemic effects of curcumin in humans, which would be gender-specific.

2.3. Curcumin and the Concept of Network Medicine

The NF-κB signaling pathway is a master regulator of inflammation-associated signaling pathways. Age-related, tissue-specific, brain inflammation mediated by NF-κB, when joined with Nitric Oxide and Reactive Oxygen Species (NOROS), in macrophages has been recognized as a most significant risk factor for developing Alzheimer's disease [48]. Activation of this pathway has been also recognized in pathogenesis of PD [49]. Thus, if we focus on the pathophysiology of these three diseases (cancer, AD and PD) and their increased incidence in older subjects, we need to take note of some shared general molecular features, of which the "inflamm-age status" represents a very important factor. It may, indeed, be the strongest indicator of perturbations which affect complex intracellular and intercellular networks which communicate at different levels, as suggested by postulates of Network Medicine. This discipline proposes a highly interconnected nature of the interactome and considers that a gene, protein or metabolite can be implicated in several disease modules. Accordingly, at the molecular level, it leads to the conclusion that diseases are not independent of one another [50].

Can this interconnective dependency explain the beneficial effects of multilevel acting pleiotropic curcumin [51] as a molecule that is considered useful for the prevention of these diseases, as recorded in various models/diseases?

First of all, surprisingly, the combined terms "curcumin" and "inflamm-age" appear in only a few research papers in the PubMed database. Secondly, there are only a few studies based on measuring cytokines in cancer-free human subjects who were taking curcumin. Different types of curcumin formulations given, in addition to various doses applied and duration of administration, makes the picture confusing. In a cohort of 72 migraine patients, only the combined daily administration of 2500 mg of ω-3 fatty acids (2 × 1250 mg) and 80 mg nano-curcumin (1 × 80 mg), led to a significant decrease of TNF-α in the serum ($p = 0.001$). Administration of curcumin alone had no significant effects [52]. However, a decrease of TNF-α was recorded (from 103.90 ± 13.29 ng/dL to 92.56 ± 8.70 ng/dL). The question is whether these subtle changes, although not statistically significant when taking into consideration the whole group of subjects, may be significant for the physiology of a particular patient. This would be in accord with the postulates of personalized medicine.

In a study which included 117 subjects suffering from metabolic syndrome, 1 g of curcumin daily and placebo were given to 59 and 58 subjects, respectively, for a period of eight weeks. In this research study, between-group comparison suggested significantly greater reductions in serum concentrations of TNF-α, IL-6, TGF-β (transforming growth factor beta) and MCP-1 in the curcumin versus the placebo group ($p < 0.001$). When adjusted for potential confounders, changes in all parameters (serum glucose and lipids, baseline serum concentration of the cytokines), except IL-6, remained statistically significant [53].

These two examples show that we are far away from firm conclusions when considering the potential beneficial effects of curcumin. The problem relating to the lack of comprehensive data associated with inflammation markers and curcumin application to healthy subjects, was very accurately addressed by Hewlings and Kalman [54], who concluded that measuring potential benefits of curcumin in healthy populations may be challenging because the benefits may not be as immediate and measurable if (bio)markers are normal at the baseline. Thus, for reaching meaningful conclusions, subjects will need to be followed over an extended time period, which would require a high level of participants' cooperation. But even if the cooperation and stringent follow-up is provided, caution in interpretation is needed.

The necessity of careful interpretation of all this data and the effects obtained must be put in the context of the most recent findings.

3. Oxidative Metabolites of Curcumin

The newest data show that the anti-inflammatory effects of curcumin, those mediated through inhibition of NF-κB [55,56], do not depend on the parent molecule, but rather on its oxidized products [57]. It was very convincingly shown that oxidative metabolites of curcumin adduct to and inhibit IKK β (inhibitor of nuclear factor kappa-B kinase subunit beta; known also as IKK2/NFKBIKB). If the cells were pretreated with N-acetylcysteine, a biosynthetic precursor of glutathione (GSH), the potency of curcumin was decreased, probably due to GSH-mediated scavenge and inactivation of curcumin-derived electrophiles. Finally, as concluded in the cited article [57], oxidative metabolites of curcumin, which occur in vitro, adduct to cellular proteins. As the authors stated, this may explain the wide range of cellular targets of curcumin identified in vitro. On the other hand, insufficient bioactivation in vivo may underlie the inconclusive data in human studies. This may mean that healthy humans who exhibit a lower level of oxidative stress, may be less likely to experience benefits from the oxidative activation of curcumin. However, the oxidative stress theory of aging, which is based on the hypothesis that age-associated functional losses are due to the accumulation of NOROS-induced damages [58], joined with recent data on age-related inflammation (inflamm-age), may strongly favor the protective effects of curcumin in older age. Thus, before coming to any final conclusion, some molecular events related to curcumin's pro-oxidative capability, obtained in vitro, need to be addressed.

Recently published data on the anti-tumorigenic effects of curcumin on CML-derived human leukemic cells, in a xenograft model and in vitro culture system [59], confirmed, mostly indirectly, data obtained in experiments with oxidized curcumin metabolites [57]. In the leukemic cells treated with curcumin, the strong cytotoxic effect was joined with the strongest increase of ROS. On the other hand, when GSH was added into the system, the level of ROS was, expectedly, lower, as was the cytotoxic effect. The most probable explanation for these phenomena may be that GSH associated decrease of ROS consequentially leads to a decreased level of oxidized curcumin metabolites. As a consequence, the binding of curcumin to its potential protein-partners decreases. In the leukemic cell model, these protein-partners were shown to be metabolic enzymes, a few of which, like NQO1 (NAD(P)H Quinone Dehydrogenase 1), are well-known targets of the NRF2 (Nuclear Factor (Erythroid-Derived 2)-Like 2) transcription factor.

In addition to NQO-1, some other enzymes discovered as curcumin-binding partners, such as CBR1 (carbonyl reductase 1), GSTP1 (glutathione-S-transferase phi 1), AKR1C1 (aldo-keto reductase family 1 member 1), GLO1 (Glyoxalase I), exert their detoxifying function in the ROS-related metabolic pathway. It is not surprising then that ectopic overexpression of these enzymes led to the same effect as was gained with GSH: decreased level of ROS accompanied by a decrease in the curcumin's cytotoxic effect.

Curcumin and ROS-Producing Compounds

When contemplating these in vitro systems, one may ask whether oxidized curcumin metabolites lay in the background of commonly-recorded synergistic effects when applied with cytotoxic drugs, for example – with cisplatin [60]. It has been shown that in cancer cells cisplatin exposure induces a mitochondria-dependent increase in ROS levels [61]. This ROS may be the fuel for occurrence of oxidized curcumin metabolites, which may block the NF-κB signaling pathway (as already described) [57] and, additionally, decrease the activity of detoxifying enzymes through direct binding. This action probably includes balancing many factors, as curcumin (or its oxidative metabolites?) can restore *NRF2* transcription through demethylation of the *NRF2* promoter (first five CpGs positioned between -1086 and -1226) [62]. Then, on the other hand, curcumin uses its oxidized metabolites for binding to at least some protein targets of NRF2 (as is the case of NQO-1, which is considered as a *bona fide* NRF2 target) [63]. This is a good example of the complexity in the field and, as already mentioned, the necessity for multilevel research approach which needs to include as many as possible explorations of various interactions.

In considering the meaning of these recent discoveries, one should remember that, traditionally, various effective combinations of curcumin are, indeed, those which are based on its combination with the ROS-producing compounds. For example, oligomeric proanthocyanidins, which are known to exhibit anticancer properties are, in some studies, shown as ROS generation activators [64]. The effect seems to be cell-type-specific [65]. The combination of proanthocyanidins and curcumin was investigated in several models of colorectal cancer (cell lines, mice xenografts, colorectal cancer patient-derived organoids), where the combined application showed superior anticancer properties. It has been again shown that the expression of some very important genes/proteins remained intact when compounds were applied separately, while combined application induced a strong change in the activity of some genes. For example, a strong decrease of glucose-6-phosphate dehydrogenase (G6PD), a key enzyme in the Pentose Phosphate Pathway (PPP) was discovered [66]. Deficiency of G6PD was recognized to be associated with a lower cancer risk already in 1965 [67]. However, metabolic reprogramming was (officially) recognized as a hallmark of cancer many years later [22]. With respect to curcumin activity, metabolic reprogramming is becoming a hot topic of scientific interest.

4. Curcumin, Cancer and Metabolic Reprogramming

"Diffuse, evolutionary and developmental processes that we diagnose as cancer" [68], comprise, through initiation and progression of the disease, dynamic, stepwise changes in fundamental physiological characteristics of cells and tissues. A variety of stresses, either extrinsic (environmental) or intrinsic (genetic, epigenetic, metabolic), induce damage to cellular components that can lead to malignant transformation. Survival of damaged, potentially dangerous cells strongly depends on stress response pathways. One of the main barriers to propagation of cells that are at risk for malignant transformation is the onset of cellular senescence, a phenomenon that closely relates to cellular metabolism.

4.1. Cellular Senescence (CS), Hypoxia and Cancer Metabolic Plasticity

Cellular senescence represents stress response which is needed for permanent arrest of division of damaged cells. It is evolutionary well conserved, highly sophisticated and extremely complex. Although CS is of utmost importance in preventing proliferation of cells that are at risk of malignant transformation, the accumulation of senescent cells in aging tissues can compromise normal tissue microenvironment and facilitate cancer progression [69,70]. We are aware that the role of CS in molecular pathophysiology of many age-associated diseases, not only cancer, is multifaceted and can be detrimental.

Senescent cells are not inert. To the contrary, they are metabolically very active, and capable to secrete a plethora of bioactive molecules - pro-inflammatory cytokines and other factors which are able to change tissue structure. In the setting of cancer, they contribute in creating a cancer permissive microenvironment. Most anti-cancer therapeutic modalities promote senescence, which is beneficial for inhibiting tumor cell proliferation. But, at the same time, it is not selective and can induce senescence of adjacent non-tumor cells with consequential local inflammation, occurrence of secondary tumors and cancer relapse.

There are two hypotheses on the protumorigenic role of cellular senescence. According to a cell non-autonomous model, senescent cells secrete a variety of cytokines and factors which modify surrounding cells that have not fully entered senescence [71]. According to cell autonomous model, some senescent cells can bypass senescence and develop stem cell properties [72]. Malignant tumors are composed of a heterogeneous population of cells. This heterogeneity is not only based on genetically distinct subpopulations of tumor cells, but also on their functional heterogeneity.

Cancer is anything but a static system in terms of metabolism. A prominent characteristic of cancer cells is uncontrolled proliferation, which requires nutrients and energy to accommodate their augmented biosynthetic activity. The difference in glucose metabolism between normal and cancer cells was first noted by Otto Warburg [73]. He observed that cancer cells from ascites "ferment" glucose into lactate, even when enough oxygen, needed for supporting mitochondrial oxidative phosphorylation (OXPHOS), is available. Proliferative cancer cells exhibit a high rate of glycolysis, for meeting their high energetic and biosynthetic requirements. Although glycolysis is less efficient in producing ATP per molecule of glucose, high glycolytic flux may provide more cellular ATP from glycolysis than from OXPHOS. This is important for supporting cellular anabolic reactions [74–76]. Otto Warburg originally postulated that cancer cells acquire a defect in the mitochondria that disturbs aerobic respiration. We now know that, although mitochondrial function is often disturbed in cancer, cancer cells retain a substantial capacity to produce energy in the mitochondria.

Considering that rapid proliferation of tumor cells is not always adequately accompanied with vascularization of tumor mass, cancer cells are forced to adapt to nutrient- and oxygen-deprived environment. To do so, cancers select metabolically plastic cells, those with the highest capacity for metabolism reprogramming. This metabolic adaptivity supports cellular survival under different types of stress.

Cellular metabolic phenotype changes considerably as malignant tumors progress. In H-RasV12/E1A transformed fibroblasts, an increase in OXPHOS activity precedes the increase of glycolytic rate [77]. The strong mediator of this switch is transcription factor HIF-1α (Hypoxia-Inducible Factor 1α).

Permanent increase of ROS, a by-product of OXPHOS, has a major role in stabilizing HIF-1α and promoting aerobic glycolysis [78–80]. The stability of cellular HIF-1α is post-translationally regulated by O_2-, Fe^{2+}- and α-ketoglutarate - dependent hydroxylation of proline residues. Hydroxylation of HIF-1α promotes its ubiquitination and degradation, thereby preventing transcription of its target genes. An elevated level of cellular ROS oxidizes Fe^{2+} to Fe^{3+}, abolishes HIF-1α hydroxylation/ ubiquitination/degradation. As a consequence, HIF-1α accumulates in the cell [79] where it promotes pseudohypoxic state, permissive of mitochondrial dysfunction.

In Hep G2 hepatocellular carcinoma cells, application of curcumin led to a significant decrease of HIF-1α protein. It also suppressed its transcriptional activity under hypoxia, which resulted in decreased expression of vascular endothelial growth factor (VEGF), known as a major HIF-1 α target [81]. The most recent data point out the strong simultaneous inhibitory effect of polymeric nano-encapsulated curcumin on HIF-1α and REL A (P65; NFKB3), in lung and breast cancer cell lines [82]. Curcumin's inhibitory effects on gastric cancer in experimental animals were also shown to be dependent not only on HIF-1α/VEGF decrease (shown immunohistochemically), but also on decrease of STAT3 (Signal Transducer and Activator of Transcription 3) transcription factor [83].

What is the role of STAT3 in cellular metabolism, how it relates to inflammation and senescence, and, finally, what kind of influence curcumin may have in relation to this potent transcription factor?

4.2. Curcumin, STAT3, and Modes of Survival

Constitutively activated in various malignancies, STAT3 has an important role in inflammation-associated tumorigenesis [84]. It has recently been reported that curcumin inhibits highly active STAT3 in H-Ras transformed breast epithelial cells (H-Ras MCF10A), through direct binding to its cysteine residue 259. This cysteine (Cys) is critical for STAT3 phosphorylation, dimerization, nuclear translocation and DNA binding [85], upon activation by various cytokines, hormones and growth factors.

In addition to inflammation-associated tumorigenesis [86], STAT3 is mandatory for the survival of cells, which, upon bypassing oncogene-induced senescence in premalignant lesions, acquire stem cell properties. This was recently shown in a model of pancreatic cancer [87]. The mechanisms by which cells circumvent senescence in tumors that spontaneously develop from premalignant lesions are still not fully elucidated.

A prominent feature of senescent cells is STAT3 decrease, due to its proteasomal degradation [88]. Considering STAT3 involvement in promoting mitochondrial functions which are needed for cancer cell stemness and metabolic reprogramming, cancer cells that bypass senescence and acquire stem cell properties are sensitive to depletion and/or inactivation of STAT3. Napabucasin, a small molecule compound which was developed to inhibit several pathways in cancer stem cell-like cells, exerts at least some of its therapeutic activity through binding to the SH2 domain of STAT3 and, consequentially, suppresses STAT3 activity [89]. Accordingly, curcumin's binding to STAT3 Cys259 will result in multiple consequences, in addition to those which were recently discovered [85].

High level of STAT3 expression and its activity was recorded in metabolically plastic, glucose deprivation-resistant, ovarian cancer cells, accompanied by increased expression of metabolic genes *G6PD*, *GLUT1* (Glucose transporter 1) and *NNMT* (nicotinamide *N*-methyltransferase) [90]. In cancer stem cells (CSC) obtained from patients with epithelial ovarian cancer, glucose deprivation leads to enrichment of cells with a high rate of OXPHOS and PPP, joined with a high level of ROS [91]. These features represent cancer stem cell properties. High expression of GLUT1 in glucose deprivation-resistant cells allows them to utilize other sugars (D-fructose, D-arabinose, mannan, maltotriose and dextrin) and ketone bodies for energy production. Ketone bodies and lactic acid enter tricarboxylic acid (TCA) cycle to produce NADH (Nicotinamide Adenine Dinucleotide) and $FADH_2$ (Flavin Adenine Dinucleotide) that feed OXPHOS to generate ATP. Elevated OXPHOS activity leads to increased levels of ROS which needs to be counterbalanced by the activity of PPP. The rate-limiting enzyme in PPP is G6PD. It generates NADPH (Nicotinamide Adenine Dinucleotide Phosphate) needed to reduce oxidized glutathione to reduced glutathione, required for reduction of ROS (Figure 1).

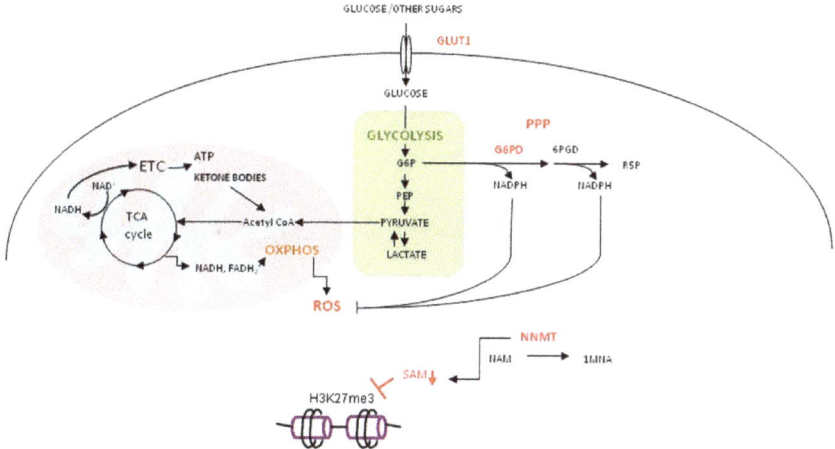

Figure 1. Derailed metabolism of cancer stem cell resistant to glucose deprivation. Metabolically plastic cancer cell, resistant to glucose deprivation, with high expression of GLUT1, G6PDH, G6PD and NNMT, reprograms metabolism to efficiently produce energy through utilization of sugars other than glucose (D-fructose, D-arabinose, mannan, maltotriose and dextrin), ketone bodies and lactate in OXPHOS. To counteract high level of ROS due to high OXPHOS, PPP is highly active. The upregulation of NNMT consumes methyl groups from S-adenosyl methionine (SAM) for methylation of nicotinamide (NAM). The level of SAM drops and hinders cellular methylation potential.

The role of NNMT in metabolic plasticity and cancer cell stemness is emerging. Contrary to the long-standing belief that the sole function of this enzyme is methylation of nicotinamide (NAM) and its excretion from the body, when in excess, NNMT is implicated in a plethora of important cellular processes [92]. This enzyme is overexpressed in various malignancies. In Hep G2 cells was shown that *NNMT* promoter activity depends on the activation of STAT3 [93]. The NNMT methylates NAM, creating a stable metabolic product 1-methylnicotinamide (1MNA). This reaction consumes methyl units from SAM. As a consequence, the methylation index (the ratio SAM/SAH; SAH - S-adenosylhomocysteine) of the cell changes. This way of acting puts NNMT in the central node involved in metabolic regulation of cellular methylation potential. Ulanovskaya et al. showed that 1MNA, rather than being an active, pro-tumorigenic metabolite, serves as "a stable sink" of methylation groups in cancer cells [94]. The NNMT activity has a strong, methionine concentration-dependent, impact on protein methylation. The effect on protein methylation has been observed only in the cells cultured with low methionine concentration (10-20 µM), while there was no effect in cells grown in high methionine concentration (100 µM) [94].

Likewise, the concentration of NAM varies in mammalian tissues and can impact the biological outcome of NNMT activity. In NAM-limited conditions, NNMT has a potential, in addition to negatively influencing methylation processes, to change the $NAD^+/NADH$ ratio. This is a consequence of the permanent loss of methylated NAM from the NAD^+ recycling process. Another very significant observation of this study [94] is that NNMT does not equally impact methylation processes of all biomolecules. Instead, the specificity of its targeting specific methylation pathways depends most probably on the relative K_m values of individual methyltransferases for SAM and SAH. Methyltransferases with higher K_m for SAM and SAH are more sensitive to the activity of NNMT [94]. Sperber et al. [95] reported high level of NNMT in naive human pluripotent stem cells (hPSC), in which it contributed to low values of SAM and H3K27me3. Down-regulation of NNMT caused naive to primed state transition in hPSC.

Considering that curcumin also has a negative effect on STAT3 phosphorylation [96], it is not surprising that it down-regulates expression of NNMT (MDA-MB-468 breast cancer cells and HT29 colon cancer cells) [93].

4.3. Oxidative Stress, Curcumin and Gerometabolite NAD⁺

The oxidative stress-induced pseudohypoxic state leads to depletion of "gerometabolites", small-molecule components of normal metabolism [97], and consequential decline in mitochondrial function [98,99]. One of the well-recognized gerometabolites is nicotinamide adenine dinucleotide, NAD^+ [97].

NAD^+ is an important co-factor in many metabolic reactions and is co-substrate for PARP-1 (Poly (ADP-Ribose) Polymerase 1) and SIRT1 (NAD-Dependent Deacetylase; Sirtuin-1), very important enzymes involved in cellular stress response [100]. We consider them as crucial nodes at the intersections of cellular metabolic and stress response pathways. For the cancer cell, adjustment of metabolic requirements must be precisely balanced with adequate stress response, as an imperative for survival. The pleiotropic activity of curcumin should be considered as a multilevel attack on this redundant cellular communication network in which "metabolic" meeting "inflammatory" and "oncogenic" serves as the basis for a unique cellular interactome, in accord with the postulates of Network Medicine [50].

4.4. Curcumin in Regulation of Metabolic and Stress Response Pathways

Curcumin supports cellular antioxidant defense through stimulating NRF2, a master regulator of ROS-scavenging enzymes. It has been shown that NRF2 may induce metabolic reprogramming by directing glucose and glutamine into the anabolic pathway. The activity of the anabolic pathway correlates with the presence of pyruvate kinase isozyme M2 (PKM2) [101]. The primary transcript of the *PKM* gene may be spliced in several different ways, and the mode of splicing is regulated by heterogeneous nuclear ribonucleoproteins (hnRNPs) [102]. The PKM1 transcript includes exon 10, while the PKM2 transcript contains part of intron 9 instead of exon 10. Of note, these two fragments are of the same length [103]. Functionally, two major protein isoforms, PKM1 (Isoform M1-PK; SwissProt Identifier P14618-2); and PKM2 (Isoform M2-PK; SwissProt Identifier P14618-1), may occur.

In contrast to the PKM1 isozyme which is normally expressed in differentiated cells, embryonic- and cancer-specific PKM2 confers a proliferative advantage to tumor cells. PKM2 can form dimers, with low activity, or active tetramers. Dimeric PKM2 diverts glucose metabolism towards aerobic glycolysis, thereby supporting biosynthetic processes, while tetrameric PKM2 promotes ATP production via OXPHOS. Since biosynthetic and energetic requirements of highly proliferative cancer cells should be simultaneously met and well adjusted, the ratio of PKM2 dimers and tetramers is critical for tumorigenesis [104]. This metabolic switch, dependent on the active axis PI3K-AKT, a part of the receptor tyrosine kinase/PI3K/AKT/mammalian target of rapamycin (RTK/PI3K/AKT/mTOR) signaling pathway, accelerates tumor proliferation and contributes to its aggressiveness [105].

Tumor cells with constitutively activated K-ras oncogenic signaling have upregulated PKM2, which is mandatory for accumulating phosphoenolpyruvate (PEP), its shunting to an alternative glycolytic pathway and utilization for anabolic processes [106]. Despite the stimulatory effect on NRF2, curcumin antagonizes metabolic reprogramming towards glycolysis (Figure 2). One of the mechanisms involved in this process is curcumin-mediated negative regulation of TNF-α, with consequent prevention of inflammatory environment-induced onset of aerobic glycolysis. Thus, curcumin makes yet another link between inflammation and metabolism. This mechanism was shown in breast epithelial cells [107]. The same negative impact of curcumin toward glycolysis was shown in Dalton's lymphoma, in mice [108].

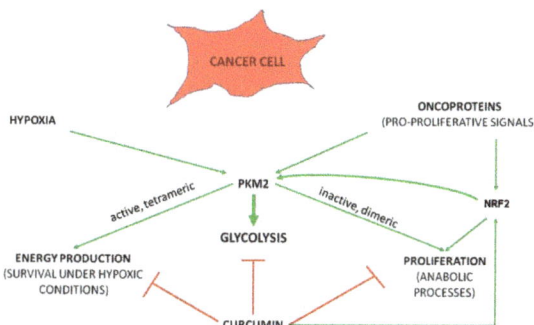

Figure 2. The principle underlying antitumorigenic effect of curcumin. Curcumin targets cellular processes central to the ability of cancer cell to survive by coordinately hindering aerobic glycolysis-dependent anabolic processes and energy production, despite of stimulating NRF2.

The unrestricted proliferative potential of cancer cells is closely dependent on PI3K/AKT/mTOR signaling pathway [109]. For example, mTOR activation in cancer cells upregulates the expression of PKM2 through HIF-1α mediated transcriptional activation of *PKM*, and Myc-hnRNPs-mediated splicing of PKM pre-mRNA, in favor of PKM2. In a nude mouse xenograft tumor model, stable knock down of PKM2 in PC3 cells (a human prostate cancer cell line with PTEN deficiency and mTOR hyperactivation) significantly extended the survival of tumor-bearing mice [110]. Silencing of PKM2 (transduction with *shPKM2*) suppresses mTOR-mediated tumorigenesis [110]. Due to the (a) dependence of PKM2 on mTOR activation and (b) mTOR-mediated cancer cell proliferation associated with PKM2 shunting PEP into alternative glycolytic pathway supporting anabolic processes, cancer cells with hyperactive mTOR are particularly sensitive to dual inhibition of mTOR and glycolysis [111].

One of the prominent features of the multifaceted antitumorigenic effects of curcumin is its ability to simultaneously inhibit glycolysis and mTOR [112]. Recently, it has been shown that 20 μM curcumin inhibits glucose uptake and down-regulates PKM2 and lactate production in various cancer cell lines (H1299, MCF-7, HeLa and PC3) [113]. In curcumin-treated cells, decreased phosphorylation of p70S6 kinase (T389) was associated with the concomitant lowering of HIF-1α protein expression. The involvement of mTOR/HIF-1α signaling inhibition, in curcumin-mediated down-regulation of PKM2 expression, was further validated by the observation that rapamycin, a well-known mTOR inhibitor, likewise down-regulates PKM2 [113]. In addition to a negative effect on PKM2 expression, curcumin treatment, in the stated cellular models, caused decreased expression of glucose transporter GLUT1 and hexokinase II (HKII) transcripts. In HCT116 and HT29 colon cancer cells, curcumin has previously been reported to down-regulate HKII, the enzyme which catalyzes the first step in glycolysis—phosphorylation of glucose to form glucose-6-phosphate [114]. Finally, in esophageal squamous cell carcinoma EC109 cells, curcumin down-regulates the expression of glycolytic enzymes, in dose- and AMPK (AMP-Activated Kinase) -dependent manner [115].

These data indicate that the actions of curcumin are highly dependent on the context of intrinsic cellular makeup, encompassing genetic, epigenetic, metabolic and cell proliferation status, together with external influences (microenvironmental cues). All these factors may also modulate its ability for binding to various cellular proteins.

4.5. Metabolic Enzymes as Targets for Curcumin Binding

Approximately 60 proteins—curcumin's binding partners, were discovered after incubating the HEI-193 human schwannoma cells with a very high concentration of biotinylated curcumin (1 mg/mL – 2.71 mM) for 30 min. The most abundant binding partners were heat shock proteins (HSPs) -70 and -90, molecular chaperones involved in the proper folding of client proteins, 3-phosphoglycerate dehydrogenase (PHDGH) and β-actin [116]. Abegg and collaborators profiled 42 proteins, covalently bound to curcumin through their cysteine residues, in HeLa cervical cancer cells [117]. A relatively small subset of Cys residues has been considered to be involved in cell signaling (contrary to "sensing") [118]. However, curcumin's binding to cysteine residues of metabolic enzymes may be very important for cellular reprogramming mechanisms.

A recently published paper [119] on in situ proteomic profiling of curcumin targets in HCT116 colon cancer cell line, reports a list of 197 curcumin-binding proteins, among which are many cancer-related metabolic enzymes: GAPDH (Glyceraldehyde 3-Phosphate Dehydrogenase), PKM isozymes M1/M2, LDHA (L-Lactate Dehydrogenase A), MDH1/2 (cytoplasmic/mitochondrial Malate Dehydrogenase), SHMT2 (Serine Hydroxymethyltransferase; mitochondrial), ADP/ATP translocase 1. Additionally, curcumin targets PARP-1, NAD^+ -consuming enzyme involved in numerous cellular processes including DNA-damage detection and repair, transcription and intracellular localization and activity of many proteins. Binding to numerous hnRNPs, including the alternative splicing repressors hnRNP A1/A2 which influence PKM splicing [103], point to the possible role of curcumin in regulating alternative splicing. So far, its influence on splicing was shown in fibroblasts from patients with SMA type II (Survival of Motor Neuron 2) in which curcumin increased the proportion of *SMN2*_exon 7-containing transcript [120].

How curcumin binding to its protein targets influences their activity is mostly unknown. The SiteMap calculation performed by Angelo et al. [116] predicted the binding of curcumin to NAD^+ binding site on PHGDH, which is crucial for PHGDH enzymatic activity. The curcumin binding enzymes, PHGDH and SHMT2, belong to the serine-glycine metabolic pathway. Both amino acids, serine and glycine, serve as intermediates for the biosynthesis of other amino acids, nucleic acids and lipids. What is the possible scenario of curcumin's binding to these enzymes?

Phosphoglycerate Dehydrogenase and Serine Hydroxymethyltransferase 2

PHGDH, the first, rate-limiting enzyme in the pathway of serine biosynthesis, catalyzes the transition of 3-phosphoglycerate (3PG) into 3-phosphohydroxypyruvate, using NAD^+/NADH as a cofactor. Shunting of the glycolytic intermediate 3PG to serine synthesis is permitted by PKM2. Low activity of PKM2 in tumor cells leads to an accumulation of its substrate PEP, which participates in phosphorylation and the catalytic activation of phosphoglycerate mutase (PGAM1) [106]. As a consequence, there is an increase of its product, 2-phosphoglycerate, which activates PHGDH and serine biosynthesis [121].

PHGDH protein level is elevated in 70% of estrogen receptor (ER)-negative breast cancers and suppression of PHGDH in breast cancer cell lines decreases cell proliferation and reduces serine synthesis [122]. In addition to increasing PHGDH, an increase of nicotinamide phosphoribosyltransferase (NAMPT), a rate-limiting enzyme of NAD^+ salvage pathway, was also shown in ER-negative breast cancer lines and patient-derived breast tumors [123]. Their interconnection was shown experimentally on $PHGDH^{high}$MDA-MB-468 and $PHGDH^{low}$ MDA-MB-231 breast cancer cells by treating them with well-established NAMPT inhibitor (FK866). This treatment caused a drop in NAD^+ level and almost completely abrogated serine synthesis in $PHGDH^{high}$MDA-MB-468 cells, while the drop in NAD^+ level and serine synthesis was insignificant in $PHGDH^{low}$ MDA-MB-231 cells [123].

Although pursued in cancer treatment, NAD^+ salvage pathway inhibitors exert various efficacy. Thus, it was suggested that NAMPT inhibitors may be effective for treating a subset of PHGDH-dependent cancers [123]. Therefore, it is possible that curcumin, in addition to inhibiting PHGDH directly by binding to its NAD^+ pocket [116], hinders its activity indirectly by down-regulating expression of NAMPT (also known as visfatin) as has been demonstrated in breast cancer cell lines (MDA-MB-231, MDA-MB-468, and MCF-7) [124]. Knocking down PHGDH in HeLa cells significantly inhibited cell proliferation and increased cisplatin chemosensitivity [125].

Serine can be directly converted to glycine by two serine hydroxymethyltransferases: cytoplasmic (SHMT1) and mitochondrial (SHMT2). SHMT2 is the main source of glycine in proliferating cells [126] and its importance for tumor cells survival in hypoxia was demonstrated in glioblastoma multiforme (GM) [127].

Competent eukaryotic SHMT2 is a tetrameric protein built as dimers of "tight" dimers which correspond to its minimal catalytic active units. A dimer-to-tetramer transition is triggered by the binding of the isozyme SHMT2 cofactor, pyridoxal 5′-phosphate (PLP) [128]. Curcumin-binding Cys80 [116] indirectly influences the formation of the binding site for PLP, through interacting with residues Arg283 and Gly284 to Arg286 (Figure 3). Cys80 also participates in protein-protein interaction of the tight dimer, through interacting with Asn93 of the other chain. Thus, covalent binding of curcumin to Cys80 may be expected to impact both, the structure and the catalytic activity of the active form of SHMT2.

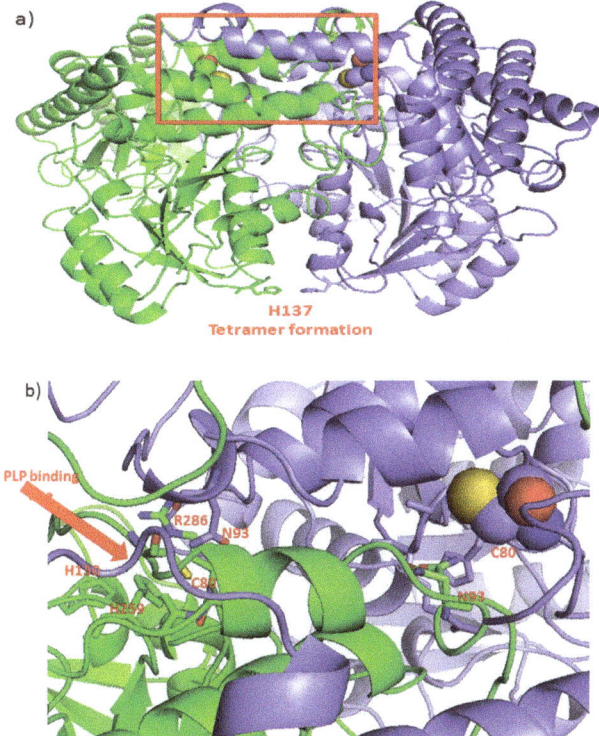

Figure 3. Possible effects of curcumin's binding to SHMT2 Cys80. (**a**) The symmetric dimer of SHMT2 (PDB: 4PVF) showing amino acid residues Cys80 (spheres) and His137 (sticks) participated in the tetramer formation [128]. Monomers are shown in green and purple. (**b**) The part of the 4PVF structure within red rectangular in (**a**), with marked amino acid residues making interactions with the nonmodified Cys80. The pyridoxal 5′-phosphate (PLP) binding site is encompassed by marked His150 and His259.

As recently described in GM, SHMT2 activity limits the activity of PKM2 and reduces oxygen consumption, thereby eliciting a metabolic state permissive of tumor cells survival in poorly vascularized tumor regions. It is plausible to expect that curcumin's binding to Cys80 may hinder formation of SHMT2 tetramers, inhibit SHMT2 activity and prevent PKM2-mediated metabolic reprogramming, needed for facilitating cell survival in hypoxia [127]. The negative effect of elevated SHMT2 activity on PKM2 may stem from the increased catabolism of serine, a known PKM2 activator [129]. Transformation of serine in the mitochondria by SHMT2 increases the cellular NADPH/NADP$^+$ ratio and decreases ROS production [130]. Consistent with its pro-survival role under hypoxia and its role in limiting ROS, SHMT2 was recently identified as a potential cancer driver gene [131].

5. Potential for Therapeutic Application?

The amplification of the chromosomal locus (1p12) containing the *PHGDH* gene, has been reported in melanomas and triple-negative breast cancers [132]. The enzyme has been recognized as a potential therapeutic target for NAD-competitive inhibitors in PHGDH-amplified breast cancer [133]. In renal carcinoma, in which PHGDH represents the key regulator of the HIF-2α pathway, targeted inactivation of PHGDH may be promising for treating patients resistant to HIF-2α antagonists [134].

When considering PHGDH prognostic significance in a broad context, bioinformatic analysis of human breast and lung cancer mRNA data sets found high *PHGDH* expression to be a negative prognostic marker in breast cancer patients in seven out of 17 breast cancer datasets [135]. However, the increased expression of the PHGDH mRNA did not appear to have any prognostic value in seven analyzed lung cancer datasets, highlighting the importance of the cell-specific molecular background as the key determinant for activating specific signaling pathways. The level of their dependency on specific molecules/enzymes should be put in the context of redundant signaling mediators, the presence of which is, again, cell-type specific.

The fact that high expression of *SHMT2* in 10 out of 17 breast cancer datasets predicted negative prognosis, seems to be in accord with this presumption. Four breast cancer datasets shared both enzymes, PHGDH and SHMT2, as negative prognostic factors. Finally, NRF2 has an important role in transcriptional regulation of genes coding for these enzymes, in ATF4-dependent fashion. As shown in the model of non-small cell lung cancer (NSCLC), high expression of NRF2, joined with high expression of both PHGDH and SHMT2, represents the clinical marker of the poor outcome [136].

Increased SHMT2 positively correlates with the breast cancer grade [137] and is associated with worse relapse-free survival (RFS), distant metastases, and overall survival (OS) in breast cancer patients ($N = 801$) [131]. Similarly, high SHMT2 expression in hepatocellular carcinoma (HCC) significantly correlates with decreased OS, lymph node metastases and HCC grade [138]. For exerting its activity, the SHMT2 must interact with sirtuin SIRT5 which desuccinylates SHMT2, at lysine 280. This modification seems to be critical for SHMT2 active involvement in tumor growth [139]. This is a good example of the complexity in the field and, as already mentioned, is necessary for the multilevel ways of research that need to include as many explorations as possible of various interactions.

6. Conclusions

The complex hierarchy in regulating inflamm-aging related pathological network is still incompletely understood, notwithstanding ever-increasing knowledge regarding every part of the process.

A recent report showing that curcumin acts as a prodrug, while its oxidative metabolites may bind to various cellular proteins, is of a great importance for understanding curcumin's action in various pathological conditions/diseases. Discovery of various proteins to which curcumin can bind adds an additional challenge for understanding all modalities resulting from its pleiotropic actions. In this review, we have dedicated a great deal of attention to cancer, which represents a disease of derailed metabolic and signaling pathways which are tightly interwoven. We have yet to discover molecules or processes which supervise and are indispensable for the establishment of an oncometabolic network comprising malignantly transformed and surrounding „normal" cells. With respect to an approach to therapy, personalized medicine has made great progress. However, developing an integrated approach, in which personalized medicine is applied as much as possible, will present a very demanding task for the future. Taking into account that the most prominent feature of cancer cells - uncontrolled division - relies on numerous, mutually and closely inter-dependent pathways, the critical nodes in this pro-proliferative, oncometabolic network must be identified and combated, according to proposed rules postulated by Network Medicine.

Since these crucial regulatory nodes are diverse and exist at several levels, the introduction of a pleiotropic molecule, as a part of the therapeutic effort, would make sense. Such a pleiotropic molecule should be able to selectively maintain the homeostatic network in normal cells, while attacking cancer cells through affecting the „unbalanced" state to which they are addicted. This is a very demanding task, asking for much knowledge and dedication to the challenge posed.

Curcumin may have features needed to help meet this challenge. In this review, we have tried to present the most current data from a perspective that would enable establishing connections and functional links between the specifics of inflamm-aging and the cancer cell's metabolism, its proliferative potential, and curcumin's pleiotropic activity. We believe that it opens the door to a wide range of therapeutic opportunities for targeting cell-type specific nodes as crucial points for targeting a functional oncometabolic signaling network, while recognizing that other aspects need to be studied.

Author Contributions: R.N.K.: wrote the sub-chapter on metabolic aspects of curcumin's action and created two illustrations related to this topic; V.S.: made the structural analysis of SHMT2, wrote the corresponding part of the text and made the corresponding figure; LM: wrote part of the sub-chapter on combined applications of curcumin; A.C.G.—wrote part of the sub-chapter on curcumin as an oxidant and sorted part of the references; M.T.—profiled the relevant statistical data and the literature related to the introductory part of the manuscript; made a partial sorting of the references; K.G.T.—developed the concept for the article, wrote the introduction and chapters on inflamm-aging and oxidative metabolites of curcumin; made relevant functional links; made a final sorting and checking of all literature and data.

Funding: This work is entirely supported by the Croatian Science Foundation under its grant: IP-2016-06-4404; NRF2 at the crossroads of epigenetic remodeling, metabolism and proliferation of cancer cells; KGT—PI.

Acknowledgments: The authors are grateful to Aaron Etra for his work on English editing, and Djurdjica Ugarkovic and Vanja Fenzl for critical reading and valuable suggestions.

Conflicts of Interest: The authors declare no conflict of interest.

Abbreviations

1MNA	1-Methylnicotinamide
3-PG	3-Phosphoglycerate
AD	Alzheimer's Disease
AMPK	AMP-Activated Kinase
ATP	Adenosine Triphosphate
CBR1	Carbonyl Reductase 1
CRP	C-Reactive Protein
CS	Cellular Senescence
CSC	Cancer Stem Cells
ER	Estrogen Receptor
$FADH_2$	Flavin Adenine Dinucleotide
G6PD	Glucose-6-Phosphate Dehydrogenase
GAPDH	Glyceraldehyde 3-Phosphate Dehydrogenase
GM	Glioblastoma Multiforme
GLUT 1	Glucose Transporter 1
GSH	Glutathione
GSTP1	Glutathione-S-Transferase Phi 1
HCC	Hepatocellular Carcinoma
HIF-1α	Hypoxia-Inducible Factor 1α
HKII	Hexokinase II
HNC	Head and Neck Carcinoma

IKK b	Inhibitor of Nuclear Factor Kappa-B Kinase Subunit Beta
IL-17R	IL-17 Receptor
LDHA	L-Lactate Dehydrogenase A
MBN	MidBrain Neuron
MCP-1	Monocyte Chemoattractant Protein-1
MDH	Malate Dehydrogenase
MMP-2	Matrix Metalloproteinase 2
NADH/NAD$^+$	Nicotinamide Adenine Dinucleotide
NADPH/NADP$^+$	Nicotinamide Adenine Dinucleotide Phosphate
NAM	Nicotinamide
NAMPT	Nicotinamide Phosphoribosyltransferase
NF-κB	Nuclear Factor Kappa-Light-Chain-Enhancer of Activated B Cells
NNMT	Nicotinamide N-Methyltransferase
NOROS	Nitric Oxide and Reactive Oxygen Species
NQO-1	NAD(P)H Quinone Dehydrogenase 1
NRF2	Nuclear Factor (Erythroid-Derived 2)-Like 2
OS	Overall Survival
OXPHOS	Oxidative Phosphorylation
PARP-1	Poly (ADP-Ribose) Polymerase 1
PD	Parkinson's Disease
PEP	Phosphoenolpyruvate
PGAM1	Phosphoglycerate Mutase
PKM	Pyruvate Kinase
PPP	Pentose Phosphate Pathway
PR	Progesterone Receptor
R5P	Ribulose 5-Phosphate
RFS	Relapse Free Survival
ROS	Reactive Oxygen Species
SAH	S-Adenosylhomocysteine
SAM	S-Adenosylmethionine
SEMF	Subepithelial Myofibroblast
SHMT2	Serine Hidroxymethyltransferase 2
STAT3	Signal Transducer and Activator of Transcription 3
TCA	Tricarboxylic Acid
TGF-b	Transforming Growth Factor Beta
TNF-a	Tumor Necrosis Factor-Alpha
VEGF	Vascular Endothelial Growth Factor

References

1. *World Health Statistics 2018: Monitoring Health for the SDGs, Sustainable Development Goals*; World Health Organization: Geneva, Switzerland, 2018; Licence: CC BY-NC-SA 3.0 IGO. Available online: https://apps.who.int/iris/bitstream/handle/10665/272596/9789241565585-eng.pdf?ua=1 (accessed on 17 January 2019).
2. United Nations, Department of Economic and Social Affairs, Population Division. *World Population Prospects: The 2017 Revision, Key Findings and Advance Tables*; Working Paper No. ESA/P/WP/248; United Nations, Department of Economic and Social Affairs, Population Division, 2017. Available online: https://esa.un.org/unpd/wpp/publications/files/wpp2017_keyfindings.pdf (accessed on 22 January 2019).
3. Virchow, R. *Die Cellularpathologie in Ihrer Begründung auf Physiologische und Pathologische Gewebelehre*; A. Hirschwald: Berlin, Germany, 1859; pp. 174, 441.
4. Balkwill, F.; Mantovani, A. Inflammation and cancer: Back to Virchow? *Lancet* **2001**, *357*, 539–545. [CrossRef]
5. Dvorak, H.F. Tumors: Wounds that do not heal. Similarities between tumor stroma generation and wound healing. *N. Engl. J. Med.* **1986**, *315*, 1650–1659. [PubMed]
6. Schäfer, M.; Werner, S. Oxidative stress in normal and impaired wound repair. *Pharmacol. Res.* **2008**, *58*, 165–171. [CrossRef] [PubMed]

7. Kasuya, A.; Tokura, Y. Attempts to accelerate wound healing. *J. Dermatol. Sci.* **2014**, *76*, 169–172. [CrossRef] [PubMed]
8. Franceschi, C.; Capri, M.; Monti, D.; Giunta, S.; Olivieri, F.; Sevini, F.; Panourgia, M.P.; Invidia, L.; Celani, L.; Scurti, M.; et al. Inflammaging and anti-inflammaging: A systemic perspective on aging and longevity emerged from studies in humans. *Mech. Ageing Dev.* **2007**, *128*, 92–105. [CrossRef] [PubMed]
9. Rea, I.M.; Gibson, D.S.; McGilligan, V.; McNerlan, S.E.; Alexander, H.D.; Ross, O.A. Age and Age-Related Diseases: Role of inflammation triggers and cytokines. *Front. Immunol.* **2018**, *9*, 586. Available online: https://www.ncbi.nlm.nih.gov/pmc/articles/PMC5900450/ (accessed on 22 November 2018). [CrossRef] [PubMed]
10. Michaud, M.; Balardy, L.; Moulis, G.; Gaudin, C.; Peyrot, C.; Vellas, B.; Cesari, M.; Nourhashemi, F. Proinflammatory cytokines, aging, and age-related diseases. *J. Am. Med. Dir. Assoc.* **2013**, *14*, 877–882. [CrossRef]
11. Bray, F.; Ferlay, J.; Soerjomataram, I.; Siegel, R.L.; Torre, L.A.; Jemal, A. Global cancer statistics 2018: GLOBOCAN estimates of incidence and mortality worldwide for 36 cancers in 185 countries. *CA Cancer J. Clin.* **2018**, *68*, 394–424. [CrossRef]
12. Ferlay, J.; Ervik, M.; Lam, F.; Colombet, M.; Mery, L.; Piñeros, M.; Znaor, A.; Soerjomataram, I.; Bray, F. *Global Cancer Observatory: Cancer Tomorrow*; International Agency for Research on Cancer: Lyon, France, 2018. Available online: https://gco.iarc.fr/tomorrow (accessed on 12 January 2019).
13. Surh, Y.J.; Lee, E.; Lee, J.M. Chemoprotective properties of some pungent ingredients present in red pepper and ginger. *Mutat. Res.* **1998**, *402*, 259–267. [CrossRef]
14. Lee, W.-H.; Loo, C.-Y.; Bebawy, M.; Luk, F.; Mason, R.S.; Rohanizadeh, R. Curcumin and its derivatives: Their application in neuropharmacology and neuroscience in the 21st century. *Curr. Neuropharmacol.* **2013**, *11*, 338–378. [CrossRef]
15. Esatbeyoglu, T.; Huebbe, P.; Ernst, I.M.A.; Chin, D.; Wagner, A.E.; Rimbach, G. Curcumin-From molecule to biological function. *Angew. Chem. Int. Ed.* **2012**, *51*, 5308–5332. [CrossRef] [PubMed]
16. Global Market Insights. Report ID: GMI788. Available online: https://www.gminsights.com/industry-analysis/curcumin-market (accessed on 20 December 2018).
17. Oppenheimer, A. Turmeric (curcumin) in biliary diseases. *Lancet* **1937**, *229*, 619–621. [CrossRef]
18. Ammon, H.P.; Wahl, M.A. Pharmacology of curcuma longa. *Planta Med.* **1991**, *57*, 1–7. [CrossRef] [PubMed]
19. Smith, B.D.; Smith, G.L.; Hurria, A.; Hortobagyi, G.N.; Buchholz, T.A. Future of cancer incidence in the United States: Burdens upon an aging, changing nation. *J. Clin. Oncol.* **2009**, *27*, 2758–2765. [CrossRef] [PubMed]
20. Siegel, R.L.; Miller, K.D.; Jemal, A. Cancer Statistics, 2019. *CA Cancer J. Clin.* **2019**, *69*, 7–34. [CrossRef] [PubMed]
21. Nolen, S.C.; Evans, M.A.; Fischer, A.; Corrada, M.M.; Kawas, C.H.; Bota, D.A. Cancer-Incidence, prevalence and mortality in the oldest-old. A comprehensive review. *Mech. Ageing Dev.* **2017**, *164*, 113–126. [CrossRef]
22. Hanahan, D.; Weinberg, R. Hallmarks of cancer: The next generation. *Cell* **2011**, *144*, 646–674. [CrossRef]
23. Varkaris, A.; Katsiampoura, A.; Davis, J.S.; Shah, N.; Lam, M.; Frias, R.L.; Ivan, C.; Shimizu, M.; Morris, J.; Menter, D.; et al. Circulating inflammation signature predicts overall survival and relapse-free survival in metastatic colorectal cancer. *Br. J. Cancer* **2019**, *120*, 340–345. [CrossRef]
24. Vainer, N.; Dehlendorff, C.; Johansen, J.S. Systematic literature review of IL-6 as a biomarker or treatment target in patients with gastric, bile duct, pancreatic and colorectal cancer. *Oncotarget* **2018**, *9*, 29820–29841. Available online: http://www.oncotarget.com/index.php?journal=oncotarget&page=article&op=view&path[]=25661&pubmed-linkout=1 (accessed on 28 December 2018). [CrossRef]
25. Sirniö, P.; Väyrynen, J.P.; Klintrup, K.; Mäkelä, J.; Karhu, T.; Herzig, K.H.; Minkkinen, I.; Mäkinen, M.J.; Karttunen, T.J.; Tuomisto, A. Alterations in serum amino-acid profile in the progression of colorectal cancer: Associations with systemic inflammation, tumour stage and patient survival. *Br. J. Cancer* **2019**, *120*, 238–246. [CrossRef]
26. Kempuraj, D.; Thangavel, R.; Natteru, P.A.; Selvakumar, G.P.; Saeed, D.; Zahoor, H.; Zaheer, S.; Iyer, S.S.; Zaheer, A. Neuroinflammation induces neurodegeneration. *J. Neurol. Neurosurg. Spine* **2016**, *1*, 1003. Available online: https://www.ncbi.nlm.nih.gov/pmc/articles/PMC5260818/ (accessed on 11 January 2019). [PubMed]

27. Giunta, B.; Fernandez, F.; Nikolic, W.V.; Obregon, D.; Rrapo, E.; Town, T.; Tan, J. Inflammaging as a prodrome to Alzheimer's Disease. *J. Neuroinflamm.* **2008**, *5*, 51. Available online: https://jneuroinflammation.biomedcentral.com/articles/10.1186/1742-2094-5-51 (accessed on 13 November 2018). [CrossRef] [PubMed]
28. Calabrese, V.; Santoro, A.; Monti, D.; Crupi, R.; Di Paola, R.; Latteri, S.; Cuzzocrea, S.; Zappia, M.; Giordano, J.; Calabrese, E.J.; et al. Aging and Parkinson's disease: Inflammaging, neuroinflammation and biological remodeling as key factors in pathogenesis. *Free Radic. Biol. Med.* **2018**, *115*, 80–91. [CrossRef] [PubMed]
29. Boyko, A.A.; Troyanova, N.I.; Kovalenko, E.I.; Sapozhnikov, A.M. Similarity and differences in inflammation-related characteristics of the peripheral immune system of patients with Parkinson's and Alzheimer's diseases. *Int. J. Mol. Sci.* **2017**, *18*, 2633. Available online: https://www.mdpi.com/1422-0067/18/12/2633 (accessed on 13 November 2018). [CrossRef] [PubMed]
30. Xia, Y.; Yeddula, N.; Leblanc, M.; Ke, E.; Zhang, Y.; Oldfield, E.; Shaw, R.J.; Verma, I.M. Reduced cell proliferation by IKK2 depletion in a mouse lung-cancer model. *Nat. Cell Biol.* **2012**, *14*, 257–265. [CrossRef] [PubMed]
31. Wang, B.; Zhao, C.-H.; Sun, G.; Zhang, Z.-W.; Qian, B.-M.; Zhu, Y.-F.; Cai, M.-Y.; Pandey, S.; Zhao, D.; Wang, Y.-W.; et al. IL-17 induces the proliferation and migration of glioma cells through the activation of PI3K/Akt1/NF-κB-p65. *Cancer Lett.* **2019**, *447*, 93–104. [CrossRef]
32. Hata, K.; Andoh, A.; Shimada, M.; Fujino, S.; Bamba, S.; Araki, Y.; Okuno, T.; Fujiyama, Y.; Bamba, T. IL-17 stimulates inflammatory responses via NF-kappaB and MAP kinase pathways in human colonic myofibroblasts. *Am. J. Physiol. Gastrointest. Liver Physiol.* **2002**, *282*, G1035–G1044. [CrossRef]
33. Sommer, A.; Maxreiter, F.; Krach, F.; Fadler, T.; Grosch, J.; Maroni, M.; Graef, D.; Eberhardt, E.; Riemenschneider, M.J.; Yeo, G.W.; et al. Th17 lymphocytes induce neuronal cell death in a human iPSC-based model of Parkinson's disease. *Cell Stem Cell* **2018**, *23*, 123–131. [CrossRef]
34. Zhang, J.; Ke, K.F.; Liu, Z.; Qiu, Y.H.; Peng, Y.P. Th17 cell-mediated neuroinflammation is involved in neurodegeneration of aβ1-42-induced Alzheimer's disease model rats. *PLoS ONE* **2013**, *8*, e75786. Available online: https://www.ncbi.nlm.nih.gov/pmc/articles/PMC3790825/ (accessed on 3 December 2018). [CrossRef]
35. Li, T.-J.; Jiang, Y.-M.; Hu, Y.-F.; Huang, L.; Yu, J.; Zhao, L.-Y.; Deng, H.-J.; Mou, T.-Y.; Liu, H.; Yang, Y.; et al. Interleukin-17-producing neutrophils link inflammatory stimuli to disease progression by promoting angiogenesis in gastric cancer. *Clin. Cancer Res.* **2017**, *23*, 1575–1585. [CrossRef]
36. Lee, M.-H.; Chang, J.T.-C.; Liao, C.-T.; Chen, Y.-S.; Kuo, M.-L.; Shen, C.-R. Interleukin 17 and peripheral IL-17-expressing T cells are negatively correlated with the overall survival of head and neck cancer patients. *Oncotarget* **2018**, *9*, 9825–9837. Available online: http://www.oncotarget.com/index.php?journal=oncotarget&page=article&op=view&path[]=23934&pubmed-linkout=1 (accessed on 4 December 2018). [CrossRef] [PubMed]
37. Latimer, B.; Ekshyyan, O.; Nathan, N.; Moore-Medlin, T.; Rong, X.; Ma, X.; Khandelwal, A.; Christy, H.T.; Abreo, F.; McClure, G.; et al. Enhanced systemic bioavailability of curcumin through transmucosal administration of a novel microgranular formulation. *Anticancer Res.* **2015**, *35*, 6411–6418. Available online: http://ar.iiarjournals.org/content/35/12/6411.long (accessed on 4 December 2018). [PubMed]
38. Verma, S.P.; Goldin, B.R.; Lin, P.S. The inhibition of the estrogenic effects of pesticides and environmental chemicals by curcumin and isoflavonoids. *Environ. Health Perspect.* **1998**, *106*, 807–812. [CrossRef] [PubMed]
39. Shao, Z.M.; Shen, Z.Z.; Liu, C.H.; Sartippour, M.R.; Go, V.L.; Heber, D.; Nguyen, M. Curcumin exerts multiple suppressive effects on human breast carcinoma cells. *Int. J. Cancer* **2002**, *98*, 234–240. [CrossRef] [PubMed]
40. Leone, B.A.; Leone, J.; Leone, J.P. Breast cancer is a systemic disease rather than an anatomical process. *Breast Cancer Res. Treat.* **2017**, *161*, 619. [CrossRef] [PubMed]
41. Morris, P.G.; Hudis, C.A.; Giri, D.; Morrow, M.; Falcone, D.J.; Zhou, X.K.; Du, B.; Brogi, E.; Crawford, C.B.; Kopelovich, L.; et al. Inflammation and increased aromatase expression occur in the breasttissue of obese women with breast cancer. *Cancer Prev. Res.* **2011**, *4*, 1021–1029. [CrossRef]
42. Brown, K.A.; Iyengar, N.M.; Zhou, X.K.; Gucalp, A.; Subbaramaiah, K.; Wang, H.; Giri, D.D.; Morrow, M.; Falcone, D.J.; Wendel, N.K.; et al. Menopause is a determinant of breast aromatase expression and its associations with BMI, inflammation, and systemic markers. *J. Clin. Endocrinol. Metab.* **2017**, *102*, 1692–1701. [CrossRef]

43. Key, T.J.; Appleby, P.N.; Reeves, G.K.; Roddam, A.; Dorgan, J.F.; Longcope, C.; Stanczyk, F.Z.; Stephenson, H.E., Jr.; Falk, R.T.; Miller, R.; et al. Body mass index, serum sex hormones, and breast cancer risk in postmenopausal women. *J. Natl. Cancer Inst.* **2003**, *95*, 1218–1226.
44. Nicklas, B.J.; Rogus, E.M.; Colman, E.G.; Goldberg, A.P. Visceral adiposity, increased adipocyte lipolysis, and metabolic dysfunction in obese postmenopausal women. *Am. J. Physiol.* **1996**, *270*, E72–E78. [CrossRef]
45. Nguyen, M.T.; Favelyukis, S.; Nguyen, A.K.; Reichart, D.; Scott, P.A.; Jenn, A.; Liu-Bryan, R.; Glass, C.K.; Neels, J.G.; Olefsky, J.M. A subpopulation of macrophages infiltrates hypertrophic tissue and is activated by free fatty acids via Toll-likereceptors 2 and 4 and JNK-dependent pathways. *J. Biol. Chem.* **2007**, *282*, 35279–35292. [CrossRef]
46. Subbaramaiah, K.; Sue, E.; Bhardwaj, P.; Du, B.; Hudis, C.A.; Giri, D.; Kopelovich, L.; Zhou, X.K.; Dannenberg, A.J. Dietary polyphenols suppress elevated levels of proinflammatory mediators and aromatase in the mammary gland of obese mice. *Cancer Prev. Res.* **2013**, *6*, 886–897. [CrossRef] [PubMed]
47. Devassy, J.G.; Nwachukwu, I.D.; Jones, P.J. Curcumin and cancer: Barriers to obtaining a health claim. *Nutr. Rev.* **2015**, *73*, 155–165. [CrossRef] [PubMed]
48. Li, X.; Long, J.; He, T.; Belshaw, R.; Scott, J. Integrated genomic approaches identify major pathways and upstream regulators in late onset Alzheimer's disease. *Sci. Rep.* **2015**, *5*, 12393. Available online: https://www.nature.com/articles/srep12393 (accessed on 5 December 2018). [CrossRef] [PubMed]
49. Ghosh, A.; Roy, A.; Liu, X.; Kordower, J.H.; Mufson, E.J.; Hartley, D.M.; Ghosh, S.; Mosley, R.L.; Gendelman, H.E.; Pahan, K. Selective inhibition of NF-kappaB activation prevents dopaminergic neuronal loss in a mouse model of Parkinson's disease. *Proc. Natl. Acad. Sci. USA* **2007**, *104*, 18754–18759. [CrossRef]
50. Barabási, A.L.; Gulbahce, N.; Loscalzo, J. Network Medicine: A network-based approach to human disease. *Nat. Rev. Genet.* **2011**, *12*, 56–68. Available online: https://www.nature.com/articles/nrg2918 (accessed on 10 January 2019). [CrossRef]
51. Kunnumakkara, A.B.; Bordoloi, D.; Padmavathi, G.; Monisha, J.; Roy, N.K.; Prasad, S.; Aggarwal, B.B. Curcumin, the golden nutraceutical: Multitargeting for multiple chronic diseases. *Br. J. Pharmacol.* **2017**, *174*, 1325–1348. Available online: https://www.ncbi.nlm.nih.gov/pmc/articles/PMC5429333/ (accessed on 26 February 2019). [CrossRef] [PubMed]
52. Abdolahi, M.; Tafakhori, A.; Togha, M.; Okhovat, A.A.; Siassi, F.; Eshraghian, M.R.; Sedighiyan, M.; Djalali, M.; Mohammadzadeh Honarvar, N.; Djalali, M. The synergistic effects of ω-3 fatty acids and nano-curcumin supplementation on tumor necrosis factor (TNF)-α gene expression and serum level in migraine patients. *Immunogenetics* **2017**, *69*, 371–378. [CrossRef]
53. Panahi, Y.; Hosseini, M.S.; Khalili, N.; Naimi, E.; Simental-Mendía, L.E.; Majeed, M.; Sahebkar, A. Effects of curcumin on serum cytokine concentrations in subjects with metabolic syndrome: A post-hoc analysis of a randomized controlled trial. *Biomed. Pharmacother.* **2016**, *82*, 578–582. [CrossRef] [PubMed]
54. Hewlings, S.J.; Kalman, D.S. Curcumin: A review of its' effects on human health. *Foods* **2017**, *6*, 92. Available online: https://www.mdpi.com/2304-8158/6/10/92 (accessed on 17 October 2018). [CrossRef] [PubMed]
55. Philip, S.; Kundu, G.C. Osteopontin induces nuclear factor B-mediated promatrix metalloproteinase-2 activation through I kappa B alpha /IKK signaling pathways, and curcumin (diferulolylmethane) down-regulates these pathways. *J. Biol. Chem.* **2003**, *278*, 14487–14497. [CrossRef] [PubMed]
56. Singh, S.; Aggarwal, B.B. Activation of transcription factor NF-kappa B is suppressed by curcumin (diferuloylmethane) [corrected]. *J. Biol. Chem.* **1995**, *270*, 24995–25000. Available online: http://www.jbc.org/content/270/42/24995.long (accessed on 1 October 2018). [CrossRef] [PubMed]
57. Edwards, R.L.; Luis, P.B.; Varuzza, P.V.; Joseph, A.I.; Presley, S.H.; Chaturvedi, R.; Schneider, C. The anti-inflammatory activity of curcumin is mediated by its oxidative metabolites. *J. Biol. Chem.* **2017**, *292*, 21243–21252. Available online: http://www.jbc.org/content/292/52/21243.long (accessed on 3 January 2019). [CrossRef] [PubMed]
58. Liochev, S.I. Reactive oxygen species and the free radical theory of aging. *Free Radic. Biol. Med.* **2013**, *60*, 1–4. [CrossRef] [PubMed]
59. Larasati, Y.A.; Yoneda-Kato, N.; Nakamae, I.; Yokoyama, T.; Meiyanto, E.; Kato, J. Curcumin targets multiple enzymes involved in the ROS metabolic pathway to suppress tumor cell growth. *Sci. Rep.* **2018**, *8*, 2039. Available online: https://www.nature.com/articles/s41598-018-20179-6 (accessed on 7 January 2019). [CrossRef] [PubMed]

60. Gall Troselj, K.; Novak Kujundzic, R. Curcumin in combined cancer therapy. *Curr. Pharm. Des.* **2014**, *20*, 6682–6696. [CrossRef]
61. Marullo, R.; Werner, E.; Degtyareva, N.; Moore, B.; Altavilla, G.; Ramalingam, S.S.; Doetsch, P.W. Cisplatin induces a mitochondrial-ROS response that contributes to cytotoxicity depending on mitochondrial redox status and bioenergetic functions. *PLoS ONE* **2013**, *8*, e81162. Available online: https://www.ncbi.nlm.nih.gov/pmc/articles/PMC3834214/ (accessed on 8 January 2019). [CrossRef] [PubMed]
62. Khor, T.O.; Huang, Y.; Wu, T.Y.; Shu, L.M.; Lee, J.; Kong, A.N.T. Pharmacodynamics of curcumin as DNA hypomethylation agent in restoring the expression of Nrf2 via promoter CpGs demethylation. *Biochem. Pharmacol.* **2011**, *82*, 1073–1078. [CrossRef]
63. Dhakshinamoorthy, S.; Jaiswal, A.K. Functional characterization and role of INrf2 in antioxidant response element-mediated expression and antioxidant induction of NAD(P)H:quinone oxidoreductase1 gene. *Oncogene* **2001**, *20*, 3906–3917. [CrossRef]
64. Singh, A.P.; Lange, T.S.; Kim, K.K.; Brard, L.; Horan, T.; Moore, R.G.; Vorsa, N.; Singh, R.K. Purified cranberry proanthocyanidines (PAC-1A) cause pro-apoptotic signaling, ROS generation, cyclophosphamide retention and cytotoxicity in high-risk neuroblastoma cells. *Int. J. Oncol.* **2012**, *40*, 99–108. [CrossRef]
65. Weh, K.M.; Aiyer, H.S.; Howell, A.B.; Kresty, L.A. Cranberry proanthocyanidins modulate reactive oxygen species in Barrett's and esophageal adenocarcinoma cell lines. *J. Berry Res.* **2016**, *6*, 125–136. Available online: https://www.ncbi.nlm.nih.gov/pmc/articles/PMC5002987/ (accessed on 7 January 2019). [CrossRef]
66. Ravindranathan, P.; Pasham, D.; Balaji, U.; Cardenas, J.; Gu, J.; Toden, S.; Goel, A. A combination of curcumin and oligomeric proanthocyanidins offer superior anti-tumorigenic properties in colorectal cancer. *Sci. Rep.* **2018**, *8*, 1–12. Available online: https://www.ncbi.nlm.nih.gov/pmc/articles/PMC6138725/ (accessed on 10 January 2019). [CrossRef] [PubMed]
67. Beaconsfield, P.; Rainsbury, R.; Kalton, G. Glucose-6-phosphate dehydrogenase deficiency and the incidence of cancer. *Oncologia* **1965**, *19*, 11–19. [CrossRef] [PubMed]
68. Foulds, L. The natural history of cancer. *J. Chronic Dis.* **1958**, *8*, 2–37. [CrossRef]
69. Campisi, J.; d'Adda di Fagagna, F. Cellular senescence: When bad things happen to good cells. *Nat. Rev. Mol. Cell Biol.* **2007**, *8*, 729–740. [CrossRef] [PubMed]
70. Lecot, P.; Alimirah, F.; Desprez, P.Y.; Campisi, J.; Wiley, C. Context-dependent effects of cellular senescence in cancer development. *Br. J. Cancer* **2016**, *114*, 1180–1184. Available online: https://www.ncbi.nlm.nih.gov/pmc/articles/PMC4891501/ (accessed on 20 November 2018). [CrossRef] [PubMed]
71. Coppé, J.P.; Desprez, P.Y.; Krtolica, A.; Campisi, J. The senescence-associated secretory phenotype: The dark side of tumor suppression. *Annu. Rev. Pathol.* **2010**, *5*, 99–118. [CrossRef] [PubMed]
72. Kuilman, T.; Michaloglou, C.; Vredeveld, L.C.; Douma, S.; van Doorn, R.; Desmet, C.J.; Aarden, L.A.; Mooi, W.J.; Peeper, D.S. Oncogene-induced senescence relayed by an interleukin-dependent inflammatory network. *Cell* **2008**, *133*, 1019–1031. Available online: https://www.sciencedirect.com/science/article/pii/S009286740800620X?via%3Dihub (accessed on 18 December 2018). [CrossRef]
73. Warburg, O. On the origin of cancer cells. *Science* **1956**, *123*, 309–314. [CrossRef]
74. Vander Heiden, M.G.; Cantley, L.C.; Thompson, C.B. Understanding the Warburg effect: The metabolic requirements of cell proliferation. *Science* **2009**, *324*, 1029–1033. Available online: http://science.sciencemag.org/content/324/5930/1029.long (accessed on 17 October 2018). [CrossRef]
75. Cairns, R.A.; Harris, I.S.; Mak, T.W. Regulation of cancer cell metabolism. *Nat. Rev. Cancer* **2011**, *11*, 85–95. [CrossRef]
76. Hamanaka, R.B.; Chandel, N.S. Cell biology. Warburg effect and redox balance. *Science* **2011**, *334*, 1219–1220. [CrossRef] [PubMed]
77. De Groof, A.J.C.; te Lindert, M.M.; van Dommelen, M.M.T.; Wu, M.; Willemse, M.; Smift, A.L.; Winer, M.; Oerlemans, F.; Pluk, H.; Fransen, J.A.M.; et al. Increased OXPHOS activity precedes rise in glycolytic rate in H-RasV12/E1A transformed fibroblasts that develop a Warburg phenotype. *Mol. Cancer* **2009**, *8*, 54. Available online: https://molecular-cancer.biomedcentral.com/articles/10.1186/1476-4598-8-54 (accessed on 20 September 2018). [CrossRef] [PubMed]
78. Chandel, N.S.; Maltepe, E.; Goldwasser, E.; Mathieu, C.E.; Simon, M.C.; Schumacker, P.T. Mitochondrial reactive oxygen species trigger hypoxia-induced transcription. *Proc. Natl. Acad. Sci. USA* **1998**, *95*, 11715–11720. Available online: https://www.pnas.org/content/95/20/11715.long (accessed on 8 October 2018). [CrossRef] [PubMed]

79. Jaakkola, P.; Mole, D.R.; Tian, Y.M.; Wilson, M.I.; Gielbert, J.; Gaskell, S.J.; von Kriegsheim, A.; Hebestreit, H.F.; Mukherji, M.; Schofield, C.J.; et al. Targeting of HIF-alpha to the von Hippel-Lindau ubiquitylation complex by O_2-regulated prolyl hydroxylation. *Science* **2001**, *292*, 468–472. [CrossRef] [PubMed]
80. Lin, X.; David, C.A.; Donnelly, J.B.; Michaelides, M.; Chandel, N.S.; Huang, X.; Warrior, U.; Weinberg, F.; Tormos, K.V.; Fesik, S.W.; et al. A chemical genomics screen highlights the essential role of mitochondria in HIF-1 regulation. *Proc. Natl. Acad. Sci. USA* **2008**, *105*, 174–179. Available online: https://www.pnas.org/content/105/1/174.long (accessed on 9 October 2018). [CrossRef] [PubMed]
81. Bae, M.-K.; Kim, S.-H.; Jeong, J.-W.; Lee, Y.M.; Kim, H.-S.; Kim, S.-R.; Yun, I.; Bae, S.-K.; Kim, K.-W. Curcumin inhibits hypoxia-induced angiogenesis via down-regulation of HIF-1. *Oncol. Rep.* **2006**, *15*, 1557–1562. [CrossRef]
82. Khan, M.N.; Haggag, Y.A.; Lane, M.E.; McCarron, P.A.; Tambuwala, M.M. Polymeric nano-encapsulation of curcumin enhances its anti-cancer activity in breast (MDA-MB231) and lung (A549) cancer cells through reduction in expression of HIF-1α and nuclear p65 (REL A). *Curr. Drug Deliv.* **2018**, *15*, 286–295. [CrossRef]
83. Wang, X.-P.; Wang, Q.-X.; Lin, H.-P.; Chang, N. Anti-tumor bioactivities of curcumin on mice loaded with gastric carcinoma. *Food Funct.* **2017**, *8*, 3319–3326. [CrossRef]
84. Grivennikov, S.; Karin, E.; Terzic, J.; Mucida, D.; Yu, G.-Y.; Vallabhapurapu, S.; Scheller, J.; Rose-John, S.; Cheroutre, H.; Eckmann, L.; et al. IL-6 and Stat3 are required for survival of intestinal epithelial cells and development of colitis-associated cancer. *Cell* **2009**, *15*, 103–113. Available online: https://www.sciencedirect.com/science/article/pii/S1535610809000026?via%3Dihub (accessed on 25 October 2018).
85. Hahn, Y.-I.; Kim, S.-J.; Choi, B.-Y.; Cho, K.-C.; Bandu, R.; Kim, K.P.; Kim, D.-H.; Kim, W.; Park, J.S.; Han, B.W.; et al. Curcumin interacts directly with the Cysteine 259 residue of STAT3 and induces apoptosis in H-Ras transformed human mammary epithelial cells. *Sci. Rep.* **2018**, *8*, 6409. Available online: https://www.nature.com/articles/s41598-018-23840-2 (accessed on 16 January 2019). [CrossRef]
86. Grivennikov, S.I.; Karin, M. Inflammation and oncogenesis: A vicious connection. *Curr. Opin. Genet. Dev.* **2010**, *20*, 65–71. Available online: https://www.sciencedirect.com/science/article/pii/S0959437X09001919?via%3Dihub (accessed on 25 October 2018). [CrossRef] [PubMed]
87. Deschênes-Simard, X.; Parisotto, M.; Rowell, M.-C.; Le Calvé, B.; Igelmann, S.; Moineau-Vallée, K.; Saint-Germain, E.; Kalegari, P.; Bourdeau, V.; Kottakis, F.; et al. Circumventing senescence is associated with stem cell properties and metformin sensitivity. *Aging Cell* **2019**, e12889. [CrossRef] [PubMed]
88. Deschênes-Simard, X.; Gaumont-Leclerc, M.-F.; Bourdeau, V.; Lessard, F.; Moiseeva, O.; Forest, V.; Igelmann, S.; Mallette, F.A.; Saba-El-Leil, M.K.; Meloche, S.; et al. Tumor suppressor activity of the ERK/MAPK pathway by promoting selective protein degradation. *Genes Dev.* **2013**, *27*, 900–915. Available online: http://genesdev.cshlp.org/content/27/8/900.long (accessed on 3 December 2018). [CrossRef] [PubMed]
89. Locken, H.; Clamor, C.; Muller, K. Napabucasin and related heterocycle-fused naphthoquinones as STAT3 inhibitors with antiproliferative activity against cancer cells. *J. Nat. Prod.* **2018**, *81*, 1636–1644. [CrossRef] [PubMed]
90. Kanska, J.; Aspuria, P.-J.P.; Taylor-Harding, B.; Spurka, L.; Funari, V.; Orsulic, S.; Karlan, B.Y.; Wiedemeyer, W.R. Glucose deprivation elicits phenotypic plasticity via ZEB1-mediated expression of NNMT. *Oncotarget* **2017**, *8*, 26200–26220. Available online: https://www.ncbi.nlm.nih.gov/pmc/articles/PMC5432250/ (accessed on 10 October 2018). [CrossRef] [PubMed]
91. Pastò, A.; Bellio, C.; Pilotto, G.; Ciminale, V.; Silic-Benussi, M.; Guzzo, G.; Rasola, A.; Frasson, C.; Nardo, G.; Zulato, E.; et al. Cancer stem cells from epithelial ovarian cancer patients privilege oxidative phosphorylation, and resist glucose deprivation. *Oncotarget* **2014**, *5*, 4305–4319. Available online: https://www.ncbi.nlm.nih.gov/pmc/articles/PMC4147325/ (accessed on 22 October 2018). [CrossRef] [PubMed]
92. Pissios, P. Nicotinamide N-Methyltransferase: More than a vitamin B3 clearance enzyme. *Trends Endocrinol. Metab.* **2017**, *28*, 340–353. [CrossRef]
93. Tomida, M.; Ohtake, H.; Yokota, T.; Kobayashi, Y.; Kurosumi, M. Stat3 up-regulates expression of nicotinamide N-methyltransferase in human cancer cells. *J. Cancer Res. Clin. Oncol.* **2008**, *134*, 551–559. [CrossRef]
94. Ulanovskaya, O.A.; Zuhl, A.M.; Cravatt, B.F. NNMT promotes epigenetic remodeling in cancer by creating a metabolic methylation sink. *Nat. Chem. Biol.* **2013**, *9*, 300–306. Available online: https://www.nature.com/articles/nchembio.1204 (accessed on 25 September 2018). [CrossRef]

95. Sperber, H.; Mathieu, J.; Wang, Y.; Ferreccio, A.; Hesson, J.; Xu, Z.; Fischer, K.A.; Devi, A.; Detraux, D.; Gu, H.; et al. The metabolome regulates the epigenetic landscape during naive-to-primed human embryonic stem cell transition. *Nat. Cell Biol.* **2015**, *17*, 1523–1535. Available online: https://www.nature.com/articles/ncb3264 (accessed on 5 December 2018). [CrossRef]
96. Xu, X.; Zhu, Y. Curcumin inhibits human non-small cell lung cancer xenografts by targeting STAT3 pathway. *Am. J. Transl. Res.* **2017**, *9*, 3633–3641. Available online: https://www.ncbi.nlm.nih.gov/pmc/articles/PMC5575177/ (accessed on 21 November 2018). [PubMed]
97. Menendez, J.A.; Alarcón, T.; Joven, J. Gerometabolites: The pseudohypoxic aging side of cancer oncometabolites. *Cell Cycle* **2014**, *13*, 699–709. [CrossRef] [PubMed]
98. Chini, C.C.S.; Tarragó, M.G.; Chini, E.N. NAD and the aging process: Role in life, death and everything in between. *Mol. Cell. Endocrinol.* **2017**, *455*, 62–74. [CrossRef] [PubMed]
99. Gomes, A.P.; Price, N.L.; Ling, A.J.Y.; Moslehi, J.J.; Montgomery, M.K.; Rajman, L.; White, J.P.; Teodoro, J.S.; Wrann, C.D.; Hubbard, B.P.; et al. Declining NAD+ induces a pseudohypoxic state disrupting nuclear-mitochondrial communication during aging. *Cell* **2013**, *155*, 1624–1638. Available online: https://www.sciencedirect.com/science/article/pii/S0092867413015213?via%3Dihub (accessed on 8 October 2018). [CrossRef] [PubMed]
100. Yaku, K.; Okabe, K.; Hikosaka, K.; Nakagawa, T. NAD metabolism in cancer therapeutics. *Front. Oncol.* **2018**, *8*, 622. [CrossRef] [PubMed]
101. Gupta, V.; Bamezai, R.N. Human pyruvate kinase M2: A multifunctional protein. *Protein Sci.* **2010**, *19*, 2031–2044. [CrossRef] [PubMed]
102. David, C.J.; Chen, M.; Assanah, M.; Canoll, P.; Manley, J.L. HnRNP proteins controlled by c-Myc deregulate pyruvate kinase mRNA splicing in cancer. *Nature* **2010**, *463*, 364–368. [CrossRef] [PubMed]
103. Clower, C.V.; Chatterjee, D.; Wang, Z.; Cantley, L.C.; Vander Heiden, M.G.; Krainer, A.R. The alternative splicing repressors hnRNP A1/A2 and PTB influence pyruvate kinase isoform expression and cell metabolism. *Proc. Natl. Acad. Sci. USA* **2010**, *107*, 1894–1899. [CrossRef] [PubMed]
104. Wong, N.; Ojo, D.; Yan, J.; Tang, D. PKM2 contributes to cancer metabolism. *Cancer Lett.* **2015**, *356 Pt A*, 184–191. [CrossRef]
105. Mitsuishi, Y.; Taguchi, K.; Kawatani, Y.; Shibata, T.; Nukiwa, T.; Aburatani, H.; Yamamoto, M.; Motohashi, H. Nrf2 redirects glucose and glutamine into anabolic pathways in metabolic reprogramming. *Cancer Cell* **2012**, *22*, 66–79. [CrossRef]
106. Vander Heiden, M.G.; Locasale, J.W.; Swanson, K.D.; Sharfi, H.; Heffron, G.J.; Amador-Noguez, D.; Christofk, H.R.; Wagner, G.; Rabinowitz, J.D.; Asara, J.M.; et al. Evidence for an alternative glycolytic pathway in rapidly proliferating cells. *Science* **2010**, *329*, 1492–1499. [CrossRef] [PubMed]
107. Vaughan, R.A.; Garcia-Smith, R.; Dorsey, J.; Griffith, J.K.; Bisoffi, M.; Trujillo, K.A. Tumor necrosis factor alpha induces Warburg-like metabolism and is reversed by anti-inflammatory curcumin in breast epithelial cells. *Int. J. Cancer* **2013**, *133*, 2504–2510. [CrossRef] [PubMed]
108. Das, L.; Vinayak, M. Long term effect of curcumin in regulation of glycolytic pathway and angiogenesis via modulation of stress activated genes in prevention of cancer. *PLoS ONE* **2014**, *9*, e99583. Available online: https://www.ncbi.nlm.nih.gov/pmc/articles/PMC4059662/ (accessed on 4 October 2018). [CrossRef] [PubMed]
109. DeBerardinis, R.J.; Lum, J.J.; Hatzivassiliou, G.; Thompson, C.B. The biology of cancer: Metabolic reprogramming fuels cell growth and proliferation. *Cell Metab.* **2008**, *7*, 11–20. Available online: https://www.sciencedirect.com/science/article/pii/S1550413107002951?via%3Dihub (accessed on 28 September 2018). [CrossRef] [PubMed]
110. Sun, Q.; Chen, X.; Ma, J.; Peng, H.; Wang, F.; Zha, X.; Wang, Y.; Jing, Y.; Yang, H.; Chen, R.; et al. Mammalian target of rapamycin up-regulation of pyruvate kinase isoenzyme type M2 is critical for aerobic glycolysis and tumor growth. *Proc. Natl. Acad. Sci. USA* **2011**, *108*, 4129–4134. [CrossRef] [PubMed]
111. Pusapati, R.V.; Daemen, A.; Wilson, C.; Sandoval, W.; Gao, M.; Haley, B.; Baudy, A.R.; Hatzivassiliou, G.; Evangelista, M.; Settleman, J. mTORC1-dependent metabolic reprogramming underlies escape from glycolysis addiction in cancer cells. *Cancer Cell* **2016**, *29*, 548–562. Available online: https://www.sciencedirect.com/science/article/pii/S1535610816300526?via%3Dihub (accessed on 30 October 2018). [CrossRef] [PubMed]

112. Beevers, C.S.; Zhou, H.; Huang, S. Hitting the golden TORget: Curcumin's effects on mTOR signaling. *Anticancer Agents Med. Chem.* **2013**, *13*, 988–994. Available online: http://www.eurekaselect.com/112990/article (accessed on 5 November 2018). [CrossRef] [PubMed]
113. Siddiqui, F.A.; Prakasam, G.; Chattopadhyay, S.; Rehman, A.U.; Padder, R.A.; Ansari, M.A.; Irshad, R.; Mangalhara, K.; Bamezai, R.N.K.; Husain, M.; et al. Curcumin decreases Warburg effect in cancer cells by down-regulating pyruvate kinase M2 via mTOR-HIF-1α inhibition. *Sci. Rep.* **2018**, *8*, 8323. Available online: https://www.nature.com/articles/s41598-018-25524-3 (accessed on 20 December 2018). [CrossRef] [PubMed]
114. Wang, K.; Fan, H.; Chen, Q.; Ma, G.; Zhu, M.; Zhang, X.; Zhang, Y.; Yu, J. Curcumin inhibits aerobic glycolysis and induces mitochondrial-mediated apoptosis through hexokinase II in human colorectal cancer cells in vitro. *Anticancer Drugs* **2015**, *26*, 15–24. [CrossRef]
115. Zhang, F.-J.; Zhang, H.-S.; Liu, Y.; Huang, Y.-H. Curcumin inhibits Ec109 cell growth via an AMPK-mediated metabolic switch. *Life Sci.* **2015**, *134*, 49–55. [CrossRef]
116. Angelo, L.S.; Maxwell, D.S.; Wu, J.Y.; Sun, D.; Hawke, D.H.; McCutcheon, I.E.; Slopis, J.M.; Peng, Z.; Bornmann, W.G.; Kurzrock, R. Binding partners for curcumin in human schwannoma cells: Biologic implications. *Bioorg. Med. Chem.* **2013**, *21*, 932–939. [CrossRef] [PubMed]
117. Abegg, D.; Frei, R.; Cerato, L.; Prasad Hari, D.; Wang, C.; Waser, J.; Adibekian, A. Proteome-wide profiling of targets of cysteine reactive small molecules by using ethynyl benziodoxolone reagents. *Angew. Chem. Int. Ed. Engl.* **2015**, *54*, 10852–10857. [CrossRef] [PubMed]
118. McBean, G.J.; Aslan, M.; Griffiths, H.R.; Torrão, R.C. Thiol redox homeostasis in neurodegenerative disease. *Redox Biol.* **2015**, *5*, 186–194. Available online: https://www.sciencedirect.com/science/article/pii/S221323171500035X?via%3Dihub (accessed on 20 December 2018). [CrossRef] [PubMed]
119. Wang, J.; Zhang, J.; Zhang, C.J.; Wong, Y.K.; Lim, T.K.; Hua, Z.C.; Liu, B.; Tannenbaum, S.R.; Shen, H.M.; Lin, Q. In situ proteomic profiling of curcumin targets in hct116 colon cancer cell line. *Sci. Rep.* **2016**, *6*, 22146. Available online: https://www.nature.com/articles/srep22146 (accessed on 3 January 2019). [CrossRef] [PubMed]
120. Feng, D.; Cheng, Y.; Meng, Y.; Zou, L.; Huang, S.; Xie, J. Multiple effects of curcumin on promoting expression of the exon 7-containing SMN2 transcript. *Genes Nutr.* **2015**, *10*, 40. Available online: https://link.springer.com/article/10.1007%2Fs12263-015-0486-y (accessed on 18 January 2019). [CrossRef] [PubMed]
121. Stine, Z.E.; Dang, C. Stress eating and tuning out: Cancer cells re-wire metabolism to counter stress. *Crit. Rev. Biochem. Mol. Biol.* **2013**, *48*, 609–619. [CrossRef] [PubMed]
122. Possemato, R.; Marks, K.M.; Shaul, Y.D.; Pacold, M.E.; Kim, D.; Birsoy, K.; Sethumadhavan, S.; Woo, H.-K.; Jang, H.G.; Jha, A.K.; et al. Functional genomics reveal that the serine synthesis pathway is essential in breast cancer. *Nature* **2011**, *476*, 346–350. [CrossRef] [PubMed]
123. Murphy, J.P.; Giacomantonio, M.A.; Paulo, J.A.; Everley, R.A.; Kennedy, B.E.; Pathak, G.P.; Clements, D.R.; Kim, Y.; Dai, C.; Sharif, T.; et al. The NAD+ salvage pathway supports PHGDH-driven serine biosynthesis. *Cell Rep.* **2018**, *24*, 2381–2391. [CrossRef] [PubMed]
124. Kim, S.R.; Park, H.J.; Bae, Y.H.; Ahn, S.C.; Wee, H.J.; Yun, I.; Jang, H.O.; Bae, M.K.; Bae, S.K. Curcumin down-regulates visfatin expression and inhibits breast cancer cell invasion. *Endocrinology* **2012**, *153*, 554–563. [CrossRef]
125. Jing, Z.; Heng, W.; Xia, L.; Ning, W.; Yafei, Q.; Yao, Z.; Shulan, Z. Downregulation of phosphoglycerate dehydrogenase inhibits proliferation and enhances cisplatin sensitivity in cervical adenocarcinoma cells by regulating Bcl-2 and caspase-3. *Cancer Biol. Ther.* **2015**, *16*, 541–548. [CrossRef]
126. Jain, M.; Nilsson, R.; Sharma, S.; Madhusudhan, N.; Kitami, T.; Souza, A.L.; Kafri, R.; Kirschner, M.W.; Clish, C.B.; Mootha, V.K. Metabolite profiling identifies a key role for glycine in rapid cancer cell proliferation. *Science* **2012**, *336*, 1040–1044. [CrossRef] [PubMed]
127. Kim, D.; Fiske, B.P.; Birsoy, K.; Freinkman, E.; Kami, K.; Possemato, R.L.; Chudnovsky, Y.; Pacold, M.E.; Chen, W.W.; Cantor, J.R.; et al. SHMT2 drives glioma cell survival in ischaemia but imposes a dependence on glycine clearance. *Nature* **2015**, *520*, 363–367. [CrossRef] [PubMed]
128. Giardina, G.; Brunotti, P.; Fiascarelli, A.; Cicalini, A.; Costa, M.G.; Buckle, A.M.; di Salvo, M.L.; Giorgi, A.; Marani, M.; Paone, A.; et al. How pyridoxal 5′-phosphate differentially regulates human cytosolic and mitochondrial serine hydroxymethyltransferase oligomeric state. *FEBS J.* **2015**, *282*, 1225–1241. [CrossRef] [PubMed]

129. Chaneton, B.; Hillmann, P.; Zheng, L.; Martin, A.C.L.; Maddocks, O.D.K.; Chokkathukalam, A.; Coyle, J.E.; Jankevics, A.; Holding, F.P.; Vousden, K.H.; et al. Serine is a natural ligand and allosteric activator of pyruvate kinase M2. *Nature* **2012**, *491*, 458–462. [CrossRef] [PubMed]
130. Ye, J.; Fan, J.; Venneti, S.; Wan, Y.W.; Pawel, B.R.; Zhang, J.; Finley, L.W.; Lu, C.; Lindsten, T.; Cross, J.R.; et al. Serine catabolism regulates mitochondrial redox control during hypoxia. *Cancer Discov.* **2014**, *4*, 1406–1417. [CrossRef] [PubMed]
131. Lee, G.Y.; Haverty, P.M.; Li, L.; Kljavin, N.M.; Bourgon, R.; Lee, J.; Stern, H.; Modrusan, Z.; Seshagiri, S.; Zhang, Z.; et al. Comparative oncogenomics identifies PSMB4 and SHMT2 as potential cancer driver genes. *Cancer Res.* **2014**, *74*, 3114–3126. [CrossRef] [PubMed]
132. Locasale, J.W.; Grassian, A.R.; Melman, T.; Lyssiotis, C.A.; Mattaini, K.R.; Bass, A.J.; Heffron, G.; Metallo, C.M.; Muranen, T.; Sharfi, H.; et al. Phosphoglycerate dehydrogenase diverts glycolytic flux and contributes to oncogenesis. *Nat. Genet.* **2011**, *43*, 869–874. [CrossRef] [PubMed]
133. Unterlass, J.E.; Baslé, A.; Blackburn, T.J.; Tucker, J.; Cano, C.; Noble, M.E.M.; Curtin, N.J. Validating and enabling phosphoglycerate dehydrogenase (PHGDH) as a target for fragment-based drug discovery in PHGDH-amplified breast cancer. *Oncotarget* **2016**, *9*, 13139–13153. Available online: https://www.ncbi.nlm.nih.gov/pmc/articles/PMC5862567/ (accessed on 17 October 2018). [CrossRef]
134. Yoshino, H.; Nohata, N.; Miyamoto, K.; Yonemori, M.; Sakaguchi, T.; Sugita, S.; Itesako, T.; Kofuji, S.; Nakagawa, M.; Dahiya, R.; et al. PHGDH as a key enzyme for serine biosynthesis in HIF2α-targeting therapy for renal cell carcinoma. *Cancer Res.* **2017**, *77*, 6321–6329. [CrossRef]
135. Antonov, A.; Agostini, M.; Morello, M.; Minieri, M.; Melino, G.; Amelio, I. Bioinformatics analysis of the serine and glycine pathway in cancer cells. *Oncotarget* **2014**, *5*, 11004–11013. Available online: https://www.ncbi.nlm.nih.gov/pmc/articles/PMC4294344/ (accessed on 17 October 2018). [CrossRef]
136. DeNicola, G.M.; Chen, P.-H.; Mullarky, E.; Sudderth, J.A.; Hu, Z.; Wu, D.; Tang, H.; Xie, Y.; Asara, J.M.; Huffman, K.E.; et al. NRF2 regulates serine biosynthesis in non–small cell lung cancer. *Nat. Genet.* **2015**, *47*, 1475–1481. [CrossRef] [PubMed]
137. Yin, K. Positive correlation between expression level of mitochondrial serine hydroxymethyltransferase and breast cancer grade. *Onco Targets Ther.* **2015**, *8*, 1069–1074. Available online: https://www.dovepress.com/positive-correlation-between-expression-level-of-mitochondrial-serine--peer-reviewed-article-OTT (accessed on 24 October 2018). [CrossRef] [PubMed]
138. Wu, X.; Deng, L.; Tang, D.; Ying, G.; Yao, X.; Liu, F.; Liang, G. miR-615-5p prevents proliferation and migration through negatively regulating serine hydromethyltransferase 2 (SHMT2) in hepatocellular carcinoma. *Tumor Biol.* **2016**, *37*, 6813–6821. [CrossRef] [PubMed]
139. Yang, X.; Wang, Z.; Li, X.; Liu, B.; Liu, M.; Liu, L.; Chen, S.; Ren, M.; Wang, Y.; Yu, M. SHMT2 desuccinylation by SIRT5 drives cancer cell proliferation. *Cancer Res.* **2018**, *78*, 372–386. [CrossRef] [PubMed]

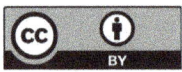

© 2019 by the authors. Licensee MDPI, Basel, Switzerland. This article is an open access article distributed under the terms and conditions of the Creative Commons Attribution (CC BY) license (http://creativecommons.org/licenses/by/4.0/).

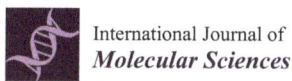

Review

The Role of Curcumin in the Modulation of Ageing

Anna Bielak-Zmijewska *, Wioleta Grabowska, Agata Ciolko, Agnieszka Bojko, Grażyna Mosieniak, Łukasz Bijoch and Ewa Sikora *

Nencki Institute of Experimental Biology, Polish Academy of Sciences, 3 Pasteur St., 02-093 Warsaw, Poland; w.grabowska@nencki.gov.pl (W.G.); a.ciolko@nencki.gov.pl (A.C.); a.bojko@nencki.gov.pl (A.B.); g.mosieniak@nencki.gov.pl (G.M.); l.bijoch@nencki.gov.pl (Ł.B.)
* Correspondence: a.bielak@nencki.gov.pl (A.B.-Z.); e.sikora@nencki.gov.pl (E.S.); Tel.: +48-22-589-2250 (A.B.-Z. & E.S.)

Received: 6 February 2019; Accepted: 6 March 2019; Published: 12 March 2019

Abstract: It is believed that postponing ageing is more effective and less expensive than the treatment of particular age-related diseases. Compounds which could delay symptoms of ageing, especially natural products present in a daily diet, are intensively studied. One of them is curcumin. It causes the elongation of the lifespan of model organisms, alleviates ageing symptoms and postpones the progression of age-related diseases in which cellular senescence is directly involved. It has been demonstrated that the elimination of senescent cells significantly improves the quality of life of mice. There is a continuous search for compounds, named senolytic drugs, that selectively eliminate senescent cells from organisms. In this paper, we endeavor to review the current knowledge about the anti-ageing role of curcumin and discuss its senolytic potential.

Keywords: ageing; anti-cancer; autophagy; microbiota; senescence; senolytics

1. Introduction

Demographic data unquestionably show that the population of elderly and very elderly people is continuously increasing. The population of people aged 65 and above represents 8.7% of the total population. However, this percentage differs between continents and is around 15–16% in North America, Europe and Central Asia, but only about 5% in the Middle East, North Africa and South Asia [1]. The increase of lifespan is not really satisfactory without an improvement of healthspan. We would like to live longer, but in good health, which is necessary to enjoy the world around us. Actually, there is a great deal of evidence that the ageing process is malleable and the rate and quality of ageing can be modulated [2]. In order to be able to postpone ageing, it is urgent to reveal the mechanisms of ageing.

It is commonly accepted that cellular senescence plays a very important role in organismal ageing and age-related diseases [3]. Namely, it has been observed that senescent cells accumulate in the tissues and organs of old animals and humans, and that proliferation potential differs among cells derived from individuals of different age [4–8]. Even though the actual number of senescent cells seems not to be very high and fluctuates between a few and a dozen percent, changes in the extracellular milieu caused by the increased production of cytokines by senescent cells, and the senescence-associated impairment of regenerative processes, can lead to spectacular organismal dysfunctions. Moreover, senescent cells contribute to the onset and progression of diseases, the frequency of which increases with age. The accumulation of senescent cells has been observed in the course of almost all age-related disorders [9]. Breakthrough experiments, which have definitely proved the involvement of cell senescence in the progression of ageing and age-related diseases, came from animal studies. It has been clearly shown that the elimination of senescent cells alleviated the symptoms of ageing and age-related disorders and improved the quality of life of genetically modified animals [10,11]. A recently proposed strategy is to protect people from ageing instead of curing particular diseases [12], and to go deeper, to eliminate cell senescence in order to prevent ageing dysfunctions. In animal models, some progress in postponing ageing has been achieved, but certain approaches cannot be transferred to humans because of the potential detrimental effects of the long-term application of anti-ageing agents (not to mention genetic manipulations). The best approach to ageing protection cannot be demanding, should be easily available, lack any risk of side effects, and should be inscribed in our lifestyle as diet or physical activity. Much hope is currently placed in natural compounds, and some promising results have already been obtained. One of such compounds is a polyphenol: curcumin. Curcumin's role in postponing ageing in animal models has already been documented, but certain data in humans must be verified in longitudinal trials.

2. Cellular Senescence

Cellular senescence was described for the first time about 60 years ago by Leonard Hayflick and Paul Moorhead [13]. Since that time, a concerted effort has been undertaken to explore the role and mechanisms of this fundamental cellular process. The role of senescence is complex and depends on the age of the organism [2]. In a young organism, cell senescence serves a beneficial function. Namely, it is essential in embryonic development (senescent cells are eliminated by immune cells as an element of body shaping), in tissue regeneration and as a cancer barrier (senescent cells are not able to proliferate). In an old organism, the number of senescent cells increases, and they generate a state of low chronic inflammation, via so called senescence-associated secretory phenotype (SASP), produce excessive reactive oxygen species (ROS) and cause microenvironmental changes, which support tumor progression. Generally, cell senescence is detrimental due to the role of senescent cells in ageing and age-related diseases. On the other hand, the role of cell senescence in organismal homeostasis should not be neglected. Moreover, senescence is a highly dynamic process induced by genetic and epigenetic changes [14]. During the lifetime of an organism, cells experience several types of intrinsic (metabolic functions with ROS production and DNA replication) and extrinsic (chemical and physical genotoxic events) stresses. Following DNA damage, cells repair their DNA to eliminate the possibility of mutations that can provoke neoplastic transformation. Cell response to a specific stress implies correct DNA repair to completely recover damaged cells or, alternatively, cells harboring unrepairable damages may enter apoptosis or senescence [15].

The most important feature of senescence is the cessation of proliferation (it concerns proliferation-competent cells), increased level of cell-cycle inhibitors (p21, p16), increased activity of a lysosomal enzyme, senescence-associated β-galactosidase (SA-β-gal), increased number of DNA double-strand breaks (DSBs) and activation of the DNA damage response (DDR) pathway, along with changes in chromatin structure due to modified gene expression and higher vulnerability to DNA damage [16]. One of the most important features of senescent cells is the appearance of senescence-associated secretory phenotype (SASP). SASP arises due to the increased production and secretion of proteins, which can act both in a paracrine and autocrine manner and are involved in the generation of low-grade inflammation. This exerts a bystander effect; that is, it induces senescence in neighboring cells. Cells can undergo senescence as a result of telomere erosion (replicative senescence) or in response to some external (chemical and physical factors) or internal (oncogene overexpression, increased ROS production, DNA damage, ER-stress, and chromatin structure dysfunction) stimuli. The latter form of senescence is termed stress-induced senescence (SIPS, stress-induced premature senescence) [17]. It seems that senescent cells are very well characterized and relatively easy to distinguish from non-senescent cells [18]. On the other hand, the sharp definition of what is cell senescence, that used to exist in the past, is not anymore so straightforward. There is a growing body of evidence showing that certain features of cell senescence and mechanisms of its induction can differ depending on the cell and senescence type [19]. This concerns, for example, different propensity of cell to respond to stress [15], some metabolic differences between stress-induced and replicative senescence [14,20] or differences in SASP components [21]. An interesting question is whether post-mitotic cells can undergo cell senescence [22], and if cancer cell senescence is reversible; in other words, whether SA-β-gal activity in these cells is indicative of their senescence or is simply unspecific [23]. Despite this dilemma, senescent cells simply identified on the basis of high level of cell cycle inhibitors, can be eliminated from a murine body leading to its rejuvenation (see [24], chapter 5.5).

3. Senescence and Age-Related Diseases

Senescent cells are linked with many age-related diseases., such as neurodegenerative diseases (Alzheimer's and Parkinson's disease; AD and PD, respectively), cataract, glaucoma, cardiovascular diseases (CVD, atherosclerosis and hypertension), chronic obstructive pulmonary disease (COPD), idiopathic pulmonary fibrosis (IPF), diabetes type II, sarcopenia, osteoarthritis, osteoporosis and certain types of tumors [9,12,25–32].

4. Anti-Ageing Intervention

The development of science and medicine has contributed to the increase in human lifespan. However, with the increase in life expectancy, an increase in the incidence of age-related diseases is observed. Therefore, it is crucial to find an approach to prevent or delay ageing and the onset of age-related diseases. Animal studies have provided us with a wealth of knowledge and cues, and several strategies to elongate the lifespan of model animals, mainly based on genetic manipulation, have been established. So far, the only non-genetic approach that can extend longevity is dietary/calorie restriction (DR/CR) [33,34]. This intervention involves a 20-40% reduction in calorie intake without causing malnutrition and has been shown to be effective in several species including yeast, fruit flies, nematodes, rats, dogs [35–37] and even primates [38]. Moreover, epidemiological studies support the positive effects of CR in humans. For example, on a Japanese island of Okinawa, the number of centenarians (people over 100 years of age) is five times higher than in any other part of the world. A study revealed that the mean calorie consumption of adult Okinawans is 17% lower than that of an average Japanese adult and 40% lower than that of an average adult citizen of the United States [39,40]. The effects of calorie restriction are not limited to lifespan extension but include also improved cardiovascular and metabolic health, decreased incidence of cancer, along with attenuated neurodegeneration and sarcopenia [39,41,42]. As sticking to a CR regime can be uncomfortable, scientists are looking for drugs, supplements or less drastic dietary intervention that could mimic CR. One of such interventions is intermittent fasting (IF), which has recently been gaining increased attention [43,44]. Goodrick's studies on rats maintained on alternative-day fasting regimen showed that, depending on the age at which the diet was started, the animals lived from 30% to 100% longer than animals fed ad libitum [45,46]. In turn, a recent study by Catterson et al. demonstrated that IF (2-day fed:5-day fasted) can extend the life of a fruit fly by 10% [47]. It has been proposed that CR acts by upregulating autophagy, as the inhibition of this process decreases the anti-ageing effects of this diet intervention [48] (see paragraph 5.3). Another research work suggests that the effects of CR are mediated by sirtuins, the expression of which increases as a result of such restriction [49]. Sirtuins are crucial for metabolism and are involved in cellular response to a variety of stresses such as oxidative or genotoxic stress. A decreased level or activity of these enzymes shortens the lifespan of different model organisms, while increased activity/level can improve both lifespan and healthspan [reviewed in 37]. There are a number of natural (quercetin, butein, curcumin, fisetin, kaempferol, catechins) [37,50] as well as synthetic [51] compounds that can induce sirtuin expression, enhancing lifespan and ameliorating age-related diseases. Besides diet intervention, mild physical activity has also been shown to improve health and lifespan. It is believed that low-intensity exercise can serve as a mild stressor, which activates stress response, preparing the organism to a greater threat. This activates antioxidant enzymes that reduce oxidative stress and can also activate sirtuins [52,53]. In summary, the potential and promising anti-ageing approaches in humans are related to the limitation of the amount of consumed food and/or the application of certain compounds or physical activity that mimic diet restriction.

5. Curcumin

Curcumin is a promising anti-ageing compound which is easily available and easy to apply in the diet, as well as being safe and not expensive. Curcumin is a widely studied nutraceutical, belonging to polyphenols, acquired from the rhizome of a plant *Curcuma longa* (turmeric), a member of the ginger family. Turmeric contains 12 active components [54], thus the percentage of curcumin (chemically known as diferuloylmethane) per dry weight of turmeric powder is no more than 3.14% [55]. Curcumin is commonly used as a spice (curry, turmeric) and yellow food dye (E100); therefore, it is consumed on a daily basis. However, curcumin is poorly absorbed by intestinal cells (low aqueous solubility and stability), rapidly metabolized by the liver (generation of less active curcumin glucuronides, see paragraph 5.6), and rapidly eliminated from an organism [56]. The highest achieved serum level of curcumin was about 1.77 µM, 1 h after administration, during the oral ingestion of 8 g of curcumin per day, or even 3.6 µM if such a dose was consumed for 3 months [57]. The Hindu people, who are the nation with the highest daily intake of curcumin (present in the turmeric spice), consume up to 100 mg/day of the active substance [58]. Due to curcumin's limited bioavailability, the potential therapeutic use of that polyphenol might be questionable. However, numerous studies have been performed to readdress these crucial issues. Moreover, numerous attempts have been made to enhance curcumin ingestion, such as the co-administration of curcumin with piperine, the active substance from pepper, which can increase curcumin's level in the blood by as much as 30 times [59]. This can also be achieved by increasing its aqueous solubility and stability by conjugation with alginate [60], improving cell targeting by self-assembling peptide nanofiber carrier [61] or creating curcumin-phospholipid complexes, microemulsions, liposomes, polymeric micelles and curcumin nanoparticles [56]. Furthermore, clinical trials showed that even extremely high daily doses of curcumin intake (12 g/day) were harmless to patients [57].

Curcumin, like other polyphenols, possesses pleiotropic activity (curcumin belongs to the PAINS, pan-assay interference compounds), which is considered as a serious disadvantage of natural compounds [62]. Indeed, due to its ability to interact simultaneously with many receptors (e.g., EGFR, CXCR4), growth factors (e.g., EGF, TGFβ), kinases (e.g., MAPK, FAK), transcription factors (e.g., NF-κβ, STAT1-5), enzymes (e.g., DNA pol, COX2), adhesion molecules (e.g., ICAM-1, VCAM-1), apoptotic regulators (e.g., survivin, Bcl-2), proinflammatory cytokines (e.g., interleukin (IL)-8, tumor necrosis factor (TNF)) and other proteins (e.g., p53, cyclin B1) [63,64], curcumin can evoke a broad cellular response to external stimuli. Furthermore, curcumin up- and down-regulates different kinds of miRNA [65] and takes part in epigenetic changes by inhibiting DNA methyltransferases and regulating histone modifications via effects on histone acetyltransferases and histone deacetylases [66–68]. However, in our opinion, this is not a disadvantage but, quite to the contrary, an advantage when one compound can affect diverse biological processes, such as the redox state, inflammation, proliferation, migration, apoptosis, wound healing and as a consequence positively affect memory, postpone ageing and age-related diseases such as atherosclerosis [63,64]. Therefore, complex, multigenic, chronic, civilization- and age-related diseases, which occur due to perturbations in multiple signaling pathways, seem to be a suitable target of curcumin-based therapy [63,64]. Due to all those properties of curcumin, it has been used in a vast amount of clinical trials as a drug or adjuvant in the treatment of various diseases [69]. Furthermore, the beneficial or detrimental effect of curcumin depends on its concentration. This phenomenon is widely described as a hormetic effect [70]: it acts as a stimulant at low and an inhibitor at high concentration. This also applies to curcumin function: in low doses, curcumin could act as a protective agent, whereas in high doses it could act as a cytostatic, cytotoxic and genotoxic agent.

5.1. Curcumin and Its Anti-Ageing Role

As ageing is characterized by chronic low-grade inflammation [71], polyphenol-rich foods, which have anti-inflammatory as well as antioxidant properties, can mitigate symptoms of ageing. There are plenty of examples to support the possible anti-ageing role of curcumin [72–75]. Curcumin supplementation in a diet extended the lifespan of fruit flies, nematodes and mice [76–79]. Moreover, in clinical trials, curcumin was proven to reduce symptoms of some age-related diseases such as atherosclerosis, diabetes and cancer [80,81]. It also serves as a neuroprotective agent [82]. Curcumin has also been shown to protect against chemotherapy-induced side effects such as cardiotoxicity elicited by doxorubicin [83] and radiation-induced dermatitis in breast cancer patients [84]. On the cellular level, curcumin protected HUVEC against peroxide-induced senescence [85], while a curcumin analogue, bis-demetoxycurcumin, inhibited the oxidative stress-induced senescence of WI38 fibroblasts [86]. Moreover, curcumin increased the ability of human epidermal keratinocytes to differentiate during replicative senescence [87]. There are some rationales suggesting that the anti-ageing function of curcumin is due to its ability to postpone cellular senescence. However, our recent results excluded such a possibility, at least for cells building the vasculature [88]. Curcumin did not postpone the replicative senescence of vascular smooth muscle cells (VSMC) and endothelial cells (EC) or the doxorubicin-induced senescence of VSMC [88]. Even though curcumin at low concentration (0.1–1.0 µM) was not able to postpone replicative senescence or protect cells from doxorubicin-induced senescence, it increased the level of sirtuins and AMPK in VSMC undergoing replicative senescence [88]. Therefore, it is possible that positive effects of curcumin supplementation, observed on the organismal level, can be attributed to sirtuin and AMPK induction rather than the inhibition of cellular senescence [88]. Others observed that curcumin supplementation in mice and rats enhanced the effect of exercise, affected the time of exhaustion and prevented fatigue, which was associated with an increased level/activity of AMPK and sirtuin 1 in muscles [89,90]. It has been shown that Sirt2 is indispensable for curcumin-induced *Caenorhabditis elegans* lifespan elongation [76].

In summary, curcumin is involved in the regulation of nutrient-sensing signaling pathways (impact on sirtuins, AMPK), and thus it is able to mimic caloric/diet restriction and increase the benefits coming from mild physical activity [37].

We have also tested concentrations of curcumin (5–7.5 µM for VSMC and 2.5–5 µM EC) which were close to those observed in serum after diet supplementation. Unexpectedly, both VSMC and EC underwent senescence upon such treatment [91]. Senescence induced by curcumin was DNA damage-independent and resulted from influencing many signaling pathways. The initial changes concerned decreased levels of sirtuins and AMPK, which suggests that the reduction of these proteins could be important for senescence induction (submitted). Altogether, these results show that curcumin, although is not able to postpone senescence per se, and can even induce it, may exert its anti-ageing effect via the ability to change the levels of proteins involved in the process of ageing (sirtuins, AMPK).

Moreover, it cannot be excluded that cell senescence induced by curcumin plays a beneficial role. Such a positive function has been shown in curcumin-senescent cancer-associated fibroblasts (CAF), which reduced the malignancy of the tumor [92], and in hepatic stellate cells (HSC), where curcumin-induced senescence protected against liver fibrosis [93].

Another important but not always direct anti-ageing function of curcumin is its anti-tumor activity [94] (detailed description in Section 5.4). Ageing is one of the most important risk factors in some types of tumor [95]. Elderly woman and men are four-fold and seven-fold, respectively, more prone to all types of cancer than their younger counterparts. Among elderly men, cancer of the prostate, lung and colon make up around half of all diagnosed cancers. The corresponding most frequent cancers among elderly women, making up 48% of all malignant cancers, are breast, colon, lung and stomach cancer. Curcumin can protect against tumorigenesis (e.g., by protection against the toxicity of some factors present in the environment or applied during therapy), reduce cancer cell number (by the induction of cancer cell apoptosis) and inhibit metastasis (anti-angiogenic properties) [72]. Some data even suggest that cancer cells are more sensitive to curcumin than normal ones. This can be explained by taking several factors into account. The first one is related to the rate of cell proliferation. Cancer cells divide more frequently than normal ones and curcumin disturbs mitosis. This is related, among other, to the impairment of the mitotic spindle [96,97], inhibition of cdk1 kinase [94] and inhibition of sirtuin 7 [98]. The second mechanism is related to curcumin's ability to inhibit NF-κB transcription factor, which is highly expressed in cancer cells. This property is due to the inhibition of IκB-IKK and also to the activation of sirtuin 1 and 6 [37], which inactivate, by deacetylation (sirtuin 1) or indirect interaction (sirtuin 6), RelA/p65, one of the NF-κB components. Yet another factor is associated with the increased activity of β-glucuronidase (responsible for deconiugation of glucuronides) and lower activity of UDP-glucuronosyltransferases (UGT) (an enzyme involved in glucuronides formation) in the tumor tissue [99]. This could lead to an increased local concentration of free, earlier glucuronized compounds, and increase the efficacy of apoptosis. Such action is also ascribed to curcumin (see also Section 5.6) and may improve its anti-cancer activity.

One of the considered strategies dedicated to tumor elimination is cell senescence induction. Curcumin is able to induce cellular senescence in cancer cells. This, which can be harmful for normal cells, could be beneficial in the context of cancer cells. Such an approach, with time, appears controversial, because some data have shown that the senescence of tumor cells can be reversible and can lead to cancer relapse [100].

5.2. Curcumin and SASP

One of the roles of curcumin in the alleviation of ageing is reduction of inflammation. Senescent cells, despite being in a non-proliferating state, remain alive, metabolically active and can influence their microenvironment. One of the most important features of senescent cells is their ability to secrete a number of proteins: mainly interleukins, chemokines and other pro-inflammatory cytokines, proteases, metalloproteinases and growth factors. This phenomenon, known as SASP, is involved in many processes such as inflammation, angiogenesis, extracellular matrix reorganization, the stimulation of proliferation and the modulation of the immune system. Depending on the cellular context, this can either be beneficial or detrimental. One of the positive aspects of SASP is that some of the secreted cytokines, such as interleukin-6 (IL-6) or interleukin-8 (IL-8), are essential in the process of inducing, maintaining and reinforcing senescence in an autocrine manner [101]. Moreover, SASP can be used as a form of communication with immune cells. Senescent cells, by secreting different chemokines (e.g., RANTES, GROα, MCP-1), may attract distinct subsets of NK cells, monocytes/macrophages, neutrophils, B cells and T cells. In consequence, these immune cells ensure the surveillance and clearance of damaged, senescent and dysfunctional cells [17,102]. This is one of the necessary steps for tissue regeneration and protection from fibrosis [103]. On the other hand, proteins secreted by senescent cells may create a tumor-promoting environment, enhance the migration of tumor cells and thus the formation of metastases, and also may induce senescence in neighboring normal cells. In addition, cytokines contribute to changes in the tissue environment and interfere with its functioning [17]. By co-culturing senescent cells with normal cells, it was shown that the senescent phenotype could be transmitted to surrounding cells via soluble SASP proteins [104].

The secretory phenotype depends on both the inducing stimulus of senescence and the cell type. Its activity can be regulated by certain proteins of the DNA damage response pathway (DDR pathway) such as ATM and CHK2 [105]. In addition, the expression of many SASP components such as IL-8 or IL-6 is regulated by the activity of the transcription factor NF-κB, responsible for the development of inflammation. It was shown that the down-regulation of a NF-κB subunit, p65, resulted in a reduced level of secreted IL-8 and lower levels of mRNAs encoding IL-8, RANTES and GROα [106]. Inflammation, in particular chronic inflammation, is associated with the pathogenesis of many diseases including those associated with age, for example Alzheimer's disease, cardiovascular diseases, cancer, diabetes and many others. Curcumin, due to its anti-inflammatory properties, can inhibit NF-κB activity and decrease the level of TNFα, which is the most effective activator of the NF-κB pathway [81,107]. We have shown that short-term cell treatment with low concentrations of curcumin has a positive effect on normal young cells by decreasing the level of secreted pro-inflammatory cytokines. Such treatment decreased IL-8 and VEGF after single application [88]. However, this effect is not observed during the permanent treatment of cells during replicative senescence. Curcumin did not reduce IL-6, IL-8 and VEGF. Quite the reverse: curcumin, due to senescence induction, increased the level of IL-6 and IL-8 [91]. Moreover, low doses of curcumin lead to increased production of sirtuin; i.e., NAD-dependent deacetylases, and sirtuin 1 reduces inflammation by inhibiting NF-κB signaling [108] (see also Section 5.1). To summarize, curcumin, depending on the concentration, is able to reduce or to elevate the level/activity of proteins involved in senescence-associated secretory phenotypes. It is believed that, besides concentration, the impact can be cell-context dependent (the type of stimuli/senescence inductor).

5.3. Curcumin and Its Role in Autophagy

The role of autophagy in ageing is evidenced by numerous studies on model organisms from yeast to mice. The expression of proteins involved in autophagy (in particular, those encoded by the ATG gene family) is required for lifespan extension. Moreover, the overexpression of some autophagy proteins is sufficient to prolong lifespan [109]. The key regulators of autophagy are mammalian target of rapamycin (mTOR) kinase and AMP-activated kinase (AMPK). Inhibition of the mTOR pathway and activation of the AMPK pathway extended the lifespan and healthspan of some model organisms [109]. Besides autophagy regulation, these signaling pathways are responsible for nutrient sensing, similarly to the insulin/IGF1 pathway, the inhibition of which was also proven to postpone ageing in animal models [110]. A number of dietary supplements and drugs can stimulate autophagy via the inhibition of mTOR or activation of AMPK pathways; e.g. resveratrol and spermidine or rapamycin and metformin, respectively. However, long-term treatment with metformin can bring about some side effects such as immunosuppression [111]. Curcumin, as mentioned before, regulates the level and activity of AMPK and, as shown in numerous studies, is able to inhibit mTOR level/activity [74,112], which suggests that it can also affect autophagy.

During cancer development, autophagy can be a double-edged sword. At benign stages of the disease, functional autophagy acts as a tumor suppressor by eliminating damaged cells and organelles and by limiting cell proliferation and maintaining genomic stability [113]. In metastasizing highly proliferating cancer cells, functional autophagy delivers much-needed energy and building blocks, thus facilitating undisturbed progression through the cell cycle [114]. Moreover, active autophagy enables cancer cells to overcome the extremely negative influence of the tumor microenvironment, such as hypoxia, inflammation and energy depletion [115]. That is why the inhibition of either induction or autophagy flux in later stages of cancer disease can have a detrimental effect on cancer cells.

Curcumin shows both activating [116] and inhibitory properties regarding autophagy [117]. The action of curcumin is highly dependent on the type of cancer cells [117]. Curcumin can modulate distinct and diverse molecular targets, including Beclin-1 and p53 [118]. Even more interestingly, curcumin can induce a non-apoptotic form of programmed cell death (PCD) called autophagy-associated cell death (type II PCD), which is caspase-independent and does not involve inflammatory response [119]. In summary, curcumin, by its modulatory impact on autophagy, is able to regulate both cancer cell senescence and tumor progression.

The deregulation of the autophagy process is also a culprit in neurodegenerative diseases. Neuronal accumulation of mutated huntingtin or misfolded amyloid beta proteins (Aβ) plays a key role in pathogenesis in Huntington's and Alzheimer's diseases, respectively. Curcumin can induce the degradation of misfolded proteins or damaged organelles due to different mechanisms. Firstly, it induces the biogenesis of lysosomes by activating TFEB [120]. Secondly, curcumin restores the physiological level of HSP70, which facilitates proper cargo loading into lysosomes [121]. Furthermore, curcumin induces mitophagy [122], thus lowering oxidative stress, which improves neuronal survival [123].

5.4. Curcumin and Cancer

Ageing is one of the factors that promotes cancer development. Among many beneficial effects exerted by curcumin on age-related diseases are its anti-cancer properties. Curcumin was shown to act at different stages of cancer development, starting from cancer initiation to tumor growth and metastasis [124]. There are many molecular targets and signaling pathways that are affected by curcumin. Among them are transcription factors, such as NF-κB and AP1, inflammatory cytokines, growth factors, receptors, kinases and many others [125]. Studies performed in vitro revealed that curcumin induced cell death in many different types of cancer cells [126,127]. Even more, curcumin is able to kill cancer cells that are resistant to commonly-used chemotherapeutic drugs by inducing apoptosis or mitotic catastrophe, as has been revealed by our studies [128–132]. Of note, we have shown that curcumin can induce atypical apoptosis, which is not accompanied either by DNA fragmentation or casapase-3 and -7 activation [132–135]. The lack of DNA fragmentation in dying cancer cells resulted from the inhibition of DNA fragmentation factor 40 (DFF40), which is a caspase-activated DNA endonuclease [136]. However, it is important to mention that, in these studies, curcumin was used in a relatively high concentration (50 µM).

Both carcinogenesis and ageing are related to increased genomic instability. Those detrimental changes that appear in DNA accumulate in the organism during ageing and favor carcinogenesis. Both increased hypomethylation and accelerated ROS production are observed during ageing. It has been demonstrated that those factors may lead to mutations that appear in protooncogenes and tumor suppressor genes [137]. According to a well-described model of cancer progression, the sequential activation or inactivation of those genes drives cancer development [138]. Importantly, curcumin can potentially decrease the probability of mutations. First of all, curcumin was shown to possess chemopreventive activity. A number of studies have demonstrated that it decreases cancer development induced by certain carcinogens simply by suppressing the mutagenic effect [124]. Curcumin acts also as an antioxidant, and in this way it can protect DNA from mutation [55]. Finally, curcumin modulates the epigenetic landscape by influencing histone acetylation, DNA methylation and miRNA expression [68]. Thus, we can speculate that, thanks to this activity, curcumin may exert anti-ageing and anti-cancer effects, although direct experimental proof is needed.

One of the examples of an oncogene is EGFR. Overexpression and/or mutation of EGFR is characteristic for numerous cancers [139]. The antiproliferative activity of curcumin in cancer cells is based, among others, on the disruption of the EGFR/EGF/TGFα autocrine loop. It inhibits both the phosphorylation of the receptor as well as expression of its ligands [125]. Furthermore, curcumin inhibits downstream signaling from the EGFR, namely PI3K/Akt/mTOR [140] and ERK/MAPK [141] cascades.

Recently, cellular senescence has been recognized as an important outcome of anticancer therapy. In that case, cell senescence results from DNA damage and DNA damage response pathway activation due to chemotherapeutic drug treatment [142–144]. Accordingly, we have demonstrated that curcumin at low, non-cytotoxic concentrations induced the senescence of human colon HCT116 cancer cells, MCF-7 human breast cancer cells and U2OS human osteosarcoma cell line [97,145]. The ability of curcumin to cause DNA damage, which is the main trigger of the senescence program, is questionable. There are some reports showing that curcumin is able to induce DNA damage [146–150] while we have revealed that even after treatment with relatively high, cytotoxic concentrations of curcumin, no DNA damage can be identified in cells [94,128,151]. However, disturbed mitosis progression due to improper mitotic spindle formation in curcumin-treated cancer cells has been shown to cause double strand DNA breaks (DSBs) in mitotic chromosomes [152]. Accordingly, we have demonstrated that DSBs remain unrepaired in cells that survived prolonged mitosis, arrest, and then progressed into the subsequent phase of the cell cycle and, finally, underwent senescence. Moreover, the inhibition of the DNA damage response pathway in curcumin-treated cancer cells attenuated senescence and increased the number of proliferating cells [97]. Thus, apart from killing cancer cells, curcumin can exert its anticancer activity also by inducing the permanent growth arrest of cancer cells due to activation of the senescence program.

Currently, the issue of the reversibility of cancer cell senescence has been raised. We have shown that the senescence of cancer cells can be accompanied by polyploidization [100,145,153]. Improper cell division of polyploid cells leads to the regaining of the proliferation potential [100]. It was also demonstrated that cancer cells undergoing senescence acquire the signature of stemness. Therefore, cells that escape senescence, due to some additional mutations, exhibit much higher tumor-initiation potential than those that were never induced to senesce [154]. Thus, the combination of prosenescent anti-cancer therapy together with senolytics seems to be the best and the safest mode of treatment.

5.5. Senolytic Activity of Curcumin

Senolytic drugs are compounds which selectively kill senescent cells. The idea to eliminate senescent cells stems from data showing a causative role of senescent cells in age and age-related diseases [3,155]. The accumulation of senescent cells increases with age, and they are found at sites of age-related pathologies [156]. As mentioned before, the selective eradication of senescent cells improved healthspan. There are also studies showing that senolytics can induce apoptosis in senescent cells in vitro [157]. Senotherapy, which aims to alleviate age-related ailments by using senolytics by improving the ability of immune cells to clear senescent cells or by reducing the low-grade inflammation state created by senescent cells is a rapidly developing branch of biogerontology [24]. Among the senolytics described so far are both small molecules, such as dasatinib, navitoclax, A1351852, A155463, and FOXO4-related peptide, and natural compounds such as piperlongumine, quercetin and fisetin [157]. Although curcumin has been shown to exert anti-ageing effects in different experimental approaches, there are only a few data displaying its capacity to modulate cell senescence. Accordingly, curcumin was applied in a mouse model of chemically-induced diabetes mellitus, which is characterized by the impairment of endothelial progenitor cells (EPCs). Results revealed that curcumin application to type I diabetic mice significantly improved blood circulation and increased capillary density in ischemic hind limbs. An in-vitro study also revealed that the angiogenesis, migration, and proliferation abilities of EPCs and the number of senescent EPCs, shown as a number of SA-β-gal-positive cells, returned to the non-pathological level following curcumin application [158].

Cell senescence refers originally to the cell cycle arrest of previously proliferation-competent cells. However, some hallmarks of cell senescence such as increased SA-β-gal activity can be found in non-proliferating neurons in the cell culture and in the brain [22]. Another feature of senescent cells, both previously proliferation-competent and non-dividing post-mitotic cells, such as neurons, is the accumulation of lipofuscin [159]. Thus, it has been revealed that in the CA1 region of rat hippocampus, in which cells were induced to senesce by treatment with d-galactose, curcumin, applied together with piperine, substantially reduced lipofuscin aggregates [160]. Another group, using the same model of rat senescence, has shown that the injection of curcumin lowered p16 mRNA level in premature ovarian failure. However, it is not known whether curcumin induced apoptosis in p16-positive cells, especially whether the overall parameters of apoptosis were increased in the ovaries [161]. Subsequently, in atherosclerotic rats, curcumin diminished SA-β-gal activity in the aorta and the level of an inflammatory marker, MCP-1, in serum [162]. Curcumin increased the survival of rat mesenchymal stem cells and decreased population-doubling time indirectly, which indicates that it can influence replicative senescence [163]. In the culture of mice embryonic fibroblasts derived from prematurely aged mice, curcumin reduced the cell number slightly less than fisetin, which is considered a strong senolytic [164]. Our results have shown that curcumin slightly diminished the survival of vascular smooth muscle cells (VSMCs) undergoing replicative but not stress-induced senescence (manuscript in preparation).

Although, originally, the term senolytic referred to agents that induced apoptosis in normal senescent cells, we are tempted to extend this definition to senescent cancer cells. We express the opinion that the induced senescence of cancer cells is harmful as it can lead to cancer recurrence due to polyploidization/depolypoidization associated with senescence and to cell regrowth [23,100,153]. Thus, it is urgent to search for drugs that would be able to kill senescent cancer cells. To our knowledge, there are no data showing that curcumin is able to selectively kill senescent cancer cells. Also, our own data do not support this possibility (manuscript in preparation). However, senescent cancer cells, as normal senescent cells, are characterized by SASP, which creates a pro-inflammatory microenvironment and reinforces cell senescence [165]. The main activator of SASP is the NF-κB transcription factor [105]. Recently, large Reed–Sternberg cells in Hodgkin's lymphoma, which display many features of cellular senescence, were shown to have an increased activity of NF-κB. Curcumin is one of the NF-κB inhibitors able to reduce the level of IL-6 secreted by senescent cells [166]. Our own results showed that there were no differences in the cytotoxicity of curcumin and SASP activity between non-senescent HCT116 cells and cells induced to senesce, or between normal replicatively and prematurely senescent VSMC (manuscript in preparation). Overall, results so far obtained by us and others do not unequivocally establish curcumin as a strong senolytic compound. However, it should be noted that no one has proved the universality of senolytic compounds. It seems that they are rather cell-type specific [157]; thus, it cannot be excluded that curcumin's usefulness as a senolytic compound is still awaiting approval.

5.6. Bioaviability and the Microbiome

A large number of controversies arise from the low bioavailability of curcumin. However, the low bioavailability of curcumin does not preclude its usage, as beneficial effects are observed in low doses [167–169]. As mentioned before, the poor bioavailability of curcumin is related to weak absorption and rapid elimination from the organism due to the high rate of metabolism. Even more, a higher curcumin concentration could be harmful. In organisms, curcumin is metabolized during transition through the digestive tract (mostly in small intestine) and in liver [170]. The most common products of curcumin metabolism are glucuronides [171,172]. Such conjugates (mono- and diglucuronides) are less active, and therefore the results obtained in cell culture can differ from those obtained in vitro. However, in organisms, there is a lysosomal enzyme responsible for the deconjugation of glucuronides, namely β-glucuronidase, and curcumin glucuronide is one of its substrates [173–175]. This protein is expressed in all cell types, with high expression in macrophages, and its activity is highest in the liver. β-glucuronidase activity increases in inflammation [176], and a low-grade inflammatory state is associated with ageing and age-related disease. It can be assumed that local concentrations of curcumin can differ from that detected in serum, as described for other polyphenols in tumor tissue [177]. It cannot be excluded that pro-inflammatory conditions associated with ageing and age-related diseases are responsible for elevated concentrations of non-metabolized curcumin in disease-affected tissue/organs. This, in turn, depending on the type of disease, may lead to adverse effects (e.g., senescence induction in neighboring non-senescent cells). Curcumin glucuronidation is only one of the many factors which affect curcumin bioavailability. The concentration in the serum and tissues depends also on numerous different elements such as low concentration in the food (curcuminoids constitute about 4% of turmeric, and curcumin constitutes 70% of curcuminoids) and interaction with other diet ingredients (the most recognized example is the already mentioned piperine). Curcumin is able to cross the blood–brain barrier (BBB) [178,179], although the permeability is limited [180]. Even though the concentration in brain tissue is lower than in serum, curcumin alleviates neuroinflammation. Nowadays, it is frequently claimed that the real activity of the majority of polyphenols, including curcumin, on the organismal level, is not direct but is mediated by microbiota [181,182]. Moreover, there are data which suggest that intestinal bacteria produce a high amount of β-glucuronidase that can elevate the level of free compounds [183]. This means that microbiota can be responsible for drug metabolism and bioavailability. The microbiome changes over the course of a lifetime [184], and ageing is associated with a reduction of microbial diversity in terms of composition, quality and quantity. It is suggested that healthy ageing correlates with microbiome diversity [185]. Microbiota can modulate certain processes, namely innate immunity, sarcopenia and cognitive dysfunction, adding up to frailty [184]. There is some indication that curcumin is able to modulate gut microbial composition (i.e., biodiversity) [186–188]. It can be assumed that, by modulating the microbiome, curcumin may reduce some adverse consequences of ageing, at least those related to frailty. In summary, curcumin, through impacts on the microbiota, might positively influence certain organismal functions, and microbiota, by their ability to metabolize curcumin, can regulate its bioavailability.

6. Conclusions

Accumulating evidence suggests that one of the causes of organismal ageing is cellular senescence. Senescent cells, besides a loss of proliferating ability, are characterized by SASP, which fuels low-grade chronic inflammation, tumor progression and hinders regeneration. The number of senescent cells increases with age, and their impact on the surrounding cells and the microenvironment escalates. Moreover, senescent cells are found in areas affected by age-related diseases. Studies on genetically modified mice showed that the removal of senescent cells (p16 positive) delayed the onset of ageing, improved tissue functioning, delayed tumorigenesis and allowed animals to reach older age, although without increasing the maximal lifespan. The mice looked younger and were fitter. These data suggest that it may be possible to mitigate age-associated diseases simply by decreasing the number of senescent cells and prompted researchers to look for senolytic drugs and supplements which can selectively induce apoptosis of such cells. Data collected by curcumin researchers showed a large number of beneficial activities for this compound. They mostly concern its anti-cancer activity, but, for several years, the amount of data showing curcumin's role in the modulation of ageing has been intensively growing, and the issue is widely discussed. Some data suggest a beneficial role, some raise a great deal of skepticism, because unexpected, and sometimes even unfavorable, effects can be observed (e.g., the induction of cell senescence). Curcumin activity depends on the concentration, formulation (pure natural or modified), cell type (differences in vulnerability) and context (organism, disease, manner of administration). Our own data shown that curcumin anti-ageing function results neither from its anti-senescent nor senolytic function, even though curcumin is able to modulate cellular senescence. Low doses activated sirtuins and AMPK, which are considered as having anti-senescent properties, but cytostatic doses inhibited sirtuins and AMPK, inducing, in this manner, cellular senescence (Figure 1).

Moreover, despite a plethora of in vitro as well as in vivo studies on model organisms which document the positive effects of curcumin treatment, human trials are not always as encouraging. For example, preclinical studies on rat models of AD-type sporadic dementia showed that curcumin supplementation was effective in counteracting cognitive decline in animals. However, in clinical studies, after 24 weeks of curcumin supplementation (4 g/day), researchers were unable to detect significant plasma levels of curcumin or any improvement in the cognitive function of AD patients [189]. One of the causes could be the low bioavailability of curcumin, which can be attributed to rapid metabolism and elimination as well as low absorption in the gastro-intestinal tract and mutual interactions with gut microbiota [190].

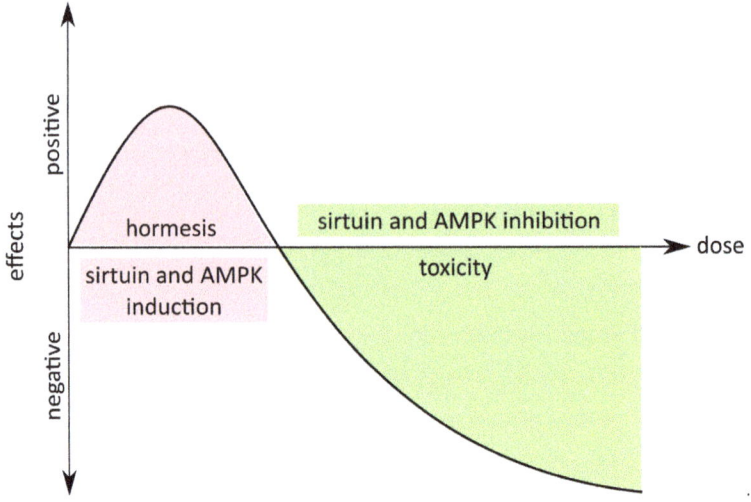

Figure 1. Hormetic properties of curcumin. Low doses of curcumin exert positive effects at the organismal (life extension) and cellular level (activation of sirtuins and AMP-activated kinase (AMPK)); however, at higher doses, curcumin can be toxic or cytostatic (inhibition of sirtuins and AMPK).

An excessive increase in bioavailability could be dangerous, especially when curcumin is used as a protective agent. As we have shown, it can induce cellular senescence in relatively low concentrations. This may be beneficial to inhibit tumor progression but could cause also adverse effects, such as the accelerated senescence of different cell types, resulting in premature loss of tissue/organ function. In turn, therapeutic doses should be much higher than protective ones. Moreover, questions arise concerning not only the dose but also when curcumin supplementation should be recommended. Additional meticulous studies are required to solve all doubts and properly exploit such an interesting and promising agent in anti-ageing research.

What is the future of curcumin in anti-ageing strategy? Curcumin possesses a substantial number of supporters and opponents. In our opinion, the positive impact of curcumin on ageing cannot be neglected. Undoubtedly, some precautions in curcumin exploitation necessarily take into account the biphasic response due to its hormetic properties. Curcumin applied in the diet is beneficial. It can act as a tumor suppressor, can lead to the reduction of low-grade inflammation, which is associated with ageing, and to the alleviation of symptoms of age-related diseases, including frailty. Moreover, the impact of curcumin on the microbiome seems to be very promising in the context of the modulation of the ageing process. This issue leaves us with many questions to consider. However, the crucial aspect is its concentration, as stated by Paracelsus, "Omnia sunt venena, nihil est sine veneno. Sola dosis facit venenum": the dose makes the poison.

An overview of the impact of curcumin on ageing and age-related diseases (ARD) at the organismal and cellular level is summarized in Figure 2.

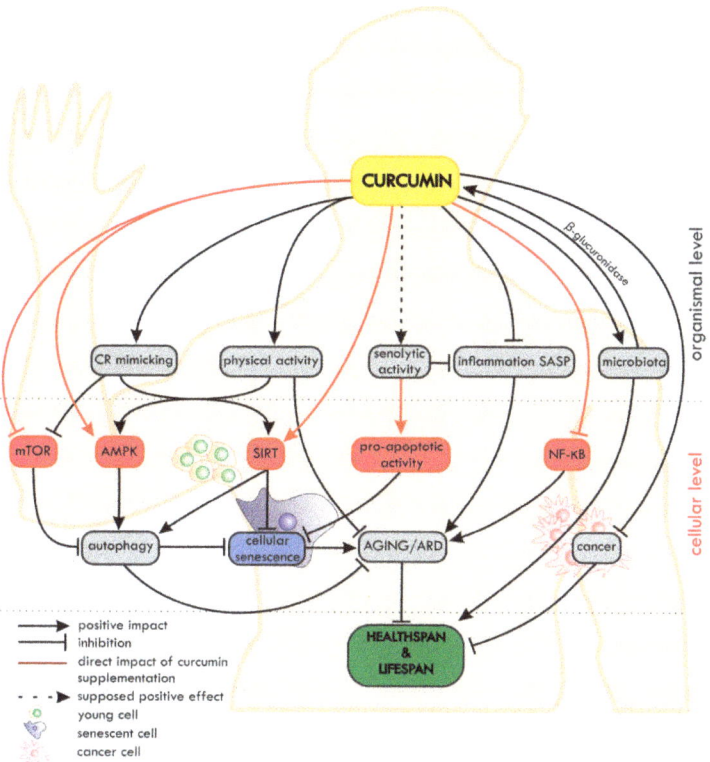

Figure 2. Overview of the impact of curcumin on ageing and age-related diseases (ARD) at the organismal and cellular level. On the organismal level, curcumin mimics caloric restriction (CR) and improves the effectiveness of physical activity (which in fact mimics CR). The potential senolytic activity of curcumin is still unclear, but curcumin can reduce inflammation and SASP, which are also considered as elements of senotherapy. Moreover, curcumin maintains the diversity of the microbiome and, in turn, the microbiota secrete β-glucuronidase, an enzyme, which, by deglucuronisation increases the level of curcumin in tissues. Curcumin is able to protect against cancer and to reduce the progression of already existing tumors. On the cellular level, curcumin elevates the level/activity of some anti-ageing proteins (e.g., sirtuins, AMPK) and inhibits pro-ageing ones (e.g., NF-κB, mTOR). Autophagy, considered as an anti-ageing mechanism, is modulated by curcumin, with the effect of preventing cell senescence. Altogether, by delaying ageing and ARD, curcumin can elongate the healthspan and probably also the lifespan.

Funding: This study was supported by National Science Centre grants: UMO-2011/01/B/NZ3/02137, UMO-2016/21/B/NZ3/00370 (to ABZ), UMO-2014/15/B/NZ3/01150 (to GM), UMO-2015/17/B/NZ3/03531 (to ES) and by the Nencki Institute statutory funds.

Conflicts of Interest: The authors declare no conflict of interest.

References

1. The World Bank. Available online: https://data.worldbank.org (accessed on 26 February 2019).
2. López-Otín, C.; Blasco, M.A.; Partridge, L.; Serrano, M.; Kroemer, G. The hallmarks of aging. *Cell* **2013**, *153*, 1194–1217. [CrossRef] [PubMed]
3. Van Deursen, J.M. The role of senescent cells in ageing. *Nature* **2014**, *509*, 439–446. [CrossRef] [PubMed]

4. Herbig, U.; Ferreira, M.; Condel, L.; Carey, D.; Sedivy, J.M. Cellular senescence in aging primates. *Science* **2006**, *311*, 1257. [CrossRef] [PubMed]
5. Wang, C.; Jurk, D.; Maddick, M.; Nelson, G.; Martin-ruiz, C.; Von Zglinicki, T. DNA damage response and cellular senescence in tissues of aging mice. *Aging Cell* **2009**, *8*, 311–323. [CrossRef] [PubMed]
6. Sedelnikova, O.A.; Horikawa, I.; Zimonjic, D.B.; Popescu, N.C.; Bonner, W.M.; Barrett, J.C. Senescing human cells and ageing mice accumulate DNA lesions with unrepairable double-strand breaks. *Nat. Cell Biol.* **2004**, *6*, 168–170. [CrossRef] [PubMed]
7. Dimri, G.P.; Lee, X.; Basile, G.; Acosta, M.; Scott, G.; Roskelley, C.; Medrano, E.E.; Linskens, M.; Rubelj, I.; Pereira-Smith, O. A biomarker that identifies senescent human cells in culture and in aging skin in vivo. *Proc Natl Acad Sci. USA* **1995**, *92*, 9363–9367. [CrossRef]
8. Jeyapalan, J.C.; Ferreira, M.; Sedivy, J.M.; Herbig, U. Accumulation of senescent cells in mitotic tissue of aging primates. *Mech. Ageing Dev.* **2007**, *128*, 36–44. [CrossRef]
9. Naylor, R.M.; Baker, D.J.; Van Deursen, J.M. Senescent cells: A novel therapeutic target for aging and age-related diseases. *Clin. Pharmacol. Ther.* **2013**, *93*, 105–116. [CrossRef]
10. Baker, D.J.; Wijshake, T.; Tchkonia, T.; Lebrasseur, N.K.; Childs, B.G.; Van De Sluis, B.; Kirkland, J.L.; Van Deursen, J.M. Clearance of p16 Ink4a-positive senescent cells delays ageing-associated disorders. *Nature* **2011**, *479*, 232–236. [CrossRef]
11. Baker, D.J.; Childs, B.G.; Durik, M.; Wijers, M.E.; Sieben, C.J.; Zhong, J.A.; Saltness, R.; Jeganathan, K.B.; Verzosa, G.C.; Pezeshki, A.; et al. Naturally occurring p16 Ink4a-positive cells shorten healthy lifespan. *Nature* **2016**, *530*, 184–189. [CrossRef]
12. Niccoli, T.; Partridge, L. Ageing as a risk factor for disease. *Curr. Biol.* **2012**, *22*, R741–R752. [CrossRef] [PubMed]
13. Hayflick, L.; Moorhead, P.S. The serial cultivation of human diploid cell strains. *Exp. Cell Res.* **1961**, *25*, 585–621. [CrossRef]
14. Capasso, S.; Alessio, N.; Squillaro, T.; Di Bernardo, G.; Melone, M.A.; Cipollaro, M.; Peluso, G.; Galderisi, U.; Capasso, S.; Alessio, N.; et al. Changes in autophagy, proteasome activity and metabolism to determine a specific signature for acute and chronic senescent mesenchymal stromal cells. *Oncotarget* **2015**, *6*, 39457–39468. [CrossRef] [PubMed]
15. Alessio, N.; Squillaro, T.; Özcan, S.; Di Bernardo, G.; Venditti, M.; Melone, M.; Peluso, G.; Galderisi, U. Stress and stem cells: Adult Muse cells tolerate extensive genotoxic stimuli better than mesenchymal stromal cells. *Oncotarget* **2018**, *9*, 19328–19341. [CrossRef] [PubMed]
16. Bielak-Zmijewska, A.; Mosieniak, G.; Sikora, E. Is DNA damage indispensable for stress-induced senescence? *Mech. Ageing Dev.* **2018**, *170*, 13–21. [CrossRef] [PubMed]
17. de Magalhães, J.P.; Passos, J.F. Stress, cell senescence and organismal ageing. *Mech. Ageing Dev.* **2018**, *170*, 2–9. [CrossRef] [PubMed]
18. Rodier, F.; Campisi, J. Four faces of cellular senescence. *J. Cell Biol.* **2011**, *192*, 547–556. [CrossRef]
19. Sikora, E.; Bielak-Żmijewska, A.; Mosieniak, G. What is and what is not cell senescence. *Postepy Biochem.* **2018**, *62*, 110–118.
20. Bielak-Zmijewska, A.; Wnuk, M.; Przybylska, D.; Grabowska, W.; Lewinska, A.; Alster, O.; Korwek, Z.; Cmoch, A.; Myszka, A.; Pikula, S.; et al. A comparison of replicative senescence and doxorubicin-induced premature senescence of vascular smooth muscle cells isolated from human aorta. *Biogerontology* **2014**, *15*, 47–64. [CrossRef]
21. Özcan, S.; Alessio, N.; Acar, M.B.; Mert, E.; Omerli, F.; Peluso, G.; Galderisi, U. Unbiased analysis of senescence associated secretory phenotype (SASP) to identify common components following different genotoxic stresses. *Aging* **2016**, *8*, 1316–1329. [CrossRef]
22. Piechota, M.; Sunderland, P.; Wysocka, A.; Nalberczak, M.; Sliwinska, M.A.; Radwanska, K.; Sikora, E. Is senescence-associated β-galactosidase a marker of neuronal senescence? *Oncotarget* **2016**, *7*, 81099–81109. [CrossRef] [PubMed]
23. Sikora, E.; Mosieniak, G.; Alicja Sliwinska, M. Morphological and Functional Characteristic of Senescent Cancer Cells. *Curr. Drug Targets* **2016**, *17*, 377–387. [CrossRef] [PubMed]
24. Schmitt, R. Senotherapy: Growing old and staying young? *Pflugers Arch. Eur. J. Physiol.* **2017**, *469*, 1051–1059. [CrossRef] [PubMed]

25. Gorenne, I.; Kavurma, M.; Scott, S.; Bennett, M. Vascular smooth muscle cell senescence in atherosclerosis. *Cardiovasc. Res.* **2006**, *72*, 9–17. [CrossRef] [PubMed]
26. Minamino, T.; Komuro, I. Vascular cell senescence: Contribution to atherosclerosis. *Circ. Res.* **2007**, *100*, 15–26. [CrossRef] [PubMed]
27. Tchkonia, T.; Morbeck, D.E.; Von Zglinicki, T.; Van Deursen, J.; Lustgarten, J.; Scrable, H.; Khosla, S.; Jensen, M.D.; Kirkland, J.L. Fat tissue, aging, and cellular senescence. *Aging Cell* **2010**, *9*, 667–684. [CrossRef]
28. Minagawa, S.; Araya, J.; Numata, T.; Nojiri, S.; Hara, H.; Yumino, Y.; Kawaishi, M.; Odaka, M.; Morikawa, T.; Nishimura, S.L.; et al. Accelerated epithelial cell senescence in IPF and the inhibitory role of SIRT6 in TGF-β-induced senescence of human bronchial epithelial cells. *Am. J. Physiol. Cell Mol. Physiol.* **2011**, *300*, L391–L401. [CrossRef] [PubMed]
29. McShea, A.; Harris, P.L.R.; Webster, K.R.; Wahl, A.F.; Smith, M.A. Abnormal Expression Of the Cell Cycle Regulators P16 and Cdk4 In Alzheimers-Disease. *Am. J. Pathol.* **1997**, *150*, 1933–1939. [CrossRef]
30. Cohen, G. The pathobiology of Parkinson's disease: Biochemical aspects of dopamine neuron senescence. *J. Neural Transm. Suppl.* **1983**, *19*, 89–103.
31. He, N.; Jin, W.L.; Lok, K.H.; Wang, Y.; Yin, M.; Wang, Z.J. Amyloid-β1-42oligomer accelerates senescence in adult hippocampal neural stem/progenitor cells via formylpeptide receptor 2. *Cell Death Dis.* **2013**, *4*, e924. [CrossRef]
32. Price, J.S.; Waters, J.G.; Darrah, C.; Pennington, C.; Edwards, D.R.; Donell, S.T.; Clark, I.M. The role of chondrocyte senescence in osteoarthritis. *Aging Cell* **2002**, *1*, 57–65. [CrossRef]
33. Balasubramanian, P.; Howell, P.R.; Anderson, R.M. Aging and Caloric Restriction Research: A Biological Perspective With Translational Potential. *EBioMedicine* **2017**, *21*, 37–44. [CrossRef]
34. Ingram, D.K.; de Cabo, R. Calorie restriction in rodents: Caveats to consider. *Ageing Res. Rev.* **2017**, *39*, 15–28. [CrossRef]
35. Weindruch, R. The retardation of aging by caloric restriction: Studies in rodents and primates. *Toxicol. Pathol.* **1996**, *24*, 742–745. [CrossRef]
36. Masoro, E.J. Overview of caloric restriction and ageing. *Mech. Ageing Dev.* **2005**, *126*, 913–922. [CrossRef]
37. Grabowska, W.; Sikora, E.; Bielak-Zmijewska, A. Sirtuins, a promising target in slowing down the ageing process. *Biogerontology* **2017**, *18*, 447–476. [CrossRef]
38. Lane, M.A.; Baer, D.J.; Rumpler, W.V.; Weindruch, R.; Ingram, D.K.; Tilmont, E.M.; Cutler, R.G.; Roth, G.S. Calorie restriction lowers body temperature in rhesus monkeys, consistent with a postulated anti-aging mechanism in rodents. *Proc Natl Acad Sci. USA* **1996**, *93*, 4159–4164. [CrossRef]
39. Most, J.; Tosti, V.; Redman, L.M.; Fontana, L. Calorie restriction in humans: An update. *Ageing Res Rev.* **2017**, *39*, 36–45. [CrossRef]
40. Suzuki, S.; Yamatoya, H.; Sakai, M.; Kataoka, A.; Furushiro, M.; Kudo, S. Oral Administration of Soybean Lecithin Transphosphatidylated Phosphatidylserine Improves Memory Impairment in Aged Rats. *J. Nutr.* **2001**, *131*, 2951–2956. [CrossRef]
41. Colman, R.J.; Anderson, R.M.; Johnson, S.C.; Kastman, E.K.; Kosmatka, K.J.; Beasley, T.M.; Allison, D.B.; Cruzen, C.; Simmons, H.A.; Kemnitz, J.W.; et al. Caloric restriction delays disease onset and mortality in rhesus monkeys. *Science* **2009**, *325*, 201–204. [CrossRef]
42. Colman, R.J.; Beasley, T.M.; Kemnitz, J.W.; Johnson, S.C.; Weindruch, R.; Anderson, R.M. Caloric restriction reduces age-related and all-cause mortality in rhesus monkeys. *Nat. Commun.* **2014**, *5*, 3557. [CrossRef]
43. Hanjani, N.; Vafa, M. Protein restriction, epigenetic diet, intermittent fasting as new approaches for preventing age-associated diseases. *Int. J. Prev. Med.* **2018**, *9*, 58. [CrossRef]
44. Mattson, M.P.; Longo, V.D.; Harvie, M. Impact of intermittent fasting on health and disease processes. *Ageing Res. Rev.* **2017**, *39*, 46–58. [CrossRef]
45. Goodrick, C.L.; Ingram, D.K.; Reynolds, M.A.; Freeman, J.R.; Cider, N.L. Effects on intermittent feeding upon growth and life span in rats. *Gerontology* **1982**, *28*, 233–241. [CrossRef]
46. Goodrick, C.L.; Ingram, D.K.; Reynolds, M.A.; Freeman, J.R.; Cider, N.L. Differential effects of intermittent feeding and voluntary exercise on body weight and lifespan in adult rats. *J. Gerontol.* **1983**, *38*, 36–45. [CrossRef]
47. Catterson, J.H.; Khericha, M.; Dyson, M.C.; Vincent, A.J.; Callard, R.; Haveron, S.M.; Rajasingam, A.; Ahmad, M.; Partridge, L. Short-Term, Intermittent Fasting Induces Long-Lasting Gut Health and TOR-Independent Lifespan Extension. *Curr. Biol.* **2018**, *28*, 1714–1724. [CrossRef]

48. Bagherniya, M.; Butler, A.E.; Barreto, G.E.; Sahebkar, A. The effect of fasting or calorie restriction on autophagy induction: A review of the literature. *Ageing Res. Rev.* **2018**, *47*, 183–197. [CrossRef]
49. Wątroba, M.; Szukiewicz, D. The role of sirtuins in aging and age-related diseases. *Adv. Med. Sci.* **2016**, *61*, 52–62. [CrossRef]
50. Jayasena, T.; Poljak, A.; Smythe, G.; Braidy, N.; Münch, G.; Sachdev, P. The role of polyphenols in the modulation of sirtuins and other pathways involved in Alzheimer's disease. *Ageing Res. Rev.* **2013**, *12*, 867–883. [CrossRef]
51. Hubbard, B.P.; Sinclair, D.A. Small molecule SIRT1 activators for the treatment of aging and age-related diseases. *Trends Pharmacol. Sci.* **2014**, *35*, 146–154. [CrossRef]
52. Greathouse, K.L.; Samuels, M.; DiMarco, N.M.; Criswell, D.S. Effects of increased dietary fat and exercise on skeletal muscle lipid peroxidation and antioxidant capacity in male rats. *Eur. J. Nutr.* **2005**, *44*, 429–435. [CrossRef]
53. Radak, Z.; Chung, H.Y.; Goto, S. Systemic adaptation to oxidative challenge induced by regular exercise. *Free Radic. Biol. Med.* **2008**, *44*, 153–159. [CrossRef]
54. Tyagi, A.K.; Prasad, S.; Yuan, W.; Li, S.; Aggarwal, B.B. Identification of a novel compound (β-sesquiphellandrene) from turmeric (*Curcuma longa*) with anticancer potential: Comparison with curcumin. *Investig. New Drugs* **2015**, *33*, 1175–1186. [CrossRef]
55. Tayyem, R.F.; Heath, D.D.; Al-Delaimy, W.K.; Rock, C.L. Curcumin content of turmeric and curry powders. *Nutr. Cancer* **2006**, *55*, 126–131. [CrossRef]
56. Liu, W.; Zhai, Y.; Heng, X.; Che, F.Y.; Chen, W.; Sun, D.; Zhai, G. Oral bioavailability of curcumin: Problems and advancements. *J. Drug Target* **2016**, *24*, 694–702. [CrossRef]
57. Cheng, A.L.; Hsu, C.H.; Lin, J.K.; Hsu, M.M.; Ho, Y.F.; Shen, T.S.; Ko, J.Y.; Lin, J.T.; Lin, B.R.; Ming-Shiang, W.; et al. Phase I clinical trial of curcumin, a chemopreventive agent, in patients with high-risk or pre-malignant lesions. *Anticancer Res.* **2001**, *21*, 2895–2900.
58. Shah, B.H.; Nawaz, Z.; Pertani, S.A.; Roomi, A.; Mahmood, H.; Saeed, S.A.; Gilani, A.H. Inhibitory effect of curcumin, a food spice from turmeric, on platelet-activating factor- and arachidonic acid-mediated platelet aggregation through inhibition of thromboxane formation and Ca2+ signaling. *Biochem. Pharmacol.* **1999**, *58*, 1167–1172. [CrossRef]
59. Shoba, G.; Joy, D.; Joseph, T.; Majeed, M.; Rajendran, R.; Srinivas, P.S.S.R. Influence of piperine on the pharmacokinetics of curcumin in animals and human volunteers. *Planta Med.* **1998**, *64*, 353–356. [CrossRef]
60. Dey, S.; Sreenivasan, K. Conjugation of curcumin onto alginate enhances aqueous solubility and stability of curcumin. *Carbohydr. Polym.* **2014**, *99*, 499–507. [CrossRef]
61. Liu, J.; Liu, J.; Xu, H.; Zhang, Y.; Chu, L.; Liu, Q.; Song, N.; Yang, C. Novel tumor-targeting, self-assembling peptide nanofiber as a carrier for effective curcumin delivery. *Int. J. Nanomed.* **2014**, *9*, 197–207. [CrossRef]
62. Nelson, K.M.; Dahlin, J.L.; Bisson, J.; Graham, J.; Pauli, G.F.; Walters, M.A. The Essential Medicinal Chemistry of Curcumin. *J. Med. Chem.* **2017**, *60*, 1620–1637. [CrossRef]
63. Kunnumakkara, A.B.; Bordoloi, D.; Padmavathi, G.; Monisha, J.; Roy, N.K.; Prasad, S.; Aggarwal, B.B. Curcumin, the golden nutraceutical: Multitargeting for multiple chronic diseases. *Br. J. Pharmacol.* **2017**, *174*, 1325–1348. [CrossRef]
64. Pulido-Moran, M.; Moreno-Fernandez, J.; Ramirez-Tortosa, C.; Ramirez-Tortosa, M.C. Curcumin and health. *Molecules* **2016**, *21*, 264. [CrossRef]
65. Gupta, S.C.; Kismali, G.; Aggarwal, B.B. Curcumin, a component of turmeric: From farm to pharmacy. *BioFactors* **2013**, *39*, 2–13. [CrossRef]
66. Boyanapalli, S.S.S.; Kong, A.N.T. "Curcumin, the King of Spices": Epigenetic Regulatory Mechanisms in the Prevention of Cancer, Neurological, and Inflammatory Diseases. *Curr. Pharmacol. Rep.* **2015**, *1*, 129–139. [CrossRef]
67. Remely, M.; Lovrecic, L.; de la Garza, A.L.; Migliore, L.; Peterlin, B.; Milagro, F.; Martinez, A.; Haslberger, A. Therapeutic perspectives of epigenetically active nutrients. *Br. J. Pharmacol.* **2015**, *172*, 2756–2768. [CrossRef]
68. Reuter, S.; Gupta, S.C.; Park, B.; Goel, A.; Aggarwal, B.B. Epigenetic changes induced by curcumin and other natural compounds. *Genes Nutr.* **2011**, *6*, 93–108. [CrossRef]
69. Salehia, B.; Stojanovc-Radcb, Z.; Matejic, J.; Sharifi-Radd, M.; Kumare, N.V.A.; Martinsf, N.; Sharifi-Rad, J. The therapeutic potential of curcumin: A review of clinical trials. *Eur. J. Med. Chem.* **2019**, *163*, 527–545. [CrossRef]

70. Moghaddam, N.S.A.; Oskouie, M.N.; Butler, A.E.; Petit, P.X.; Barreto, G.E.; Sahebkar, A. Hormetic effects of curcumin: What is the evidence? *J. Cell. Physiol.* **2018**, *1*, 1–12. [CrossRef]
71. Calder, P.C.; Bosco, N.; Bourdet-Sicard, R.; Capuron, L.; Delzenne, N.; Doré, J.; Franceschi, C.; Lehtinen, M.J.; Recker, T.; Salvioli, S.; et al. Health relevance of the modification of low grade inflammation in ageing (inflammageing) and the role of nutrition. *Ageing Res. Rev.* **2017**, *40*, 95–119. [CrossRef]
72. Sandur, S.K.; Ichikawa, H.; Pandey, M.K.; Kunnumakkara, A.B.; Sung, B.; Sethi, G.; Aggarwal, B.B. Role of pro-oxidants and antioxidants in the anti-inflammatory and apoptotic effects of curcumin (diferuloylmethane). *Free Radic. Biol. Med.* **2007**, *43*, 568–580. [CrossRef]
73. Sikora, E.; Scapagnini, G.; Barbagallo, M. Curcumin, inflammation, ageing and age-related diseases. *Immun. Ageing* **2010**, *7*, 1. [CrossRef]
74. Sikora, E.; Bielak-Zmijewska, A.; Mosieniak, G.; Piwocka, K. The Promise of Slow Down Ageing May Come from Curcumin. *Curr. Pharm. Des.* **2010**, *16*, 884–892. [CrossRef]
75. Salvioli, S.; Sikora, E.; Cooper, E.L.; Franceschi, C. Curcumin in cell death processes: A challenge for CAM of age-related pathologies. *Evid.-Based Complement. Altern. Med.* **2007**, *4*, 181–190. [CrossRef]
76. Liao, V.H.C.; Yu, C.W.; Chu, Y.J.; Li, W.H.; Hsieh, Y.C.; Wang, T.T. Curcumin-mediated lifespan extension in Caenorhabditis elegans. *Mech. Ageing Dev.* **2011**, *132*, 480–487. [CrossRef]
77. Lee, K.-S.; Lee, B.-S.; Semnani, S.; Avanesian, A.; Um, C.-Y.; Jeon, H.-J.; Seong, K.-M.; Yu, K.; Min, K.-J.; Jafari, M. Curcumin Extends Life Span, Improves Health Span, and Modulates the Expression of Age-Associated Aging Genes in Drosophila melanogaster. *Rejuvenation Res.* **2010**, *13*, 561–570. [CrossRef]
78. Soh, J.W.; Marowsky, N.; Nichols, T.J.; Rahman, A.M.; Miah, T.; Sarao, P.; Khasawneh, R.; Unnikrishnan, A.; Heydari, A.R.; Silver, R.B.; et al. Curcumin is an early-acting stage-specific inducer of extended functional longevity in Drosophila. *Exp. Gerontol.* **2013**, *48*, 229–239. [CrossRef]
79. Shen, L.R.; Parnell, L.D.; Ordovas, J.M.; Lai, C.Q. Curcumin and aging. *BioFactors* **2013**, *39*, 133–140. [CrossRef]
80. Olszanecki, R.; Jawień, J.; Gajda, M.; Mateuszuk Gębska, A.; Korabiowska, M.; Chłopicki, S.; Korbut, R. Effect of curcumin on atherosclerosis in apoE/LDLR—Double knockout mice. *J. Physiol. Pharmacol.* **2005**, *56*, 627–635.
81. He, Y.; Yue, Y.; Zheng, X.; Zhang, K.; Chen, S.; Du, Z. Curcumin, inflammation, and chronic diseases: How are they linked? *Molecules* **2015**, *20*, 9183–9213. [CrossRef]
82. Sun, Q.; Jia, N.; Wang, W.; Jin, H.; Xu, J.; Hu, H. Activation of SIRT1 by curcumin blocks the neurotoxicity of amyloid-β25-35 in rat cortical neurons. *Biochem. Biophys. Res. Commun.* **2014**, *448*, 89–94. [CrossRef]
83. Swamy, A.; Gulliaya, S.; Thippeswamy, A.; Koti, B.; Manjula, D. Cardioprotective effect of curcumin against doxorubicin-induced myocardial toxicity in albino rats. *Indian J. Pharmacol.* **2012**, *44*, 73. [CrossRef]
84. Ryan, J.L.; Heckler, C.E.; Ling, M.; Katz, A.; Williams, J.P.; Pentland, A.P.; Morrow, G.R. Curcumin for Radiation Dermatitis: A Randomized, Double-Blind, Placebo-Controlled Clinical Trial of Thirty Breast Cancer Patients. *Radiat. Res.* **2013**, *180*, 34–43. [CrossRef]
85. Sun, Y.; Hu, X.; Hu, G.; Xu, C.; Jiang, H. Curcumin Attenuates Hydrogen Peroxide-Induced Premature Senescence via the Activation of SIRT1 in Human Umbilical Vein Endothelial Cells. *Biol. Pharm. Bull.* **2015**, *38*, 1134–1141. [CrossRef]
86. Kitani, K.; Osawa, T.; Yokozawa, T. The effects of tetrahydrocurcumin and green tea polyphenol on the survival of male C57BL/6 mice. *Biogerontology* **2007**, *8*, 567–573. [CrossRef]
87. Berge, U.; Kristensen, P.; Rattan, S.I.S. Hormetic modulation of differentiation of normal human epidermal keratinocytes undergoing replicative senescence in vitro. *Exp. Gerontol.* **2008**, *43*, 658–662. [CrossRef]
88. Grabowska, W.; Suszek, M.; Wnuk, M.; Lewinska, A.; Wasiak, E.; Sikora, E.; Bielak-Zmijewska, A. Curcumin elevates sirtuin level but does not postpone in vitro senescence of human cells building the vasculature. *Oncotarget* **2016**, *7*, 19201–19213. [CrossRef]
89. Huang, W.C.; Chiu, W.C.; Chuang, H.L.; Tang, D.W.; Lee, Z.M.; Li, W.; Chen, F.A.; Huang, C.C. Effect of curcumin supplementation on physiological fatigue and physical performance in mice. *Nutrients* **2015**, *7*, 905–921. [CrossRef]
90. Ray Hamidie, R.D.; Yamada, T.; Ishizawa, R.; Saito, Y.; Masuda, K. Curcumin treatment enhances the effect of exercise on mitochondrial biogenesis in skeletal muscle by increasing cAMP levels. *Metabolism* **2015**, *64*, 1334–1347. [CrossRef]

91. Grabowska, W.; Kucharewicz, K.; Wnuk, M.; Lewinska, A.; Suszek, M.; Przybylska, D.; Mosieniak, G.; Sikora, E.; Bielak-Zmijewska, A. Curcumin induces senescence of primary human cells building the vasculature in a DNA damage and ATM-independent manner. *Age* **2015**, *37*, 1–17. [CrossRef]
92. Hendrayani, S.-F.; Al-Khalaf, H.H.; Aboussekhra, A. Curcumin Triggers p16-Dependent Senescence in Active Breast Cancer-Associated Fibroblasts and Suppresses Their Paracrine Procarcinogenic Effects. *Neoplasia* **2013**, *15*, 631–640. [CrossRef] [PubMed]
93. Jin, H.; Jia, Y.; Yao, Z.; Huang, J.; Hao, M.; Yao, S.; Lian, N.; Zhang, F.; Zhang, C.; Chen, X.; et al. Hepatic stellate cell interferes with NK cell regulation of fibrogenesis via curcumin induced senescence of hepatic stellate cell. *Cell Signal.* **2017**, *33*, 79–85. [CrossRef] [PubMed]
94. Bielak-Zmijewska, A.; Sikora-Polaczek, M.; Nieznanski, K.; Mosieniak, G.; Kolano, A.; Maleszewski, M.; Styrna, J.; Sikora, E. Curcumin disrupts meiotic and mitotic divisions via spindle impairment and inhibition of CDK1 activity. *Cell Prolif.* **2010**, *43*, 354–364. [CrossRef] [PubMed]
95. Hansen, J. Common cancers in the elderly. *Drugs Aging* **1998**, *13*, 467–478. [CrossRef] [PubMed]
96. Holy, J. Curcumin inhibits cell motility and alters microfilament organization and function in prostate cancer cells. *Cell Motil. Cytoskelet.* **2004**, *58*, 253–268. [CrossRef]
97. Mosieniak, G.; Sliwinska, M.A.; Przybylska, D.; Grabowska, W.; Sunderland, P.; Bielak-Zmijewska, A.; Sikora, E. Curcumin-treated cancer cells show mitotic disturbances leading to growth arrest and induction of senescence phenotype. *Int. J. Biochem. Cell Biol.* **2016**, *74*, 33–43. [CrossRef] [PubMed]
98. Lewinska, A.; Wnuk, M.; Grabowska, W.; Zabek, T.; Semik, E.; Sikora, E.; Bielak-Zmijewska, A. Curcumin induces oxidation-dependent cell cycle arrest mediated by SIRT7 inhibition of rDNA transcription in human aortic smooth muscle cells. *Toxicol. Lett.* **2015**, *233*, 227–238. [CrossRef] [PubMed]
99. Albin, N.; Massaad, L.; Toussaint, C.; Mathieu, M.C.; Morizet, J.; Parise, O.; Gouyette, A.; Chabot, G.G. Main Drug-metabolizing Enzyme Systems in Human Breast Tumors and Peritumoral Tissues. *Cancer Res.* **1993**, *53*, 3541–3546.
100. Mosieniak, G.; Sliwinska, M.A.; Alster, O.; Strzeszewska, A.; Sunderland, P.; Piechota, M.; Was, H.; Sikora, E. Polyploidy Formation in Doxorubicin-Treated Cancer Cells Can Favor Escape from Senescence. *Neoplasia* **2015**, *17*, 882–893. [CrossRef]
101. Kuilman, T.; Michaloglou, C.; Vredeveld, L.C.W.; Douma, S.; van Doorn, R.; Desmet, C.J.; Aarden, L.A.; Mooi, W.J.; Peeper, D.S. Oncogene-Induced Senescence Relayed by an Interleukin-Dependent Inflammatory Network. *Cell* **2008**, *133*, 1019–1031. [CrossRef]
102. Sagiv, A.; Krizhanovsky, V. Immunosurveillance of senescent cells: The bright side of the senescence program. *Biogerontology* **2013**, *14*, 617–628. [CrossRef] [PubMed]
103. Krizhanovsky, V.; Yon, M.; Dickins, R.A.; Hearn, S.; Simon, J.; Miething, C.; Yee, H.; Zender, L.; Lowe, S.W. Senescence of Activated Stellate Cells Limits Liver Fibrosis. *Cell* **2008**, *134*, 657–667. [CrossRef] [PubMed]
104. Acosta, J.C.; Banito, A.; Wuestefeld, T.; Georgilis, A.; Janich, P.; Morton, J.P.; Athineos, D.; Kang, T.W.; Lasitschka, F.; Andrulis, M.; et al. A complex secretory program orchestrated by the inflammasome controls paracrine senescence. *Nat. Cell Biol.* **2013**, *15*, 978–990. [CrossRef] [PubMed]
105. Rodier, F.; Coppé, J.P.; Patil, C.K.; Hoeijmakers, W.A.M.; Muñoz, D.P.; Raza, S.R.; Freund, A.; Campeau, E.; Davalos, A.R.; Campisi, J. Persistent DNA damage signalling triggers senescence-associated inflammatory cytokine secretion. *Nat. Cell Biol.* **2009**, *11*, 973–979. [CrossRef] [PubMed]
106. Strzeszewska, A.; Alster, O.; Mosieniak, G.; Ciolko, A.; Sikora, E. Insight into the role of PIKK family members and NF-kB in DNAdamage-induced senescence and senescence-associated secretory phenotype of colon cancer cells article. *Cell Death Dis.* **2018**, *9*, 44. [CrossRef] [PubMed]
107. Aggarwal, S.; Ichikawa, H.; Takada, Y.; Sandur, S.K.; Shishodia, S.; Aggarwal, B.B. Curcumin (diferuloylmethane) down-regulates expression of cell proliferation and antiapoptotic and metastatic gene products through suppression of IkappaBalpha kinase and Akt activation. *Mol. Pharmacol.* **2006**, *69*, 195–206. [CrossRef]
108. Chung, S.; Yao, H.; Caito, S.; Hwang, J.; Arunachalam, G.; Rahman, I. Regulation of SIRT1 in cellular functions: Role of polyphenols. *Arch. Biochem. Biophys.* **2010**, *501*, 79–90. [CrossRef]
109. Hansen, M.; Rubinsztein, D.C.; Walker, D.W. Autophagy as a promoter of longevity: Insights from model organisms. *Nat. Rev. Mol. Cell Biol.* **2018**, *19*, 579–593. [CrossRef]
110. Brown-Borg, H.M.; Bartke, A. GH and IGF1: Roles in energy metabolism of long-living GH mutant mice. *J. Gerontol. Ser. A Biol. Sci. Med. Sci.* **2012**, *67*, 652–660. [CrossRef]

111. Hartford, C.M.; Ratain, M.J. Rapamycin: Something old, something new, sometimes borrowed and now renewed. *Clin. Pharmacol. Ther.* **2007**, *82*, 381–388. [CrossRef]
112. Jiao, D.; Wang, J.; Lu, W.; Tang, X.; Chen, J.; Mou, H.; Chen, Q.Y. Curcumin inhibited HGF-induced EMT and angiogenesis through regulating c-Met dependent PI3K/Akt/mTOR signaling pathways in lung cancer. *Mol. Ther. Oncolytics* **2016**, *3*, 16018. [CrossRef]
113. Onorati, A.V.; Dyczynski, M.; Ojha, R.; Amaravadi, R.K. Targeting autophagy in cancer. *Cancer* **2018**, *124*, 3307–3318. [CrossRef] [PubMed]
114. Saha, S.; Panigrahi, D.P.; Patil, S.; Bhutia, S.K. Autophagy in health and disease: A comprehensive review. *Biomed. Pharmacother.* **2018**, *104*, 485–495. [CrossRef] [PubMed]
115. Yun, C.W.; Lee, S.H. The Roles of Autophagy in Cancer. *Int. J. Mol. Sci.* **2018**, *19*, 3466. [CrossRef] [PubMed]
116. Lin, S.R.; Fu, Y.S.; Tsai, M.J.; Cheng, H.; Weng, C.F. Natural compounds from herbs that can potentially execute as autophagy inducers for cancer therapy. *Int. J. Mol. Sci.* **2017**, *18*, 1412. [CrossRef]
117. Shakeri, A.; Cicero, A.F.G.; Panahi, Y.; Mohajeri, M.; Sahebkar, A. Curcumin: A naturally occurring autophagy modulator. *J. Cell Physiol.* **2018**, *234*, 5643–5654. [CrossRef]
118. Zhang, X.; Chen, L.X.; Ouyang, L.; Cheng, Y.; Liu, B. Plant natural compounds: Targeting pathways of autophagy as anti-cancer therapeutic agents. *Cell Prolif.* **2012**, *45*, 466–476. [CrossRef]
119. Hasima, N.; Ozpolat, B. Regulation of autophagy by polyphenolic compounds as a potential therapeutic strategy for cancer. *Cell Death Dis.* **2014**, *5*, e1509. [CrossRef]
120. Zhang, J.; Wang, L.; Jiang, J.; Lu, Y.; Shen, H.-M.; Xia, D.; Wang, J.; Xu, J. Curcumin targets the TFEB-lysosome pathway for induction of autophagy. *Oncotarget* **2016**, *7*, 75659–75671. [CrossRef]
121. Maiti, P.; Rossignol, J.; Dunbar, G.L. Curcumin Modulates Molecular Chaperones and Autophagy-Lysosomal Pathways In Vitro after Exposure to Aβ42. *J. Alzheimer's Dis.* **2017**, *7*, 1000299. [CrossRef]
122. de Oliveira, M.R.; Jardim, F.R.; Setzer, W.N.; Nabavi, S.M.; Nabavi, S.F. Curcumin, mitochondrial biogenesis, and mitophagy: Exploring recent data and indicating future needs. *Biotechnol. Adv.* **2016**, *34*, 813–826. [CrossRef]
123. Giordano, S.; Darley-Usmar, V.; Zhang, J. Autophagy as an essential cellular antioxidant pathway in neurodegenerative disease. *Redox. Biol.* **2014**, *2*, 82–90. [CrossRef]
124. Kunnumakkara, A.B.; Anand, P.; Aggarwal, B.B. Curcumin inhibits proliferation, invasion, angiogenesis and metastasis of different cancers through interaction with multiple cell signaling proteins. *Cancer Lett.* **2008**, *269*, 199–225. [CrossRef]
125. Shanmugam, M.K.; Rane, G.; Kanchi, M.M.; Arfuso, F.; Chinnathambi, A.; Zayed, M.E.; Alharbi, S.A.; Tan, B.K.H.; Kumar, A.P.; Sethi, G. The multifaceted role of curcumin in cancer prevention and treatment. *Molecules* **2015**, *20*, 2728–2769. [CrossRef]
126. Mortezaee, K.; Salehi, E.; Mirtavoos-Mahyari, H.; Motevaseli, E.; Najafi, M.; Farhood, B.; Rosengren, R.J.; Sahebkar, A. Mechanisms of apoptosis modulation by curcumin: Implications for cancer therapy. *J. Cell Physiol.* **2019**, *1*. [CrossRef]
127. Shehzad, A.; Lee, J.; Lee, Y.S. Curcumin in various cancers. *BioFactors* **2013**, *39*, 56–68. [CrossRef]
128. Mosieniak, G.; Sliwinska, M.; Piwocka, K.; Sikora, E. Curcumin abolishes apoptosis resistance of calcitriol-differentiated HL-60 cells. *FEBS Lett.* **2006**, *580*, 4653–4660. [CrossRef]
129. Wolanin, K.; Magalska, A.; Mosieniak, G.; Klinger, R.; McKenna, S.; Vejda, S.; Sikora, E.; Piwocka, K. Curcumin Affects Components of the Chromosomal Passenger Complex and Induces Mitotic Catastrophe in Apoptosis-Resistant Bcr-Abl-Expressing Cells. *Mol. Cancer Res.* **2006**, *4*, 457–469. [CrossRef]
130. Magalska, A.; Sliwinska, M.; Szczepanowska, J.; Salvioli, S.; Franceschi, C.; Sikora, E. Resistance to apoptosis of HCW-2 cells can be overcome by curcumin- or vincristine-induced mitotic catastrophe. *Int. J. Cancer* **2006**, *119*, 1811–1818. [CrossRef]
131. Bielak-Zmijewska, A.; Piwocka, K.; Magalska, A.; Sikora, E. P-glycoprotein expression does not change the apoptotic pathway induced by curcumin in HL-60 cells. *Cancer Chemother. Pharmacol.* **2004**, *53*, 179–185. [CrossRef]
132. Piwocka, K.; Bielak-Zmijewska, A.; Sikora, E. Curcumin induces caspase-3-independent apoptosis in human multidrug-resistant cells. *Ann. N. Y. Acad Sci.* **2002**, *973*, 250–254. [CrossRef]
133. Piwocka, K.; Zablocki, K.; Wieckowski, M.R.; Skierski, J.; Feiga, I.; Szopa, J.; Drela, N.; Wojtczak, L.; Sikora, E. A novel apoptosis-like pathway, independent of mitochondria and caspases, induced by curcumin in human lymphoblastoid T (Jurkat) cells. *Exp. Cell Res.* **1999**, *249*, 299–307. [CrossRef]

134. Bielak-Żmijewska, A.; Koronkiewicz, M.; Skierski, J.; Piwocka, K.; Radziszewska, E.; Sikora, E. Effect of curcumin on the apoptosis of rodent and human nonproliferating and proliferating lymphoid cells. *Nutr. Cancer* **2000**, *38*, 131–138. [CrossRef]
135. Piwocka, K.; Jaruga, E.; Skierski, J.; Gradzka, I.; Sikora, E. Effect of glutathione depletion on caspase-3 independent apoptosis pathway induced by curcumin in Jurkat cells. *Free Radic. Biol. Med.* **2001**, *31*, 670–678. [CrossRef]
136. Sikora, E.; Bielak-Zmijewska, A.; Magalska, A.; Piwocka, K.; Mosieniak, G.; Kalinowska, M.; Widlak, P.; Cymerman, I.; Bujnicki, J. Curcumin induces caspase-3-dependent apoptotic pathway but inhibits DNA fragmentation factor 40/caspase-activated DNase endonuclease in human Jurkat cells. *Mol. Cancer Ther.* **2006**, *5*, 927–934. [CrossRef]
137. Anisimov, V.N. The relationship between aging and carcinogenesis: A critical appraisal. *Crit. Rev. Oncol. Hematol.* **2003**, *10*, 323–338. [CrossRef]
138. Vogelstein, B.; Papadopoulos, N.; Velculescu, V.E.; Zhou, S.; Diaz, L.A.; Kinzler, K.W. Cancer genome landscapes. *Science* **2013**, *339*, 1546–1558. [CrossRef]
139. Wee, P.; Wang, Z. Epidermal growth factor receptor cell proliferation signaling pathways. *Cancers* **2017**, *9*, 52. [CrossRef]
140. Rahmani, A.H.; Al Zohairy, M.A.; Aly, S.M.; Khan, M.A. Curcumin: A Potential Candidate in Prevention of Cancer via Modulation of Molecular Pathways. *Biomed. Res. Int.* **2014**, *2014*, 761608. [CrossRef]
141. Hatcher, H.; Planalp, R.; Cho, J.; Torti, F.M.; Torti, S.V. Curcumin: From ancient medicine to current clinical trials. *Cell. Mol. Life Sci.* **2008**, *65*, 1631–1652. [CrossRef]
142. Gonzalez, L.C.; Ghadaouia, S.; Martinez, A.; Rodier, F. Premature aging/senescence in cancer cells facing therapy: Good or bad? *Biogerontology* **2016**, *17*, 71–87. [CrossRef]
143. Lee, S.; Schmitt, C.A. The dynamic nature of senescence in cancer. *Nat. Cell Biol.* **2019**, *21*, 94–101. [CrossRef]
144. Lee, S.; Lee, J.-S. Cellular senescence: A promising strategy for cancer therapy. *BMR Rep.* **2019**, *52*, 35–41. [CrossRef]
145. Mosieniak, G.; Adamowicz, M.; Alster, O.; Jaskowiak, H.; Szczepankiewicz, A.A.; Wilczynski, G.M.; Ciechomska, I.A.; Sikora, E. Curcumin induces permanent growth arrest of human colon cancer cells: Link between senescence and autophagy. *Mech. Ageing Dev.* **2012**, *133*, 444–455. [CrossRef]
146. Kocyigit, A.; Guler, E.M. Curcumin induce DNA damage and apoptosis through generation of reactive oxygen species and reducing mitochondrial membrane potential in melanoma cancer cells. *Cell. Mol. Biol.* **2017**, *63*, 97–105. [CrossRef]
147. Shang, H.S.; Chang, C.H.; Chou, Y.R.; Yeh, M.Y.; Au, M.K.; Lu, H.F.; Chu, Y.L.; Chou, H.M.; Chou, H.C.; Shih, Y.L.; et al. Curcumin causes DNA damage and affects associated protein expression in HeLa human cervical cancer cells. *Oncol. Rep.* **2016**, *36*, 2207–2215. [CrossRef]
148. Kumar, D.; Basu, S.; Parija, L.; Rout, D.; Manna, S.; Dandapat, J.; Debata, P.R. Curcumin and Ellagic acid synergistically induce ROS generation, DNA damage, p53 accumulation and apoptosis in HeLa cervical carcinoma cells. *Biomed. Pharmacother.* **2016**, *81*, 31–37. [CrossRef]
149. Bojko, A.; Cierniak, A.; Adamczyk, A.; Ligeza, J. Modulatory Effects of Curcumin and Tyrphostins (AG494 and AG1478) on Growth Regulation and Viability of LN229 Human Brain Cancer Cells. *Nutr. Cancer* **2015**, *67*, 1170–1182. [CrossRef]
150. Lu, J.J.; Cai, Y.J.; Ding, J. Curcumin induces DNA damage and caffeine-insensitive cell cycle arrest in colorectal carcinoma HCT116 cells. *Mol. Cell. Biochem.* **2011**, *354*, 247–252. [CrossRef]
151. Korwek, Z.; Bielak-Zmijewska, A.; Mosieniak, G.; Alster, O.; Moreno-Villanueva, M.; Burkle, A.; Sikora, E. DNA damage-independent apoptosis induced by curcumin in normal resting human T cells and leukaemic Jurkat cells. *Mutagenesis* **2013**, *28*, 411–416. [CrossRef]
152. Blakemore, L.M.; Boes, C.; Cordell, R.; Manson, M.M. Curcumin-induced mitotic arrest is characterized by spindle abnormalities, defects in chromosomal congression and DNA damage. *Carcinogenesis* **2013**, *34*, 351–360. [CrossRef] [PubMed]
153. Sliwinska, M.A.; Mosieniak, G.; Wolanin, K.; Babik, A.; Piwocka, K.; Magalska, A.; Szczepanowska, J.; Fronk, J.; Sikora, E. Induction of senescence with doxorubicin leads to increased genomic instability of HCT116 cells. *Mech. Ageing Dev.* **2009**, *130*, 24–32. [CrossRef] [PubMed]

154. Milanovic, M.; Fan, D.N.Y.; Belenki, D.; Däbritz, J.H.M.; Zhao, Z.; Yu, Y.; Dörr, J.R.; Dimitrova, L.; Lenze, D.; Monteiro Barbosa, I.A.; et al. Senescence-associated reprogramming promotes cancer stemness. *Nature* **2018**, *553*, 96–100. [CrossRef] [PubMed]
155. Sikora, E.; Arendt, T.; Bennett, M.; Narita, M. Impact of cellular senescence signature on ageing research. *Ageing Res. Rev.* **2011**, *10*, 146–152. [CrossRef] [PubMed]
156. Childs, B.G.; Durik, M.; Baker, D.J.; Van Deursen, J.M. Cellular senescence in aging and age-related disease: From mechanisms to therapy. *Nat. Med.* **2015**, *21*, 1424–1435. [CrossRef]
157. Kirkland, J.L.; Tchkonia, T. Cellular Senescence: A Translational Perspective. *EBioMedicine* **2017**, *21*, 21–28. [CrossRef]
158. You, J.; Sun, J.; Ma, T.; Yang, Z.; Wang, X.; Zhang, Z.; Li, J.; Wang, L.; Ii, M.; Yang, J.; et al. Curcumin induces therapeutic angiogenesis in a diabetic mouse hindlimb ischemia model via modulating the function of endothelial progenitor cells. *Stem. Cell Res. Ther.* **2017**, *8*, 182. [CrossRef]
159. Evangelou, K.; Lougiakis, N.; Rizou, S.V.; Kotsinas, A.; Kletsas, D.; Muñoz-Espín, D.; Kastrinakis, N.G.; Pouli, N.; Marakos, P.; Townsend, P.; et al. Robust, universal biomarker assay to detect senescent cells in biological specimens. *Aging Cell* **2017**, *16*, 192–197. [CrossRef]
160. Banji, D.; Banji, O.J.F.; Dasaroju, S.; Annamalai, A.R. Piperine and curcumin exhibit synergism in attenuating D-galactose induced senescence in rats. *Eur. J. Pharmacol.* **2013**, *703*, 91–99. [CrossRef]
161. Yan, Z.; Dai, Y.; Fu, H.; Zheng, Y.; Bao, D.; Yin, Y.; Chen, Q.; Nie, X.; Hao, Q.; Hou, D.; et al. Curcumin exerts a protective effect against premature ovarian failure in mice. *J. Mol. Endocrinol.* **2018**, *60*, 261–271. [CrossRef]
162. Takano, K.; Tatebe, J.; Washizawa, N.; Morita, T. Curcumin inhibits age-related vascular changes in aged mice fed a high-fat diet. *Nutrients* **2018**, *10*, 1476. [CrossRef]
163. Pirmoradi, S.; Fathi, E.; Farahzadi, R.; Pilehvar-Soltanahmadi, Y.; Zarghami, N. Curcumin Affects Adipose Tissue-Derived Mesenchymal Stem Cell Aging Through TERT Gene Expression. *Drug Res.* **2018**, *68*, 213–221. [CrossRef]
164. Yousefzadeh, M.J.; Zhu, Y.; McGowan, S.J.; Angelini, L.; Fuhrmann-Stroissnigg, H.; Xu, M.; Ling, Y.Y.; Melos, K.I.; Pirtskhalava, T.; Inman, C.L.; et al. Fisetin is a senotherapeutic that extends health and lifespan. *EBioMedicine* **2018**, *36*, 18–28. [CrossRef]
165. Kuilman, T.; Michaloglou, C.; Mooi, W.J.; Peeper, D.S. The essence of senescence. *Genes Dev.* **2010**, *24*, 2463–2479. [CrossRef]
166. Gopas, J.; Stern, E.; Zurgil, U.; Ozer, J.; Ben-Ari, A.; Shubinsky, G.; Braiman, A.; Sinay, R.; Ezratty, J.; Dronov, V.; et al. Reed-Sternberg cells in Hodgkin's lymphoma present features of cellular senescence. *Cell Death Dis.* **2016**, *7*, e2457. [CrossRef]
167. Calabrese, E.J. Hormesis: From mainstream to therapy. *J. Cell Commun. Signal.* **2014**, *8*, 289–291. [CrossRef]
168. Demirovic, D.; Rattan, S.I.S. Curcumin induces stress response and hormetically modulates wound healing ability of human skin fibroblasts undergoing ageing in vitro. *Biogerontology* **2011**, *12*, 437–444. [CrossRef]
169. Rattan, S.I.S.; Ali, R.E. Hormetic prevention of molecular damage during cellular aging of human skin fibroblasts and keratinocytes. *Ann. N. Y. Acad. Sci.* **2007**, *1100*, 424–430. [CrossRef]
170. Anand, P.; Kunnumakkara, A.B.; Newman, R.A.; Aggarwal, B.B. Bioavailability of curcumin: Problems and promises. *Mol. Pharm.* **2007**, *4*, 807–818. [CrossRef]
171. Vareed, S.K.; Kakarala, M.; Ruffin, M.T.; Crowell, J.A.; Normolle, D.P.; Djuric, Z.; Brenner, D.E. Pharmacokinetics of curcumin conjugate metabolites in healthy human subjects. *Cancer Epidemiol. Biomark. Prev.* **2008**, *17*, 1411–1417. [CrossRef]
172. Szymusiak, M.; Hu, X.; Leon Plata, P.A.; Ciupinski, P.; Wang, Z.J.; Liu, Y. Bioavailability of curcumin and curcumin glucuronide in the central nervous system of mice after oral delivery of nano-curcumin. *Int. J. Pharm.* **2016**, *511*, 415–423. [CrossRef]
173. Takahashi, M.; Uechi, S.; Takara, K.; Asikin, Y.; Wada, K. Evaluation of an oral carrier system in rats: Bioavailability and antioxidant properties of liposome-encapsulated curcumin. *J. Agric. Food Chem.* **2009**, *57*, 9141–9146. [CrossRef]
174. Sasaki, H.; Sunagawa, Y.; Takahashi, K.; Imaizumi, A.; Fukuda, H.; Hashimoto, T.; Wada, H.; Katanasaka, Y.; Kakeya, H.; Fujita, M.; et al. Innovative Preparation of Curcumin for Improved Oral Bioavailability. *Biol. Pharm. Bull.* **2011**, *34*, 660–665. [CrossRef]

175. Kanai, M.; Imaizumi, A.; Otsuka, Y.; Sasaki, H.; Hashiguchi, M.; Tsujiko, K.; Matsumoto, S.; Ishiguro, H.; Chiba, T. Dose-escalation and pharmacokinetic study of nanoparticle curcumin, a potential anticancer agent with improved bioavailability, in healthy human volunteers. *Cancer Chemother. Pharmacol.* **2012**, *69*, 65–70. [CrossRef]
176. Peyrol, J.; Meyer, G.; Obert, P.; Dangles, O.; Pechère, L.; Amiot, M.J.; Riva, C. Involvement of bilitranslocase and beta-glucuronidase in the vascular protection by hydroxytyrosol and its glucuronide metabolites in oxidative stress conditions. *J. Nutr. Biochem.* **2018**, *51*, 8–15. [CrossRef]
177. Mukkavilli, R.; Yang, C.; Tanwar, R.S.; Saxena, R.; Gundala, S.R.; Zhang, Y.; Ghareeb, A.; Floyd, S.D.; Vangala, S.; Kuo, W.-W.; et al. Pharmacokinetic-pharmacodynamic correlations in the development of ginger extract as an anticancer agent. *Sci. Rep.* **2018**, *8*, 3056. [CrossRef]
178. Yang, F.; Lim, G.P.; Begum, A.N.; Ubeda, O.J.; Simmons, M.R.; Ambegaokar, S.S.; Chen, P.; Kayed, R.; Glabe, C.G.; Frautschy, S.A.; et al. Curcumin inhibits formation of amyloid β oligomers and fibrils, binds plaques, and reduces amyloid in vivo. *J. Biol. Chem.* **2005**, *280*, 5892–5901. [CrossRef]
179. Yuan, J.; Liu, W.; Zhu, H.; Zhang, X.; Feng, Y.; Chen, Y.; Feng, H.; Lin, J. Curcumin attenuates blood-brain barrier disruption after subarachnoid hemorrhage in mice. *J. Surg. Res.* **2017**, *207*, 85–91. [CrossRef]
180. Tsai, Y.M.; Chien, C.F.; Lin, L.C.; Tsai, T.H. Curcumin and its nano-formulation: The kinetics of tissue distribution and blood-brain barrier penetration. *Int. J. Pharm.* **2011**, *416*, 331–338. [CrossRef]
181. Tomás-Barberán, F.A.; Selma, M.V.; Espín, J.C. Interactions of gut microbiota with dietary polyphenols and consequences to human health. *Curr. Opin. Clin. Nutr. Metab. Care* **2016**, *19*, 471–476. [CrossRef]
182. Zam, W. Gut Microbiota as a Prospective Therapeutic Target for Curcumin: A Review of Mutual Influence. *J. Nutr. Metab.* **2018**, *2018*, 1367984. [CrossRef] [PubMed]
183. McIntosh, F.M.; Maison, N.; Holtrop, G.; Young, P.; Stevens, V.J.; Ince, J.; Johnstone, A.M.; Lobley, G.E.; Flint, H.J.; Louis, P. Phylogenetic distribution of genes encoding β-glucuronidase activity in human colonic bacteria and the impact of diet on faecal glycosidase activities. *Environ. Microbiol.* **2012**, *14*, 1876–1887. [CrossRef] [PubMed]
184. O'Toole, P.W.; Jeffery, I.B. Gut microbiota and aging. *Science* **2015**, *350*, 1214–1215. [CrossRef]
185. Biagi, E.; Rampelli, S.; Turroni, S.; Quercia, S.; Candela, M.; Brigidi, P. The gut microbiota of centenarians: Signatures of longevity in the gut microbiota profile. *Mech. Ageing Dev.* **2017**, *165*, 180–184. [CrossRef] [PubMed]
186. Ohno, M.; Nishida, A.; Sugitani, Y.; Nishino, K.; Inatomi, O.; Sugimoto, M.; Kawahara, M.; Andoh, A. Nanoparticle curcumin ameliorates experimental colitis via modulation of gut microbiota and induction of regulatory T cells. *PLoS ONE* **2017**, *12*, e0185999. [CrossRef] [PubMed]
187. Zhang, Z.; Chen, Y.; Xiang, L.; Wang, Z.; Xiao, G.G.; Hu, J. Effect of curcumin on the diversity of gut microbiota in ovariectomized rats. *Nutrients* **2017**, *9*, 1146. [CrossRef] [PubMed]
188. Shen, L.; Liu, L.; Ji, H.-F. Regulative effects of curcumin spice administration on gut microbiota and its pharmacological implications. *Food Nutr. Res.* **2017**, *61*, 1361780. [CrossRef]
189. Squillaro, T.; Schettino, C.; Sampaolo, S.; Galderisi, U.; Di Iorio, G.; Giordano, A.; Melone, M.A.B. Adult-onset brain tumors and neurodegeneration: Are polyphenols protective? *J. Cell. Physiol.* **2018**, *233*, 3955–3967. [CrossRef]
190. Finicelli, M.; Squillaro, T.; Di Cristo, F.; Di Salle, A.; Melone, M.A.B.; Galderisi, U.; Peluso, G. Metabolic syndrome, Mediterranean diet, and polyphenols: Evidence and perspectives. *J. Cell. Physiol.* **2018**, *234*, 5807–5826. [CrossRef]

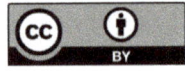

© 2019 by the authors. Licensee MDPI, Basel, Switzerland. This article is an open access article distributed under the terms and conditions of the Creative Commons Attribution (CC BY) license (http://creativecommons.org/licenses/by/4.0/).

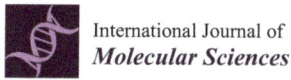

Review

Curcumin: A Potent Protectant against Esophageal and Gastric Disorders

Slawomir Kwiecien, Marcin Magierowski, Jolanta Majka, Agata Ptak-Belowska, Dagmara Wojcik, Zbigniew Sliwowski, Katarzyna Magierowska and Tomasz Brzozowski *

Department of Physiology, Faculty of Medicine, Jagiellonian University Medical College, 16 Grzegorzecka Street, 31-531 Cracow, Poland; skwiecien@cm-uj.krakow.pl (S.K.); m.magierowski@uj.edu.pl (M.M.); jolmaj@poczta.fm (J.M.); agata.ptak-belowska@uj.edu.pl (A.P.-B.); dagmara1.wojcik@uj.edu.pl (D.W.); AgaZS@poczta.fm (Z.S.); katarzyna.magierowska@uj.edu.pl (K.M.)
* Correspondence: mpbrzozo@cyf-kr.edu.pl; Tel.: +48-12-421-10-06

Received: 28 February 2019; Accepted: 19 March 2019; Published: 24 March 2019

Abstract: Turmeric obtained from the rhizomes of Curcuma longa has been used in the prevention and treatment of many diseases since the ancient times. Curcumin is the principal polyphenol isolated from turmeric, which exhibits anti-inflammatory, antioxidant, antiapoptotic, antitumor, and antimetastatic activities. The existing evidence indicates that curcumin can exert a wide range of beneficial pleiotropic properties in the gastrointestinal tract, such as protection against reflux esophagitis, Barrett's esophagus, and gastric mucosal damage induced by nonsteroidal anti-inflammatory drugs (NSAIDs) and necrotizing agents. The role of curcumin as an adjuvant in the treatment of a *Helicobacter pylori* infection in experimental animals and humans has recently been proposed. The evidence that this turmeric derivative inhibits the invasion and proliferation of gastric cancer cells is encouraging and warrants further experimental and clinical studies with newer formulations to support the inclusion of curcumin in cancer therapy regimens. This review was designed to analyze the existing data from in vitro and in vivo animal and human studies in order to highlight the mechanisms of therapeutic efficacy of curcumin in the protection and ulcer healing of the upper gastrointestinal tract, with a major focus on addressing the protection of the esophagus and stomach by this emerging compound.

Keywords: curcumin; reflux esophagitis; gastroprotection; gastric ulcer; *Helicobacter pylori*; gastric cancer

1. Introduction

Curcumin, the natural phenolic active ingredient of turmeric (Curcuma longa) rhizome, has been used in Asia as an herbal remedy for a variety of diseases [1]. Similar to chili, turmeric is commonly used in Asian cuisine to add a yellow color, both as a flavor and as a preservative [2]. In addition to the use of curcumin as an anti-inflammatory in ancient times, it has also been used to treat gastrointestinal (GI) diseases such as indigestion, flatulence, diarrhea, and even gastric and duodenal ulcers [1–3]. Recently, great attention has been paid to the medical applications of curcumin in the treatment of human diseases associated with oxidative stress and inflammation, including different cancers [3]. Curcumin treatment has also led to the improvement of metabolic parameters involving aging-associated diseases such as atherosclerosis, diabetes, cardiovascular disease, and chronic kidney diseases [4,5]. Interestingly, some promising effects of curcumin have been observed in the alleviation by this turmeric derivative of the chronic inflammatory conditions such as arthritis, uveitis, and inflammatory bowel disease [6]. In some instances, curcumin has been found to aid in the prevention and treatment of various cancers [7]. Recently, the anticarcinogenic activity of curcumin has been documented in the GI tract because this compound has proven to exert a therapeutic effect on different human GI cancers such as esophageal, gastric, and small and large intestinal cancer [8,9]. This overview was aimed to document the beneficial and emerging effects of curcumin in the upper GI tract, focusing on the mechanism of local, systemic, and molecular actions of this compound in the esophagus and stomach.

2. Curcumin in the Protection of the Esophagus against Reflux Esophagitis, Barrett's Esophagus, and Esophageal Carcinoma

The esophagus, which carries food and liquid from the mouth to the stomach, undergoes transient lower esophageal sphincter relaxation (TLESR), which is considered the main mechanism of gastroesophageal reflux disease (GERD) [10]. Under physiological conditions, these TLESRs are induced spontaneously without swallowing and allow for the "physiological" contact of gastric juice containing hydrochloric acid (HCl) with the esophageal wall [10]. Interestingly, this acid reflux occurs at a higher frequency during TLESR in patients with GERD than in healthy subjects [10,11]. Furthermore, the anatomical abnormalities in the structure of the lower esophageal sphincter or its dysfunction can result in more frequent or sometimes prolonged exposure of the esophageal mucosa to gastric acid, resulting in esophageal damage due to reflux esophagitis. If this mucosal contact of epithelial cells with acid or acid and bile (mixed reflux) is prolonged, GERD develops [12]. Thus, human esophageal epithelial cells are a direct target and play a key role in esophageal inflammation in response to acidic pH in the course of GERD development. Complications of GERD development include Barrett's esophagus with an increased risk for esophageal adenocarcinoma formation [13]. In a study designed to mimic the acid exposure experienced by GERD patients, treatment with curcumin prevented the expression of inflammatory cytokines in human esophageal tissue [14]. This anti-inflammatory effect of curcumin has been confirmed by an in vitro study, testing the protective potential of curcumin in esophageal epithelial cell lines exposed to exogenous acid [15]. That study examined the HET-1A cell lines exposed to hydrochloric acid in relation to the role of PKC, MAPK, and NFκB signaling pathways and the transcriptional regulation of IL-6 and IL-8 expression [15]. This HET-1A cell line appears to be suitable for investigating the cellular action of putative esophageal metaplasia development, and both acid and bile are considered potent carcinogenic factors in the mechanism of esophageal dysplasia and adenocarcinoma formation [15–17]. The exposure of HET-1A cells to pH 4.5 induced the activity of the transcription factor NF-κB while enhancing IL-6 and IL-8 secretion and their mRNA and protein expression [15]. Among the kinases system tested in their study [17], particularly the MAPKs and PKC (alpha and epsilon) activity were activated when HET-1A cells were exposed to acid. Curcumin was equally potent as SN-50 (an NF-κB inhibitor), chelerythrine (a PKC inhibitor), and PD-098059 (a p44/42 MAPK inhibitor), yet all of them efficiently abolished the acid-induced mucosal expression of IL-6 and IL-8 [17].

In in vivo studies, curcumin was compared with lansoprazole, the proton pump inhibitor (PPI) commonly used as the recommended standard drug against GI-tract disorders including GERD [18,19]. In these reports, curcumin was shown to effectively prevent the esophageal mucosal damage induced by acute reflux esophagitis [18,19]. Although curcumin was documented as less potent than the proton pump inhibitor (PPI) lansoprazole in the inhibition of acid reflux esophagitis, it became superior to lansoprazole in the inhibition of mixed acid-bile reflux-induced esophagitis. This protective mechanism caused by curcumin in the esophagus has been attributed to the antioxidant nature of this turmeric derivative [18,19].

Gastroesophageal reflux is a major mechanism responsible for Barrett's metaplasia, which develops from the cellular reprogramming of the esophageal squamous epithelium due to the reflux of acidic or acidic-bile content to the esophagus [20]. The protection against oxidative stress and the preservation of the antioxidative activity induced by esophageal protectants play an important role in the strategy against the pathogenesis of acid-induced esophageal mucosa damage. Thus, the anti-reflux therapy alternative to PPIs is widely expected. In line with this notion, the anti-inflammatory properties of curcumin and the relationship between bile-reflux and the expression of antioxidative enzymes and the reactive oxygen metabolites (ROM) scavenging enzyme MnSOD have been investigated [21]. The molecular approach was to examine therapies effective in the preservation of both the expression of the antioxidative enzyme MnSOD at the level of the protein and the enzymatic activity of MnSOD [21]. Curcumin applied in the form of oil exerted an esophagoprotective activity against acidic reflux injury through its ability to maintain mitochondrial function, as documented by the preservation of both the MnSOD expression and activity by this turmeric compound [21]. These authors concluded that curcumin oil prevented the loss of MnSOD expression in the rat esophageal epithelium caused by bile [21]. In addition, the treatment with curcumin oil prior to acid or bile salt exposure prevented the loss of MnSOD activity in an esophageal HET-1A cell line. Notably, when cells were treated with curcumin oil, the highest level of MnSOD enzyme activity was observed [19]. However, it is worth to mention that besides curcumin, MnTBAP and other nutraceuticals including certain berry extracts also offered the efficient preservation of MnSOD expression in HET-1A cells [21].

Curcumin may offer a benefit over the single pathway-targeted anticancer therapy, and this effect could be due to its pleiotropic properties [20]. Figure 1 summarizes the pleiotropic effects of curcumin resulting in the amelioration of inflammation and cell death, which protects the tissue against injury.

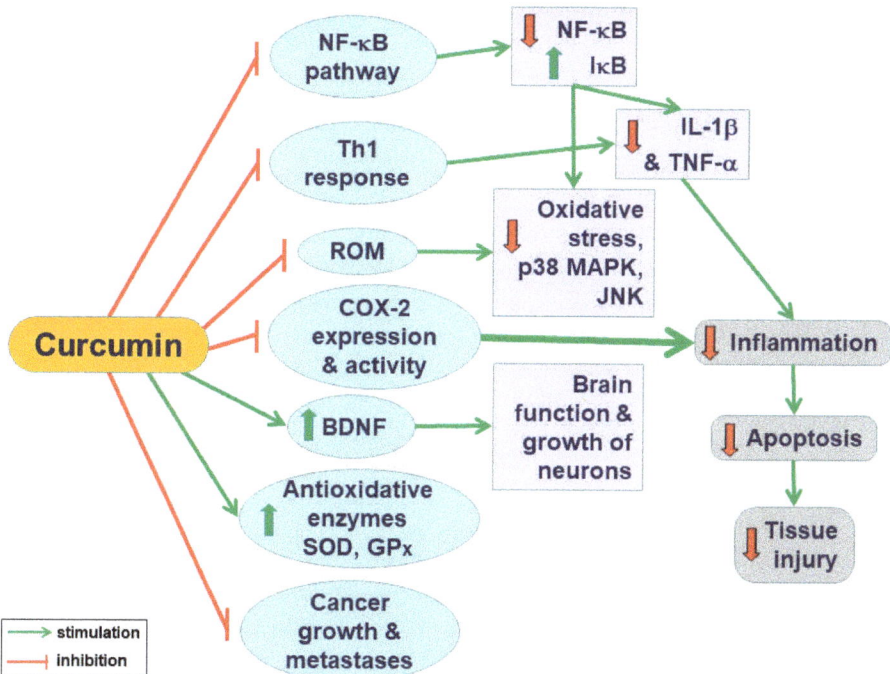

Figure 1. A conclusive summary of the pleiotropic action of curcumin in the body system: Curcumin exhibits anti-inflammatory, antioxidant, antiapoptotic, antitumor, and antimetastatic activities and suppresses multiple signalling pathways responsible for inflammation, apoptosis, and cellular death. Curcumin improves the growth of neurons and the functions of the brain in addition to the downregulation of reactive oxygen species, oxidative stress, and proinflammatory factors (NF-κB and cytokines).

Considerable evidence indicates that curcumin can efficiently prevent the acid- and bile-induced NF-κB changes from the normal mRNA phenotype into the oncogenic phenotype of human hypopharyngeal primary cells (HHPC) in culture [22]. Curcumin inhibited the bile acid-induced genes dependent on the NF-κB signalling pathway in this HHPC culture. This turmeric was capable in selectively inhibiting Bcl-2 overexpression induced in HHPC exposed to bile at both acidic (pH 4.0) and neutral (pH 7.0) environments [22]. This evidence clearly indicates that curcumin might be superior over NF-κB inhibitors. Furthermore, its beneficial anti-inflammatory and anticarcinogenic effects are independent of pH status and can be explained either by the promotion of cell apoptosis or the inhibition of antiapoptotic pathway in these HHPC cells [22]. In another study, the efficacy of curcumin in the prevention of bile acid-induced DNA damage using micronucleus assay was investigated [23]. Moreover, these authors tested the effect of curcumin on NF-κB and NF-κB p65 activities in the curcumin-pretreated esophageal cell line (OE33) exposed to deoxycholic acid (DCA) using real-time PCR of the extracted RNA. In their study, the bile-induced DNA damage and the activation of NF-κB activity in vitro were completely abolished by curcumin [23]. An important part of this translational study has been run in human subjects and dealt with the curcumin efficacy to treat patients with Barrett's esophagus [23]. These patients with Barrett's esophagus took a daily dose of 500 mg of curcumin tablets for 7 days prior to endoscopy [23]. Interestingly, curcumin-supplemented patients presented a slightly reduced expression of IL-8 as compared to the squamous control tissue non-treated with curcumin. However, this treatment resulted in an almost doubled apoptotic frequency compared to the non-supplemented control patients [23]. To reiterate, the data has clearly indicated that curcumin exerted a beneficial effect against bile-driven deleterious effects on the mucosal esophageal cells. Although curcumin was poorly delivered to the esophagus, the supplementation of patients with Barrett's esophagus with curcumin not only reduced NF-κB activity and inflammatory features in esophagi but also increased apoptosis in the Barrett's esophageal tissues. This confirms that apoptosis could be one of the potentially important mechanisms of the curcumin-beneficial effect on squamous esophageal mucosa.

3. Curcumin-Induced Gastric Protection against NSAID-Induced Gastric Damage: Experimental and Clinical Evidence

It is well-known that the ingestion of NSAIDs is associated with the risk of GI adverse effects including gastric micro bleeding, damage to the epithelial structure, cessation of GI blood flow, decline in gastric mucus and alkaline secretion, and alteration in GI motility [24]. The mechanism of NSAID-induced gastropathy involves an impairment of the gastric mucosal barrier mainly due to the inhibition of endogenous prostaglandins (PGs), which are considered prototypes of the cytoprotective agents with the ability to protect the gastric mucosa against a variety of topical and non-topical ulcerogenes [25,26]. The therapy with NSAIDs which includes aspirin, the most popular and widely used world-wide, and other drugs, such as indomethacin, diclofenac or naproxen, have especially brought great attention towards their anti-inflammatory potential and efficacy to treat rheumatoid arthritis [24–27]. The most common adverse effects of NSAIDs documented in experimental animals and confirmed in humans include potent ulcerogenic activity and the enhancement of oxidative stress [27–29]. Therefore, the reduction of oxidative stress may be an effective curative strategy for preventing and treating NSAIDs-induced gastric mucosal complications, such as micro bleedings and hemorrhagic lesions. The alternative therapy by phytochemicals such as supplementation by the dietary phenolic compounds including curcumin, could exert antioxidant, anti-inflammatory, and antibacterial benefits, thus preventing digestive diseases of upper GI tract including the ulcerogenic activity of NSAIDs [30].

In rodents, the NSAID-induced gastric mucosal damage is mainly localized to the oxyntic mucosa of the stomach's corpus region. These lesions are recognized as bleeding erosions or lesions rather than typical ulcers [28]. This is contrary to the situation in humans, where NSAID-induced gastric ulceration occurs mainly in the gastric antrum [31]. For instance, naproxen is the most common and frequent NSAID used in rheumatoid arthritis patients, and the naproxen-induced gastropathy occurs mainly in the gastric antrum [31]. Using this experimental antral model of gastric ulcerations in rats to mimic the human scenario of complication risk after naproxen ingestion, Kim et al. [32] have shown that the administration of naproxen caused the macro- and microscopic antral lesions and increased the tissue lipid peroxidation levels. When curcumin was combined with naproxen, the size of the gastric antral ulcers had diminished, followed by the restoration of the activity of antioxidative enzymes SOD, catalase, and glutathione peroxidase (GPx), which are all recognized as ROM scavengers in the gastric mucosa [32]. Notably, curcumin protection was accompanied by the fall in the lipid peroxides, suggesting that the mechanism of curcumin-induced attenuation of gastric mucosal injury caused by NSAIDs such as naproxen can involve the inhibition of lipid peroxidation and activation of radical scavenging enzymes [32]. Thus, the data clearly indicates that curcumin possesses protective anti-antral ulcer properties due to its capability to decrease the damage of antral gastric mucosa. Therefore, the future clinical utility of curcumin may offer an attractive strategy and an encouraging opportunity for curing gastric lesions induced by NSAIDs in humans.

Recent studies confirmed that curcumin is an effective antioxidant and anti-inflammatory compound in the upper GI-tract and a scavenger of ROM and nitrogen metabolites [33]. There is considerable evidence that curcumin, which is not associated with significant adverse effects, exhibits a comparable anti-inflammatory efficacy with those presented by some derivatives of NSAIDs [33–35]. Nowadays, it seems obvious that the mechanism of curcumin-induced gastroprotection against indomethacin injury depends on the curcumin-mediated downregulation of pro-inflammatory mediator expression, the decline in free nitrogen radical generation in addition to the enhanced resistance of mucosal epithelium due to the inhibition of apoptosis, and the increased cell proliferation in the gastric mucosa [33]. Ganguly et al. [34] have shown that curcumin is similar to melatonin with regards to its down regulatory action against the activity of metalloproteinase-2 (MMP-2) generated by ROM in animal models of gastric damage and during the course of ulcer healing. In addition, the suppression of MMP-2 activity by H_2O_2 in a dose- and time-dependent manner in vitro was blocked by antioxidants including curcumin [34]. Curcumin, similarly to melatonin and omeprazole, afforded gastroprotection in vivo against indomethacin-induced gastric damage by the suppression of gastric mucosal biosynthesis and expression of MMP-2 [34]. Interestingly, they have proposed that the protection of curcumin, melatonin, and the PPI omeprazole against H_2O_2-mediated inactivation depends on the downregulation of MMP-2 and TIMP-2 expression and the upregulation of MT1-MMP during the onset of indomethacin-induced ulceration [34].

Morsy et al. [35] have confirmed the protective efficacy of curcumin against the damaging activity of indomethacin in the rat stomach. Indomethacin administered intraperitoneally at a dose of 30 mg/kg produced gastric bleeding erosions, predominantly due to the profound inhibition of endogenous PG in the gastric mucosa evoked by this agent [24,25]. The pretreatment with a single dose of curcumin reduced the index of indomethacin-induced gastric lesions and the malondialdehyde (MDA) concentration, which is considered the index of ROM-induced lipid peroxidation [35,36]. Along with the attenuation of the indomethacin-induced gastric mucosal damage, the concomitant increase in mucin content of gastric juice and the gastric mucosal nitric oxide (NO) levels in rats pretreated with curcumin have been observed [36]. Furthermore, the treatment with curcumin raised the antioxidant enzyme catalase and SOD activities and decreased the expression of pro-inflammatory stimuli such as inducible nitric oxide synthase (iNOS) and NF-κB. Curcumin attenuated gastric acid secretory activity, an important component implicated in the pathogenesis of gastrointestinal peptic ulcer disease, and inhibited the activity of caspase-3. This finding suggests that the mechanism of this protection depends on the strengthening of the mucosal barrier and the antioxidant and antiapoptotic activities of this compound. Of note, this beneficial gastroprotective effect of curcumin against NSAIDs could be attributed, at least in part, to the antisecretory activity of this turmeric compound [37]. Interestingly, the addition of microelements such as zinc (Zn) to curcumin enhanced the gastroprotective and ulcer healing activities compared with those exhibited by curcumin alone [37]. Such a complex of Zn(II)-curcumin dose-dependently reduced the severity of the indomethacin-induced gastric damage, as reflected by the lower gastric ulcer index in animals treated with this combination [37]. Using rats with chronic preexisting gastric ulcers, Mei and coworkers concluded that the Zn(II)-curcumin complex efficiently enhanced the mucosal barrier defence activity by the attenuation of oxidative stress and MMP-9-mediated inflammation to a greater extent than curcumin alone [38]. Indeed, the treatment with curcumin raised SOD activity and GSH levels and markedly inhibited the MDA content and the expression of MMP-9 in the ulcerated mucosa [38]. In another report, curcumin-mediated gastric mucosal healing has been associated with the upregulation of genes for MMP-2, TGF-β, and VEGF. These effects were considered essential for an angiogenic modulatory role of this turmeric as documented by its stimulatory effect on the vascular sprout formation and collagen fiber restoration in ulcerated tissues [39]. In nineteen-hour animal ulcer models, Tuorkey and Karolin [40] have shown that the mechanism of anti-ulcer activity of curcumin depends upon the attenuating effect of this compound on gastric acid hypersecretion, total peroxides, MPO activity, IL-6 levels, and apoptotic incidence. This observation was in keeping with the earlier study by Mathattanadul et al., who have also indicated that both curcumin and bisdemethoxycurcumin can inhibit the basal gastric acid secretion in pylorus-ligated rat model and that this antisecretory effect can contribute to an acceleration of the healing of chronic gastric ulcerations of the mucosa [19].

To date, only a few studies mentioned above have been conducted—in vitro and especially in vivo—on the inhibitory properties of curcumin affecting gastric secretion. Kim et al. demonstrated that the *Curcuma longa* extract protected the gastric mucosa against ulceration with an extent similar to ranitidine and inhibited gastric acid secretion in rats with pylorus ligation procedure, thus preventing gastric mucosa from gastric ulcerations [41]. Zinc(II)-curcumin complex A also shared similar antisecretory properties because this combination of zinc and curcumin provided protection against indomethacin injury, in part, by the inhibition of gastric acid secretion [42].

The question remains whether the bioavailability of NSAIDs is affected by curcumin or if turmeric shows the genuine gastroprotective action in the stomach. Zazueta-Beltran et al. have demonstrated that the concurrent administration of indomethacin and curcumin resulted in a significant reduction of gastric damage when compared to indomethacin alone [43]. However, the bioavailability parameters of indomethacin and the prodrug acemetacin co-administered with curcumin was not significantly altered after the administration of either the active compound or the prodrug. This important evidence indicates that curcumin exhibits a protective effect against indomethacin-induced gastric damage without marked change in bioavailability or through the pharmacokinetics of NSAIDs such as indomethacin [43].

4. Role of Curcumin in the Protection against Gastric Mucosal Injury Induced by Strong Necrotizing Agents and Stress-Induced Gastric Mucosal Bleeding Erosions

Despite the proven multi-target, anti-inflammatory properties of curcumin, the potential protective action of this turmeric derivative against the gastric mucosal damage induced by noxious agents has not been extensively studied. As a consequence, the mediating factors and mechanisms of the potential protective effects of curcumin in the stomach injured by necrotizing agents such as ethanol are poorly understood. Despite ethanol being known as a strong gastric-damaging agent causing mucosal injury due to its direct contact with the gastric mucosa, ethanol-induced gastropathy constitutes a serious clinical entity in humans [44]. In the original report, Mei et al. [37] have demonstrated that the oral administration of a complex of zinc and curcumin (zinc(II)-curcumin) dose-dependently reduced the severity of ethanol-induced gastric lesions while suppressing the gastric acid secretory activity as reflected by the H^+/K^+-ATPase activity comparable with that exhibited by the PPI, lansoprazole. Furthermore, Zn(II)-curcumin significantly inhibited TNF-α and IL-6 mRNA expression, increased the activity of SOD and GPx, and reduced MDA levels in gastric mucosa of rats when compared to the respective controls. These findings suggest that the gastroprotective activity of the Zn(II)-curcumin complex might be important for stimulating cell proliferation and adjusting the pro-inflammatory cytokine-mediated oxidative damage caused by ethanol insult of the gastric mucosa [37].

Previous studies have demonstrated that endogenous NO and other gaseous molecules such as H_2S and CO can cooperate with PG and sensory nerve neuropeptides such as calcitonin gene-related peptide (CGRP) in the mechanism of gastric mucosal integrity and gastroprotection [45,46]. The recent study by Czekaj et al. revealed that some of these factors, such as PG and NO, may contribute to the mechanism of curcumin-induced gastric protection against ethanol injury [47]. They have demonstrated that curcumin given intragastrically provided a dose-dependent gastroprotection against gastric lesions induced by ethanol while increasing both the GBF and the plasma gastrin levels [47]. Furthermore, they proposed that curcumin-induced protection may depend upon the reduced mRNA expression of pro-inflammatory mediators HIF-1α and caudal type home box 2 (Cdx-2), both also recognized as tumour markers in the gastric mucosa [47]. The evidence that curcumin enhanced the gastric mucosal expression of antioxidative enzymes HO-1 and SOD2 indicated that the mechanism of gastroprotection-induced by this turmeric compound involves the enhancement of the antioxidative status of gastric mucosa challenged by ethanol [47]. Interestingly, the mechanism of curcumin-induced protection against ethanol injury could also depend upon the endogenous bioavailability of PG because nonselective and selective COX-1 and COX-2 inhibitors (indomethacin, rofecoxib, and SC-560) reversed this protection and the accompanying rise in GBF evoked by this polyphenolic compound. Furthermore, the concurrent treatment with the synthetic analogue of PGE$_2$ combined with these COX-1 and COX-2 inhibitors restored the protective and hyperaemic activities of curcumin against ethanol damage [47]. This clearly indicates that PG can be an important downstream effector of curcumin-evoked beneficial protective action in the stomach. NO, which is an important endogenous mediator of gastroprotection and ulcer healing, could be involved in the mechanisms underlying the gastroprotective activity of curcumin because the L-NNA-induced depletion of NO biosynthesis in the gastric mucosa abolished the gastroprotective effects of curcumin. Moreover, this gastroprotective effect was accompanied by a marked reduction in the GBF. The concurrent treatment with L-arginine together with L-NNA not only restored the protective and hyperaemic activities of curcumin against ethanol injury but also abrogated an increase in the mRNA expression of HIF-1α and Cdx-2 induced by L-NNA. Nowadays it seems likely that CGRP released from sensory afferents as well as vanilloid receptor TRPV1 can cooperate with PG and NO in the mechanism of the gastroprotective action of curcumin against ethanol injury [48–51]. This notion is supported by the observation that the protection and gastric hyperaemic response induced by curcumin were lost in animals with deactivated sensory nerves by capsaicin and were further restored when exogenous CGRP was concurrently administered with curcumin in rats with capsaicin-deactivated sensory nerves compromised by ethanol (Figure 2) [47].

Recent evidence indicates that curcumin can be effective as a protective substance against the formation of stress-induced gastric lesions in rats [52], in part due to the inhibition of gastric secretory activity mediated by a strong inhibitory action on H$^+$/K$^+$ATPase activity in parietal cells of the rat stomach. Using a chromatin immunoprecipitation assay, He et al. have demonstrated that curcumin inhibited the H$^+$/K$^+$ATPase promoter via histone acetylation, the gene and protein expression of the gastric H$^+$/K-ATPase α subunit, thus resulting in the rise in pH and the amelioration of stress-induced gastric ulcerogenesis [52]. In another study, the anti-ulcer activity of curcumin in rats exposed to either chronic stress and/or unpredictable stressors was observed simultaneously with an evident improvement in memory deficit assessed in their study by the elevated plus maze test and by the overall improvement of homeostatic functions [53]. The pretreatment of stressed rats with curcumin via the oral route attenuated chronic stress and chronic unpredictable stress-associated memory deficits and counteracted the increase in TBARS generation and the decrease in GSH content and markers of oxidative stress (corticosterone, glucose, and creatine kinase) [53]. These authors concluded that the curcumin-mediated antioxidant actions help the body to regulate corticosterone secretion and the stress-induced ulcerative action and possibly to play an important central and peripheral adaptive role against chronic and unpredictable stressors [53].

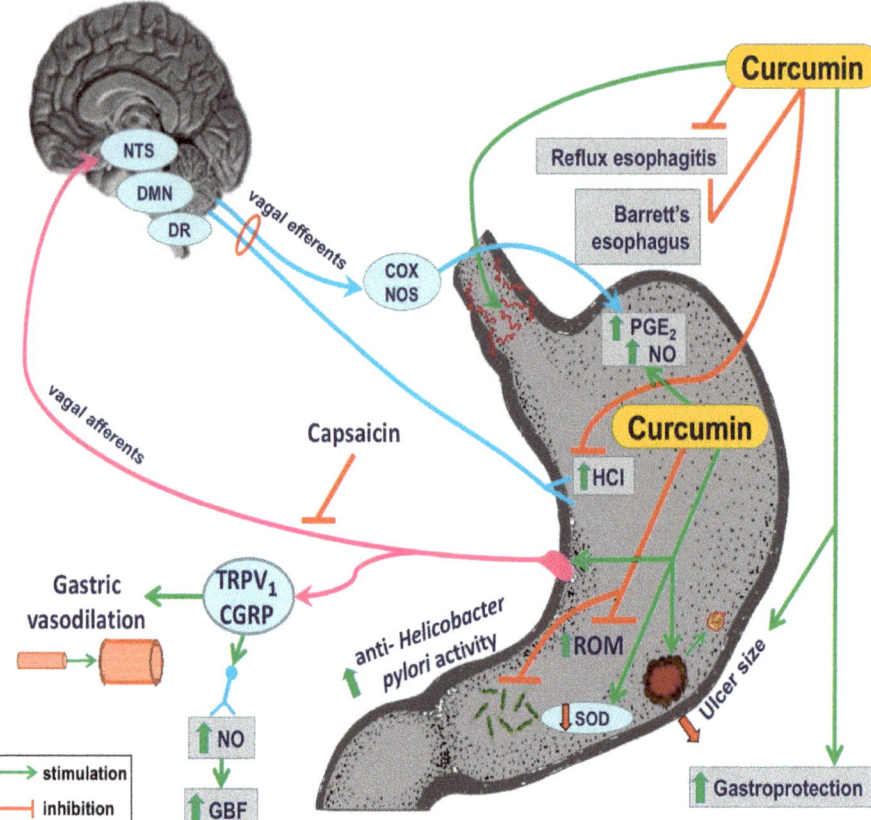

Figure 2. The complex summary of the beneficial effect of treatment with curcumin in esophageal and gastric protection: It involves the amelioration of damage induced by reflux esophagitis and incidence of Barrett's esophagus, attenuation of inflammation, prevention of gastric damage formation, the anti-*Helicobacter pylori* activity, and an improvement of communication between gut function and the brain (gut–brain axis) by this turmeric derivative to facilitate local microvascular vasodilation and an increase in organ blood flow, gastroprotection, and ulcer healing.

The protective activity of curcumin against stress ulcerogenesis can involve the cooperation of endogenous prostaglandins and NO and the activity of capsaicin-sensitive afferent fibers releasing CGRP and capsaicin receptors TRPV1 [54]. Recent studies revealed that the intragastric administration of curcumin dose-dependently prevented the formation of gastric bleeding erosions in gastric mucosa compromised by cold stress. Furthermore, it inhibited basal and histamine- and pentagastrin-stimulated gastric acid secretion, recognized as one of the major pathogenic factors in stress ulcerogenesis [54,55]. Interestingly, the gastroprotective effects of curcumin raised the plasma concentration of gastrin in rats exposed to cold stress [55]. Gastrin is a hormone secreted by the G cells of the APUD cells of the antral gastric mucosa known to exhibit a trophic effect on mucosa, resulting in increasing cell proliferation and gastroprotection against the damaging effects of ethanol and aspirin [56]. Exposure to stress increased the gastric mucosal expression of mRNA for pro-inflammatory markers TNF-α, COX-2, and iNOS, but these effects were inhibited by curcumin administered in graded dosages [55]. The functional ablation of sensory afferent nerves with capsaicin or pretreatment with capsazepine blunted the curcumin-induced decrease in the lesion index and the increase in GBF evoked by cold stress [55]. This vasoactive activity of curcumin corroborates the recent observation that the turmeric derivative, as well as other curcuminoids, can exert vasodilatory activity even in isolated organs [57]. These effects of curcumin in rats with capsaicin denervation were restored by the concomitant treatment with exogenous CGRP combined with curcumin in rats subsequently exposed to cold stress, therefore supporting the role of sensory afferent vasodilatory neuropeptides in gastroprotection by this turmeric derivative against stress-induced gastric damage [55].

5. Efficacy of Curcumin to Treat the Impairment the Gastric Mucosa Infected by *Helicobacter pylori* (*H. pylori*)

According to the World Health Organization (WHO), *H. pylori* has been accepted as a first-class human pathogen implicated in the pathogenesis of major disorders of the upper GI-tract such as the development of gastritis, peptic ulcers, MALT lymphoma, and in some cases, gastric adenocarcinoma. The problem of an infection with *H. pylori* is nowadays important in the general population since epidemiological studies have shown that over 50% of the populations is infected with H. pylori, with a much higher rate in developing countries. Therefore, various drugs including antibiotics have been routinely used for the eradication of this infection. However, steadily increasing resistance to antibiotics, undesirable side effects, the raising costs, and the impaired *H. pylori*-infected patient's quality of life have given rise to the recent surge of interest in alternative approaches [58].

Recent evidence revealed that treatment with curcumin can attenuate oxidative stress and the histological changes accompanying chronic gastritis associated with *H. pylori*. In a randomized clinical trial, patients were divided into two groups: a standard triple therapy group and a group treated with triple therapy with the concurrent administration of curcumin [58]. Endoscopic and histological examinations were performed for all patients before and after 8 weeks of treatments [58]. Triple therapy with curcumin adjuvant as a treatment group significantly decreased the MDA markers and glutathione peroxides and increased the total antioxidant capacity of the gastric mucosa at the end of study, compared to the baseline and triple regimen groups without curcumin [58]. In addition, the oxidative damage to DNA was significantly decreased in triple therapy with the curcumin group at the end of study, compared to the baseline and the triple therapy [58]. This important study has documented that curcumin added to the triple therapy markedly attenuated the inflammation scores (active, chronic, and endoscopic) of patients, compared to the baseline and triple therapy group without combination with curcumin [58]. These authors have concluded that curcumin added to the triple anti-*H. pylori* therapy considerably increased the eradication rate, which was superior as compared to triple therapy alone [58]. Using an experimental mouse model, the effects of curcumin on lipid peroxidation level, MPO and urease activity, number of colonized bacteria, levels of anti-*H. pylori* antibodies, biofilm formation, IFN-γ, IL-4, and gastrin and somatostatin levels in serum have been studied [59]. While all parameters were increased in *H. pylori*-infected mice, the treatment with curcumin notably reduced the number of bacteria colonizing gastric mucosa and attenuated the activity of lipid peroxide, MPO and urease strongly supporting the hypothesis that curcumin can reduce the effects of *H. pylori* infection due to its potent antioxidizing properties. Curcumin also exhibited a potent antimicrobial activity against *H. pylori* isolates in mice infected with this bacterium [59]. In contrast, the level of anti-IgG antibodies and somatostatin was increased following curcumin treatment, suggesting that this compound possessed immunomodulation properties resulting in the normalization of the feedback inhibition of gastrin by somatostatin disturbed in *H. pylori*-infected gastric mucosa [59]. Both pro-inflammatory NF-κB and the motogenic response in *H. pylori*-infected epithelial cells were inhibited by curcumin [60]. In recent trials, the addition of curcumin to triple therapy regimes ameliorated the oxidative stress and histopathologic changes in chronic gastritis-associated *H. pylori* infections [61–63]. All together, these studies suggest that curcumin can be a useful supplement to improve the gastric mucosal protection against chronic inflammation and may prevent the carcinogenic changes in patients with chronic gastritis associated with *H. pylori* (Figure 2).

6. Conclusions and Future Perspectives

The poor water solubility, dissolution, and retention time of curcumin in the stomach limits its practical usefulness in the treatment of peptic ulcer disease and neoplastic alterations including oral, esophageal, and gastric cancers in humans [62–64]. However, the therapeutic effect of curcumin might be exerted by its metabolites. For instance, Jamil et al. [57] have studied the spasmolytic, inotropic, and chronotropic activity of major curcumin metabolite tetrahydrocurcumin and the nonenzymatic curcumin hydrolysis products ferulic acid, feruloyl methane, and vanillin. They concluded that demethoxycurcumin and bisdemethoxycurcumin showed more pronounced spasmolytic effects in guinea pig ileum as well as vasodilation and negative inotropic activity in guinea pig arteries and atria, respectively, than those exhibited by a parent curcumin. This evidence seems to indicate that both curcuminoids derivatives can contribute to the observed pharmacological effects of the *C. longa* extract [57]. Thus, future studies are required to prove if the enrichment of extracts of *C. longa* with curcumin metabolites demethoxycurcumin and bisdemethoxycurcumin could potently enhance the therapeutic efficacy of curcumin. Recently, Chen et al. (65) have shown that plasma curcumin was below the detection limit of 0.1 ng/ml after oral curcumin administration in healthy volunteers; instead, only the curcumin metabolite, curcumin glucuronide, has been detected as early as 30 min after curcumin administration and achieved a maximal concentration within 2.7 hours. This suggests a rapid metabolism of curcumin which form the glucuronide conjugate (65). More importantly Chen et al. (65) have revealed that the gene expression of antioxidative genes NRF2, HO-1, and NQO1 was increased and the epigenetic genes for histone deacetylases HDAC1, HADAC2, HADAC3, and HADFAC4 have been suppressed by curcumin glucuronide. They concluded that despite the absence of the parent curcumin in the blood/plasma, the antioxidant and epigenetic modulatory effects of curcumin glucuronide can explain the potential overall health beneficial effect of this herbal medicinal product [65]. Thus, it is reasonable to believe that most of the curcumin effects in vivo may be due to local and direct effects rather than systemic effects of this turmeric compound after absorption. This notion which is supported by the pharmacokinetics and pharmacodynamics of curcumin regulating antioxidant and epigenetic gene expression in humans could be of interest for basic researchers and clinicians.

However, a recent study with a controlled release therapy of curcumin to treat gastric ulcers by novel raft forming systems incorporating curcumin-Eudragit® EPO solid dispersions has triggered attention with a great hope to develop a curcumin carrier with improved solubility and the dissolution of this compound and its prolonged gastric residence time [66]. Importantly, these authors have demonstrated a curative effect of this curcumin raft on the acetic acid-induced chronic gastric ulcer in rats. The curcumin raft forming formulations at the dose of 40 mg/kg administered once daily showed a superior effect in terms of the acceleration of the ulcer healing, as compared with the standard antisecretory therapy with the PPI lansoprazole (1 mg/kg, twice daily) and a curcumin suspension (40 mg/kg, twice daily) [66]. These studies have indicated that this new raft-forming system containing curcumin solid dispersions could serve as a promising carrier for the specific delivery of poorly soluble lipophilic compounds, such as curcumin, to treat upper GI tract disorders in humans.

Author Contributions: Conceptualization, T.B. and S.K.; Methodology, M.M., Z.S., A.P.-B.; Software, T.B., M.M. and D.W.; Validation, A.P.-B., T.B., K.M., Y.Y. and Z.Z.; Formal Analysis, S.K., J.M., M.M. X.X.; Investigation, Z.S., K.M., D.W. X.X.; Resources, X.X.; Data; Writing-Original Draft Preparation, T.B., S.K., J.M.; Writing-Review & Editing, T.B., S.K., M.M.

Funding: This work was supported by the statutory grant to S.K. (K/ZDS/006422) from the Jagiellonian University Medical College. M.M. received financial support from Foundation for Polish Science (START 62.2018).

Acknowledgments: The authors express their best gratitude to Ms. Katherine Kreciwilk for her linguistic suggestions and helpful discussion in the preparation of this manuscript.

Conflicts of Interest: The authors declare no conflict of interest.

References

1. Hatcher, H.; Planalp, R.; Cho, J.; Torti, F.M.; Torti, S.V. Curcumin: From ancient medicine to current clinical trials. *Cell. Mol. Life Sci.* **2008**, *65*, 1631–1652. [CrossRef] [PubMed]
2. Goel, A.; Kunnumakkara, A.B.; Aggarwal, B.B. Curcumin as "Curecumin": From kitchen to clinic. *Biochem. Pharmacol.* **2008**, *75*, 787–809. [CrossRef]
3. Menon, V.P.; Sudheer, A.R. Antioxidant and anti-inflammatory properties of curcumin. *Adv. Exp. Med. Biol.* **2007**, *595*, 105–125.
4. Kunnumakkara, A.B.; Anad, P.; Aggarwal, B.B. Curcumin inhibits proliferation, invasion, angiogenesis and metastasis of different cancers trough interaction with multiple cell signalling proteins. *Cancer Lett.* **2008**, *269*, 199–225. [CrossRef] [PubMed]
5. Anand, P.; Sundaram, C.; Jhurani, S.; Kunnumakkara, A.B.; Aggarwal, B.B. Curcumin and cancer: An "old-age" disease with an "age-old" solution. *Cancer Lett.* **2008**, *267*, 133–164. [CrossRef] [PubMed]
6. Lang, A.; Salomon, N.; Wu, J.C.; Kopylov, U.; Lahat, A.; Har-Noy, O.; Ching, J.Y.; Cheong, P.K.; Avidan, B.; Gamus, D.; et al. Curcumin in combination with mesalamine induces remission in patients with mild-to-moderate ulcerative colitis in a randomized controlled trial. *Clin. Gastroenterol. Hepatol.* **2015**, *13*, 1444–1449. [CrossRef]
7. Adiwidjaja, J.; McLachlan, A.J.; Boddy, A.V. Curcumin as a clinically-promising anti-cancer agent: Pharmacokinetics and drug interactions. *Expert Opin. Drug Metab. Toxicol.* **2017**, *13*, 953–972. [CrossRef]
8. Sundar Dhilip Kumar, S.; Houreld, N.N.; Abrahamse, H. Therapeutic potential and recent advances of curcumin in the treatment of aging-associated diseases. *Molecules* **2018**, *23*, 835. [CrossRef]
9. Morris, J.; Fang, Y.; De Mukhopdhyay, K.; Wargovich, M.J. Natural agents used in chemoprevention of aerodigestive and GI cancers. *Curr. Pharmacol. Rep.* **2016**, *2*, 11–20. [CrossRef]
10. Simental-Mendía, L.E.; Caraglia, M.; Majeed, M.; Sahebkar, A. Impact of curcumin on the regulation of microRNAs in colorectal cancer. *Expert Rev. Gastroenterol. Hepatol.* **2017**, *11*, 99–101. [CrossRef] [PubMed]
11. Kim, H.I.; Hong, S.J.; Han, J.P.; Seo, J.Y.; Hwang, K.H.; Maeng, H.J.; Lee, T.H.; Lee, J.S. Specific movement of esophagus during transient lower esophageal sphincter relaxation in gastroesophageal reflux disease. *J. Neurogastroenterol. Motil.* **2013**, *19*, 332–337. [CrossRef] [PubMed]
12. Souza, R.F. Reflux esophagitis and its role in the pathogenesis of Barrett's metaplasia. *J. Gastroenterol.* **2017**, *52*, 767–776. [CrossRef] [PubMed]
13. Tack, J.; Pandolfino, J.E. Pathophysiology of gastroesophageal reflux disease. *Gastroenterology* **2018**, *154*, 277–288. [CrossRef]
14. Souza, R.F. From reflux esophagitis to esophageal adenocarcinoma. *Dig. Dis.* **2016**, *34*, 483–490. [CrossRef] [PubMed]
15. Schlottmann, F.; Molena, D.; Patti, M.G. Gastroesophageal reflux and Barrett's esophagus: A pathway to esophageal adenocarcinoma. *Updates Surg.* **2018**, *70*, 339–342. [CrossRef]
16. Patrick, L. Gastroesophageal reflux disease (GERD): A review of conventional and alternative treatments. *Altern. Med. Rev.* **2011**, *16*, 116–133. [PubMed]
17. Rafiee, P.; Nelson, V.M.; Manley, S.; Wellner, M.; Floer, M.; Binion, D.G.; Shaker, R. Effect of curcumin on acidic pH-induced expression of IL-6 and IL-8 in human esophageal epithelial cells (HET-1A): Role of PKC, MAPKs and NF-kappaB. *Am. J. Physiol. Gastrointest. Liver Physiol.* **2009**, *296*, G388–G398. [CrossRef] [PubMed]
18. Mahattanadul, S.; Radenahmad, N.; Phadoongsombut, N.; Chuchom, T.; Panichayupakaranant, P.; Yano, S.; Reanmongkol, W. Effects of curcumin on reflux esophagitis in rats. *J. Nat. Med.* **2006**, *60*, 198–205. [CrossRef]
19. Mahattanadul, S.; Nakamura, T.; Panichayupakaranant, P.; Phdoongsombut, N.; Tungsinmunkong, K.; Bouking, P. Comparative antiulcer effect of bisdemethoxycurcumin and curcumin in a gastric ulcer model system. *Phytomedicine* **2009**, *16*, 342–351. [CrossRef]
20. Minacapelli, C.D.; Bajpai, M.; Geng, X.; Cheng, C.L.; Chouthai, A.A.; Souza, R.; Spechler, S.J.; Das, K.M. Barrett's metaplasia develops from cellular reprograming of esophageal squamous epithelium due to gastroesophageal reflux. *Am. J. Physiol. Gastrointest. Liver Physiol.* **2017**, *312*, G615–G622. [CrossRef]
21. Schiffman, S.C.; Li, Y.; Martin, R.C. The association of manganese superoxide dismutase expression in Barrett's esophageal progression with MnTBAP and curcumin oil therapy. *J. Surg. Res.* **2012**, *176*, 535–541. [CrossRef] [PubMed]

22. Vageli, D.P.; Doukas, S.G.; Spock, T.; Sasaki, C.T. Curcumin prevents the bile reflux-induced NF-κB-related mRNA oncogenic phenotype in human hypopharyngeal cells. *J. Cell. Mol. Med.* **2018**, *22*, 4209–4220. [CrossRef] [PubMed]
23. Rawat, N.; Alhamdani, A.; McAdam, E.; Cronin, J.; Eltahir, Z.; Lewis, P.; Griffiths, P.; Baxter, J.N.; Jenkins, G.J. Curcumin abrogates bile-induced NF-κB activity and DNA damage in vitro and suppresses NF-κB activity whilst promoting apoptosis in vivo, suggesting chemopreventive potential in Barrett's oesophagus. *Clin. Transl. Oncol.* **2012**, *14*, 302–311. [CrossRef] [PubMed]
24. Wallace, J.L. Prostaglandins, NSAIDs and gastric mucosal protection: Why doesn't the stomach digest itself? *Physiol. Rev.* **2008**, *88*, 1547–1565. [CrossRef] [PubMed]
25. Laine, L.; Takeuchi, K.; Tarnawski, A. Gastric mucosal defence and cytoprotection: Bench to bedside. *Gastroenterology* **2008**, *135*, 41–60. [CrossRef]
26. Brzozowski, T.; Konturek, P.C.; Konturek, S.J.; Brzozowska, I.; Pawlik, W. Role of prostaglandins in gastroprotection and gastric adaptation. *J. Physiol. Pharmacol.* **2005**, *56* (Suppl. 5), 33–55.
27. Tsujimoto, S.; Mokuda, S.; Matoba, K.; Yamada, A.; Jouyama, K.; Murata, Y.; Ozaki, Y.; Ito, T.; Nomura, S.; Okuda, Y. The prevalence of endoscopic gastric mucosal damage in patients with rheumatoid arthritis. *PLoS ONE* **2018**, *13*, e0200023. [CrossRef]
28. Wallace, J.L. Mechanisms, prevention and clinical implications of nonsteroidal anti-inflammatory drug-enteropathy. *World J. Gastroenterol.* **2013**, *28*, 1861–1876. [CrossRef]
29. Sinha, M.; Gautam, L.; Shukla, P.K.; Kaur, P.; Sharma, S.; Singh, T.P. Current perspectives in NSAID-induced gastropathy. *Mediat. Inflamm.* **2013**, *2013*, 258209. [CrossRef]
30. Cheng, Y.T.; Lu, C.C.; Yen, G.C. Phytochemicals enhance antioxidant enzyme expression to protect against NSAID-induced oxidative damage of the gastrointestinal mucosa. *Mol. Nutr. Food Res.* **2017**, *61*. [CrossRef]
31. Desai, J.C.; Goo, T.; Fukata, M.; Sanyal, S.; Dikman, A.; Miller, K.; Cohen, L.; Brooks, A.; Wang, Q.; Abreu, M.T.; et al. NSAID-induced antral ulcers are associated with distinct changes in mucosal gene expression Aliment. *Pharmacol. Ther.* **2009**, *30*, 71–81.
32. Kim, J.H.; Jin, S.; Kwon, H.J.; Kim, B.W. Curcumin blocks naproxen-induced gastric antral ulcerations through inhibition of lipid peroxidation and activation of enzymatic scavengers in rats. *J. Microbiol. Biotechnol.* **2016**, *26*, 1392–1397. [CrossRef] [PubMed]
33. Chattopadhyay, I.; Bandyopadhyay, U.; Biswas, K.; Maity, P.; Banerjee, R.K. Indomethacin inactivates gastric peroxidase to induce reactive-oxygen-mediated gastric mucosal injury and curcumin protects it by preventing peroxidase inactivation and scavenging reactive oxygen. *Free Radic. Biol. Med.* **2006**, *40*, 1397–1408. [CrossRef]
34. Ganguly, K.; Kundu, P.; Banerjee, A.; Reiter, R.J.; Swarnakar, S. Hydrogen peroxide-mediated downregulation of matrix metalloprotease-2 in indomethacin-induced acute gastric ulceration is blocked by melatonin and other antioxidants. *Free Radic. Biol. Med.* **2006**, *41*, 911–925. [CrossRef] [PubMed]
35. Thong-Ngam, D.; Choochuai, S.; Patumraj, S.; Chayanupatkul, M.; Klaikeaw, N. Curcumin prevents indomethacin-induced gastropathy in rats. *World J. Gastroenterol.* **2012**, *18*, 1479. [CrossRef] [PubMed]
36. Morsy, M.A.; El-Moselhy, M.A. Mechanisms of the protective effects of curcumin against indomethacin-induced gastric ulcer in rats. *Pharmacology* **2013**, *91*, 267–274. [CrossRef]
37. Mei, X.; Hu, D.; Xu, S.; Zheng, Y.; Xu, S. Novel role of Zn(II)-curcumin in enhancing cell proliferation and adjusting proinflammatory cytokine-mediated oxidative damage of ethanol-induced acute gastric ulcers. *Chem. Biol. Interact.* **2012**, *197*, 31–39. [CrossRef]
38. Mei, X.T.; Xu, D.H.; Xu, S.K.; Zheng, Y.P.; Xu, S.B. Zinc(II)-curcumin accelerates the healing of acetic acid-induced chronic gastric ulcers in rats by decreasing oxidative stress and downregulation of matrix metalloproteinase-9. *Food Chem. Toxicol.* **2013**, *60*, 448–454. [CrossRef]
39. Sharma, A.V.; Ganguly, K.; Paul, S.; Maulik, N.; Swarnakar, S. Curcumin heals indomethacin-induced gastric ulceration by stimulation of angiogenesis and restitution of collagen fibers via VEGF and MMP-2 mediated signaling. *Antioxid. Redox. Signal.* **2012**, *16*, 351–362. [CrossRef] [PubMed]
40. Tourkey, M.; Karolin, K. Antiulcer activity of curcumin on experimental gastric ulcer in rats and its effect on oxidative stress/antioxidant, IL-6 and enzyme activities. *Biomed. Environ. Sci.* **2009**, *22*, 488–495. [CrossRef]
41. Kim, D.C.; Kim, S.H.; Choi, B.H.; Baek, M.I.; Kim, D.; Kim, M.J.; Kim, K.T. Curcuma longa extracts protects against gastric ulcers by blocking H_2 histamine receptors. *Boil. Pharm. Bull.* **2005**, *28*, 2220–2224. [CrossRef]

42. Mei, X.T.; Luo, H.J.; Xu, S.K.; Xu, D.; Zheng, Y.; Xu, S.; Lv, J. Gastroprotective effects of new zinc(II)-curcumin complex against pylorus-ligature-induced gastric ulcer in rats. *Chem. Biol. Interact.* **2009**, *18*, 316–321. [CrossRef] [PubMed]
43. Zazueta-Beltran, L.; Medina-Aymerich, L.; Estela Diaz-Triste, N.; Chavez-Pina, A.E.; Castaneda-Hernandez, G.; Cruz-Antonio, L. Evidence against the participation of a pharmacokinetic interaction in the protective effect of single-dose curcumin against gastrointestinal damage induced by indomethacin in rats. *J. Integr. Med.* **2017**, *15*, 151–157. [CrossRef]
44. Takeuchi, K. Gastric cytoprotection by prostaglandin E_2 and prostacyclin: Relationship to EP1 and IP receptors. *J. Physiol. Pharmacol.* **2014**, *65*, 3–14. [PubMed]
45. Magierowska, K.; Wojcik, D.; Chmura, A.; Bakalarz, D.; Wierdak, M.; Kwiecien, S.; Sliwowski, Z.; Brzozowski, T.; Magierowski, M. Alterations in gastric mucosal expression of calcitonin gene-related peptides, vanilloid receptors, and heme oxygenase-1 mediate gastroprotective action of carbon monoxide against ethanol-induced gastric mucosal lesions. *Int. J. Mol. Sci* **2018**, *19*. [CrossRef]
46. Bronowicka-Adamska, P.; Wróbel, M.; Magierowski, M.; Magierowska, K.; Kwiecień, S.; Brzozowski, T. Hydrogen Sulphide Production in Healthy and Ulcerated Gastric Mucosa of Rats. *Molecules* **2017**, *22*, 530. [CrossRef]
47. Czekaj, R.; Majka, J.; Magierowska, K.; Sliwowski, Z.; Magierowski, M.; Pajdo, R.; Ptak-Belowska, A.; Surmiak, M.; Kwiecien, S.; Brzozowski, T. Mechanisms of curcumin-induced gastroprotection against ethanol-induced gastric mucosal lesions. *J. Gastroenterol.* **2018**, *53*, 618–630. [CrossRef] [PubMed]
48. Brzozowski, T.; Konturek, S.J.; Sliwowski, Z.; Pytko-Polończyk, J.; Szlachcic, A.; Drozdowicz, D. Role of capsaicin-sensitive sensory nerves in gastroprotection against acid-independent and acid-dependent ulcerogens. *Digestion* **1996**, *57*, 424–432. [CrossRef] [PubMed]
49. Holzer, P. Role of visceral afferent neurons in mucosal inflammation and defence. *Curr. Opin. Pharmacol.* **2007**, *7*, 563–569. [CrossRef] [PubMed]
50. Szallasi, A.; Blumberg, P.M. Vanilloid (Capsaicin) receptors and mechanisms. *Pharmacol. Rev.* **1999**, *51*, 159–212. [PubMed]
51. Lam, P.M.; McDonald, J.; Lambert, D.G. Characterization and comparison of recombinant human and rat TRPV1 receptors: Effects of exo- and endocannabinoids. *Br. J. Anaesth.* **2005**, *94*, 649–656. [CrossRef] [PubMed]
52. He, P.; Zhou, R.; Hu, G.; Liu, Z.; Jin, Y.; Yang, G.; Li, M.; Lin, Q. Curcumin-induced histone acetylation inhibition improves stress-induced gastric ulcer disease in rats. *Mol. Med. Rep.* **2015**, *11*, 1911–1916. [CrossRef] [PubMed]
53. Bhatia, N.; Jaggi, A.S.; Singh, N.; Anand, P.; Dhawan, R. Adaptogenic potential of curcumin in experimental chronic stress and chronic unpredictable stress-induced memory deficits and alterations in functional homeostasis. *J. Nat. Med.* **2011**, *65*, 532–543. [PubMed]
54. Konturek, P.C.; Brzozowski, T.; Konturek, S.J. Stress and the gut: Pathophysiology, clinical consequences, diagnostic approach and treatment options. *J. Physiol. Pharmacol.* **2011**, *62*, 591–599. [PubMed]
55. Czekaj, R.; Majka, J.; Ptak-Belowska, A.; Szlachcic, A.; Targosz, A.; Magierowska, K.; Strzalka, M.; Magierowski, M.; Brzozowski, T. Role of curcumin in protection of gastric mucosa against stress-induced gastric mucosal damage. Involvement of hypoacidity, vasoactive mediators and sensory neuropeptides. *J. Physiol. Pharmacol.* **2016**, *67*, 261–275.
56. Konturek, S.J.; Brzozowski, T.; Bielanski, W.; Schally, A.V. Role of endogenous gastrin in gastroprotection. *Eur. J. Pharmacol.* **1995**, *278*, 203–212. [CrossRef]
57. Jamil, Q.U.A.; Iqbal, S.M.; Jaeger, W.; Studenik, C. Vasodilating, spasmolytic, inotropic and chronotropic activities of curcuminoids from Curcuma longa in isolated organ preparations of guinea pigs. *J. Physiol. Pharmacol.* **2018**, *69*. [CrossRef]
58. Khonche, A.; Biglarian, O.; Panahi, Y.; Valizadegan, G.; Soflaei, S.S.; Ghamarchehreh, M.E.; Majeed, M.; Sahebkar, A. Adjunctive therapy with curcumin for peptic ulcer: A randomized controlled trial. *Drug. Res. (Stuttg.)* **2016**, *66*, 444–448. [CrossRef]
59. De, R.; Kundu, P.; Swarnakar, S.; Ramamurthy, T.; Chowdhury, A.; Nair, G.B.; Mukhopadhyay, A.K. Antimicrobial activity of curcumin against Helicobacter pylori isolates from India and during infections in mice. *Antimicrob. Agents Chemother.* **2009**, *53*, 1592–1597. [CrossRef]

60. Foryst-Ludwig, A.; Neumann, M.; Schneider-Brachert, W.; Naumann, M. Curcumin blocks NF-kappaB and the motogenic response in Helicobacter pylori-infected epithelial cells. *Biochem. Biophys. Res. Commun.* **2004**, *316*, 1065–1072. [CrossRef]
61. Vetvicka, V.; Vetvickova, J.; Fernandez-Botran, R. Effects of curcumin on Helicobacter pylori infection. *Ann. Transl. Med.* **2016**, *4*, 479. [CrossRef] [PubMed]
62. Sarkar, A.; De, R.; Mukhopadhyay, A.K. Curcumin as a potential therapeutic candidate for Helicobacter pylori associated diseases. *World J. Gastroenterol.* **2016**, *22*, 2736–2748. [CrossRef]
63. Judaki, A.; Rahmani, A.; Feizi, J.; Asadollahi, K.; Hafezi Ahmadi, M.R. Curcumin in combination with triple therapy regimes ameliorates oxidative stress and histopathologic changes in chronic gastritis-associated Helicobacter pylori infection. *Arq. Gastroenterol.* **2017**, *54*, 177–182. [CrossRef] [PubMed]
64. Scrobota, I.; Bolfa, P.; Filip, A.G.; Catoi, C.; Alb, C.; Pop, O.; Tatomir, C.; Baciut, G. Natural chemopreventive alternatives in oral cancer chemoprevention. *J. Physiol. Pharmacol.* **2016**, *67*, 161–172. [PubMed]
65. Cheng, D.; Li, W.; Wang, L.; Lin, T.; Poiani, G.; Wassef, A.; Hudlikar, R.; Ondar, P.; Brunetti, L.; Kong, A.N. Pharmacokinetics, pharmacodynamics and PKPD modeling of curcumin in regulating antioxidant and epigenetic gene expression in human healthy volunteers. *Mol. Pharm.* **2019**. [CrossRef] [PubMed]
66. Kerdsakundee, N.; Mahattanadul, S.; Wiwattanapatapee, R. Development and evaluation of gastroretentive raft forming systems incorporating curcumin-Eudragit® EPO solid dispersions for gastric ulcer treatment. *Eur. J. Pharm. Biopharm.* **2015**, *94*, 513–520. [CrossRef] [PubMed]

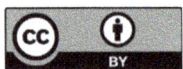

© 2019 by the authors. Licensee MDPI, Basel, Switzerland. This article is an open access article distributed under the terms and conditions of the Creative Commons Attribution (CC BY) license (http://creativecommons.org/licenses/by/4.0/).

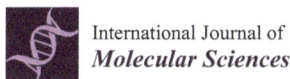

Review

Curcumin and Intestinal Inflammatory Diseases: Molecular Mechanisms of Protection

Kathryn Burge, Aarthi Gunasekaran, Jeffrey Eckert and Hala Chaaban *

Department of Pediatrics, Division of Neonatology, University of Oklahoma Health Sciences Center, 1200 North Everett Drive, ETNP7504, Oklahoma City, OK 73104, USA; Kathryn-Burge@ouhsc.edu (K.B.); Aarthi-Gunasekaran@ouhsc.edu (A.G.); Jeffrey-Eckert@ouhsc.edu (J.E.)
* Correspondence: Hala-Chaaban@ouhsc.edu

Received: 22 March 2019; Accepted: 17 April 2019; Published: 18 April 2019

Abstract: Intestinal inflammatory diseases, such as Crohn's disease, ulcerative colitis, and necrotizing enterocolitis, are becoming increasingly prevalent. While knowledge of the pathogenesis of these related diseases is currently incomplete, each of these conditions is thought to involve a dysfunctional, or overstated, host immunological response to both bacteria and dietary antigens, resulting in unchecked intestinal inflammation and, often, alterations in the intestinal microbiome. This inflammation can result in an impaired intestinal barrier allowing for bacterial translocation, potentially resulting in systemic inflammation and, in severe cases, sepsis. Chronic inflammation of this nature, in the case of inflammatory bowel disease, can even spur cancer growth in the longer-term. Recent research has indicated certain natural products with anti-inflammatory properties, such as curcumin, can help tame the inflammation involved in intestinal inflammatory diseases, thus improving intestinal barrier function, and potentially, clinical outcomes. In this review, we explore the potential therapeutic properties of curcumin on intestinal inflammatory diseases, including its antimicrobial and immunomodulatory properties, as well as its potential to alter the intestinal microbiome. Curcumin may play a significant role in intestinal inflammatory disease treatment in the future, particularly as an adjuvant therapy.

Keywords: ulcerative colitis; Crohn's disease; necrotizing enterocolitis; curcumin; inflammatory bowel disease

1. Introduction

The incidence of intestinal inflammatory diseases, such as necrotizing enterocolitis (NEC), Crohn's disease (CD), and ulcerative colitis (UC), is increasing worldwide. NEC is the most common gastrointestinal emergency affecting premature infants, and is associated with a high mortality rate and significant morbidity. The disease is multifactorial with, currently, poorly understood pathogenesis. A number of risk factors have been identified for developing the condition, including prematurity, hypoxic-ischemic injury, altered microbiome, and formula feeding [1]. NEC is largely characterized by intestinal inflammation and necrosis of the gut. To date, limited treatments for NEC are available, consisting of supportive treatment, surgical resection of damaged tissue, antibiotics, and rest of the bowels [1]. Many infants surviving NEC are subsequently subject to additional morbidity in the form of short-gut syndrome and neurodevelopmental impairments [2].

CD and UC, together referred to as inflammatory bowel disease (IBD), are chronic, relapsing inflammatory diseases with no cure and significant morbidity, most often affecting young adults [3]. Much like NEC, the etiology of IBD is, as yet, unexplained, but is thought to involve an overstimulation and excessive response of the intestinal mucosal immune system to resident luminal microorganisms [4]. In Crohn's disease, inflammation is discontinuous and manifests as distinct granulomas, with inflammation often permeating transmurally and even affecting adjacent lymph nodes [5]. In contrast, ulcerative colitis, occasionally a milder condition, is characterized by continuous mucosal inflammation localized to the colon. Both CD and UC result in extensive epithelial damage. Treatment options for both diseases, including drugs such as cyclosporine, corticosteroids, 5-aminosalicylic acid (mesalamine), mercaptopurines, anti-tumor necrosis factor-alpha (TNF-α), and azathioprine, are costly, often involve significant side effects, and are limited in effectiveness and specificity [6].

The intestinal barrier is critical to health and is one of the most metabolically dynamic systems in the body. The intestines must constantly balance allowing molecules in (e.g., water, electrolytes, nutrients) while keeping inflammatory environmental antigens out [7]. Additionally, the intestinal barrier must manage the prevention of invading and translocating luminal bacteria, but also not become hyperreactive to these commensal or symbiotic microorganisms [1]. The intestinal barrier is composed of both an external physical and biochemical barrier and a complementary inner immunological barrier [7]. Wang et al. [8] have described the physical intestinal barrier as a four-layered system, where a strengthening in any one of these layers serves to strengthen the barrier as a whole. The four integral components of the physical barrier consist of (1) a lipopolysaccharide (LPS)-detoxifying alkaline phosphatase layer, (2) a physical mucin barrier that inhibits bacterial interaction with the intestine, (3) tight junctions, and (4) Paneth cell-secreted antimicrobial proteins (AMPs) [8].

The cells comprising the physical intestinal barrier are intestinal epithelial cells (IECs), a group encompassing mucus-secreting goblet cells, AMP-secreting Paneth cells, enteroendocrine cells, and absorptive enterocytes, among others [9,10]. IECs can not only sense microbes and microbial products, but they can respond by further reinforcement of their own physical barrier and coordination of the response by the intestinal immune system, becoming more or less tolerogenic as dictated by the intestinal luminal contents [11]. Commensal bacteria signal the development of tolerogenic dendritic cells (DCs) and macrophages by spurring IEC-derived production of retinoic acid (RA), transforming growth factor-beta (TGF-β), and thymic stromal lymphopoietin (TSLP) [11]. A tolerogenic immune population allows for the production of interleukin (IL)-10 and RA, both immunomodulatory compounds that can suppress pro-inflammatory cytokine production and promote the function of regulatory T cells [12]. Intestinal epithelial cells sense pathogenic microbes and microbial products via transmembrane pattern recognition receptors (PRRs). One class of PRRs expressed in IECs is toll-like receptors (TLRs). TLR4, in particular, a PRR recognizing LPS from gram-negative bacteria [13], is thought to play an important role in intestinal inflammatory diseases [4,14]. IECs can also respond to luminal bacteria by producing reactive oxygen species (ROS), which can both eliminate bacteria and signal for cell migration and epithelial repair [15].

The functional immunological barrier of the intestines lies largely underneath the physical barrier of IECs. The immune system of the intestine is composed of both innate and adaptive arms. As a newborn, adaptive immunity is less effective, so the infant relies primarily on innate immunity [16]. Innate immunity is comprised of primarily physical barriers (e.g., IEC mucus and AMP production), and a reactive component (e.g., resident and patrolling immune cells) [1]. Adaptive immunity is reliant upon antigen-presenting cells (APC), largely dendritic cells, which direct T and B cell differentiation and activation. Both goblet cells and specialized IECs, microfold cells (M cells), can present antigens to dendritic cells, priming the adaptive immune system [11]. From here, naïve T helper (Th) cells are differentiated into subsets (e.g., Th1 or Th2) with varying characteristics and cytokine profiles depending upon the local environment.

The pathogenesis of intestinal inflammatory diseases likely involves both IECs and intestinal immune cells. When the highly complex, bilayered intestinal barrier is either underdeveloped or disturbed, intestinal inflammatory diseases may result [17,18]. The breakdown of the intestinal barrier is most often attributed to overproduction of pro-inflammatory cytokines, such as TNF-α, IL-1β, and interferon-gamma (IFN-γ) [7], triggered by activation of the nuclear factor-kappaB (NF-κB) and activator protein 1/mitogen-activated protein kinase (AP-1/MAPK) pathways.

2. Intestinal Microbiome in Intestinal Inflammatory Diseases

2.1. Microbiome in NEC

The status of the microbiome in NEC has been widely investigated, but is inherently complex, involving frequent interindividual differences and temporal variability in microbial populations with development and progression of the disease and maturation of the intestine [19]. Intestinal microbes are known to play a role in NEC, as germ-free animal models are protected from development of the disease [20,21]. Preterm infants are recognized to harbor suppressed bacterial diversity, increased percentage of likely pathogenic flora, and reduced bacterial species compared to term infants [22,23]. The development of NEC has been correlated to relative increases in Proteobacteria phylum microbiota, while microbes in Firmicutes, Bacteroides, and Negativicutes are found in reduced proportions [24,25]. The role of microbial species diversity in NEC has been questioned, however, as meta-analyses have failed to find differences in either alpha or beta diversity indices when comparing babies developing NEC to healthy infants [26]. These changes in the NEC preterm infant microbiome may be innate to the maturity of the intestine, but may also be predicated on a number of risk factors for NEC development. For example, antibiotic usage predisposes preterm infants to the development of NEC [27,28], likely through increases in Proteobacteria and reductions in Firmicutes and Actinobacteria [26]. Interestingly, the microbial environment of the placenta and amniotic fluid, both previously thought to be sterile environments, clearly impacts the infant, as the meconium of babies developing NEC differs from those not developing the disease [29]. Additionally, higher intestinal luminal pH is associated with the development of NEC [30], and studies in babies prescribed H2 blockers demonstrated increases in Proteobacteria and a reduction in Firmicutes microbes [30,31], mimicking changes seen in NEC babies [25]. Finally, the role of breastfeeding in the development of NEC has been well established, and the microbiome of the milk appears to be highly individualized [32]. Breastmilk is known to reduce the incidence of NEC [33], potentially through oligosaccharide-associated increases in Bifidobacteria microbial growth [34].

Functional changes associated with shifts in the microbiome are increasingly recognized to be important, and will likely be a point of emphasis in future research. For example, short chain fatty acids (SCFAs), such as butyrate, are produced by gut bacteria and enhance the barrier function of the intestinal epithelium [35]. Host metabolism of butyrate leads to an environment less conducive to intestinal dysbiosis [36]. Intestinal microbial metabolites are also known to affect gut motility via indirect influences on serotonin production [37], a process which may influence the development or progression of NEC [35].

2.2. Microbiome in IBD

As with NEC, the development of IBD is thought to involve intestinal dysbiosis [38]. In IBD, a shift in the intestinal microbiota occurs, resulting in overall decreased diversity, reduced percentages of Firmicutes, and increased percentages of Actinobacteria and Proteobacteria [39]. In particular, pro-inflammatory *Escherichia* and *Fusobacterium* species are increased, while anti-inflammatory *Roseburia* and *Faecalibacterium* species are decreased [39]. Additionally, the microbial composition of IBD patients in remission compared to those with active disease differs, with those with active disease demonstrating higher levels of *Clostridium*, *Faecalibacterium*, and *Bifidobacterium* species [40]. Despite these general trends, human studies of microbial shifts in the context of IBD show very individualized differences [41].

Many of the risk factors for developing IBD-associated intestinal dysbiosis are similar to those of NEC, such as a lack of breastfeeding or caesarean instead of vaginal delivery [38]. However, the composition of the diet in IBD patients also appears to be highly relevant [42]. For example, diets low in fiber have been associated with an increase in the development of colitis, while high-fiber diets have been linked to protection from the disease [43]. Increased dietary fiber leads to the production of butyrate by commensal bacteria [44], known for its beneficial role in immunomodulation of regulatory T cells [45]. Both pre- and probiotics have also been studied in the context of IBD, but clinical trials have shown largely inconsistent results from these supplements [38].

3. Signal Transduction in Intestinal Inflammatory Diseases

3.1. NF-κB Signaling

Both NF-κB and AP-1/MAPK pathways (Figure 1) are thought to play a role in intestinal inflammatory diseases [4,46–48]. NF-κB and AP-1 are ubiquitous transcription factors that bind DNA to regulate gene expression of inflammatory, differentiating, proliferative, and apoptotic genes. The NF-κB pathway can be stimulated via cytokine receptor ligands, PRRs, ROS, TNF receptor proteins, T cell receptors, and B cell receptors [49]. NF-κB is likely the dominant transcription factor involved in intestinal inflammatory diseases, and involves five subunits: p50, p65 (RelA), p52, cRel, and RelB [50–52]. These NF-κB components either homo- or heterodimerize to form active NF-κB [52]. In unstimulated cells, NF-κB resides in the cytoplasm, bound to inhibitory molecules of the IκB family that deem the proteins inactive [53]. Once stimulated, however, IκB proteins are degraded by the IκB kinase (IKK) complex [49]. The IKK complex includes the subunits IKKα and IKKβ, as well as the regulatory protein, NEMO (NF-κB essential modulator) [53]. IKK activation can be triggered by cytokines, microbial components, generalized cellular stress, and growth factors [49]. Following release into the cytoplasm, NF-κB proteins can translocate to the nucleus to bind to DNA promoters and initiate transcription of inflammatory genes, such as IL-1β, TNF-α, IL-12, inducible nitric oxide synthase (iNOS), cyclooxygenase-2 (COX-2), IL-23, and IL-6, as well as genes related to the function and activation of T cells [49,51,54]. Negative regulation of NF-κB signaling largely occurs through IκBα, which is able to translocate to the nucleus and negatively regulate NF-κB activation [55], interleukin-1 receptor-associated kinase-M (IRAK-M), a negative regulator of TLR signaling upstream of NF-κB, and through TNF receptor-associated factor 1 (TRAF1), which blocks the IKK complex [56].

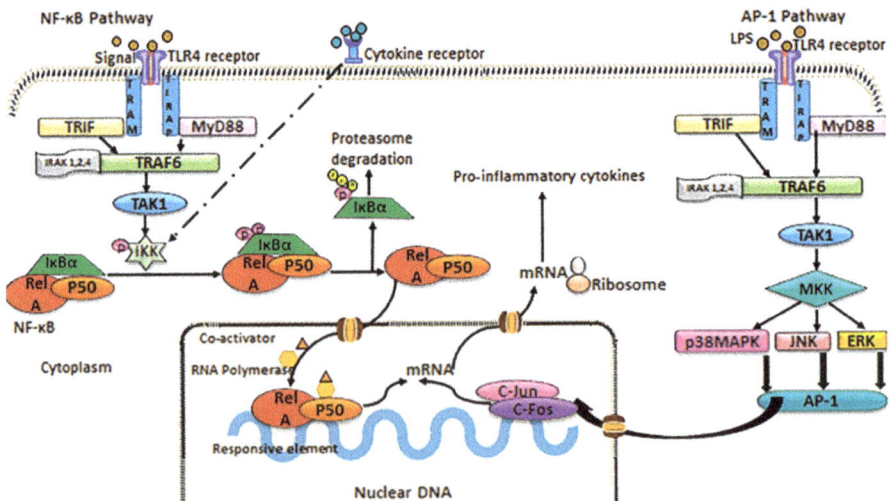

Figure 1. Schematic of TLR4/NF-κB/AP-1 signaling.

Inflammation is a necessary defensive reaction of the host to both microbial infections and tissue damage, and is normally an acute and short-lived process. Dysregulated NF-κB signaling, however, can quickly lead to chronic inflammation and tissue damage. However, NF-κB plays a necessary role in healthy physiology. Interestingly, though NF-κB signaling occurs in both immune and IECs of the intestine [57,58], some evidence suggests NF-κB is protective in IECs, where it is necessary for the integrity of the epithelium, but inflammatory in intestinal myeloid cells. For example, studies in NEMO-deficient [59] and gastrointestinally infected [60] mice have indicated that an absence of NF-κB signaling in IECs leads to severe inflammation, indicating NF-κB can also play an anti-inflammatory role, depending on the context. Clearly, however, NF-κB is critical to IEC-driven lymphocyte development and host defense, particularly against pathogenic bacteria [55].

3.2. AP-1 Signaling

The AP-1 pathway, much like NF-κB, can be stimulated by LPS-activated TLR4 [61–63], growth factors [64], ROS [65], inflammatory cytokines [66], and generalized cellular stress. AP-1 consists of four DNA-binding families, the Fos, Jun, ATF/cyclic AMP-response element-binding (CREB), and Maf families, which homo- or heterodimerize [67,68]. The AP-1 pathway is also dependent on activation of MAPKs, which include extracellular signal-regulated kinases (ERK1/2), Jun N-terminal kinases (JNK), c-Fos-regulating kinases, and p38 [69,70]. The regulation of the AP-1 pathway is complex, with dimer composition, transcriptional and translational activity, and various protein interactions playing multiple roles [71]. When activated via pro-inflammatory cytokines and oxidative stress, as is most common in intestinal inflammatory diseases, the MAPK JNK translocates to the nucleus, phosphorylating c-Jun, activating transcription upon dimerization with c-Fos [71,72]. Target genes include pro-inflamatory mediators such as IL-1β, IL-6, IL-12, IL-23, iNOS, COX-2, and TNF-α [73–75], as well as matrix metalloproteinase 9 (MMP9) [76]. Adding to the complexity, though NF-κB and AP-1 are often differentiated as two separate signaling pathways, they are capable of modulating each other, with multiple overlapping downstream target genes [67]. For example, Mishra et al. [77] have demonstrated that c-Jun, a member of the DNA-binding families of AP-1, is necessary in NF-κB-dependent LPS signaling for transcription in macrophages.

The AP-1 pathway is active in both IECs [78] and immune cells [79] of the intestine. As with NF-κB, AP-1 signaling is believed to be necessary for healthy intestinal homeostasis and microbiota crosstalk [80]. For example, Wang et al. [81] have demonstrated that c-Jun is important in the resolution of intestinal wounds. However, dysregulated or unabated AP-1 signaling can lead to a number of physiological abnormalities, including excessive inflammation, and is believed to contribute to the development of intestinal inflammatory diseases [82–85].

3.3. TLR4 Induction

TLR4 is an upstream regulator of both NF-κB and AP-1, and its induction is critical to intestinal inflammatory diseases [14,86,87]. The TLR4 pathways aid in host immunity by allowing the host to distinguish between self and non-self molecules [6]. TLR4 signaling occurs in both IECs and intestinal immune cells [49], and is unique in that it operates, in both NF-κB and AP-1 signaling, through myeloid differentiation factor 88 (MyD88)-dependent and -independent mechanisms. In both MyD88-dependent and -independent mechanisms, ligand-induced dimerization of TLR4 is necessary to signal downstream [88]. In NF-κB, MyD88-dependent signaling, TLR4 ligand-binding recruits Toll/interleukin-1 receptor domain-containing adaptor protein (TIRAP), which then recruits MyD88 to the site. MyD88 interacts with and activates IRAK4, which then phosphorylates IRAK1. These IRAKs then detach from MyD88 and bind with TRAF6. TRAF6 activates transforming growth factor-beta-activated kinase 1 (TAK1), and TAK1, through TAK1-binding proteins, TAB1 and TAB2, activates IKK, initializing the NF-κB pathway [75]. In NF-κB, MyD88-independent signaling, TLR4 recruits the adaptor proteins TIR-domain-containing adaptor protein inducing interferon-β (TRIF) and translocation associated membrane protein (TRAM) [11,75]. Receptor-interacting protein (RIP1) associates with TRIF and TANK-binding kinase (TBK1) to form a signaling complex, which then regulates the downstream IκBα degradation [75]. RIP1 is also capable of signaling through a PI3K-Akt-dependent mechanism, negatively regulating mammalian target of rapamycin (mTOR) through NF-κB [89].

Alternatively, in AP-1, MyD88-dependent signaling, ligand-binding recruits TIRAP, and subsequently MyD88. Signaling progresses similar to that of NF-κB, MyD88-dependent (above) through the activation of TAK1. While in NF-κB signaling, TAK1 activates IKK, in AP-1 transduction, TAK1 activates MAPK family members (ERK1/2, JNK, and p38), leading to the activation and nuclear translocation of of AP-1 proteins (c-Fos, c-Jun, ETS domain-containing protein 2 (ELK-2), activating transcription factor 2 (ATF-2)) and gene transcription [77]. In AP-1, MyD88-independent signaling, ligand-binding recruits TRAM, and subsequently TRIF [75]. TRIF binds to TRAF6, leading to the activation of TAK1 [75]. From here, phosphorylation of MAPKs occurs similarly to the AP-1, MyD88-dependent pathway. TLR4 signaling is generally regulated by vascular endothelial growth factor-C (VEGF-C), nerve growth factor 1B (Nur-77), and selective androgen receptor modulators (SARMs), which negatively feedback to control this inflammatory pathway [75,90,91].

TLR4 signaling is important in that it primes the immune system, leading to the maturation of DCs and differentiation of Th1 and Th2 T cell subsets [4]. Additionally, TLR4 signaling promotes the differentiation of macrophages to an M1 phenotype, characterized by the production of pro-inflammatory cytokines [92]. Because TLR4 is upstream of both NF-κB and AP-1, however, denotes that a disproportionate TLR4 induction begets excessive inflammation [4].

4. Molecular Mechanisms of Injury in Intestinal Inflammatory Diseases

4.1. Pathogenesis of NEC

The pathogenesis of NEC is thought to involve the underdeveloped intestinal motility and barrier functions of the infant [93], an altered microbiome [94,95], and an immature, but hypersensitive, immune system [96]. Both innate and adaptive immune factors contribute to susceptibility to NEC, but the exact sequence of events in development of the disease is poorly understood.

In NEC, induction of the TLR4 pathway is not only implicated in the disease, but is thought to potentially be required for its development [87,97–102]. In normal physiology, IECs express very low levels of TLR4 [103]. However, in both mice and humans, prematurity is denoted by an unusually high expression of TLR4 [97,98,101,104–106]. Activation of TLR4 signaling in this environment not only leads to excessive inflammation, but also increased apoptosis of IECs, reduced migration and proliferation of IECs to replace those lost to apoptotic events, and the destruction of the intestinal epithelium [10]. The impaired intestinal barrier now allows the immature immune system greater and more frequent access to microbial antigens [107]. Dendritic cells residing in the intestine begin presenting antigens, and T cells, monocytes, and macrophages activate and initiate the production of a wealth of pro-inflammatory cytokines and chemokines [1,108]. This inflammatory cascade leads to recruitment of neutrophils, release of ROS, and further intestinal inflammation and necrosis [52]. Endothelial nitric oxide synthase (eNOS) is also reduced by TLR4 activation, potentially resulting in intestinal ischemia and necrosis [102,109]. A vicious cycle ensues, where inflammation begets more inflammation, overriding any attempts by the host of counterregulation. This inflammation spreads systemically, affecting organs as remote as the brain [2].

Evidence of the upregulation of TLR4/NF-κB/AP-1 signaling in NEC is robust. Preterm infants are likely developmentally predisposed to excessive NF-κB activation. In vitro and fetal cell explant studies of IECs have revealed that immature enterocytes display lower levels of the NF-κB-inhibiting IκBα compared to mature cells [110], resulting in elevated IL-8 production in response to LPS [111]. De Plaen et al. [52] demonstrated persistent NF-κB activation in intestinal epithelial cells in a rat model of NEC, while additional animal models have established that levels of NF-κB positively correlate with disease severity [14,112]. Managlia et al. [107] demonstrated that NF-κB activation occurs before the onset of intestinal injury, and that monocytes are differentiated into inflammatory intestinal macrophages during the very early stages of NEC via IKKβ. Fusunyan et al. [106] examined small intestinal histology from preterm infants with NEC and denoted both increased TLR4 and reduced IκB expression. Additionally, the neonatal intestine is also characterized by higher levels of c-Jun and c-Fos, important mediators in the AP-1 pathway [78]. Thus, the immature intestinal environment of the premature infant predisposes it to chronic inflammatory signaling.

A number of differences beyond the hyperinduction of TLR4/NF-κB/AP-1 have been noted between normal physiology and NEC, in both animal models and humans. IECs not only express PRRs, such as TLR4, but also present major histocompatibility class (MHC) I and II molecules [10], information presented to the adaptive immune system for future identification of foreign compounds. In NEC, infants generally show a lower expression of MHC II molecules [113], potentially allowing pathogenic bacteria to more easily translocate the intestinal epithelium. Goblet cells in the epithelium, characterized by protective mucin 2 (MUC2) production, are reduced in number and show decreased MUC2 production in both mice and humans [87,114–116].

The importance of neutrophils in the development of NEC is still unclear. Neutrophils, among the first cells recruited to the site of injury, release bactericidal compounds and ROS, and attract further immune cell recruitment [117]. Some animal studies have demonstrated a protective effect of neutrophil recruitment in NEC [118], while others have shown the oxidative metabolites from neutrophils may further degrade tissue impacted by NEC [119]. However, limited studies in humans have indicated that neutropenia is a significant risk factor for NEC [120], and immature human neutrophils show a reduced ability to phagocytize [121]. Meanwhile, macrophages in the immature intestine are hyperactive, demonstrating an increased sensitivity to microbial products [122–124], but the presence of TGF-β can suppress this immune activity [122]. Patients with NEC show increased tissue macrophage infiltration and suppressed levels of TGF-β2, an embryonic isoform [2,125]. Additionally, these macrophages may not be fully functional, as they, like immature neutrophils, show a reduced ability to phagocytize [121]. Dendritic cells, while not studied much in the context of NEC, may also contribute to the breakdown of the intestinal barrier [126].

Though adaptive immunity is less pronounced in neonates [16], T cells are still believed to contribute to NEC pathogenesis in a number of ways. For example, neonatal γδ intraepithelial lymphocytes (IELs), the first subset of intestinal T cells present during embryogenesis [127], produce higher levels of the cytokines IFN-γ and IL-10 compared to adult populations [128]. γδ IELs are thought to protect against bacterial invasion if mucosal injury occurs [129]. However, these γδ IELs are significantly less abundant in preterm infants with NEC compared to age-matched controls [127]. Tregs, T cells that regulate immune responses and promote tolerance, in both mice and humans, are found in lower levels in NEC infants compared to controls [98,130]. Th17 cells, a pro-inflammatory subset of T helper cells credited with tissue inflammation and destruction, are present in higher concentrations in the context of NEC [98]. The primary cytokine produced by Th17 cells, IL-17A, is believed to contribute significantly to NEC development by disrupting tight junctions, reducing IEC proliferation, and increasing IEC apoptosis [98]. Another subset of T helper cells, Th1, mediate, in large part, the cellular response to intracellular pathogens and microbial products. In NEC, there is some evidence these inflammatory mediators have a reduced ability to respond to pathogens and produce their signature cytokine, IFN-γ [131].

As expected given the upregulation of TLR4/NF-κB/AP-1 signaling in NEC, cytokine and pro-inflammatory ROS-associated enzyme levels drastically differ compared to age-matched controls [132]. For example, levels of inducible nitric oxide synthase (iNOS), an enzyme responsible for the production of nitric oxide (NO) and involved in inflammatory immune defense and oxidative tissue damage, are upregulated in NEC, both in tissue and serum [133]. TNF-α, a pro-inflammatory cytokine known to increase IL-1, provoke leukocyte migration, spur angiogenesis [134], and associated with shock [135], is increased in NEC [136–139]. TNF-α also increases levels of matrix metalloproteinases, such as MMP9, MMP12 [140,141], and MMP19 [142], destructive proteins which serve in the breakdown of the intestinal extracellular matrix [143]. Interestingly, the inhibitor of MMPs, tissue inhibitor of metalloproteinases (TIMPs), is also upregulated in NEC, likely indicating an attempt by the body at repair [144].

IL-1, a pro-inflammatory cytokine stimulated by TNF-α [134], is associated with leukocyte adhesion, macrophage and neutrophil activation [145], and the upregulation of IL-8 [146]. Levels of both IL-1α and IL-1β are upregulated in the NEC intestine [130,147]. Additionally, evidence suggests the neonatal intestine has enhanced sensitivity to IL-1β compared to more mature enterocytes [78]. IL-1 receptor antagonist (IL-1Ra), an anti-inflammatory protein competitively inhibiting both IL-1 isoforms, is also upregulated in NEC, though this upregulation is clearly not enough to counteract the rampant inflammation induced by IL-1 [148].

IL-6, a cytokine stimulated by a variety of pro-inflammatory cytokines including IL-1 and TNF-α, can act in both pro-inflammatory and anti-inflammatory means, and is an activator of lymphocytes in the adaptive immune system [149]. Levels of IL-6 are elevated in NEC [150]. Plasma IL-6, in particular, is significantly associated with higher NEC morbidity and mortality [151]. IL-8, a neutrophil and monocyte chemokine [152], is found in greater abundance in premature infants [111], but levels are upregulated further still in NEC, though often with a temporal delay [130,148]. IL-12, IL-18, and IFN-γ, which work simultaneously to increase inflammation via ROS [153,154], are upregulated in NEC [155–157]. Serum levels of IL-2 and IL-5 are also increased in the disease [158]. Finally, levels of IL-4 and IL-10, counterregulatory anti-inflammatory cytokines, are increased in NEC [130,148,158], while serum and tissue levels of the immune suppressor TGF-β are reduced [159]. The upregulation of IL-10, again, may demonstrate an attempt by the host at repair [1].

4.2. Pathogenesis of IBD

Whereas in NEC, pathogenesis of the disease is strongly predicated on prematurity, the development of IBD is thought to be dependent upon genetic susceptibility [160], lifestyle factors, such as diet and antibiotic use [161], intestinal barrier dysfunction [162], and, potentially, altered microbiome [163–165]. These factors, altogether, result in a heightened mucosal inflammatory response to luminal microbiota and breakdown of the intestinal barrier, likely through disruption of tight junctions [163,166–168]. Interestingly, increased intestinal permeability is often used clinically to predict relapse of Crohn's disease, in particular [142,143], but intestinal permeability is, itself, not enough to initiate CD development, as first-degree relatives of CD patients, though asymptomatic, also demonstrate increased intestinal permeability [169–172]. As with NEC, the succession of events leading to development of IBD is not known.

Both the innate and adaptive immune systems contribute to IBD pathology. In a genetically susceptible individual, a small break in the intestinal epithelium, such as through bacterial translocation, activates the innate immune system, most likely through upregulated TLR4 activity. Activation of TLR4, and subsequently NF-κB and AP-1, promotes the enlistment of monocyte-derived macrophages, initializing production of pro-inflammatory cytokines, leukocyte-attracting chemokines, such as IL-8, monocyte chemoattractant protein 1 (MCP-1) and MCP-3, and macrophage inflammatory proteins (MIP) [163,173]. When inflammation is not constrained [174], APCs then enter mesenteric lymph nodes and drive T helper cell differentiation and the proliferation of macrophages, resulting in heightened sensitivity to luminal commensal bacteria [175]. Neutrophils then infiltrate damaged tissue and excessive pro-inflammatory cytokine release ensues, as well as the release of additional pro-inflammatory mediators, such as eicosanoids, MMPs, platelet-activating factor (PAF), reactive nitrogen species (RNS), and ROS [176–181]. MAPK activation in IECs spurs the upregulation of both COX-2 and iNOS, which can cause additional damage to the intestinal epithelium [182]. Furthermore, levels of vascular cell adhesion molecule 1 (VCAM-1), E-selectins, very late antigen 4 (VLA-4), macrophage 1 antigen (Mac-1), lymphocyte function-associated antigen 1 (LFA-1), and intercellular adhesion molecule 1 (ICAM-1) increase, attracting further recruitment and activation of lymphocytes [183]. Levels of counterregulatory mediators, meanwhile, such as TGF-β1 and IL-10, are reduced [184,185]. Thus, a vicious cycle of chronic inflammation ensues, resulting in the apoptosis of IECs [162], the prevention of apoptosis in, and accumulation of, T cells [5], and further compromise of intestinal barrier function. In the long-term, excessive signaling and inflammation resulting from microbial recognition by IECs has also been shown to drive colorectal cancer development in individuals suffering from IBD [186,187].

There is significant evidence of the upregulation of TLR4/NF-κB/AP-1 signaling in IBD. Levels of TLR4 are upregulated in the intestinal tissue of both humans [188] and animal models [189] of IBD. In both CD and UC, levels of tissue NF-κB are positively correlated with intestinal inflammation severity [51,190]. Intestinal mucosal macrophages of both UC and CD patients demonstrate increased levels of NF-κB, resulting in increased capacity for inflammatory TNF-α, IL-1 and IL-6 cytokine production [191]. In IBD, the p65 subunit of NF-κB is increased, particularly in Crohn's disease [51,53]. Additionally, in an extensively utilized mouse model of IBD, trinitrobenzene sulfonic acid (TNBS)/ethanol-induced colitis, activation of the p65 subunit is a requisite step in the pathogenesis of the disease model [191]. AP-1 signaling has been deemed dysfunctional in IBD through increased JNK activity in both macrophages [192] and IECs [83,193]. Several studies have also indicated increased JNK activity in the inflamed mucosa of IBD patients [194].

IBD intestinal physiology vastly differs from that of healthy individuals, in both humans and animal models. For example, Paneth cells in IBD are known to release fewer AMPs, potentially allowing more bacteria to translocate the intestinal epithelium [195]. Recent research has also pointed to potential differences in autophagy in IBD, both of pathogens (xenophagy), as well as damaged mitochondria (mitophagy), leading to more microbial invasion and reduced clearance of damaged tissue [196]. Monocytes in IBD also show reduced MHC II expression, which has been shown to correlate with disease activity [197].

T cells contribute significantly to inflammatory bowel disease, and therapy aimed at T cell reduction has been shown to abrogate the disease [198]. In Crohn's disease, in particular, T cells are extremely prevalent, and often form distinctive granulomas [5]. These T cells, primarily naïve, are recruited via the blood to the intestinal mucosa, largely through the production of adhesion molecules and pro-inflammatory cytokines [160]. An upregulation of IL-6 during IBD development leads to activation of the STAT3 pathway, preventing T cell apoptosis, and allowing for the abnormal accumulation of these cells in the intestine [199]. These T cells secrete large amounts of pro-inflammatory cytokines, permitting IBD disease progression.

In IBD, T helper cell profiles differ by disease. In CD, the profile of T helper cells is strongly skewed toward that of the Th1 and Th17 phenotypes [200,201], driven by LPS-associated IL-12 production [202]. Th1 cells, important in pathogen clearance, produce large amounts of IFN-γ, TNF-α, and IL-2 [5,203], and active CD lesions show high levels of these cytokines [204] and their associated T cells [205]. Th1 cells, much like naïve T cells in IBD, appear to be protected from apoptosis [206]. Th17 cells, the differentiation of which is spurred by IL-6 and TGF-β [207], are maintained via IL-12-associated release of IL-23 [208]. Th17 cells, native to the intestinal barrier and important in the elimination of extracellular pathogens, produce IL-17, an inflammatory cytokine aiding in neutrophil and monocyte recruitment [49,209]. Unlike in NEC, the role of IL-17 in IBD is not clear, as it plays a protective [210,211] and pathogenic role [212,213], depending upon the model. In UC, however, the T helper cell profile leans towards Th2, Th9, and Th17 phenotypes, producing large amounts of IL-5 and IL-13 [214]. Th2 cell differentiation is driven by IL-4, and when this pathway becomes dysregulated, upregulated Th2-associated production of IL-13 contributes to tissue destruction, as it induces apoptosis in IECs [215]. Th9 cells, meanwhile, driven simultaneously by IL-4 and TGF-β, produce IL-9, a pleotropic cytokine thought to impair the intestinal barrier function and exacerbate UC-associated tissue damage [216]. Additionally, the production of IL-21 may also play a role in IBD by driving both Th1 and Th17 responses [217].

T regulatory cells (Tregs) also play an important role in intestinal inflammatory disease pathogenesis, as they can inhibit effector T cells from functioning, promoting a more tolerogenic immune phenotype [218]. There is some indication the balance between effector T cells and Tregs is altered in intestinal inflammatory diseases [219], allowing for disease progression via inflammatory cytokine production and T cell activation positive feedback loops [220]. Further evidence of this imbalance is provided by studies denoting transfusions of Tregs into animal models of experimental colitis ameliorate the disease [221,222]. Treg function and Th17 differentiation is, in part, due to regulation by IL-18 [223,224], a cytokine found in higher levels in IBD patients [225].

Another group of lymphocytes thought to be important in IBD are the innate lymphoid cells, a population of lymphocytes which lack typical adaptive lymphocyte markers [226]. Patients with IBD, particularly CD, show significant mucosal infiltration of innate lymphoid cells, group 1 (ILC1), demarcated by production of IFN-γ and TNF [227,228], and mouse studies mirror this finding [229]. Type 3 innate lymphoid cells (ILC3s) also play a role, producing both IL-22 and IL-17. IL-22 is important in intestinal repair, and in mouse models, blocking this pathway leads directly to colitis [230,231]. IBD patients are known to have an increase in the IL-22 binding protein, an antagonist to IL-22 [232].

With increased TLR4/NF-κB/AP-1 signaling comes excessive production of inflammatory cytokines and oxidative molecules, some of which have already been discussed. Both CD and UC are characterized by increased synthesis of IL-1β, IL-6, IL-8, TNF-α, and IL-16, a T cell chemoattractant [51,160,233–235]. In the context of IBD, TNF-α and IL-1β are particularly important. TNF-α can activate resident tissue macrophages, spur further proinflammatory cytokine and oxidative inflammatory mediator release, as well as induce adhesion molecule expression, further driving leukocyte recruitment to areas of inflammation [160,233]. IL-1β, a pro-inflammatory cytokine associated with the innate immune response, has been found in high levels in the tissues of patients with IBD [236], as well as in monocytes from these patients [237]. In both humans and animal models, the balance of IL-1 and IL-1Ra plays a determinative role in IBD [238,239]. The IL-1Ra/IL-1 ratio is decreased in IBD, and this ratio correlates negatively with clinical severity of the disease [238,240]. In Crohn's disease, the activity of inositol polyphosphate 5′-phosphatase D (SHIP), a negative regulator of IL-1β expression [241], is reduced, furthering the imbalance of IL-1Ra/IL-1. Both IL-1β and TNF-α can induce production of MMPs, further destroying the intestinal scaffolding [176,242]. MMP3, in particular, has been found in high levels in the tissues of IBD patients [243–245]. Overproduction of IL-6 is also thought to be important in IBD, where in mouse models, elevated IL-6 levels are directly involved in disease pathogenesis and can result in the abnormal accumulation of T cells in the intestine [199]. IFN-γ production, in the context of CD, is important in driving further production of IL-1, IL-6, and TNF-α [198]. Finally, the negative regulator of the immune-calming TGF-β, mothers against decapentaplegic homolog 7 (SMAD7), is increased in IBD [246], thereby blocking one counterregulatory measure to the excessive inflammation induced by these cytokines.

Pro-inflammatory cytokine release may result in tight junction disruption in IBD, further damaging the intestinal barrier [162]. For example, claudin-2, a pore-forming protein, is known to be upregulated in IBD, particularly in crypts where the protein is not normally present [235,247]. Additionally, the loss of tight junction strands and physical severing of these strands is associated with IBD-associated intestinal barrier defects [162]. Alterations in tight junctions, however, are thought to be a consequence of upregulated cytokine production, rather than a causative factor in IBD.

5. The Effects of Curcumin on Intestinal Inflammatory Diseases

Curcumin, the biologically active, hydrophobic, phenolic component of turmeric (*Curcuma longa*), is a natural product commonly utilized in Ayurdevic and traditional medicine, both topically and orally, for its potent effects on multiple body systems [248]. Four compounds, collectively termed curcuminoids and imparting a yellow color, are derived from turmeric, including curcumin, bisdemethoxycurcumin, demethoxycurcumin, and cyclocurcumin, with curcumin found in the highest concentration by weight [214,249]. Commercially purchased curcumin is often an impure mixture of approximately three-quarters curcumin, 17% demethoxycurcumin, 3% bisdemethyoxycurcumin, and little to no cyclocurcumin [248], and human curcumin clinical trial results have been complicated by the fact that multiple, heterogeneous mixtures of curcuminoids have been used in these studies [250]. Curcumin is characterized by the inclusion of two aromatic rings, and its phenolic hydrogens are believed to impart antioxidant activity to the molecule [214,248]. Curcumin, also known as diferuloylmethane, has been a popular supplement largely because of its affordability and safety, with no known toxic side effects in humans up to doses of 12 g/day [251].

5.1. Antibacterial and Microbiome Effects

Curcumin demonstrates a wide range of effects on the gastrointestinal system. In in vitro and in vivo models of *Helicobacter pylori* infection, curcumin inhibited bacterial growth on agar plates, and eradicated the bacteria from mice, respectively [252]. The bactericidal effect of curcumin appears to occur through an inhibition of bacterial cell division, resulting in the inappropriate assembly of the bacterial protofilament [253]. Further, Niamsa and Sittiwet [254] demonstrated the antimicrobial activity of curcumin against a number of commonly encountered pathogenic Gram-negative and Gram-positive bacteria.

Curcumin is also capable of regulating the gut microbiota, as a whole. Intestinal inflammatory diseases are defined, in part, by an altered, frequently pathogenic, microbiome [163–165,255]. In IBD, the microbiome is often enriched by a population of adherent invasive *E. coli* (AIEC), which can promote inflammation in the gut [256,257]. Studies investigating the effects of curcumin on the microbiome have attained different results depending upon the disease characteristics of the studied population. For example, in mice living in specific-pathogen-free conditions, curcumin supplementation decreased the microbial richness and diversity [258]. In a rat model of hepatic steatosis, curcumin administration reduced species richness and diversity, shifted the structure of the gut microbiota, and induced significant microbiota compositional changes compared to both high-fat diet and control groups, reversing the buildup of fat in the liver [259]. Importantly, curcumin favored the maintenance of short-chain fatty acid-producing bacteria, which are known to provide intestinal mucosal protection and inhibit intestinal inflammation [260,261].

In rats that have been ovariectomized, estrogen-deficiency-associated gut microbial shift is partially reversed by supplementation with curcumin [262]. Ohno et al. [263] showed, in a mouse model of colitis, an immunological and microbiological shift towards improved intestinal barrier function and reduced intestinal inflammation with nanoparticle curcumin supplementation. Curcumin administration in these mice significantly increased butyrate-producing microbiota, which are associated with colonic induction of Tregs, tolerance-promoting T cells [264,265]. McFadden et al. [266] utilized an IL-10-deficient model of murine colitis to demonstrate that curcumin supplementation prevented age-associated decreases in bacterial alpha diversity, increased bacterial richness, decreased *Coriobacterales*, increased *Lactobacillales*, and prevented development of colorectal cancer.

Studies on the effects of curcumin on the human gut microbiota are generally lacking, potentially due to the widely acknowledged absorption issues of the compound. Peterson et al. [250], in a pilot study, compared whole turmeric or curcumin extracts to placebo, and showed an increase in species and a trend toward increased alpha diversity with turmeric or curcumin supplementation. While individual responses to treatment varied, the patterns within the groups were very similar in both turmeric and curcumin, suggesting that curcumin, the most significant bioactive component of turmeric, was driving the observed changes. Interestingly, in subjects supplementing with turmeric or curcumin, the relative abundance of *Blautia* spp., believed to be the major metabolizers of curcumin [267], was reduced compared to controls [250]. While more complete studies on the effects of curcumin on the human microbiota are warranted, curcumin may be able to both simultaneously eradicate some pathogenic bacteria while globally shifting the composition of the intestinal microbiome.

5.2. Effects on Signal Transduction

Inflammation in intestinal inflammatory diseases is largely driven through upregulated TLR4/NF-κB/AP-1 signaling. Activation of TLR4 initiates an innate immune response and subsequent inflammation, in both NEC [14] and IBD [86]. Treatments abrogating TLR4-dependent signal transduction have been shown to lead to an amelioration of intestinal inflammatory disease [268]. Curcumin has been shown to inhibit both MyD88-dependent and -independent signaling mechanisms [88,269]. Additionally, curcumin can bind to myeloid differentiation protein 2 (MD-2), a protein bound to the extracellular TLR4 domain, thereby suppressing the innate immune response to LPS [270]. Additionally, should this initial inhibition not occur, curcumin can inhibit TLR4 signaling at a number of downstream steps, including TRAF6 and IRAK1, as well as through immune-modulating (e.g., MCP-1, MIP-2) and signaling-associated cytokine blockades [269,271]. In a Caco-2 model of the intestinal epithelium, treatment with curcumin resulted in diminished LPS-induced pro-inflammatory cytokine release and tight junction protein disruption [8], likely through a TLR4-dependent reduction in signaling. In TNBS-induced colitis rodent models, curcumin has been shown to ameliorate the disease through a reduction in TLR4 signal transduction [6,272].

Eckert et al. [273] treated T84 intestinal epithelial monolayers with FLLL32, an analog of curcumin with greater solubility and potency. FLLL32 treatment reduced paracellular permeability associated with IL-6-induced inflammation, denoted as an alleviation of the IL-6-induced drop in transepithelial electrical resistance (TEER) (Figure 2). This same group, in a dithizone/*Klebsiella* Paneth cell ablation animal model of NEC, showed mouse pups treated with 25 mg/kg FLLL32 developed NEC less frequently, and at a significantly reduced severity, compared to pups with untreated NEC (Figure 3A–D; 20× magnification). Additionally, a fluorescein isothiocyanate (FITC)-dextran in vivo intestinal barrier assay demonstrated enhanced preservation of the intestinal barrier in FLLL32-treated animals compared to those with untreated NEC (Figure 3E). Finally, FLLL32 treatment decreased levels of the inflammatory cytokines IL-1β, IL-6, TNF-α, and growth-regulated oncogene-alpha (GRO-α) compared to levels in pups with untreated NEC, thereby inhibiting NEC-associated inflammation, likely through a TLR4/NF-κB-dependent reduction in signaling (Figure 3F–I).

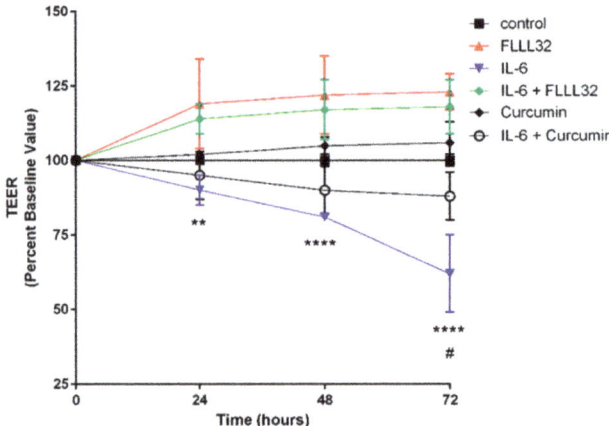

Figure 2. (Reprinted with permission from Dove Medical Press, Ltd.). Effect of FLLL32 and curcumin on IL-6-induced reduction of TEER in T84 monolayer. TEER value of T84 monolayers incubated with cell culture medium for 0–72 h in the presence of IL-6 (10 ng/mL) with FLLL32 (50 μM), curcumin (50 μM), or carrier (dimethyl sulfoxide) for 1 h in serum-free medium. ** $p = 0.001$ (IL-6 vs. IL-6 + FLLL32 at 24 h), **** $p < 0.0001$ (IL-6 vs. IL-6 + FLLL32 at 48 and 72 h), and # $p = 0.003$ (IL-6 vs. IL-6 + curcumin).

Downstream of TLR4, signaling continues through either NF-κB or AP-1, both of which are upregulated in, and critical to, intestinal inflammatory diseases [4,46–48]. In both NEC and IBD, inhibition of NF-κB signaling has been shown to reduce injuries to the bowel [52,274,275]. Additionally, p38 MAPK inhibitors have established some success against colitis [192], including potentially in human IBD [276]. Curcumin inhibition of NF-κB activation appears to be through inhibition of IKKβ [277], thus reducing IκB kinase activity [278], and preventing NF-κB subunit movement to the nucleus. The mechanism of curcumin therapy in intestinal inflammatory diseases mimics that of steroids, blocking IκBα degradation in the cytoplasm and inhibiting nuclear translocation of the p65 subunit, in particular [51]. In AP-1 signaling, curcumin can inhibit MAPK [269], ERK1/2, JNK, and p38, both directly and indirectly, thereby limiting transcription of inflammatory target genes [279].

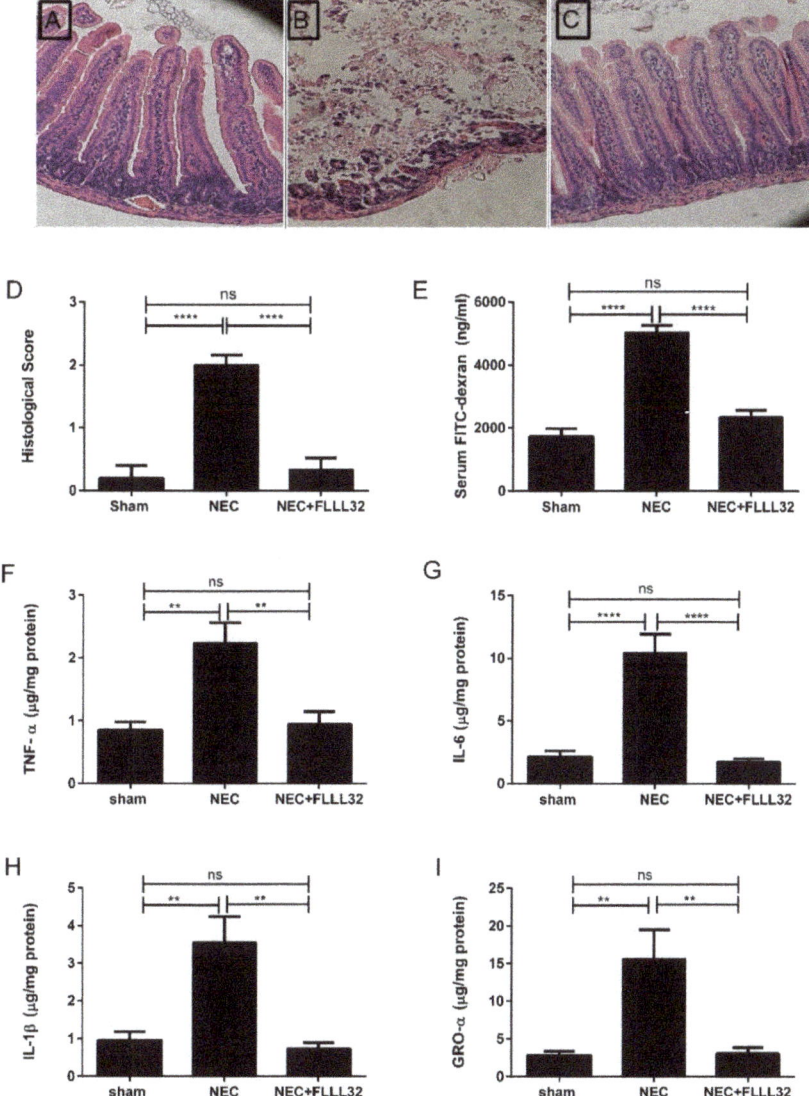

Figure 3. (Reprinted with permission from Dove Medical Press, Ltd.). FLLL32 attenuates intestinal inflammation and injury in DK NEC model. Representative H&E pictures from pups in the sham group (**A**), untreated NEC group (**B**), and NEC + FLLL32 group (**C**) (20× magnification). (**D**) Histological NEC scoring was obtained by two pathologists blinded to the groups (**** $p < 0.0001$). (**E**) FLLL32 preserved intestinal permeability in the NEC + FLLL32 group compared to the untreated group and control group (**** $p < 0.0001$). FLLL32 pretreatment reduced the levels of proinflammatory cytokines, TNF-α (**F**, $p = 0.001$), IL-6 (**G**, $p < 0.001$), IL-1β (**H**, $p = 0.009$), and GRO-α levels (**I**, $p = 0.034$) compared to pups in the untreated NEC group. Data are mean ± SEM. Results are representative of at least three separate experiments.

Numerous studies, in both animal models and humans, have documented curcumin inhibition of NF-κB and AP-1 signaling [280–285]. For example, in a variety of IEC lines, Jobin et al. [278] showed curcumin can inhibit NF-κB-binding to DNA, degradation of IκBα, translocation to the nucleus of RelA, serine phosphorylation of IκB, and activity of IKK. In HT29 IECs, in vitro treatment with curcumin inhibited TNF-α- and IL-1β-induced activation of p38 and JNK, while also inhibiting IκB degradation [286]. In a rat model of TNBS-colitis, curcumin treatment significantly reduced protein expression of MyD88 and NF-κB [6], prevented the degradation of IκB [287], and also alleviated symptoms of colitis via a reduction in p38 MAPK [288]. Sugimoto et al. [289] showed an amelioration of experimental TNBS-colitis in mice via a reduction in NF-κB activity. Additionally, curcumin pretreatment of mouse dendritic cells suppressed NF-κB translocation to the nucleus, as well as decreased phosphorylation of ERK, p38, and JNK [290].

5.3. Effects on Inflammation and Immunomodulation

The effects of curcumin on inflammation and immunomodulation are widely touted. Curcumin affects the function, differentiation, and maturation of a number of immune cells actively engaged in the pathogenesis or progression of intestinal inflammatory diseases. Dendritic cells treated with curcumin tend to promote the induction of intestinal T cells with a hyporesponsive phenotype, and these dendritic cells also demonstrate inhibited antigen presenting ability, leading to reduced stimulation of the adaptive immune system [291]. Curcumin-treated DCs also stimulate the differentiation of intestinal Tregs, and in a mouse model of colitis, these Tregs prevented the development of the disease [291]. Other studies have indicated that curcumin pretreatment suppresses LPS-induced NF-κB p65 translocation and MAPK phosphorylation in dendritic cells, leading to a reduction in inflammation [290]. Curcumin treatment of DCs reduces pro-inflammatory cytokine expression (IL-1, IL-6, TNF-α), and importantly that of IL-12, inhibiting the ability of these DCs to induce Th1-type responses [290]. Additionally, curcumin can reduce the dendritic cell expression of ICAM-1 (intercellular adhesion molecule-1) and CD11c, proteins related to both cellular adhesion and T cell activation [292], likely through an AP-1-dependent pathway. However, potentially the most important effect of curcumin on dendritic cells is to prevent their maturation via a suppression of indoleamine 2,3-dioxygenase (IDO), with an anti-inflammatory effect similar to that of corticosteroids [290,293].

Curcumin has been demonstrated to inhibit T cell-mediated immune functions playing a significant role in chronic intestinal inflammatory diseases [2,294], such as the ability to reduce the proliferative response of lymphocytes. This reduction in proliferation may occur due to both the antioxidant properties of curcumin, reducing ROS-related proliferation, and inhibition of ribonucleotide reductase and DNA polymerase activation, important in the cell cycle [294,295]. In addition, curcumin has been shown to reduce NF-κB-induced, T cell-initiated cytokine production [294], including the Th1-type cytokines, IL-2 and IFN-γ, further inhibiting lymphocyte proliferation [294,296]. In CD, Th1 cells predominate and are thought to drive much of the adaptive immune-related inflammation [200,201]. Curcumin can block production of the Th1 subset by suppressing macrophage production of IL-12, while also enhancing proliferation of the Th2 subclass [297,298], characterized by a more anti-inflammatory cytokine profile. For example, in a rat model of TNBS-induced colitis, curcumin at a dose of 30 mg/kg enhanced Th2 synthesis and suppressed Th1 proliferation, leading to a less inflammatory T helper profile [298]. Curcumin may also inhibit Th17 development, important in NEC [98], reducing production of the pro-inflammatory cytokines IL-6, IL-21, and IL-17 [299].

Dysregulation or hyperstimulation of the macrophage response [300], and alterations in function (e.g., decreased phagocytic ability in premature infant macrophages) [121] are critical in intestinal inflammatory diseases. Both monocytes and monocyte-derived macrophages in NEC infants exhibit an elevated expression of TLR4, TNF-α, and IL-6 compared to age-, sex-, and weight-matched controls, as well as lower levels of TGF-β1 [2]. Curcumin has been shown to inhibit TLR4 activation [6] and enhance production of TGF-β1, particularly in areas of active inflammation [301], such as the disrupted intestinal barrier. In rat macrophages, curcumin treatment at 30 mg/kg reduces the ability of cells to generate ROS and secrete lysosomal breakdown enzymes [302,303], leading to a potential reduction in mucosal inflammation. Curcumin can also inhibit NF-κB-induced macrophage and monocyte production of IL-12, IFN-γ, iNOS, MIP-2, IL-1β, IL-8, MCP-1, MIP-1α, and TNF-α [294,297,304,305]. Inhibition of IL-12 is particularly important in the context of adaptive immune cell differentiation and further progression of intestinal inflammation. In addition, several studies have indicated treatment with curcumin enhances the phagocytic activity of macrophages [298,306–309].

Intestinal inflammatory diseases are characterized by neutrophil recruitment and activation to the site(s) of injury, an early step providing a major source of ROS [310] for further mucosal and epithelial degradation. Curcumin is known to prevent neutrophil recruitment [288,311,312], largely accomplished through downregulation of NF-κB- and PI3K-Akt-induced chemotaxis [313,314], as well as a reduction in superoxide release [304]. Curcumin also inhibits neutrophils from aggregating, degranulating, and producing superoxide radicals [315]. In both B cells and natural killer cells, curcumin has been shown to enhance activity [295,316,317] or suppress activation [294,318], depending upon the dose and context [296]. Both B cells and natural killer cells have been identified as a potential general source of inflammation in the intestine [319], particularly in the context of microbial infection [320].

In addition to the effects on specific immune cells, curcumin alters the generalized production of cytokines across the entire intestinal immune system. Curcumin inhibits production of TNF-α [321], IFN-γ [322], IL-1 [323], IL-2 [294], IL-6 [290], and IL-8 [269], while elevating that of IL-10 [324] and TGF-β [325]. For instance, in both rat methotrexate-colitis and LPS-treated IEC-6 models, curcumin decreases levels of TNF-α and IL-1β, as well as increases levels of the anti-inflammatory cytokine, IL-10 [324]. In HT29 IECs, in vitro treatment with curcumin inhibited TNF-α- and IL-1β-induced IL-8 release [286]. In mice, curcumin has also been shown to suppress LPS-induced IL-12, IL-1β, IL-6, and TNF-α production [290].

Finally, COX-2, an inflammatory enzyme induced by NF-κB and AP-1 signaling, is an important mediator in prostaglandin synthesis. Levels of COX-2 are known to be upregulated in the context of intestinal inflammatory diseases [288,311]. In BV2 microglial cells, curcumin treatment abrogated COX-2 gene expression through reduction of both AP-1 and NF-κB signaling [326]. In addition to inhibiting the production of COX-2, curcumin can inhibit the receptors for COX-2 [311]. In a rat model of TNBS-induced colitis, curcumin reduced COX-2 expression, as well as the expression of several inflammatory cytokines, but increased levels of prostaglandin E_2 (PGE_2) [311]. In human colon epithelial cells [327], as well as HT-29 colonocytes [328], COX-2 has also been shown to be blocked by curcumin, likely through inhibition of NF-κB and IKK activity. Clinical trials with curcumin treatment have been largely successful, but the mechanisms of action have not been well-studied in these trials. For example, in quiescent ulcerative colitis patients, 2 g curcumin effectively maintained remission [329]. In UC patients with mild-to-moderate disease, 3 g curcumin, in combination with the anti-inflammatory drug, mesalamine, induced remission in over 50% of the study population [330]. Both clinical trials likely depend on the anti-inflammatory effects of curcumin.

5.4. Antioxidant Effects

Curcumin is characterized by extensive antioxidant activity. Profligate oxidative stress plays a pathogenic role in intestinal inflammatory diseases [331–333], primarily through the breakdown of intact tight junctions [334–336]. Physiological levels of nitric oxide protect the intestinal mucosa [337,338], but the large amounts of NO released via iNOS, and potentially eNOS, during intestinal inflammatory disease progression can lead to tissue injury and necrosis [339,340]. Unabated generation of ROS and RNS can result in the peroxidation of membrane lipids, DNA damage, and the denaturing of cellular proteins [288]. In the intestinal mucosa, curcumin reduces levels of ROS, such as NO, superoxide anions, and malondialdehyde (MDA) [283].

During inflammatory events, iNOS produces nitric oxide in pathogenic amounts. In intestinal inflammatory diseases, chronic iNOS stimulation likely leads to the breakdown of the intestinal integrity due to this generation of RNS. In vitro experiments have demonstrated iNOS works in tandem with

COX-2 through MAPK-dependent signaling, resulting in synergistic levels of inflammation and tissue destruction. In human tissues, increased levels of NO and iNOS expression have been demonstrated in intestinal inflammatory diseases [156,341]. iNOS expression appears to be a critical step in experimental colitis models, as iNOS-deficient mice do not develop the disease [341]. iNOS production is inhibited by curcumin [300,305]. In vitro studies have demonstrated curcumin can scavenge excess NO effectively [342,343], and in rat colitis models, curcumin can downregulate iNOS expression and decrease tissue levels of nitrite [288,321,344]. Finally, in a mouse model of TNBS-colitis, curcumin inhibits production of iNOS and peroxidation of lipids via reducing the Th1 cytokine response, leading to diminished tissue damage [283].

Myeloperoxidase (MPO), a component of monocyte and neutrophil granules, produces high levels of ROS. MPO is often used clinically as a marker of neutrophil infiltration into the intestinal mucosa [345]. Curcumin has been shown to decrease intestinal inflammatory disease-associated MPO activity in animal models of colitis, thereby limiting oxidative tissue damage [288,298,311]. For example, in an immune-mediated model of mouse colitis, Mouzaoui et al. [321] demonstrated curcumin is capable of reducing neutrophil intestinal infiltration, thereby reducing MPO activity, as well as returning NO levels to baseline via inhibition of iNOS and reduced inflammatory cell infiltration. In a rat model of TNBS-colitis, treatment with curcumin significantly reduced activity of MPO [6]. Additionally, in a rat methotrexate-colitis model, curcumin decreased intestinal MPO and increased levels of free radical-scavenging superoxide dismutase (SOD) [324]. These effects appeared to occur via a mitogen-activated protein kinase phosphatase 1 (MKP1)-induced reduction in p38 phosphorylation, as well as inhibition of IκB cytoplasmic degradation [324].

Matrix metalloproteinases (MMPs) are enzymes required in the degradation of the extracellular matrix. MMPs are upregulated in intestinal inflammatory diseases largely due to pro-inflammatory cytokine production. Research in humans suffering from IBD has established the intestinal epithelium overexpresses levels of MMP1, MMP3, MMP7, MMP9, MMP10, and MMP12 [346]. Infiltrating leukocytes and vascular endothelial cells were determined to be the source of MMP7 and MMP13 [347], while macrophages produced MMP8, MMP9, and MMP10 [348]. Neutrophils were largely responsible for MMP9 [348,349]. Matrix metalloproteinases have not been well studied in NEC; however, MMP3 is known to be upregulated in the disease [143]. Curcumin is known to inhibit the large majority of these matrix metalloproteinases, though their inhibition has not been extensively investigated in the context of intestinal inflammatory diseases. For example, in human umbilical vein endothelial cells (HUVEC), curcumin inhibits the expression of MMP9 [350], while, in cartilage explants, curcumin reduces MMP3 [351]. In human fibroblasts, curcumin downregulates MMP1 and MMP3 expression through a MAPK-dependent pathway [352], and in HT29 cells, curcumin reduced production of MMP7 [353].

Finally, curcumin can upregulate phase II enzymes related to the metabolism and detoxification of xenobiotics [354], as well as additional antioxidant proteins, such as nuclear factor (erythroid-derived 2)-related factor (Nrf2) [354], a transcription factor functioning as a master regulator of antioxidant proteins, and heme oxygenase-1 (HO-1) [355,356], a redox-sensitive, stress-induced protein capable of degrading heme to iron, biliverdin, and carbon monoxide (CO) [357]. In an in vitro model of rat hepatic stellate cells, Liu et al. [358] showed curcumin upregulates the nuclear translocation of Nrf2, thereby protecting the cells from oxidative stress. HO-1 can be induced by a variety of ROS, including H_2O_2. In a Caco-2 model of the intestinal epithelium, Wang et al. [359] indicated curcumin reduced the oxidative stress and cytotoxicity induced by H_2O_2 production. Additionally, curcumin was protective against H_2O_2-induced tight junction disruption, and its associated increase in paracellular permeability [359].

6. Conclusions

In this review, we discussed the potential protective effects of curcumin on intestinal inflammatory diseases. IBD and NEC are characterized by hyperstimulation of the immune system to luminal bacteria and dietary antigens, resulting in rampant intestinal inflammation. This inflammation impairs the functioning of the intestinal barrier, allowing for increased bacterial translocation, systemic inflammation, and in very severe cases, sepsis. Recent research has focused on the effects of natural anti-inflammatories, such as curcumin, on intestinal inflammatory diseases, largely due to their safety profile and affordability. Curcumin is characterized by beneficial effects on the microbiome, antimicrobial properties, inhibition of TLR4/NF-κB/AP-1 signal transduction, changes in cytokine profiles, and alterations to immune cell maturation and differentiation. The culmination of the vast number of effects of curcumin on the intestinal epithelium and immune system is to strengthen the intestinal barrier through a reduction in bacterial translocation and inflammation. While curcumin looks promising in the treatment of intestinal inflammatory diseases, further controlled clinical trials are needed.

Author Contributions: Conceptualization, K.B., A.G., J.E., H.C.; writing—original draft preparation, K.B.; writing—review and editing, K.B., A.G., J.E., H.C.; visualization, A.G.; supervision, H.C.; funding acquisition, H.C.

Funding: This research received funding from NIH (K08GM127308), provided to Hala Chaaban.

Acknowledgments: The authors acknowledge support from the Division of Neonatology at the University of Oklahoma Health Sciences Center (OUHSC) and K08GM127308 National Institute of General Medical Sciences (H.C.).

Conflicts of Interest: The authors declare no conflict of interest.

Abbreviations

AIEC	adherent invasive *E. coli*
AMP	antimicrobial protein
APC	antigen-presenting cell
AP-1	activator protein 1
ATF-2	activating transcription factor 2
CD	Crohn's disease
CO	carbon monoxide
COX-2	cyclooxygenase-2
CREB	ATF/cyclic AMP-response element-binding
DC	dendritic cell
eNOS	endothelial nitric oxide synthase
ELK-2	ETS domain-containing protein 2
ERK	extracellular signal-regulated kinases
FITC	fluorescein isothiocyanate
GRO-α	growth-regulated oncogene-alpha
H&E	hematoxylin and eosin
HO-1	heme oxygenase-1
HUVEC	human umbilical vein endothelial cells
IBD	inflammatory bowel disease
ICAM	intercellular adhesion molecule
IDO	indoleamine 2,3-dioxygenase
IEC	intestinal epithelial cell
IEL	intraepithelial lymphocyte
IFN-γ	interferon-gamma
IKK	IκB kinase
IL	interleukin
ILC	innate lymphoid cell
IL-1Ra	IL-1 receptor antagonist
iNOS	inducible nitric oxide synthase
IRAK-M	interleukin-1 receptor-associated kinase-M
JNK	jun N-terminal kinases
LFA	lymphocyte function-associated antigen
LPS	lipopolysaccharide

M	microfold
Mac-1	macrophage 1 antigen
MAPK	mitogen-activated protein kinase
MCP	monocyte chemoattractant protein
MD	myeloid differentiation protein
MDA	malondialdehyde
MDPI	Multidisciplinary Digital Publishing Institute
MHC	major histocompatibility class
MIP	macrophage inflammatory protein
MKP-1	mitogen-activated protein kinase phosphatase 1
MMP	matrix metalloproteinase
MPO	myeloperoxidase
mTOR	mammalian target of rapamycin
MyD88	myeloid differentiation factor 88
MUC	mucin
NEC	necrotizing enterocolitis
NEMO	NF-κB essential modulator
NF-κB	nuclear factor-kappaB
NO	nitric oxide
Nrf2	nuclear factor (erythroid-derived 2)-related factor
ns	not significant
Nur-77	nerve growth factor 1B
PAF	platelet-activating factor
PGE_2	prostaglandin E_2
PRR	pattern-recognition receptor
RA	retinoic acid
RIP	receptor-interacting protein
RNS	reactive nitrogen species
ROS	reactive oxygen species
SARM	selective androgen receptor modulator
SCFA	short chain fatty acid
SEM	standard error of mean
SHIP	inositol polyphosphate 5'-phosphatase D
SMAD7	mothers against decapentaplegic homolog 7
SOD	superoxide dismutase
TAB	TAK1-binding
TAK	transforming growth factor-beta-activated kinase
TBK	TANK-binding kinase
TEER	transepithelial electrical resistance
TGF-β	transforming growth factor-beta
Th	T helper
TIMP	tissue inhibitor of metalloproteinase
TIRAP	toll/interleukin-1 receptor domain-containing adaptor protein
TLR	toll-like receptor
TNBS	trinitrobenzene sulfonic acid
TNF-α	tumor necrosis factor-alpha
TRAF	TNF receptor-associated factor
TRAM	translocation associated membrane
Treg	regulatory T cell
TRIF	TIR-domain-containing adaptor protein inducing interferon-β
TSLP	thymic stromal lymphopoietin
UC	ulcerative colitis
VCAM	vascular cell adhesion molecule
VEGF-C	vascular endothelial growth factor-C
VLA	very late antigen

References

1. Cho, S.X.; Berger, P.J.; Nold-Petry, C.A.; Nold, M.F. The immunological landscape in necrotising enterocolitis. *Expert Rev. Mol. Med.* **2016**, *18*, e12. [CrossRef] [PubMed]
2. Pang, Y.; Du, X.; Xu, X.; Wang, M.; Li, Z. Monocyte activation and inflammation can exacerbate Treg/Th17 imbalance in infants with neonatal necrotizing enterocolitis. *Int. Immunopharmacol.* **2018**, *59*, 354–360. [CrossRef]
3. Dias, A.M.; Correia, A.; Pereira, M.S.; Almeida, C.R.; Alves, I.; Pinto, V.; Catarino, T.A.; Mendes, N.; Leander, M.; Oliva-Teles, M.T.; et al. Metabolic control of T cell immune response through glycans in inflammatory bowel disease. *Proc. Natl. Acad. Sci. USA* **2018**, *115*, E4651–E4660. [CrossRef] [PubMed]
4. Lu, Y.; Li, X.; Liu, S.; Zhang, Y.; Zhang, D. Toll-like receptors and inflammatory bowel disease. *Front. Immunol.* **2018**, *9*, 72. [CrossRef] [PubMed]
5. Pallone, F.; Monteleone, G. Mechanisms of tissue damage in inflammatory bowel disease. *Curr. Opin. Gastroenterol.* **2001**, *17*, 307–312. [CrossRef] [PubMed]
6. Lubbad, A.; Oriowo, M.A.; Khan, I. Curcumin attenuates inflammation through inhibition of TLR-4 receptor in experimental colitis. *Mol. Cell. Biochem.* **2009**, *322*, 127–135. [CrossRef]
7. Bischoff, S.C.; Barbara, G.; Buurman, W.; Ockhuizen, T.; Schulzke, J.-D.; Serino, M.; Tilg, H.; Watson, A.; Wells, J.M. Intestinal permeability—A new target for disease prevention and therapy. *BMC Gastroenterol.* **2014**, *14*, 189. [CrossRef]
8. Wang, J.; Ghosh, S.S.; Ghosh, S. Curcumin improves intestinal barrier function: Modulation of intracellular signaling, and organization of tight junctions. *Am. J. Physiol. Cell Physiol.* **2017**, *312*, C438–C445. [CrossRef]
9. Santaolalla, R.; Fukata, M.; Abreu, M.T. Innate immunity in the small intestine. *Curr. Opin. Gastroenterol.* **2011**, *27*, 125–131. [CrossRef]
10. Mara, M.A.; Good, M.; Weitkamp, J.-H. Innate and adaptive immunity in necrotizing enterocolitis. *Semin. Fetal Neonatal Med.* **2018**, *23*, 394–399. [CrossRef] [PubMed]
11. Peterson, L.W.; Artis, D. Intestinal epithelial cells: Regulators of barrier function and immune homeostasis. *Nat. Rev. Immunol.* **2014**, *14*, 141–153. [CrossRef] [PubMed]
12. Murai, M.; Turovskaya, O.; Kim, G.; Madan, R.; Karp, C.L.; Cheroutre, H.; Kronenberg, M. Interleukin 10 acts on regulatory T cells to maintain expression of the transcription factor Foxp3 and suppressive function in mice with colitis. *Nat. Immunol.* **2009**, *10*, 1178–1184. [CrossRef] [PubMed]
13. Krappmann, D.; Wegener, E.; Sunami, Y.; Esen, M.; Thiel, A.; Mordmuller, B.; Scheidereit, C. The IκB kinase complex and NF-κB act as master regulators of lipopolysaccharide-induced gene expression and control subordinate activation of AP-1. *Mol. Cell. Biol.* **2004**, *24*, 6488–6500. [CrossRef] [PubMed]
14. Le Mandat Schultz, A.; Bonnard, A.; Barreau, F.; Aigrain, Y.; Pierre-Louis, C.; Berrebi, D.; Peuchmaur, M. Expression of TLR-2, TLR-4, NOD2 and pNF-kappaB in a neonatal rat model of necrotizing enterocolitis. *PLoS ONE* **2007**, *2*, e1102. [CrossRef]
15. Swanson, P.A., 2nd; Kumar, A.; Samarin, S.; Vijay-Kumar, M.; Kundu, K.; Murthy, N.; Hansen, J.; Nusrat, A.; Neish, A.S. Enteric commensal bacteria potentiate epithelial restitution via reactive oxygen species-mediated inactivation of focal adhesion kinase phosphatases. *Proc. Natl. Acad. Sci. USA* **2011**, *108*, 8803–8808. [CrossRef] [PubMed]
16. Dowling, D.J.; Levy, O. Ontogeny of early life immunity. *Trends Immunol.* **2014**, *35*, 299–310. [CrossRef] [PubMed]
17. Brandtzaeg, P. The gut as communicator between environment and host: Immunological consequences. *Eur. J. Pharmacol.* **2011**, *668* (Suppl. 1), S16–S32. [CrossRef] [PubMed]
18. Hering, N.A.; Fromm, M.; Schulzke, J.D. Determinants of colonic barrier function in inflammatory bowel disease and potential therapeutics. *J. Physiol.* **2012**, *590*, 1035–1044. [CrossRef]
19. Neu, J.; Pammi, M. Pathogenesis of NEC: Impact of an altered intestinal microbiome. *Semin. Perinatol.* **2017**, *41*, 29–35. [CrossRef]
20. Afrazi, A.; Sodhi, C.P.; Richardson, W.; Neal, M.; Good, M.; Siggers, R.; Hackam, D.J. New insights into the pathogenesis and treatment of necrotizing enterocolitis: Toll-like receptors and beyond. *Pediatr. Res.* **2011**, *69*, 183–188. [CrossRef]
21. Musemeche, C.A.; Kosloske, A.M.; Bartow, S.A.; Umland, E.T. Comparative effects of ischemia, bacteria, and substrate on the pathogenesis of intestinal necrosis. *J. Pediatr. Surg.* **1986**, *21*, 536–538. [CrossRef]

22. Carlisle, E.M.; Morowitz, M.J. The intestinal microbiome and necrotizing enterocolitis. *Curr. Opin. Pediatr.* **2013**, *25*, 382–387. [CrossRef] [PubMed]
23. Wang, Y.; Hoenig, J.D.; Malin, K.J.; Qamar, S.; Petrof, E.O.; Sun, J.; Antonopoulos, D.A.; Chang, E.B.; Claud, E.C. 16S rRNA gene-based analysis of fecal microbiota from preterm infants with and without necrotizing enterocolitis. *ISME J.* **2009**, *3*, 944–954. [CrossRef] [PubMed]
24. Warner, B.B.; Deych, E.; Zhou, Y.; Hall-Moore, C.; Weinstock, G.M.; Sodergren, E.; Shaikh, N.; Hoffmann, J.A.; Linneman, L.A.; Hamvas, A.; et al. Gut bacteria dysbiosis and necrotising enterocolitis in very low birthweight infants: A prospective case-control study. *Lancet* **2016**, *387*, 1928–1936. [CrossRef]
25. Neu, J.; Walker, W.A. Necrotizing enterocolitis. *N. Engl. J. Med.* **2011**, *364*, 255–264. [CrossRef] [PubMed]
26. Pammi, M.; Cope, J.; Tarr, P.I.; Warner, B.B.; Morrow, A.L.; Mai, V.; Gregory, K.E.; Kroll, J.S.; McMurty, V.; Ferris, M.J.; et al. Intestinal dysbiosis in preterm infants preceding necrotizing enterocolitis: A systematic review and meta-analysis. *Microbiome* **2017**, *5*, 31. [CrossRef] [PubMed]
27. Cotton, C.M.; Taylor, S.; Stoll, B.; Goldberg, R.N.; Hansen, N.I.; Sanchez, P.J.; Ambalavanan, N.; Benjamin, D.K., Jr.; NICHD Neonatal Research Network. Prolonged duration of initial empirical antibiotic treatment is associated with increased rates of necrotizing enterocolitis and death for extremely low birth weight infants. *Pediatrics* **2009**, *123*, 58–66. [CrossRef] [PubMed]
28. Alexander, V.N.; Northrup, V.; Bizzarro, M.J. Antibiotic exposure in the newborn intestive care unit and the risk of necrotizing enterocolitis. *J. Pediatr.* **2011**, *159*, 392–397. [CrossRef]
29. Heida, F.H.; van Zoonen, A.G.J.F.; Hulscher, J.B.F.; Te Kiefte, B.J.C.; Wessels, R.; Kooi, E.M.W.; Bos, A.F.; Harmsen, H.J.M.; de Goffau, M.C. A necrotizing enterocolitis-associated gut microbiota is present in the meconium: Results of a prospective study. *Clin. Infect. Dis.* **2016**, *62*, 863–870. [CrossRef]
30. Terrin, G.; Passariello, A.; De Curtis, M.; Manguso, F.; Salvia, G.; Lega, L.; Messina, F.; Paludetto, R.; Canani, R.B. Ranatidine is associated with infections, necrotizing enterocolitis, and fatal outcome in newborns. *Pediatrics* **2012**, *129*, e40–e45. [CrossRef]
31. Bilali, A.; Galanis, P.; Bartsocas, C.; Sparos, L.; Velonakis, E. H2-blocker therapy and incidence of necrotizing enterocolitis in preterm infants: A case-control study. *Pediatr. Neonatol.* **2013**, *54*, 141–142. [CrossRef]
32. Zivkovic, A.M.; German, J.B.; Lebrilla, C.B.; Mills, D.A. Human milk glycobiome and its impact on the infant gastrointestinal microbiota. *Proc. Natl. Acad. Sci. USA* **2011**, *108* (Suppl. 1), 4653–4658. [CrossRef]
33. Good, M.; Sodhi, C.P.; Hackam, D.J. Evidence-based feeding strategies before and after the development of necrotizing enterocolitis. *Expert Rev. Clin. Immunol.* **2014**, *10*, 875–884. [CrossRef]
34. Sela, D.A. Bifidobacterial utilization of human milk oligosaccharides. *Int. J. Food Microbiol.* **2011**, *149*, 58–64. [CrossRef]
35. Niemarkt, H.J.; De Meij, T.G.; van Ganzewinkel, C.-J.; de Boer, N.K.H.; Andriessen, P.; Hutten, M.C.; Kramer, B.W. Necrotizing enterocolitis, gut microbiota, and brain development: Role of the brain-gut axis. *Neonatology* **2019**, *115*, 423–431. [CrossRef]
36. Byndloss, M.X.; Olsan, E.E.; Rivera-Chavez, F.; Tiffany, C.R.; Cevallos, S.A.; Lokken, K.L.; Torres, T.P.; Byndloss, A.J.; Faber, F.; Gao, Y.; et al. Microbiota-activated PPAR-γ signaling inhibits dysbiotic Enterobacteriaceae expansion. *Science* **2017**, *357*, 570–575. [CrossRef]
37. Ge, X.; Pan, J.; Liu, Y.; Wang, H.; Zhou, W.; Wang, X. Intestinal crosstalk between microbiota and serotonin and its impact on gut motility. *Curr. Pharm. Biotechnol.* **2018**, *19*, 190–195. [CrossRef]
38. Aleksandrova, K.; Romero-Mosquera, B.; Hernandez, V. Diet, gut microbiome and epigenetics: Emerging links with inflammatory bowel diseases and prospects for management and prevention. *Nutrients* **2017**, *9*, 962. [CrossRef]
39. Kostic, A.D.; Xavier, R.J.; Gevers, D. The microbiome in inflammatory bowel disease: Current status and the future ahead. *Gastroenterology* **2014**, *146*, 1489–1499. [CrossRef]
40. Prosberg, M.; Bendtsen, F.; Vind, I.; Petersen, A.M.; Gluud, L.L. The association between the gut microbiota and the inflammatory bowel disease activity: A systematic review and meta-analysis. *Scand. J. Gastroenterol.* **2016**, *51*, 1407–1415. [CrossRef]
41. Wills, E.S.; Jonkers, D.M.A.E.; Savelkoul, P.H.; Masclee, A.A.; Pierik, M.J.; Penders, J. Fecal microbial composition of ulcerative colitis and Crohn's disease patients in remission and subsequent exacerbation. *PLoS ONE* **2014**, *9*, e90981. [CrossRef]
42. Malavia, D.; Crawford, A.; Wilson, D. Nutritional immunity and fungal pathogenesis: The struggle for micronutrients and the host-pathogen interface. *Adv. Microb. Phys.* **2017**, *70*, 85–103. [CrossRef]

43. Macia, L.; Tan, J.; Vieira, A.T.; Leach, K.; Stanley, D.; Luong, S.; Maruya, M.; Ian McKenzie, C.; Hijikata, A.; Wong, C.; et al. Metabolite-sensing receptors GPR43 and GPR109A facilitate dietary fibre-induced gut homeostasis through regulation of the inflammasome. *Nat. Commun.* **2015**, *6*, 6734. [CrossRef]
44. Koh, A.; De Vadder, F.; Kovatcheva-Datchary, P.; Backhed, F. From dietary fiber to host physiology: Short-chain fatty acids as key bacterial metabolites. *Cell* **2016**, *165*, 1332–1345. [CrossRef]
45. Atarashi, K.; Tanoue, T.; Oshima, K.; Suda, W.; Nagano, Y.; Nishikawa, H.; Fukuda, S.; Saito, T.; Narushima, S.; Hase, K.; et al. Treg induction by a rationally selected mixture of Clostridia stains from the human microbiota. *Nature* **2013**, *500*, 232–236. [CrossRef]
46. Gao, Y.; Huang, Y.; Zhao, Y.; Hu, Y.; Li, Z.; Guo, Q.; Zhao, K.; Lu, N. LL202 protects against dextran sulfate sodium-induced experimental colitis in mice by inhibiting MAPK/AP-1 signaling. *Oncotarget* **2016**, *7*, 63981–63994. [CrossRef]
47. Grishin, A.V.; Wang, J.; Potoka, D.A.; Hackam, D.J.; Upperman, J.S.; Boyle, P.; Zamora, R.; Ford, H.R. Lipopolysaccharide induces cyclooxygenase-2 in intestinal epithelium via a noncanonical p38 MAPK pathway. *J. Immunol.* **2006**, *176*, 580–588. [CrossRef]
48. Nanthakumar, N.N.; Young, C.; Ko, J.S.; Meng, D.; Chen, J.; Buie, T.; Walker, W.A. Glucocorticoid responsiveness in developing human intestine: Possible role in prevention of necrotizing enterocolitis. *Am. J. Physiol. Gastrointest. Liver Physiol.* **2005**, *288*, G85–G92. [CrossRef]
49. Liu, T.; Zhang, L.; Joo, D.; Sun, S.-C. NF-κB signaling in inflammation. *Signal Transduct. Target Ther.* **2017**, *2*, e17023. [CrossRef]
50. Baldwin, A.S. The NF-KB and I-KB proteins: New discoveries and insights. *Annu. Rev. Immunol.* **1996**, *14*, 649–681. [CrossRef]
51. Schreiber, S.; Nikolaus, S.; Hampe, J. Activation of nuclear factor κB in inflammatory bowel disease. *Gut* **1998**, *42*, 477–484. [CrossRef]
52. De Plaen, I.G.; Liu, S.X.; Tian, R.; Neequaye, I.; May, M.J.; Han, X.B.; Hsueh, W.; Jilling, T.; Lu, J.; Caplan, M.S. Inhibition of nuclear factor-kappaB ameliorates bowel injury and prolongs survival in a neonatal rat model of necrotizing enterocolitis. *Pediatr. Res.* **2007**, *62*, 716–721. [CrossRef]
53. Atreya, I.; Atreya, R.; Neurath, M.F. NF-κB in inflammatory bowel disease. *J. Intern. Med.* **2008**, *263*, 591–596. [CrossRef] [PubMed]
54. Brown, K.; Gerstberger, S.; Carlson, L.; Franzoso, G.; Siebenlist, U. Control of IκB-α proteolysis by site-specific signal induced phosphorylation. *Science* **1995**, *267*, 1485–1487. [CrossRef]
55. Siebenlist, U.; Brown, K.; Claudio, E. Control of lymphocyte development by nuclear factor-κB. *Nat. Rev. Immunol.* **2005**, *5*, 435–445. [CrossRef]
56. Afonina, I.S.; Zhong, Z.; Karin, M.; Beyaert, R. Limiting inflammation—the negative regulation of NF_κB and NLRP3 inflammasome. *Nat. Immunol.* **2017**, *18*, 861–869. [CrossRef]
57. Abreu, M.T. Toll-like receptor signaling in the intestinal epithelium: How bacterial recognition shapes intestinal function. *Nat. Rev. Immunol.* **2010**, *10*, 131–144. [CrossRef]
58. Wullaert, A.; Bonnet, M.C.; Pasparakis, M. NF-κB in the regulation of epithelial homeostasis and inflammation. *Cell Res.* **2011**, *21*, 146–158. [CrossRef]
59. Nenci, A.; Becker, C.; Wullaert, A.; Gareus, R.; van Loo, G.; Danese, S.; Huth, M.; Nikolaev, A.; Neufert, C.; Madison, B.; et al. Epithelial NEMO links innate immunity to chronic intestinal inflammation. *Nature* **2007**, *446*, 557–561. [CrossRef]
60. Zaph, C.; Troy, A.E.; Taylor, B.C.; Berman-Booty, L.D.; Guild, K.J.; Du, Y.; Yost, E.A.; Gruber, A.D.; May, M.J.; Greten, F.R.; et al. Epithelial-cell-intrinsic IKK-beta expression regulates intestinal immune homeostasis. *Nature* **2007**, *446*, 552–556. [CrossRef]
61. Guha, M.; Mackman, N. LPS induction of gene expression in human monocytes. *Cell. Signal.* **2001**, *13*, 85–94. [CrossRef]
62. Granet, C.; Miossec, P. Combination of the pro-inflammatory cytokines IL-1, TNF-alpha and IL-17 leads to enhanced expression and additional recruitment of AP-1 family members, Egr-1 and NF-κB in osteoblast-like cells. *Cytokine* **2004**, *26*, 169–177. [CrossRef]
63. Dokter, W.H.A.; Koopmans, S.B.; Vellenga, E. Effects of IL-10 and IL-4 on LPS-induced transcription factors (AP-1, NF-IL6 and NF-kappaB) which are involved in IL-6 regulation. *Leukemia* **1996**, *10*, 1038–1316.
64. Eferl, R.; Wagner, E.F. AP-1: A double-edged sword in tumorigenesis. *Nat. Rev. Cancer* **2003**, *3*, 859–868. [CrossRef]

65. Karin, M.; Takahashi, T.; Kapahi, P.; Delhase, M.; Chen, Y.; Makris, C.; Rothwarf, D.; Baud, V.; Natoli, G.; Guido, F.; et al. Oxidative stress and gene expression: The AP-1 and NF-κB connections. *Biofactors* **2001**, *15*, 87–89. [CrossRef]
66. Verma, I.M.; Stevenson, J.K.; Schwarz, E.M.; Van Antwerp, D.; Miyamoto, S. Rel/NF-kappa B/I kappa B family: Intimate tales of association and dissociation. *Genes Dev.* **1995**, *9*, 2723–2735. [CrossRef]
67. Fujioka, S.; Niu, J.; Schmidt, C.; Sclabas, G.M.; Peng, B.; Uwagawa, T.; Li, Z.; Evans, D.B.; Abbruzzese, J.L.; Chiao, P.J. NF-κB and AP-1 connection: Mechanism of NF-κB-dependent regulation of AP-1 activity. *Mol. Cell Biol.* **2004**, *24*, 7806–7819. [CrossRef]
68. Angel, P.; Karin, M. The role of Jun, Fos and the AP-1 complex in cell-proliferation and transformation. *Biochim. Biophys. Acta* **1991**, *1072*, 129–157. [CrossRef]
69. Chang, L.; Karin, M. Mammalian MAP kinase signalling cascades. *Nature* **2001**, *410*, 37–40. [CrossRef] [PubMed]
70. Johnson, G.L.; Lapadat, R. Mitogen-activated protein kinase pathways mediated by ERK, JNK, and p38 protein kinases. *Science* **2002**, *298*, 1911–1912. [CrossRef]
71. Gazon, H.; Barbeau, B.; Mesnard, J.-M.; Peloponese, J.-M., Jr. Hijacking of the AP-1 signaling pathway during development of ATL. *Front. Microbiol.* **2018**, *8*, 2686. [CrossRef] [PubMed]
72. Chen, Y.; Currie, R.W. Small interfering RNA knocks down heat shock factor-1 (HSF-1) and exacerbates pro-inflammatory activation of NF-kappa B and AP-1 in vascular smooth muscle cells. *Cardiovasc. Res.* **2006**, *69*, 66–75. [CrossRef] [PubMed]
73. Riesenberg, S.; Groetchen, A.; Siddaway, R.; Bald, T.; Reinhardt, J.; Smorra, D.; Kohlmeyer, J.; Renn, M.; Phung, B.; Aymans, P.; et al. MITF and c-Jun antagonism interconnects melanoma dedifferentiation with pro-inflammatory cytokine responsiveness and myeloid cell recruitment. *Nat. Commun.* **2015**, *6*, 8755. [CrossRef]
74. Tremblay, L.; Valenza, F.; Ribeiro, S.P.; Li, J.F.; Slutsky, A.S. Injurious ventilatory strategies increase cytokines and c-fos m-RNA expression in an isolated rat lung model. *J. Clin. Investig.* **1997**, *99*, 944–952. [CrossRef]
75. Roy, A.; Srivastava, M.; Saqib, U.; Liu, D.; Faisal, S.M.; Sugathan, S.; Bishnoi, S.; Baig, M.S. Potential therapeutic targets for inflammation in toll-like receptor 4 (TLR4)-mediated signaling pathways. *Int. Immunopharmacol.* **2016**, *40*, 79–89. [CrossRef] [PubMed]
76. Fanjul-Fernández, M.; Folgueras, A.R.; Cabrera, S.; López-Otín, C. Matrix metalloproteinases: Evolution, gene regulation and functional analysis in mouse models. *Cell Res.* **2010**, *1803*, 3–19. [CrossRef] [PubMed]
77. Mishra, R.K.; Potteti, H.R.; Tamatam, C.R.; Elangovan, I.; Reddy, S.P. c-Jun is required for nuclear factor-κB-dependent, LPS-stimulated Fos-related Antigen-1 transcription in alveolar macrophages. *Am. J. Respir. Cell Mol. Biol.* **2016**, *55*, 667–674. [CrossRef] [PubMed]
78. Cahill, C.M.; Zhu, W.; Oziolor, E.; Yang, Y.-J.; Tam, B.; Rajanala, S.; Rogers, J.T.; Walker, W.A. Differential expression of the activator protein 1 transcription factor regulates interleukin-1β induction of interleukin 6 in the developing enterocyte. *PLoS ONE* **2016**, *11*, e0145184. [CrossRef]
79. Kwon, D.-J.; Ju, S.M.; Youn, G.S.; Choi, S.Y.; Park, J. Suppression of iNOS and COX-2 expression by flavokawain A via blockade of NF-κB and AP-1 activation in RAW 264.7 macrophages. *Food Chem. Toxicol.* **2013**, *58*, 479–486. [CrossRef]
80. Nepelska, M.; Cultrone, A.; Béguet-Crespel, F.; Le Roux, K.; Doré, J.; Arulampalam, V.; Blottière, H.M. Butyrate produced by commensal bacteria potentiates phorbol esters induced AP-1 response in human intestinal epithelial cells. *PLoS ONE* **2012**, *7*, e52869. [CrossRef]
81. Wang, P.-Y.; Wang, S.R.; Xiao, L.; Chen, J.; Wang, J.-Y.; Rao, J.N. c-Jun enhances intestinal epithelial restitution after wounding by increasing phospholipase C-γ1 transcription. *Am. J. Physiol. Cell Physiol.* **2017**, *312*, C367–C375. [CrossRef] [PubMed]
82. Ishiguro, Y.; Yamagata, K.; Sakuraba, H.; Munakata, A.; Nakane, A.; Morita, T.; Nishihira, J. Macrophage migration inhibitory factor and activator protein-1 in ulcerative colitis. *Ann. N. Y. Acad. Sci.* **2006**, *1029*, 348–349. [CrossRef]
83. Zingarelli, B.; Yang, Z.; Hake, P.W.; Denenberg, A.; Wong, H.R. Absence of endogenous interleukin-10 enhances early stress response during postischemic injury in mice intestine. *Gut* **2001**, *5*, 610–622. [CrossRef]
84. Nicolaou, F.; Teodoridis, J.M.; Park, H.; Georgakis, A.; Farokhzad, O.C.; Böttinger, E.P.; Da Silva, N.; Rousselot, P.; Chomienne, C.; Ferenczi, K.; et al. CD11c gene expression in hairy cell leukemia is dependent upon activation of the proto-oncogenes ras and junD. *Blood* **2003**, *101*, 4033–4041. [CrossRef]

85. Moriyama, I.; Ishihara, S.; Rumi, M.A.; Aziz, M.D.; Mishima, Y.; Oshima, N.; Kadota, C.; Kadowaki, Y.; Amano, Y.; Kinoshita, Y. Decoy oligodeoxynucleotide targeting activator protein-1 (AP-1) attenuates intestinal inflammation in murine experimental colitis. *Lab. Investig.* **2008**, *88*, 652–663. [CrossRef] [PubMed]
86. Boone, D.L.; Ma, A. Connecting the dots from Toll-like receptors to innate immune cells and inflammatory bowel disease. *J. Clin. Investig.* **2003**, *111*, 1284–1286. [CrossRef] [PubMed]
87. Sodhi, C.P.; Neal, M.D.; Siggers, R.; Sho, S.; Ma, C.; Branca, M.F.; Prindle, T., Jr.; Russo, A.M.; Afrazi, A.; Good, M.; et al. Intestinal epithelial Toll-like receptor 4 regulates goblet cell development and is required for necrotizing enterocolitis in mice. *Gastroenterology* **2012**, *143*, 708–718. [CrossRef]
88. Youn, H.S.; Saitoh, S.I.; Miyake, K.; Hwang, D.H. Inhibition of homodimerization of Toll-like receptor 4 by curcumin. *Biochem. Pharmacol.* **2006**, *72*, 62–69. [CrossRef]
89. Park, H.H.; Lo, Y.C.; Lin, S.C.; Wang, L.; Yang, J.K.; Wu, H. The death domain superfamily in intracellular signaling of apoptosis and inflammation. *Annu. Rev. Immunol.* **2007**, *25*, 561–586. [CrossRef]
90. Zhang, Y.; Lu, Y.; Ma, L.; Cao, X.; Xiao, J.; Chen, J.; Jiao, S.; Gao, Y.; Liu, C.; Duan, Z.; et al. Activation of vascular endothelial growth factor receptor-3 in macrophages restrains TLR4-NF-κB signaling and protects against endotoxin shock. *Immunity* **2014**, *40*, 501–514. [CrossRef]
91. Li, L.; Liu, Y.; Chen, H.Z.; Li, F.W.; Wu, J.F.; Zhang, H.K.; He, J.P.; Xing, Y.Z.; Chen, Y.; Wang, W.J.; et al. Impeding the interaction between Nur77 and p38 reduces LPS-induced inflammation. *Nat. Chem. Biol.* **2015**, *11*, 339–346. [CrossRef] [PubMed]
92. Gohda, J.; Matsumura, T.; Inoue, J. Cutting edge: TNFR-associated factor (TRAF) 6 is essential for MyD88-dependent pathway but not toll/IL-1 receptor domain-containing adaptor-inducing IFN-beta (TRIF)-dependent pathway in TLR signaling. *J. Immunol.* **2004**, *173*, 2913–2917. [CrossRef] [PubMed]
93. Neu, J. Gastrointestinal development and meeting the nutritional needs to premature infants. *Am. J. Clin. Nutr.* **2007**, *85*, 629S–634S. [CrossRef]
94. Papillon, S.; Castle, S.L.; Gayer, C.P.; Ford, H.R. Necrotizing enterocolitis: Contemporary management and outcomes. *Adv. Pediatr.* **2013**, *60*, 263–279. [CrossRef] [PubMed]
95. Niño, D.F.; Sodhi, C.P.; Hackam, D.J. Necrotizing enterocolitis: New insights into pathogenesis and mechanisms. *Nat. Rev. Gastroenterol. Hepatol.* **2016**, *13*, 590–600. [CrossRef] [PubMed]
96. Battersby, A.J.; Gibbons, D.L. The gut mucosal immune system in the neonatal period. *Ped. Allergy Immunol.* **2013**, *24*, 414–421. [CrossRef] [PubMed]
97. Leaphart, C.L.; Cavallo, J.C.; Gribar, S.C.; Cetin, S.; Li, J.; Branca, M.F.; Dubowski, T.D.; Sodhi, C.P.; Hackam, D.J. A critical role for TLR4 in the pathogenesis of necrotizing enterocolitis by modulating intestinal injury and repair. *J. Immunol.* **2007**, *179*, 4808–4820. [CrossRef] [PubMed]
98. Egan, C.E.; Sodhi, C.P.; Good, M.; Lin, J.; Jia, H.; Yamaguchi, Y.; Lu, P.; Ma, C.; Branca, M.F.; Weyandt, S.; et al. Toll-like receptor 4-mediated lymphocyte influx induces neonatal necrotizing enterocolitis. *J. Clin. Investig.* **2016**, *126*, 495–508. [CrossRef]
99. Good, M.; Siggers, R.H.; Sodhi, C.P.; Afrazi, A.; Alkhudari, F.; Egan, C.E.; Neal, M.D.; Yazji, I.; Jia, H.; Lin, J.; et al. Amniotic fluid inhibits Toll-like receptor 4 signaling in the fetal and neonatal intestinal epithelium. *Proc. Natl. Acad. Sci. USA* **2012**, *109*, 11330–11335. [CrossRef]
100. Good, M.; Sodhi, C.P.; Egan, C.E.; Afrazi, A.; Jia, H.; Yamaguchi, Y.; Lu, P.; Branca, M.F.; Ma, C.; Prindle, T., Jr.; et al. Breast milk protects against the development of necrotizing enterocolitis through inhibition of Toll-like receptor 4 in the intestinal epithelium via activation of the epidermal growth factor. *Mucosal Immunol.* **2015**, *8*, 1166–1179. [CrossRef]
101. Neal, M.D.; Sodhi, C.P.; Dyer, M.; Craig, B.T.; Good, M.; Jia, H.; Yazji, I.; Afrazi, A.; Richardson, W.M.; Beer-Stolz, D.; et al. A critical role for TLR4 induction of autophagy in the regulation of enterocyte migration and the pathogenesis of necrotizing enterocolitis. *J. Immunol.* **2013**, *190*, 3541–3551. [CrossRef]
102. Good, M.; Sodhi, C.P.; Yamaguchi, Y.; Jia, H.; Lu, P.; Fulton, W.B.; Martin, L.Y.; Prindle, T.; Nino, D.F.; Zhou, Q.; et al. The human milk oligosaccharide 2′-fucosyllactose attenuates the severity of experimental necrotising enterocolitis by enhancing mesenteric perfusion in the neonatal intestine. *Br. J. Nutr.* **2016**, *116*, 1175–1187. [CrossRef] [PubMed]
103. Toiyama, Y.; Araki, T.; Yoshiyama, S.; Hiro, J.; Miki, C.; Kusonoki, M. The expression patterns of toll-like receptors in the ileal pouch mucosa of postoperative ulcerative colitis patients. *Surg. Today* **2006**, *36*, 287–290. [CrossRef]

104. Lu, P.; Sodhi, C.P.; Hackam, D.J. Toll-like receptor regulation of intestinal development and inflammation in the pathogenesis of necrotizing enterocolitis. *Pathophysiology* **2014**, *21*, 81–93. [CrossRef]
105. Nanthakumar, N.N.; Meng, D.; Goldstein, A.M.; Zhu, W.; Lu, L.; Uauy, R.; Llanos, A.; Claud, E.C.; Walker, W.A. The mechanism of excessive intestinal inflammation in necrotizing enterocolitis: An immature innate immune response. *PLoS ONE* **2011**, *6*, e17776. [CrossRef]
106. Fusunyan, R.D.; Nanthakumar, N.N.; Baldeon, M.E.; Walker, W.A. Evidence for an innate immune response in the immature human intestine: Toll-like receptors on fetal enterocytes. *Pediatr. Res.* **2001**, *49*, 589–593. [CrossRef] [PubMed]
107. Managlia, E.; Liu, S.X.L.; Yan, X.; Tan, X.-D.; Chou, P.M.; Barrett, T.A.; De Plaen, I.G. Blocking NF-κB activation in Ly6c$^+$ monocytes attenuates necrotizing enterocolitis. *Am. J. Pathol.* **2019**, *189*, 604–618. [CrossRef] [PubMed]
108. Martinez, F.O.; Gordon, S.; Locati, M.; Mantovani, A. Transcriptional profiling of the human monocyte-to-macrophage differentiation and polarization: New molecules and patterns of gene expression. *J. Immunol.* **2006**, *177*, 7303–7311. [CrossRef] [PubMed]
109. Yazji, I.; Sodhi, C.P.; Lee, E.K.; Good, M.; Egan, C.E.; Afrazi, A.; Neal, M.D.; Jia, H.; Lin, J.; Ma, C.; et al. Endothelial TLR4 activation impairs intestinal microcirculatory perfusion in necrotizing enterocolitis via eNOS-NO-nitrite signaling. *Proc. Natl. Acad. Sci. USA* **2013**, *110*, 9451–9456. [CrossRef] [PubMed]
110. Claud, E.C.; Lu, L.; Anton, P.M.; Savidge, T.; Walker, W.A.; Cherayil, B.J. Developmentallly regulated IkappaB expression in intestinal epithelium and susceptibility to flagellin-induced inflammation. *Proc. Natl. Acad. Sci. USA* **2004**, *101*, 7404–7408. [CrossRef]
111. Nanthakumar, N.N.; Fusunyan, R.D.; Sanderson, I.; Walker, W.A. Inflammation in the developing human intestine: A possible pathophysiologic contribution to necrotizing enterocolitis. *Proc. Natl. Acad. Sci. USA* **2000**, *97*, 6043–6048. [CrossRef] [PubMed]
112. Rentea, R.M.; Welak, S.R.; Fredrich, K.; Donohoe, D.; Pritchard, K.A.; Oldham, K.T.; Gourlay, D.M.; Liedel, J.L. Early enteral stressors in newborns increase inflammatory cytokine expression in a neonatal necrotizing enterocolitis rat model. *Eur. J. Ped. Surg.* **2013**, *23*, 39–47. [CrossRef]
113. Jones, C.A.; Holloway, J.A.; Warner, J.O. Phenotype of fetal monocytes and B lymphocytes during the third trimester of pregnancy. *J. Reprod. Immunol.* **2002**, *56*, 45–60. [CrossRef]
114. Hackam, D.J.; Upperman, J.S.; Grishin, A.; Ford, H.R. Disordered enterocyte signaling and intestinal barrier dysfunction in the pathogenesis of necrotizing enterocolitis. *Semin. Pediatr. Surg.* **2005**, *14*, 49–57. [CrossRef] [PubMed]
115. Clark, J.A.; Doelle, S.M.; Halpern, M.D.; Saunders, T.A.; Holubee, H.; Dvorak, D.; Boitano, S.A.; Dvorak, B. Intestinal barrier failure during experimental necrotizing enterocolitis: Protective effect of EGF treatment. *Am. J. Physiol.* **2006**, *291*, G938–G949. [CrossRef] [PubMed]
116. Martin, N.A.; Mount Patrick, S.K.; Estrada, T.E.; Frisk, H.A.; Rogan, D.T.; Dvorak, B.; Halpern, M.D. Active transport of bile acids decreases mucin 2 in neonatal ileum: Implications for development of necrotizing enterocolitis. *PLoS ONE* **2011**, *6*, e27191. [CrossRef]
117. Nathan, C. Neutrophils and immunity: Challenges and opportunities. *Nat. Rev. Immunol.* **2006**, *6*, 173–182. [CrossRef] [PubMed]
118. Emami, C.N.; Mittal, R.; Wang, L.; Ford, H.R.; Prasadarao, N.V. Role of neutrophils and macrophages in the pathogenesis of necrotizing enterocolitis caused by *Cronobacter sakazakii*. *J. Surg. Res.* **2012**, *172*, 18–28. [CrossRef] [PubMed]
119. Musemeche, C.; Caplan, M.; Hsueh, W.; Sun, X.; Kelly, A. Experimental necrotizing enterocolitis: The role of polymorphonuclear neutrophils. *J. Pediatr. Surg.* **1991**, *26*, 1047–1049. [CrossRef]
120. Christensen, R.D.; Yoder, B.A.; Baer, V.L.; Snow, G.L.; Butler, A. Early-onset neutropenia in small-for-gestational-age infants. *Pediatrics* **2015**, *136*, e1259–e1267. [CrossRef]
121. Strunk, T.; Temming, P.; Gembruch, U.; Reiss, I.; Bucsky, P.; Schultz, C. Differential maturation of the innate immune response in human fetuses. *Ped. Res.* **2004**, *56*, 219–226. [CrossRef] [PubMed]
122. Maheshwari, A.; Kelly, D.R.; Nicola, T.; Ambalavanan, N.; Jain, S.K.; Murphy-Ullrich, J.; Athar, M.; Shimamura, M.; Bhandari, V.; Aprahamian, C.; et al. TFG-beta2 suppresses macrophage cytokine production and mucosal inflammatory responses in the developing intestine. *Gastroenterology* **2011**, *140*, 242–253. [CrossRef] [PubMed]

123. MohanKumar, K.; Namachivayam, K.; Chapalamadugu, K.C.; Garzon, S.A.; Premkumar, M.H.; Tipparaju, S.M.; Maheshwari, A. Smad7 interrupts TGF-beta signaling in intestinal macrophages and promotes inflammatory activation of these cells during necrotizing enterocolitis. *Pediatr. Res.* **2016**, *79*, 951–961. [CrossRef] [PubMed]
124. Namachivayam, K.; Blanco, C.L.; MohanKumar, K.; Jagadeeswaran, R.; Vasquez, M.; McGill-Vargas, L.; Garzon, S.A.; Jain, S.K.; Gill, R.K.; Freitag, N.E.; et al. Smad7 inhibits autocrine expression of TGF-beta2 in intestinal epithelial cells in baboon necrotizing enterocolitis. *Am. J. Physiol. Gastrointest. Liver Physiol.* **2013**, *304*, G167–G180. [CrossRef] [PubMed]
125. MohanKumar, K.; Kaza, N.; Jagadeeswaran, R.; Garzon, S.A.; Bansal, A.; Kurundkar, A.R.; Namachivayam, K.; Remon, J.I.; Bandepalli, C.R.; Feng, X.; et al. Gut mucosal injury in neonates is marked by macrophage infiltration in contrast to pleomorphic infiltrates in adult: Evidence from an animal model. *Am. J. Physiol. Gastrointest. Liver Physiol.* **2012**, *303*, G93–G102. [CrossRef] [PubMed]
126. Emami, C.N.; Mittal, R.; Wang, L.; Ford, H.R.; Prasadarao, N.V. Recruitment of dendritic cells is responsible for intestinal epithelial damage in the pathogenesis of necrotizing enterocolitis by *Cronobacter sakazakii*. *J. Immunol.* **2011**, *186*, 7067–7079. [CrossRef] [PubMed]
127. Weitkamp, J.H.; Rosen, M.J.; Zhao, Z.; Koyama, T.; Geem, D.; Denning, T.L.; Rock, M.T.; Moore, D.J.; Halpern, M.D.; Matta, P.; et al. Small intestinal intraepithelial TCRgammadelta+ T lymphocytes are present in the premature intestine but selectively reduced in surgical necrotizing enterocolitis. *PLoS ONE* **2014**, *9*, e99042. [CrossRef]
128. Gibbons, D.L.; Haque, S.F.; Silberzahn, T.; Hamilton, K.; Langford, C.; Ellis, P.; Carr, R.; Hayday, A.C. Neonates harbour highly active gammadelta T cells with selective impairments in preterm infants. *Eur. J. Immunol.* **2009**, *39*, 1794–1806. [CrossRef] [PubMed]
129. Ismail, A.S.; Behrendt, C.L.; Hooper, L.V. Reciprocal interactions between commensal bacteria and gamma delta intraepithelial lymphocytes during mucosal injury. *J. Immunol.* **2009**, *182*, 3047–3054. [CrossRef]
130. Weitkamp, J.H.; Koyama, T.; Rock, M.T.; Correa, H.; Goettel, J.A.; Matta, P.; Oswald-Richter, K.; Rosen, M.J.; Engelhardt, B.G.; Moore, D.J.; et al. Necrotising enterocolitis is characterised by disrupted immune regulation and diminished mucosal regulatory (FOXP3)/effector (CD4, CD8) T cell ratios. *Gut* **2013**, *62*, 73–82. [CrossRef]
131. Basha, S.; Surendran, N.; Pichichero, M. Immune responses in neonates. *Exp. Rev. Clin. Immunol.* **2014**, *10*, 1171–1184. [CrossRef] [PubMed]
132. Markel, T.A.; Crisostomo, P.R.; Wairiuko, G.M.; Pitcher, J.; Tsai, B.M.; Meldrum, D.R. Cytokines in necrotizing enterocolitis. *Shock* **2006**, *25*, 329–337. [CrossRef]
133. Kling, K.M.; Kirby, L.; Kwan, K.Y.; Kim, F.; McFadden, D.W. Interleukin-10 inhibits inducible nitric oxide synthase in an animal model of necrotizing enterocolitis. *Int. J. Surg. Investig.* **1999**, *1*, 337–342. [PubMed]
134. Baud, V.; Karin, M. Signal transduction by tumor necrosis factor and its relatives. *Trends Cell Biol.* **2001**, *11*, 372–377. [CrossRef]
135. Tracey, K.J.; Fong, Y.; Hesse, D.G.; Manogue, K.R.; Lee, A.T.; Kuo, G.C.; Lowry, S.F.; Cerami, A. Anti-cachectin/TNF monoclonal antibodies prevent septic shock during lethal bacteremia. *Nature* **1987**, *330*, 662–664. [CrossRef]
136. Baregamian, N.; Song, J.; Bailey, C.E.; Papaconstantinou, J.; Evers, B.M.; Chung, D.H. Tumor necrosis factor-alpha and apoptosis signal-regulating kinase 1 control reactive oxygen species release, mitochondrial autophagy, and C-Jun N-terminal kinase/p38 phosphorylation during necrotizing enterocolitis. *Oxid. Med. Cell. Longev.* **2009**, *2*, 297–306. [CrossRef]
137. Caplan, M.S.; Hsueh, W. Necrotizing enterocolitis: Role of platelet activating factor, endotoxin, and tumor necrosis factor. *J. Pediatr.* **1990**, *117*, S47–S51. [CrossRef]
138. Harris, M.C.; Costarino, A.T., Jr.; Sullivan, J.S.; Dulkerian, S.; McCawley, L.; Corcoran, L.; Butler, S.; Kilpatrick, L. Cytokine elevations in critically ill infants with sepsis and necrotizing enterocolitis. *J. Pediatr.* **1994**, *124*, 105–111. [CrossRef]
139. Morecroft, J.A.; Spitz, L.; Hamilton, P.A.; Holmes, S.J. Plasma cytokine levels in necrotizing enterocolitis. *Acta Paediatr. Suppl.* **1994**, *396*, 18–20. [CrossRef]
140. Churg, A.; Wang, R.D.; Tai, H.; Wang, X.; Xie, C.; Dai, J.; Shapiro, S.D.; Wright, J.L. Macrophage metalloelastase mediates acute cigarette smoke-induced inflammation via tumor necrosis factor-alpha release. *Am. J. Respir. Crit. Care Med.* **2003**, *167*, 1083–1089. [CrossRef]

141. Saren, P.; Welgus, H.G.; Kovanen, P.T. TNF-α and IL-1β selectively induce expression of 92 kDa gelatinase by human macrophages. *J. Immunol.* **1996**, *157*, 4159–4165. [PubMed]
142. Impola, U.; Toriseva, M.; Suomela, S.; Jeskanen, L.; Hieta, N.; Jahkola, T.; Grenman, R.; Kähäri, V.; Saarialho-Kere, U. Matrix metalloproteinase-19 is expressed by proliferating epithelium but disappears with neoplastic dedifferentiation. *Int. J. Cancer* **2003**, *103*, 709–716. [CrossRef]
143. Pender, S.L.; Braegger, C.; Gunther, C.; Monteleone, G.; Meuli, M.; Schuppan, D.; MacDonald, T.T. Matrix metalloproteinases in necrotising enterocolitis. *Pediatr. Res.* **2003**, *54*, 160–164. [CrossRef] [PubMed]
144. Birkedal-Hansen, H.; Moore, W.G.; Bodden, M.K.; Windsor, L.J.; Birkedal-Hansen, B.; DeCarlo, A.; Engler, J.A. Matrix metalloproteinases: A review. *Crit. Rev. Oral Biol. Med.* **1993**, *4*, 197–250. [CrossRef]
145. Male, D. *Immunology: An Illustrated Outline*, 3rd ed.; Mosby: London, UK, 1998; pp. 1–146.
146. Minekawa, R.; Takeda, T.; Sakata, M.; Hayashi, M.; Isobe, A.; Yamamoto, T.; Tasaka, K.; Murata, Y. Human breast milk suppresses the transcriptional regulation of IL-1β induced NF-κB signaling in human intestinal cells. *Am. J. Physiol. Cell Physiol.* **2004**, *287*, C1401–C1411. [CrossRef] [PubMed]
147. Viscardi, R.M.; Lyon, N.H.; Sun, C.C.; Hebel, J.R.; Hasday, J.D. Inflammatory cytokine mRNAs in surgical specimens of necrotizing enterocolitis and normal newborn intestine. *Pediatr. Pathol. Lab. Med.* **1997**, *17*, 547–559. [CrossRef] [PubMed]
148. Edelson, M.B.; Bagwell, C.E.; Rozycki, H.J. Circulating pro- and counterinflammatory cytokine levels and severity in necrotizing enterocolitis. *Pediatrics* **1999**, *103*, 766–771. [CrossRef]
149. Romagnoli, C.; Freeza, S.; Cingolani, A.; De Luca, A.; Puopolo, M.; De Carolis, M.P.; Vento, G.; Antinori, A.; Tortorolo, G. Plasma levels of interleukin-6 and interleukin-10 in preterm neonates evaluated for sepsis. *Eur. J. Pediatr.* **2001**, *160*, 345–350. [CrossRef]
150. Ren, Y.; Lin, C.L.; Chen, X.Y.; Huang, X.; Lui, V.; Nicholls, J.; Lan, H.Y.; Tam, P.K. Up-regulation of macrophage migration inhibitory factor in infants with acute neonatal necrotizing enterocolitis. *Histopathology* **2005**, *46*, 659–667. [CrossRef]
151. Goepfert, A.R.; Andrews, W.W.; Waldemar, C.; Ramsey, P.S.; Cliver, S.P.; Goldenber, R.L.; Hauth, J.C. Umbilical cord plasma interleukin-6 concentrations in preterm infants and risk of neonatal morbidity. *Am. J. Obstet. Gynecol.* **2004**, *191*, 1375–1381. [CrossRef]
152. Luster, A.D. Chemokines—Chemotactic cytokines that mediate inflammation. *N. Engl. J. Med.* **1998**, *338*, 436–445. [CrossRef]
153. Chikano, S.; Sawada, K.; Shimoyama, T.; Kashiwamura, S.I.; Sugihara, A.; Sekikawa, K.; Terada, N.; Nakanishi, K.; Okamura, H. IL-18 and IL-12 induce intestinal inflammation and fatty liver in mice in an IFN-gamma dependent manner. *Gut* **2000**, *47*, 779–786. [CrossRef]
154. Kashiwamura, S.; Ueda, H.; Okamura, H. Roles of interleukin-18 in tissue destruction and compensatory reactions. *J. Immunol.* **2002**, *25* (Suppl. 1), S4–S11. [CrossRef]
155. Halpern, M.D.; Holubec, H.; Dominguez, J.A.; Williams, C.S.; Meza, Y.G.; McWilliam, D.L.; Payne, C.M.; McCuskey, R.S.; Besselsen, D.G.; Dvorak, B. Upregulation of IL-18 and Il-12 in the ileum of neonatal rats with necrotizing enterocolitis. *Pediatr. Res.* **2002**, *51*, 733–739. [CrossRef]
156. Nadler, E.P.; Dickinson, E.; Knisely, A.; Zhang, X.R.; Boyle, P.; Beer-Stolz, D.; Watkins, S.C.; Ford, H.R. Expression of inducible nitric oxide synthase and interleukin 12 in experimental necrotizing enterocolitis. *J. Surg. Res.* **2000**, *92*, 71–77. [CrossRef]
157. Ford, H.R.; Sorrells, D.L.; Knisely, A.S. Inflammatory cytokines, nitric oxide, and necrotizing enterocolitis. *Semin. Pediatr. Surg.* **1996**, *5*, 155–159.
158. Benkoe, T.; Baumann, S.; Weninger, M.; Pones, M.; Reck, C.; Rebhandl, W.; Oehler, R. Comprehensive evaluation of 11 cytokines in premature infants with surgical necrotizing enterocolitis. *PLoS ONE* **2013**, *8*, e58720. [CrossRef]
159. Maheshwari, A.; Schelonka, R.L.; Dimmitt, R.A.; Carlo, W.A.; Munoz-Hernandez, B.; Das, A.; McDonald, S.A.; Thorsen, P.; Skogstrand, K.; Hougaard, D.M.; et al. Cytokines associated with necrotizing enterocolitis in extremely-low-birth-weight infants. *Pediatr. Res.* **2014**, *76*, 100–108. [CrossRef]
160. Fiocchi, C. Inflammatory bowel disease: Etiology and pathogenesis. *Gastroenterology* **1998**, *115*, 182–205. [CrossRef]
161. Uhlig, H.H.; Powrie, F. Translating immunology into therapeutic concepts for inflammatory bowel disease. *Annu. Rev. Immunol.* **2018**, *36*, 755–781. [CrossRef]

162. Zeissig, S.; Bürgel, N.; Günzel, D.; Richter, J.; Mankertz, J.; Wahnschaffe, U.; Kroesen, A.J.; Zeitz, M.; Fromm, M.; Schulzke, J.D. Changes in expression and distribution of claudins 2, 5 and 8 lead to discontinuous tight junctions and barrier dysfunction in active Crohn's disease. *Gut* **2007**, *56*, 61–72. [CrossRef] [PubMed]
163. Vezza, T.; Rodríguez-Nogales, A.; Algieri, F.; Utrilla, M.P.; Rodriguez-Cabezas, M.E.; Galvez, J. Flavonoids in inflammatory bowel disease: A review. *Nutrients* **2016**, *8*, 211. [CrossRef]
164. Cao, Y.; Shen, J.; Ran, Z.H. Association between *Faecalibacterium prausnitzii* reduction and inflammatory bowel disease: A meta-analyis and systematic review of the literature. *Gastroenterol. Res. Pract.* **2014**, *2014*, 872725. [CrossRef] [PubMed]
165. Levy, M.; Kolodziejezyk, A.A.; Thaiss, C.A.; Elinav, E. Dysbiosis and the immune system. *Nat. Rev. Immunol.* **2017**, *17*, 219–232. [CrossRef] [PubMed]
166. Weber, C.R.; Turner, J.R. Inflammatory bowel disease: Is it really just another break in the wall? *Gut* **2007**, *56*, 6–8. [CrossRef] [PubMed]
167. Hollander, D. Crohn's disease—A permeability disorder of the tight junction? *Gut* **1988**, *29*, 1621–1624. [CrossRef] [PubMed]
168. Xavier, R.J.; Podolsky, D.K. Unravelling the pathogenesis of inflammatory bowel disease. *Nature* **2007**, *448*, 427–434. [CrossRef]
169. Arnott, I.D.; Kingstone, K.; Ghosh, S. Abnormal intestinal permeability predicts relapse in inactive Crohn disease. *Scand. J. Gastroenterol.* **2000**, *35*, 1163–1170.
170. Wyatt, J.; Vogelsang, H.; Hubl, W.; Waldhoer, T.; Lochs, H. Intestinal permeability and the prediction of relapse in Crohn's disease. *Lancet* **1993**, *341*, 1437–1439. [CrossRef]
171. Katz, K.D.; Hollander, D.; Vadheim, C.M.; McElree, C.; Delahunty, T.; Dadufalza, V.D.; Krugliak, P.; Rotter, J.I. Intestinal permeability in patients with Crohn's disease and their healthy relatives. *Gastroenterology* **1989**, *97*, 927–931. [CrossRef]
172. Peeters, M.; Geypens, B.; Claus, D.; Nevens, H.; Ghoos, Y.; Verbeke, G.; Baert, F.; Vermeire, S.; Vlietinck, R.; Rutgeerts, P. Clustering of increased small intestinal permeability in families with Crohn's disease. *Gastroenterology* **1997**, *113*, 802–807. [CrossRef]
173. Smith, P.D.; Smythies, L.E.; Shen, R.; Greenwell-Wild, T.; Gliozzi, M.; Wahl, S.M. Intestinal macrophages and response to microbial environment. *Mucosal Immunol.* **2011**, *4*, 31–42. [CrossRef] [PubMed]
174. Schreiber, S.; Heinig, T.; Panzer, U.; Reinking, R.; Bouchard, A.; Stahl, P.D.; Raedler, A. Impaired response of activated mononuclear phagocytes to interleukin-4 in inflammatory bowel disease. *Gastroenterology* **1995**, *108*, 21–33. [CrossRef]
175. Podolsky, D.K. Inflammatory bowel disease. *N. Engl. J. Med.* **2002**, *347*, 417–429. [CrossRef]
176. Holtmann, M.H.; Neurath, M.F. Differential TNF-signaling in chronic inflammatory disorders. *Curr. Mol. Med.* **2004**, *4*, 439–444. [CrossRef]
177. Sartor, R.B. Mechanisms of disease: Pathogenesis of Crohn's disease and ulcerative colitis. *Nat. Clin. Pract. Gastroenterol. Hepatol.* **2006**, *3*, 390–407. [CrossRef]
178. Shih, D.Q.; Targan, S.R. Insights into IBD pathogenesis. *Curr. Gastroenterol. Rep.* **2009**, *11*, 473–480. [CrossRef]
179. Strober, W.; Fuss, I.; Mannon, P. The fundamental basis of inflammatory bowel disease. *J. Clin. Investig.* **2007**, *117*, 514–521. [CrossRef]
180. Cerovic, V.; Houston, S.A.; Scott, C.L.; Aumeunier, A.; Yrlid, U.; Mowat, A.M.; Milling, S.W. Intestinal cd103(-) dendritic cells migrate in lymph and prime effector T cells. *Mucosal Immunol.* **2013**, *6*, 104–113. [CrossRef]
181. Laing, K.J.; Secombes, C.J. Chemokines. *Dev. Comp. Immunol.* **2004**, *28*, 443–460. [CrossRef]
182. Kim, J.M.; Jung, H.Y.; Lee, J.Y.; Youn, J.; Lee, C.H.; Kim, K.H. Mitogen-activated protein kinase and activator protein-1 dependent signals are essential for *Bacteroides fragilis* enterotoxin-induced enteritis. *Eur. J. Immunol.* **2005**, *35*, 2648–2657. [CrossRef] [PubMed]
183. Vainer, B. Intercellular adhesion molecule-1 (ICAM-1) in ulcerative colitis: Presence, visualization, and significance. *APMIS Suppl.* **2010**, *129*, 1–43. [CrossRef]
184. Steidler, L.; Hans, W.; Schotte, L.; Neirynck, S.; Obermeier, F.; Falk, W.; Fiers, W.; Remaut, E. Treatment of murine colitis by Lactococcus lactis secreting interleukin-10. *Science* **2000**, *289*, 1352–1355. [CrossRef] [PubMed]

185. Kitani, A.; Fuss, U.; Nakamura, K.; Schwartz, O.M.; Usui, T.; Strober, W. Treatment of experimental (trinitrobenzene sulfonic acid) colitis by intranasal administration of transforming growth factor (TGF)-β1 plasmid: TGF-β1-mediated suppression of T helper cell type 1 response occurs by interleukin (IL)-10 induction and IL-12 receptor β2 chain downregulation. *J. Exp. Med.* **2000**, *192*, 41–52. [PubMed]
186. Fukata, M.; Chen, A.; Vamadevan, A.S.; Cohen, J.; Breglio, K.; Krishnareddy, S.; Hsu, D.; Xu, R.; Harpaz, N.; Dannenberg, A.J.; et al. Toll-like receptor-4 promotes the development of colitis-associated colorectal tumors. *Gastroenterology* **2007**, *133*, 1869–1881. [CrossRef] [PubMed]
187. Vlantis, K.; Wullaert, A.; Sasaki, Y.; Schmidt-Supprian, M.; Rajewsky, K.; Roskams, T.; Pasparakis, M. Constitutive IKK2 activation in intestinal epithelial cells induces intestinal tumors in mice. *J. Clin. Investig.* **2011**, *121*, 2781–2793. [CrossRef]
188. Cario, E.; Podolsky, D.K. Differential alteration in intestinal epithelial cells expression of toll-like receptor 3 (TLR3) and TLR4 in inflammatory bowel disease. *Infect. Immun.* **2000**, *68*, 7010–7017. [CrossRef] [PubMed]
189. Ortegea-Cava, C.F.; Ishihara, S.; Rumi, M.A.; Kawashima, K.; Ishimura, N.; Kazumori, H.; Udagawa, J.; Kadowaki, Y.; Kinoshita, Y. Strategic compartmentalization of Toll-like receptor 4 in the mouse gut. *J. Immunol.* **2003**, *170*, 3977–3985. [CrossRef]
190. Rogler, G.; Brand, K.; Vogl, D.; Page, S.; Hofmeister, R.; Andus, T.; Knuechel, R.; Baeuerle, P.A.; Scholmerich, J.; Gross, V. Nuclear factor kappaB is activated in macrophages and epithelial cells of inflamed intestinal mucosa. *Gastroenterology* **1998**, *115*, 357–369. [CrossRef]
191. Neurath, M.F.; Petterson, S.; Meyer zum Büschenfelde, K.H.; Strober, W. Local administration of antisense phosphorothioate oligonucleotides to the p65 subunit of NF-κB abrogates established experimental colitis in mice. *Nat. Med.* **1996**, *2*, 998–1004. [CrossRef]
192. Waetzig, G.H.; Seegert, D.; Rosenstiel, P.; Nikolaus, S.; Schreiber, S. p38 mitogen-activated protein kinase is activated and linked to TNF-alpha signaling in inflammatory bowel disease. *J. Immunol.* **2002**, *168*, 5342–5351. [CrossRef]
193. Abreu-Martin, M.T.; Palladino, A.A.; Faris, M.; Carramanzana, N.M.; Nel, A.E.; Targan, S.R. Fas activates the JNK pathway in human colonic epithelial cells: Lack of a direct role in apoptosis. *Am. J. Physiol.* **1999**, *276*, G599–G605. [CrossRef] [PubMed]
194. Bantel, H.; Schmitz, M.L.; Raible, A.; Gregor, M.; Schulze-Osthoff, K. Critical role of NF-κB and stress-activated protein kinases in steroid unresponsiveness. *FASEB J.* **2002**, *16*, 1832–1834. [CrossRef]
195. Salzman, N.H.; Underwood, M.A.; Bevins, C.L. Paneth cells, defensins, and the commensal microbiota: A hypothesis on intimate interplay at the intestinal mucosa. *Semin. Immunol.* **2007**, *19*, 70–83. [CrossRef]
196. Iida, T.; Onodera, K.; Nakase, H. Role of autophagy in the pathogenesis of inflammatory bowel disease. *World J. Gastroenterol.* **2017**, *23*, 1944–1953. [CrossRef] [PubMed]
197. Gardiner, K.R.; Crockard, A.D.; Halliday, M.I.; Rowlands, B.J. Class II major histocompatibility complex antigen expression on peripheral blood monocytes in patients with inflammatory bowel disease. *Gut* **1994**, *35*, 511–516. [CrossRef] [PubMed]
198. MacDonald, T.T.; Monteleone, G.; Pender, S.L.F. Recent developments in the immunology of inflammatory bowel disease. *Scand. J. Immunol.* **2000**, *51*, 2–9. [CrossRef] [PubMed]
199. Atreya, R.; Mudter, J.; Finotto, S.; Müllberg, J.; Jostock, T.; Wirtz, S.; Schütz, M.; Bartsch, B.; Holtmann, M.; Becker, C.; et al. Blockade of interleukin 6 trans signaling suppresses T-cell resistance against apoptosis in chronic intestinal inflammation: Evidence in Crohn's disease and experimental colitis in vivo. *Nat. Med.* **2000**, *6*, 583–588. [CrossRef] [PubMed]
200. Fuss, I.J.; Neurath, M.; Boirivant, M.; Klein, J.S.; de la Motte, C.; Strong, S.A.; Fiocchi, C.; Strober, W. Disparate CD4+ lamina propria (LP) lymphokine secretion profiles in inflammatory bowel disease. Crohn's disease LP cells manifest increased secretion of IFN-gamma, whereas ulcerative colitis LP cells manifest increased secretion of IL-5. *J. Immunol.* **1996**, *157*, 1261–1270.
201. Parronchi, P.; Romagnani, P.; Annunziato, F.; Sampognaro, S.; Becchio, A.; Giannarini, L.; Maggi, E.; Pupilli, C.; Tonelli, F.; Romagnani, S. Type 1 T-helper cell predominance and interleukin-12 expression in the gut of patients with Crohn's disease. *Am. J. Pathol.* **1997**, *150*, 823–832. [PubMed]
202. Romagnani, S. Lymphokine production by human T cells in disease states. *Annu. Rev. Immunol.* **1994**, *12*, 227–257. [CrossRef] [PubMed]

203. Ebrahimpour, S.; Shahbazi, M.; Khalili, A.; Tahoori, M.T.; Zavaran Hosseini, A.; Amari, A.; Aghili, B.; Abediankenari, S.; Mohammadizad, H.; Mohammadnia-Afrouzi, M. Elevated levels of IL-2 and IL-21 produced by CD4+ T cells in inflammatory bowel disease. *J. Biol. Regul. Homeost. Agents* **2017**, *31*, 279–287.
204. Breese, E.; Braegger, C.P.; Corrigan, C.J.; Walker-Smith, J.A.; MacDonald, T.T. Interleukin-2 and interferon-γ secreting T cells in normal and diseased human intestinal mucosa. *Immunology* **1993**, *78*, 127–131. [PubMed]
205. Mariani, P.; Bachetoni, A.; D'Alessandro, M.; Lomanto, D.; Mazzocchi, P.; Speranza, V. Effector Th-1 cells with cytotoxic function in the intestinal lamina propria of patients with Crohn's disease. *Dig. Dis. Sci.* **2000**, *45*, 2029–2035. [CrossRef] [PubMed]
206. Fuss, I.J.; Marth, T.; Neurath, M.F.; Pearlstein, G.R.; Jain, A.; Strober, W. Anti-interleukin 12 treatment regulates apoptosis of Th1 cells in experimental colitis in mice. *Gastroenterology* **1999**, *117*, 1078–1088. [CrossRef]
207. Stockinger, B.; Veldhoen, M. Differentiation and function of Th17 T cells. *Curr. Opin. Immunol.* **2007**, *19*, 281–286. [CrossRef]
208. Schmidt, C.; Giese, T.; Ludwig, B.; Mueller-Molaian, I.; Marth, T.; Zeuzem, S.; Meuer, S.C.; Stallmach, A. Expression of interleukin-12-related cytokine transcripts in inflammatory bowel disease: Elevated interleukin-23p19 and interleukin-27p28 in Crohn's disease but not in ulcerative colitis. *Inflamm. Bowel Dis.* **2005**, *11*, 16–23. [CrossRef]
209. Korn, T.; Bettelli, E.; Oukka, M.; Kuchroo, V.K. IL-17 and Th17 cells. *Annu. Rev. Immunol.* **2009**, *27*, 485–517. [CrossRef]
210. O'Connor, W., Jr.; Kamanaka, M.; Booth, C.J.; Town, T.; Nakae, S.; Iwakura, Y.; Kolls, J.K.; Flavell, R.A. A protective function for interleukin 17A in T cell-mediated intestinal inflammation. *Nat. Immunol.* **2009**, *10*, 603–609. [CrossRef]
211. Song, X.; Dai, D.; He, X.; Zhu, S.; Yao, Y.; Gao, H.; Wang, J.; Qu, F.; Qiu, J.; Wang, H.; et al. Growth factor FGF2 cooperates with interleukin-17 to repair intestinal epithelial damage. *Immunity* **2015**, *43*, 488–501. [CrossRef]
212. Yen, D.; Cheung, J.; Scheerens, H.; Poulet, F.; McClanahan, T.; McKenzie, B.; Kleinschek, M.A.; Owyang, A.; Mattson, J.; Blumenschein, W.; et al. IL-23 is essential for T cell-mediated colitis and promotes inflammation via IL-17 and IL-6. *J. Clin. Investig.* **2006**, *116*, 1310–1316. [CrossRef] [PubMed]
213. Khor, B.; Gardet, A.; Xavier, R.J. Genetics and pathogenesis of inflammatory bowel disease. *Nature* **2011**, *474*, 307–317. [CrossRef] [PubMed]
214. Mazieiro, R.; Frizon, R.R.; Barbalho, S.M.; de Alvares Goulart, R. Is curcumin a possibility to treat inflammatory bowel diseases? *J. Med. Food* **2018**, *21*, 1077–1085. [CrossRef] [PubMed]
215. Bamias, G.; Cominelli, F. Role of Th2 immunity in intestinal inflammation. *Curr. Opin. Gastroenterol.* **2015**, *31*, 471–476. [CrossRef] [PubMed]
216. Shohan, M.; Elahi, S.; Shirzad, H.; Rafieian-Kopaei, M.; Bagheri, N.; Soltani, E. Th9 cells: Probably players in ulcerative colitis pathogenesis. *Int. Rev. Immunol.* **2018**, *37*, 192–205. [CrossRef] [PubMed]
217. Fina, D.; Caruso, R.; Pallone, F.; Monteleone, G. Interleukin-21 (IL-21) controls inflammatory pathways in the gut. *Endocr. Metab. Immune Disord. Drug Targets* **2007**, *7*, 288–291. [CrossRef]
218. Rivas, M.N.; Koh, Y.T.; Chen, A.; Nguyen, A.; Lee, Y.H.; Lawson, G.; Chatila, T.A. MyD88 is critically involved in immune tolerance breakdown at environmental interfaces of Foxp3-deficient mice. *J. Clin. Investig.* **2012**, *122*, 1933–1947. [CrossRef]
219. Mayne, C.G.; Williams, C.B. Induced and natural regulatory T cells in the development of inflammatory bowel disease. *Inflamm. Bowel Dis.* **2013**, *19*, 1772–1788. [CrossRef]
220. De Souza, H.S.; Fiocchi, C. Immunopathogenesis of IBD: Current state of the art. *Nat. Rev. Gastroenterol. Hepatol.* **2016**, *13*, 13–27. [CrossRef]
221. Veltkamp, C.; Anstaett, M.; Wahl, K.; Möller, S.; Gangl, S.; Bachmann, O.; Hardtke-Wolenski, M.; Länger, F.; Stremmel, W.; Manns, M.P.; et al. Apoptosis of regulatory T lymphocytes is increased in chronic inflammatory bowel disease and reversed by anti-TNFα treatment. *Gut* **2011**, *60*, 1345–1353. [CrossRef]
222. Liu, Z.; Geboes, K.; Colpaert, S.; Overbergh, L.; Mathieu, C.; Heremans, H.; de Boer, M.; Boon, L.; D'Haens, G.; Rutgeerts, P.; et al. Prevention of experimental colitis in SCID mice reconstituted with CD45RBhigh CD4+ T cells by blocking the CD40-CD154 interactions. *J. Immunol.* **2000**, *164*, 6005–6014. [CrossRef]
223. Harrison, O.J.; Srinivasan, N.; Pott, J.; Schiering, C.; Krausgruber, T.; Ilott, N.E.; Maloy, K.J. Epithelial-derived IL-18 regulates Th17 cell differentiation and Foxp3+ Treg cell function in the intestine. *Mucosal Immunol.* **2015**, *8*, 1226–12236. [CrossRef]

224. Nowarski, R.; Jackson, R.; Gagliani, N.; de Zoete, M.R.; Palm, N.W.; Bailis, W.; Low, J.S.; Harman, C.C.; Graham, M.; Elinav, E.; et al. Epithelial IL-18 equilibrium controls barrier function in colitis. *Cell* **2015**, *163*, 1444–14456. [CrossRef]
225. Ludwiczek, O.; Kaser, A.; Novick, D.; Dinarello, C.A.; Rubinstein, M.; Tilg, H. Elevated systemic levels of free interleukin-18 (IL-18) in patients with Crohn's disease. *Eur. Cytokine Netw.* **2005**, *16*, 27–33.
226. Artis, D.; Spits, H. The biology of innate lymphoid cells. *Nature* **2015**, *517*, 293–301. [CrossRef]
227. Elemam, N.M.; Hannawi, S.; Maghazachi, A.A. Innate lymphoid cells (ILCs) as mediators of inflammation, release of cytokines and lytic molecules. *Toxins* **2017**, *9*, 398. [CrossRef]
228. Bernink, J.H.; Peters, C.P.; Munneke, M.; te Velde, A.A.; Meijer, S.L.; Weijer, K.; Hreggvidsdottir, H.S.; Heinsbroek, S.E.; Legrand, N.; Buskens, C.J.; et al. Human type 1 innate lymphoid cells accumulate in inflamed mucosal tissues. *Nat. Immunol.* **2013**, *14*, 221–229. [CrossRef]
229. Fuchs, A.; Vermi, W.; Lee, J.S.; Lonardi, S.; Gilfillan, S.; Newberry, R.D.; Cella, M.; Colonna, M. Intraepithelial type 1 innate lymphoid cells are a unique subset of IL-12- and IL-15-responsive IFN-gamma-producing cells. *Immunity* **2013**, *38*, 769–781. [CrossRef]
230. Sugimoto, K.; Ogawa, A.; Mizoguchi, E.; Shimomura, Y.; Andoh, A.; Bhan, A.K.; Blumberg, R.S.; Xavier, R.J.; Mizoguchi, A. IL-22 ameliorates intestinal inflammation in a mouse model of ulcerative colitis. *J. Clin. Investig.* **2008**, *118*, 534–544. [CrossRef]
231. Zenewicz, L.A.; Yancopoulos, G.D.; Valenzuela, D.M.; Murphy, A.J.; Stevens, S.; Flavell, R.A. Innate and adaptive interleukin-22 protects mice from inflammatory bowel disease. *Immunity* **2008**, *29*, 947–957. [CrossRef]
232. Pelczar, P.; Witkowski, M.; Perez, L.G.; Kempski, J.; Hammel, A.G.; Brockmann, L.; Kleinschmidt, D.; Wende, S.; Haueis, C.; Bedke, T.; et al. A pathogenic role for T cell-derived IL-22BP in inflammatory bowel disease. *Science* **2016**, *354*, 358–362. [CrossRef]
233. Van Deventer, S.J.H. Tumour necrosis factor and Crohn's disease. *Gut* **1997**, *40*, 443–448. [CrossRef]
234. Keates, A.C.; Castagnuolo, I.; Crickshank, W.W.; Qiu, B.; Arseneau, K.O.; Brazer, W.; Kelly, C.P. Interleukin 16 is upregulated in Crohn's disease and participates in TNBS colitis in mice. *Gastroenterology* **2000**, *119*, 972–982. [CrossRef]
235. Prasad, S.; Mingrino, R.; Kaukinen, K.; Hayes, K.L.; Powell, R.M.; MacDonald, T.T.; Collins, J.E. Inflammatory processes have differential effects on claudins 2, 3 and 4 in colonic epithelial cells. *Lab. Investig.* **2005**, *85*, 1139–1162. [CrossRef]
236. McCabe, R.P.; Secrist, H.; Botney, M.; Egan, M.; Peters, M.G. Cytokine mRNA expression in intestine from normal and inflammatory bowel disease patients. *Clin. Immunol. Immunopathol.* **1993**, *66*, 52–58. [CrossRef]
237. Nakamura, M.; Saito, H.; Kasanuki, J.; Tamura, Y.; Yoshida, S. Cytokine production in patients with inflammatory bowel disease. *Gut* **1992**, *33*, 55–58. [CrossRef]
238. Arend, W.P. The balance between IL-1 and IL-1Ra in disease. *Cytokine Growth Factor Rev.* **2002**, *13*, 323–340. [CrossRef]
239. Maeda, S.; Ohno, K.; Nakamura, K.; Uchida, K.; Nakashima, K.; Fukushima, K.; Tsukamoto, A.; Goto-Koshino, Y.; Fujino, Y.; Tsujimoto, H. Mucosal imbalance of interleukin-1β and interleukin-1 receptor antagonist in canine inflammatory bowel disease. *Vet. J.* **2012**, *194*, 66–70. [CrossRef]
240. Casini-Raggi, V.; Kam, L.; Chong, Y.J.T.; Fiocchi, C.; Pizarro, T.T.; Cominelli, F. Mucosal imbalance of IL-1 and IL-1 receptor antagonist in inflammatory bowel disease. A novel mechanism of chronic intestinal inflammation. *J. Immunol.* **1995**, *154*, 2434–2440.
241. Ngoh, E.N.; Weisser, S.B.; Lo, Y.; Kozicky, L.K.; Jen, R.; Brugger, H.K.; Menzies, S.C.; McLarren, K.W.; Nackiewicz, D.; van Rooijen, N.; et al. Activity of SHIP, which prevents expression of interleukin 1β, is reduced in patients with Crohn's disease. *Gastroenterology* **2016**, *150*, 465–476. [CrossRef]
242. MacDonald, T.T.; Bajaj-Elliott, M.; Pender, S.L.F. T cells orchestrate intestinal mucosal shape and integrity. *Immunol. Today* **1999**, *20*, 505–510. [CrossRef]
243. Louis, E.; Ribberns, C.; Godon, A.; I Franchimont, D.; De Groote, D.; Hardy, N.; Boniver, J.; Belaiche, J.; Malaise, M. Increased production of matrix metalloproteinase-3 and tissue inhibitor of metalloproteinase-1 by inflamed mucosa in inflammatory bowel disease. *Clin. Exp. Immunol.* **2000**, *120*, 241–246. [CrossRef] [PubMed]

244. Heuschkel, R.B.; MacDonald, T.T.; Monteleone, G.; Bajaj-Elliott, M.; Smith, J.A.; Pender, S.L. Imbalance of stromelysin-1 and TIMP-1 in the mucosal lesions of children with inflammatory bowel disease. *Gut* **2000**, *47*, 57–62. [CrossRef]
245. Saarialho-Kere, U.; Vaalamo, M.; Puolakkainen, P.; Airola, K.; Parks, W.C.; Karjalainen-Lindsberg, M.L. Enhanced expression of matrilysin, collagenase, and stromelysin-1 in gastrointestinal ulcers. *Am. J. Pathol.* **1996**, *148*, 519–526.
246. Monteleone, G.; Kumberova, A.; Croft, N.M.; McKenzie, C.; Steer, H.W.; MacDonald, T.T. Blocking Smad7 restores TGF-β1 signaling in chronic inflammatory bowel disease. *J. Clin. Investig.* **2001**, *108*, 601–609. [CrossRef] [PubMed]
247. Heller, F.; Florian, P.; Bojarski, C.; Richter, J.; Christ, M.; Hillenbrand, B.; Mankertz, J.; Gitter, A.H.; Bürgel, N.; Fromm, M.; et al. Interleukin-13 is the key effector th2 cytokine in ulcerative colitis that affects epithelial tight junctions, apoptosis, and cell restitution. *Gastroenterology* **2005**, *129*, 550–564. [CrossRef] [PubMed]
248. Pari, L.; Tewas, D.; Eckel, J. Role of curcumin in health and disease. *Arch. Physiol. Biochem.* **2008**, *114*, 127–149. [CrossRef] [PubMed]
249. Gupta, S.C.; Patchva, S.; Aggarwal, B.B. Therapeutic roles of curcumin: Lessons learned from clinical trials. *AAPS J.* **2013**, *15*, 195–218. [CrossRef] [PubMed]
250. Peterson, C.T.; Vaughn, A.R.; Sharma, V.; Chopra, D.; Mills, P.J.; Peterson, S.N.; Sivamani, R.K. Effects of turmeric and curcumin dietary supplementation on human gut microbiota: A double-blind, randomized, placebo-controlled pilot study. *J. Evid. Based Integr. Med.* **2018**, *23*, 1–8. [CrossRef]
251. Lao, C.D.; Ruffin, M.T.; Normolle, D.; Heath, D.D.; Murray, S.I.; Bailey, J.M.; Boggs, M.E.; Crowell, J.; Rock, C.L.; Brenner, D.E. Dose escalation of a curcuminoid formulation. *BMC Complement. Altern. Med.* **2006**, *6*, 10. [CrossRef]
252. De, R.; Kundu, P.; Swarnakar, S.; Ramamurthy, T.; Chowdhury, A.; Nair, G.B.; Mukhopadhyay, A.K. Antimicrobial activity of curcumin against Helicobacter pylori isolates from India and during infections in mice. *Antimicrob. Agents Chemother.* **2009**, *53*, 1592–1597. [CrossRef] [PubMed]
253. Rai, D.; Singh, J.K.; Roy, N.; Panda, D. Curcumin inhibits FtsZ assembly: An attractive mechanism for its antibacterial activity. *Biochem. J.* **2008**, *410*, 147–155. [CrossRef] [PubMed]
254. Niamsa, N.; Sittiwet, C. Antimicrobial activity of *Curcuma longa* aqueous extract. *J. Pharmacol. Toxicol.* **2009**, *4*, 173–177.
255. Patole, S. Microbiota and necrotizing enterocolitis. *Nestle Nutr. Inst. Workshop Ser.* **2017**, *88*, 81–94. [CrossRef]
256. Chassaing, B.; Darfeuille-Michaud, A. The commensal microbiota and enteropathogens in the pathogenesis of inflammatory bowel diseases. *Gastroenterology* **2011**, *140*, 1720–1728. [CrossRef] [PubMed]
257. Chow, J.; Tang, H.; Mazmanian, S.K. Pathobionts of the gastrointestinal microbiota and inflammatory disease. *Curr. Opin. Immunol.* **2011**, *23*, 473–480. [CrossRef] [PubMed]
258. Shen, L.; Liu, L.; Ji, H.-F. Regulative effects of curcumin spice administration on gut microbiota and its pharmacological implications. *Food Nutr. Res.* **2017**, *61*, 1361780. [CrossRef] [PubMed]
259. Feng, W.; Wang, H.; Zhang, P.; Gao, C.; Tao, J.; Ge, Z.; Zhu, D.; Bi, Y. Modulation of gut microbiota contributes to curcumin-mediated attenuation of hepatic steatosis in rats. *Biochim. Biophys. Acta* **2017**, *1861*, 1801–1812. [CrossRef]
260. Maslowski, K.M.; Vieira, A.T.; Ng, A.; Kranich, J.; Sierro, F.; Yu, D.; Schilter, H.C.; Rolph, M.S.; Mackay, F.; Artis, D.; et al. Regulation of inflammatory responses by gut microbiota and chemoattractant receptor GPR43. *Nature* **2009**, *461*, 1282–1286. [CrossRef]
261. De Filippo, C.; Cavalieri, D.; Di Paola, M.; Ramazzotti, M.; Poullet, J.B.; Massart, S.; Collini, S.; Pieraccini, G.; Lionetti, P. Impact of diet in shaping gut microbiota revealed by a comparative study in children from Europe and rural Africa. *Proc. Natl. Acad. Sci. USA* **2010**, *107*, 14691–14696. [CrossRef]
262. Zhang, Z.; Chen, Y.; Xiang, L.; Wang, Z.; Xiao, G.C.; Hu, J. Effect of curcumin on the diversity of gut microbiota in ovariectomized rats. *Nutrients* **2017**, *9*, 1146. [CrossRef] [PubMed]
263. Ohno, M.; Nishida, A.; Sugitani, Y.; Nishino, K.; Inatomi, O.; Sugimoto, M.; Kawahara, M.; Andoh, A. Nanoparticle curcumin ameliorates experimental colitis via modulation of gut microbiota and induction of regulatory T cells. *PLoS ONE* **2017**, *12*, e0185999. [CrossRef] [PubMed]
264. Law, I.K.; Bakirtzi, K.; Polytarchou, C.; Oikonomopoulos, A.; Hommes, D.; Iliopoulos, D.; Pothoulakis, C. Neurotensin—regulated miR-133alpha is involved in proinflammatory signaling in human colonic epithelial cells and in experimental colitis. *Gut* **2015**, *64*, 1095–1104. [CrossRef] [PubMed]

265. Narushima, S.; Sugiura, Y.; Oshima, K.; Atarashi, K.; Hattori, M.; Suematsu, M.; Honda, K. Characterization of the 17 strains of regulatory T cell-inducing human-derived Clostridia. *Gut Microbes* **2014**, *5*, 333–339. [CrossRef]
266. McFadden, R.M.; Larmonier, C.B.; Shehab, K.W.; Midura-Kiela, M.; Ramalingam, R.; Harrison, C.A.; Besselsen, D.G.; Chase, J.H.; Caporaso, J.G.; Jobin, C.; et al. The role of curcumin in modulating colonic microbiota during colitis and colon cancer prevention. *Inflamm. Bowel Dis.* **2015**, *21*, 2483–2494. [CrossRef]
267. Burapan, S.; Kim, M.; Han, J. Curcuminoid demethylation as an alternative metabolism by human intestinal microbiota. *J. Agric. Food Chem.* **2017**, *65*, 3305–3310. [CrossRef]
268. Hwang, S.W.; Kim, J.H.; Lee, C.; Im, I.P.; Kim, J.S. Intestinal alkaline phosphatase ameliorates experimental colitis via toll-like receptor 4-dependent pathway. *Eur. J. Pharmacol.* **2018**, *820*, 156–166. [CrossRef] [PubMed]
269. Boozari, M.; Butler, A.E.; Sahebkar, A. Impact of curcumin on toll-like receptors. *J. Cell. Physiol.* **2019**. Preprint. [CrossRef] [PubMed]
270. Gradišar, H.; Keber, M.M.; Pristovšek, P.; Jerala, R. MD-2 as the target of curcumin in the inhibition of response to LPS. *J. Leukoc. Biol.* **2007**, *82*, 968–974. [CrossRef]
271. Peng, L.; Li, X.; Song, S.; Wang, Y.; Xu, L. Effects of curcumin on mRNA expression of cytokines related to toll-like receptor 4 signaling in THP-1 cells. *Chin. J. Dermatol.* **2010**, *43*, 493–496.
272. Baliga, M.S.; Joseph, N.; Venkataranganna, M.V.; Saxena, A.; Ponemone, V.; Fayad, R. Curcumin, an active component of turmeric in the prevention and treatment of ulcerative colitis: Preclinical and clinical observations. *Food Funct.* **2012**, *3*, 1109–1117. [CrossRef] [PubMed]
273. Eckert, J.; Scott, B.; Lawrence, S.M.; Ihnat, M.; Chaaban, H. FLLL32, a curcumin analog, ameliorates intestinal injury in necrotizing enterocolitis. *J. Inflamm. Res.* **2017**, *10*, 75–81. [CrossRef] [PubMed]
274. Murano, M.; Maemura, K.; Hirata, I.; Toshina, K.; Nishikawa, T.; Hamamoto, N.; Sasaki, S.; Saitoh, O.; Katsu, K. Therapeutic effect of intracolonically administered nuclear factor kappa B (p65) antisense oligonucleotide on mouse dextran sulphate sodium (DSS)-induced colitis. *Clin. Exp. Immunol.* **2000**, *120*, 51–58. [CrossRef] [PubMed]
275. Gan, H.T.; Chen, Y.Q.; Ouyang, Q. Sulfasalazine inhibits activation of nuclear factor-kappaB in patients with ulcerative colitis. *J. Gastroenterol. Hepatol.* **2005**, *20*, 1016–1024. [CrossRef]
276. Hommes, D.; van den Blink, B.; Plasse, T.; Bartelsman, J.; Xu, C.; Macpherson, B.; Tytgat, G.; Peppelenbosch, M.; Van Deventer, S. Inhibition of stress-activated MAP kinases induces clinical improvement in moderate to severe Crohn's disease. *Gastroenterology* **2002**, *122*, 7–14. [CrossRef] [PubMed]
277. Pan, M.H.; Lin-Shiau, S.Y.; Lin, J.K. Comparative studies on the suppression of nitric oxide synthase by curcumin and its hydrogenated metabolites through down-regulation of IkappaB kinase and NFkappaB activation in macrophages. *Biochem. Pharmacol.* **2000**, *60*, 1665–1676. [CrossRef]
278. Jobin, C.; Bradham, C.A.; Russo, M.P.; Juma, B.; Narula, A.S.; Brenner, D.A.; Sartor, R.B. Curcumin blocks cytokine-mediated NF-κB activation and proinflammatory gene expression by inhibiting inhibitory factor I-κB kinase activity. *J. Immunol.* **1999**, *163*, 3474–3483.
279. Shishodia, S.; Singh, T.; Chaturvedi, M.M. Modulation of transcription factors by curcumin. *Adv. Exp. Med. Biol.* **2007**, *595*, 127–148. [CrossRef]
280. Hahm, E.R.; Cheon, G.; Lee, J.; Kim, B.; Park, C.; Yang, C.H. New and known symmetrical curcumin derivatives inhibit the formation of Fos-Jun-DNA complex. *Cancer Lett.* **2002**, *184*, 89–96. [CrossRef]
281. Huang, T.S.; Lee, S.C.; Lin, J.K. Suppression of c-Jun/AP-1 activation by an inhibitor of tumor promotion in mouse fibroblast cells. *Proc. Natl. Acad. Sci. USA* **1991**, *88*, 5292–5296. [CrossRef]
282. Huang, M.T.; Smart, R.C.; Wong, C.Q.; Conney, A.H. Inhibitory effect of curcumin, chlorogenic acid, caffeic acid, and ferulic acid on tumor promotion in mouse skin by 12-O-tetradecanoylphorbol-13-acetate. *Cancer Res.* **1988**, *48*, 5941–5946. [PubMed]
283. Ukil, A.; Maity, S.; Karmakar, S.; Datta, N.; Vedasiromoni, J.R.; Das, P.K. Curcumin, the major component of food flavour turmeric, reduces mucosal injury in trinitrobenzene sulphonic acid-induced colitis. *Br. J. Pharmacol.* **2003**, *139*, 209–2018. [CrossRef] [PubMed]
284. Salh, B.; Assi, K.; Templeman, V.; Parhar, K.; Owen, D.; Gomez-Munoz, A.; Jacobson, K. Curcumin attenuates DNB-induced murine colitis. *Am. J. Physiol. Gastrointest. Liver Physiol.* **2003**, *285*, G235–G243. [CrossRef] [PubMed]
285. Holt, P.R.; Katz, S.; Kirshoff, R. Curcumin therapy in inflammatory bowel disease: A pilot study. *Dig. Dis. Sci.* **2005**, *50*, 2191–2193. [CrossRef] [PubMed]

286. Moon, D.O.; Jin, C.Y.; Lee, J.D.; Choi, Y.H.; Ahn, S.C.; Lee, C.M.; Jeong, S.C.; Park, Y.M.; Kim, G.Y. Curcumin decreases binding of Shiga-like toxin-1B on human intestinal epithelial cell line HT29 stimulated with TNF-alpha and Il-1beta: Suppression of p38, JNK and NF-kappaB p65 as potential targets. *Biol. Pharm. Bull.* **2006**, *29*, 1470–1475. [CrossRef]
287. Jian, Y.T.; Mai, G.F.; Wang, J.D.; Zhang, Y.L.; Luo, R.C.; Fang, Y.X. Preventive and therapeutic effects of NF-κB inhibitor curcumin in rats colitis induced by trinitrobenzene sulfonic acid. *World J. Gastroenterol.* **2005**, *11*, 1747–1752. [CrossRef] [PubMed]
288. Camacho-Barquero, L.; Villegas, I.; Sánchez-Fidalgo, S.; Motilva, V.; de la Lastra, C.A. Curcumin, a Curcuma longa constituent, acts on MAPK p38 pathway modulating COX-2 and iNOS expression in chronic experimental colitis. *Int. Immunopharmacol.* **2007**, *7*, 333–342. [CrossRef] [PubMed]
289. Sugimoto, K.; Hanai, H.; Tozawa, K.; Aoshi, T.; Uchijima, M.; Nagata, T.; Koide, Y. Curcumin prevents and ameliorates trinitrobenzene sulfonic acid-induced colitis in mice. *Gastroenterology* **2002**, *123*, 1912–1922. [CrossRef]
290. Kim, G.Y.; Kim, K.H.; Lee, S.H.; Yoon, M.S.; Lee, H.J.; Moon, D.O.; Lee, C.M.; Ahn, S.C.; Park, Y.C.; Park, Y.M. Curcumin inhibits immunostimulatory function of dendritic cells: MAPKs and translocation of NF-kappa B as potential targets. *J. Immunol.* **2005**, *174*, 8116–8124. [CrossRef]
291. Cong, Y.; Wang, L.; Konrad, A.; Schoeb, T.; Elson, C.O. Curcumin induces the tolerogenic dendritic cell that promotes differentiation of intestine-protective regulatory T cells. *Eur. J. Immunol.* **2009**, *39*, 3134–3146. [CrossRef]
292. Abdollahi, E.; Momtazi, A.A.; Johnston, T.P.; Sahebkar, A. Therapeutic effects of curcumin in inflammatory and immune-mediated diseases: A nature-made jack-of-all-trades? *J. Cell Physiol.* **2018**, *233*, 830–848. [CrossRef] [PubMed]
293. Jung, I.D.; Jeong, Y.-I.; Lee, C.-M.; Noh, K.T.; Jeong, S.K.; Chun, S.H.; Choi, O.H.; Park, W.S.; Han, J.; Shin, Y.K.; et al. COX-2 and PGE2 signaling is essential for the regulation of IDO expression by curcumin in murine bone marrow-derived dendritic cells. *Int. Immunopharmacol.* **2010**, *10*, 760–768. [CrossRef] [PubMed]
294. Gao, X.; Kuo, J.; Jiang, H.; Deeb, D.; Liu, Y.; Divine, G.; Chapman, R.A.; Dulchavsky, S.A.; Gautam, S.C. Immunomodulatory activity of curcumin: Suppression of lymphocyte proliferation, development of cell-mediated cytotoxicity, and cytokine production in vitro. *Biochem. Pharmacol.* **2004**, *68*, 51–61. [CrossRef] [PubMed]
295. Yadav, V.S.; Mishra, K.P.; Singh, D.P.; Mehrota, S.; Singh, V.K. Immunomodulatory effects of curcumin. *Immunopharmacol. Immunotoxicol.* **2005**, *27*, 485–497. [CrossRef] [PubMed]
296. Jagetia, G.C.; Aggarwal, B.B. "Spicing up" of the immune system by curcumin. *J. Clin. Immunol.* **2007**, *27*, 19–35. [CrossRef]
297. Kang, B.Y.; Chung, S.W.; Chung, W.-J.; Im, S.-Y.; Hwang, S.Y.; Kim, T.S. Inhibition of interleukin-12 production in lipopolysaccharide-activated macrophages by curcumin. *Eur. J. Pharmacol.* **1999**, *384*, 191–195. [CrossRef]
298. Zhang, M.; Deng, C.S.; Zheng, J.J.; Xia, J. Curcumin regulated shift from Th1 to Th2 in trinitrobenzene sulphonic acid-induced chronic colitis. *Acta Pharmacol.* **2006**, *27*, 1071–1077. [CrossRef] [PubMed]
299. Bakır, B.; Yetkin Ay, Z.; Büyükbayram, H.İ.; Kumbul Doğuç, D.; Bayram, D.; Candan, I.A.; Uskun, E. Effect of curcumin on systemic T helper 17 cell response: Gingival expression of interleukin-17 and retinoic acid receptor-related orphan receptor γt and alveolar bone loss in experimental periodontitis. *J. Periodontol.* **2016**, *87*, e183–e191. [CrossRef]
300. Brouet, I.; Ohshima, H. Curcumin, an anti-tumour promoter and anti-inflammatory agent, inhibits induction of nitric oxide synthase in activated macrophages. *Biochem. Biophys. Res. Commun.* **1995**, *206*, 533–540. [CrossRef]
301. Mani, H.; Sidhu, G.S.; Kumari, R.; Gaddipati, J.P.; Seth, P.; Maheshwari, R.K. Curcumin differentially regulates TGF-β1, its receptors and nitrix oxide synthase during impaired wound healing. *BioFactors* **2002**, *16*, 29–43. [CrossRef]
302. Joe, B.; Lokesh, B.R. Role of capsaicin, curcumin and dietary *n*-3 fatty acids in lowering the generation of reactive oxygen species in rat peritoneal macrophages. *Biochim. Biophys. Acta* **1994**, *1224*, 255–263. [CrossRef]
303. Joe, B.; Lokesh, B.R. Dietary *n*-3 fatty acids, curcumin and capsaicin lower the release of lysosomal enzymes and eicosanoids in rat peritoneal macrophages. *Mol. Cell. Biochem.* **2000**, *203*, 153–161. [CrossRef] [PubMed]

304. Billerey-Larmonier, C.; Uno, J.K.; Larmonier, N.; Midura, A.J.; Timmermann, B.; Ghishan, F.K.; Kiela, P.R. Protective effects of dietary curcumin in mouse model of chemically induced colitis are strain dependent. *Inflamm. Bowel Dis.* **2008**, *14*, 780–793. [CrossRef] [PubMed]
305. Chan, M.M.; Huang, H.I.; Fenton, M.R.; Fong, D. In vivo inhibition of nitric oxide synthase gene expression by curcumin, a cancer preventive natural produce with anti-inflammatory properties. *Biochem. Pharmacol.* **1998**, *55*, 1955–1962. [CrossRef]
306. Li, X.; Liu, X. Effect of curcumin on immune function of mice. *J. Huazhong Univ. Sci. Technol. Med. Sci.* **2005**, *25*, 137–140. [PubMed]
307. Antony, S.; Kuttan, R.; Kuttan, G. Immunomodulatory activity of curcumin. *Immunol. Investig.* **1999**, *28*, 291–303. [CrossRef]
308. Bai, X.; Oberley-Deegan, R.E.; Bai, A.; Ovrutsky, A.R.; Kinney, W.H.; Weaver, M.; Zhang, G.; Honda, J.R.; Chan, E.D. Curcumin enhances human macrophage control of *Mycobacterium tuberculosis* infection. *Respirology* **2016**, *21*, 951–957. [CrossRef]
309. Mimche, P.N.; Thompson, E.; Taramelli, D.; Vivas, L. Curcumin enhances non-opsonic phagocytosis of *Plasmodium falciparum* through up-regulation of CD36 surface expression on monocytes/macrophages. *J. Antimicrob. Chemother.* **2012**, *67*, 1895–1904. [CrossRef]
310. Martin, A.R.; Villegas, I.; La Casa, C.; de la Lastra, C.A. Resveratrol, a polyphenol found in grapes, suppresses oxidative damage and stimulates apoptosis during early colonic inflammation in rats. *Biochem. Pharmacol.* **2004**, *67*, 1399–1410. [CrossRef]
311. Jiang, H.; Deng, C.S.; Zhang, M.; Xia, J. Curcumin-attenuated trinitrobenzene sulphonic acid induces chronic colitis by inhibiting expression of cyclooxygenase-2. *World J. Gastrolenterol.* **2006**, *12*, 3848–3853. [CrossRef]
312. Zhang, M.; Denc, C.; Zheng, J.; Xia, J.; Sheng, D. Curcumin inhibits trinitrobenzene sulphonic acid-induced colitis in rats by activation of peroxisome proliferator-activated receptor gamma. *Int. Immunopharmacol.* **2006**, *6*, 1233–1242. [CrossRef]
313. Larmonier, C.B.; Midura-Kiela, M.T.; Ramalingam, R.; Laubitz, D.; Janikashvili, N.; Larmonier, N.; Ghishan, F.K.; Kiela, P.R. Modulation of neutrophil motility by curcumin: Implications for inflammatory bowel disease. *Inflamm. Bowel Dis.* **2011**, *17*, 503–515. [CrossRef] [PubMed]
314. Larmonier, C.B.; Uno, J.K.; Lee, K.M.; Karrasch, T.; Laubitz, D.; Thurston, R.; Midura-Kiela, M.T.; Ghishan, F.K.; Sartor, R.B.; Jobin, C.; et al. Limited effects of dietary curcumin on Th-1 driven colitis in IL-10 deficient mice suggest an IL-10-dependent mechanism of protection. *Am. J. Physiol. Gastrointest. Liver Physiol.* **2008**, *295*, G1079–G1091. [CrossRef] [PubMed]
315. Srivastava, R. Inhibition of neutrophil response by curcumin. *Agents Actions* **1989**, *28*, 298–303. [CrossRef] [PubMed]
316. Okazaki, Y.; Han, Y.; Kayahara, M.; Watanabe, T.; Arishige, H.; Kato, N. Consumption of curcumin elevates fecal immunoglobulin A, an index of intestinal immune function, in rats fed a high-fat diet. *J. Nutr. Sci. Vitaminol.* **2010**, *56*, 68–71. [CrossRef] [PubMed]
317. Churchill, M.; Chadburn, A.; Bilinski, R.T.; Bertagnolli, M.M. Inhibition of intestinal tumors by curcumin is associated with changes in the intestinal immune cell profile. *J. Surg. Res.* **2000**, *89*, 169–175. [CrossRef]
318. Decoté-Ricardo, D.; Chagas, K.; Rocha, J.; Redner, P.; Lopes, U.; Cambier, J.; Pecanha, L. Modulation of in vitro murine B-lymphocyte response by curcumin. *Phytomedicine* **2009**, *16*, 982–988. [CrossRef]
319. Timmermans, W.M.C.; van Laar, J.A.M.; van der Houwen, T.B.; Kamphuis, L.S.J.; Bartol, S.J.W.; Lam, K.H.; Ouwendijk, R.J.; Sparrow, M.P.; Gibson, P.R.; van Hagen, P.M.; et al. B-cell dysregulation in Crohn's disease is partially restored with infliximab therapy. *PLoS ONE* **2016**, *11*, e0160103. [CrossRef] [PubMed]
320. Harrington, L.; Srikanth, C.V.; Antony, R.; Shi, H.N.; Cherayil, B.J. A role for natural killer cells in intestinal inflammation caused by infection with *Salmonella enterica* serovar Typhimurium. *FEMS Immunol. Med. Microbiol.* **2007**, *51*, 372–380. [CrossRef]
321. Mouzaoui, S.; Rahim, I.; Djerdjouri, B. Aminoguanidine and curcumin attenuated tumor necrosis factor (TNF)-alpha induced oxidative stress, colitis and hepatotoxicity in mice. *Int. Immunopharmacol.* **2012**, *12*, 302–311. [CrossRef]
322. Midura-Kiela, M.T.; Radhakrishnan, V.M.; Larmonier, C.B.; Laubitz, D.; Ghishan, F.K.; Kiela, P.R. Curcumin inhibits interferon-γ signaling in colonic epithelial cells. *Am. J. Physiol. Gastrointest. Liver Physiol.* **2012**, *302*, G85–G96. [CrossRef]

323. Kim, Y.S.; Young, M.R.; Bobe, G.; Colburn, N.H.; Milner, J.A. Bioactive food components, inflammatory targets, and cancer prevention. *Cancer Prev. Res.* **2009**, *2*, 200–208. [CrossRef] [PubMed]

324. Song, W.-B.; Wang, Y.-Y.; Meng, F.-S.; Zhang, Q.-H.; Zeng, J.-Y.; Xiao, L.-P.; Yu, X.-P.; Peng, D.-D.; Su, L.; Xiao, B.; et al. Curcumin protects intestinal mucosal barrier function of rat enteritis via activation of MKP-1 and attenuation of p38 and NF-κB activation. *PLoS ONE* **2010**, *5*, e12969. [CrossRef] [PubMed]

325. Zhang, X.; Wu, J.; Ye, B.; Wang, Q.; Xie, X.; Shen, H. Protective effect of curcumin on TNBS-induced intestinal inflammation is mediated through the JAK/STAT pathway. *BMC Complement. Altern. Med.* **2016**, *16*, 299. [CrossRef]

326. Kang, G.; Kong, P.J.; Yuh, Y.J.; Lim, S.Y.; Yim, S.V.; Chun, W.; Kim, S.S. Curcumin suppresses lipopolysaccharide-induced cyclooxygenase-2 expression by inhibiting activator protein 1 and nuclear factor kappaB bindings in BV2 microglial cells. *J. Pharmacol. Sci.* **2004**, *94*, 325–328. [CrossRef]

327. Plummer, S.M.; Holloway, K.A.; Manson, M.M.; Munks, R.J.; Kaptein, A.; Farrow, S.; Howells, L. Inhibition of cyclo-oxygenase 2 expression in colon cells by the chemoprotective agent curcumin involves inhibition of NF-kappaB activation via the NIK/IKK signaling complex. *Oncogene* **1999**, *18*, 6013–6020. [CrossRef] [PubMed]

328. Goel, A.; Boland, C.R.; Chauhan, D.P. Specific inhibition of cyclooxygenase-2 (COX-2) expression by dietary curcumin in HT-29 human colon cancer cells. *Cancer Lett.* **2001**, *172*, 111–118. [CrossRef]

329. Hanai, H.; Iida, T.; Takeuchi, K.; Watanabe, F.; Maruyama, Y.; Andoh, A.; Tsujikawa, T.; Fujiyama, Y.; Mitsuyama, K.; Sata, M.; et al. Curcumin maintenance therapy for ulcerative colitis: Randomized, multicenter, double-blind, placebo-controlled trial. *Clin. Gastroenterol. Hepatol.* **2006**, *4*, 1502–1506. [CrossRef]

330. Lang, A.; Salomon, N.; Wu, J.C.Y.; Kopylov, U.; Lahat, A.; Har-Noy, O.; Ching, J.Y.L.; Cheong, P.K.; Avidan, B.; Gamus, D.; et al. Curcumin in combination with mesalamine induces remission in patients with mild-to-moderate ulcerative colitis in randomized controlled trial. *Clin. Gastroenterol. Hepatol.* **2015**, *13*, 1444–1449. [CrossRef] [PubMed]

331. Babbs, C.F. Oxygen radicals in ulcerative colitis. *Free Radic. Biol. Med.* **1992**, *13*, 169–181. [CrossRef]

332. Grisham, M.B. Oxidants and free radicals in inflammatory bowel disease. *Lancet* **1994**, *344*, 859–861. [CrossRef]

333. Aceti, A.; Beghetti, I.; Martini, S.; Faldella, G.; Corvaglia, L. Oxidative stress and necrotizing enterocolitis: Pathogenetic mechanisms, opportunities for intervention, and the role of human milk. *Oxid. Med. Cell. Longev.* **2018**, *2018*, 7397659. [CrossRef] [PubMed]

334. Chen, M.L.; Ge, Z.; Fox, J.G.; Schauer, D.B. Disruption of tight junctions and induction of proinflammatory cytokine responses in colonic epithelial cells by *Campylobacter jejuni*. *Infect. Immun.* **2006**, *74*, 6581–6589. [CrossRef] [PubMed]

335. Tanida, S.; Mizoshita, T.; Mizushima, T.; Sasaki, M.; Shimura, T.; Kamiya, T.; Kataoka, H.; Joh, T. Involvement of oxidative stress and mucosal address in cell adhesion molecule-1 (MAdCAM-1) in inflammatory bowel disease. *J. Clin. Biochem. Nutr.* **2011**, *48*, 112–116. [CrossRef]

336. Basuroy, S.; Seth, A.; Elias, B.; Naren, A.P.; Rao, R. MAPK interacts with occluding and mediates EGF-induced prevention of tight junction disruption by hydrogen peroxide. *Biochem. J.* **2006**, *393 (Pt 1)*, 69–77. [CrossRef]

337. Grisham, M.B.; Yamada, T. Neutrophils, nitrogen oxides, and inflammatory bowel disease. *Ann. N. Y. Acad. Sci.* **1992**, *664*, 103–115. [CrossRef] [PubMed]

338. Lundberg, J.O.; Hellstrom, P.M.; Lundberg, J.M.; Alving, K. Greatly increased luminal nitric oxide in ulcerative colitis. *Lancet* **1994**, *344*, 1673–1674. [CrossRef]

339. Wallace, J.L.; Miller, M.J.S. Nitric oxide in mucosal defense: A little goes a long way. *Gastroenterology* **2000**, *119*, 512–520. [CrossRef]

340. Stroes, E.; Hijmering, M.; van Zandvoort, M.; Wever, R.; Rabelink, T.J.; Van Faassen, E.E. Origin of superoxide production by endothelial nitric oxide synthase. *FEBS Lett.* **1998**, *438*, 161–164. [CrossRef]

341. Cross, R.K.; Wilson, K.T. Nitric oxide in inflammatory bowel disease. *Inflamm. Bowel Dis.* **2003**, *9*, 179–189. [CrossRef]

342. Sreejayan; Rao, M.N. Curcuminoids as potent inhibitors of lipid peroxidation. *J. Pharm. Pharmacol.* **1994**, *46*, 1013–1016. [CrossRef] [PubMed]

343. Onoda, M.; Inano, H. Effect of curcumin on the production of nitric oxide by cultured rat mammary gland. *Nitric Oxide* **2000**, *4*, 505–515. [CrossRef]

344. Venkataranganna, M.V.; Rafiq, M.; Gopumadhavan, S.; Peer, G.; Babu, U.V.; Mitra, S.K. NCB-02 (standardized Curcumin preparation) protects dinitrochlorobenzene-induced colitis through down-regulation of NFkappa-B and iNOS. *World J. Gastroenterol.* **2007**, *13*, 1103–1107. [CrossRef]
345. Sanchez-Munoz, F.; Dominguez-Lopez, A.; Yamamoto-Furusho, J.K. Role of cytokines in inflammatory bowel disease. *World J. Gastroenterol.* **2008**, *14*, 4280–4288. [CrossRef] [PubMed]
346. Pedersen, G.; Saermark, T.; Kirkegaard, T.; Brynskov, J. Spontaneous and cytokine induced expression and activity of matrix metalloproteinases in human colonic epithelium. *Clin. Exp. Immunol.* **2009**, *155*, 257–265. [CrossRef] [PubMed]
347. Rath, T.; Roderfeld, M.; Halwe, J.M.; Tschuschner, A.; Roeb, E.; Graf, J. Cellular sources of MMP-7, MMP-13 and MMP-28 in ulcerative colitis. *Scand. J. Gastroenterol.* **2010**, *45*, 1186–1196. [CrossRef]
348. Koelink, P.J.; Overbeek, S.A.; Braber, S.; Morgan, M.E.; Henricks, P.A.; Abdul Roda, M.; Verspaget, H.W.; Wolfkamp, S.C.; te Velde, A.A.; Jones, C.W.; et al. Collagen degradation and neutrophilic infiltration: A vicious circle in inflammatory bowel disease. *Gut* **2014**, *63*, 578–587. [CrossRef]
349. Vandooren, J.; van den Steen, P.E.; Opdenakker, G. Biochemistry and molecular biology of gelatinase B or matrix metalloproteinase-9 (MMP-9): The next decade. *Crit. Rev. Biochem. Mol. Biol.* **2013**, *48*, 222–272. [CrossRef]
350. Thaloor, D.; Singh, A.K.; Sidhu, G.S.; Prasad, P.V.; Kleinman, H.K.; Maheshwari, R.K. Inhibition of angiogenic differentiation of human umbilical vein endothelial cells by curcumin. *Cell Growth Differ.* **1998**, *9*, 305–312.
351. Clutterbuck, A.L.; Allaway, D.; Harris, P.; Mobasheri, A. Curcumin reduces prostaglandin E2, matrix metalloproteinase-3 and proteoglycan release in the secretome of interleukin 1β-treated articular cartilage. *F1000 Res.* **2013**, *2*, 147. [CrossRef]
352. Hwang, B.M.; Noh, E.M.; Kim, J.S.; Kim, J.M.; You, Y.O.; Hwang, J.K.; Kwon, K.B.; Lee, Y.R. Curcumin inhibits UVB-induced matrix metalloproteinase-1/3 expression by suppressing the MAPK-p38/JNK pathways in human dermal fibroblasts. *Exp. Dermatol.* **2013**, *22*, 371–374. [CrossRef] [PubMed]
353. Kim, M.; Murakami, A.; Ohigashi, H. Modifying effects of dietary factors on (-)-epigallocatechin-3-galalte-induced pro-matrix metalloproteinase-7 production in HT-29 human colorectal cancer cells. *Biosci. Biotechnol. Biochem.* **2007**, *71*, 2442–2450. [CrossRef] [PubMed]
354. Li, W.; Kong, A.N. Molecular mechanisms of Nrf2-mediated antioxidant response. *Mol. Carcinog.* **2009**, *48*, 91–104. [CrossRef] [PubMed]
355. Motterlini, R.; Foresti, R.; Bassi, R.; Green, C.J. Curcumin, an antioxidant and anti-inflammatory agent, induces heme oxygenase-1 and protects endothelial cells against oxidative stress. *Free Radic. Biol. Med.* **2000**, *28*, 1303–1312. [CrossRef]
356. McNally, S.J.; Harrison, E.M.; Ross, J.A.; Garden, O.J.; Wigmore, S.J. Curcumin induces heme oxygenase 1 through generation of reactive oxygen species, p38 activation and phosphatase inhibition. *Int. J. Mol. Med.* **2007**, *19*, 165–172. [CrossRef] [PubMed]
357. Pedersen, C.B.; Gregersen, N. Stress response profiles in human fibroblasts exposed to heat shock or oxidative stress. *Methods Mol. Biol.* **2010**, *648*, 161–173. [CrossRef] [PubMed]
358. Liu, Z.; Dou, W.; Zheng, Y.; Wen, Q.; Qin, M.; Wang, X.; Tang, H.; Zhang, R.; Lv, D.; Wang, J.; Zhao, S. Curcumin upregulates Nrf2 translocation and protects rat hepatic stellate cells against oxidative stress. *Mol. Med. Rep.* **2016**, *13*, 1717–1724. [CrossRef]
359. Wang, N.; Wang, G.; Hao, J.; Ma, J.; Wang, Y.; Jiang, X.; Jiang, H. Curcumin ameliorates hydrogen peroxide-induced epithelial barrier disruption by upregulating heme oxygenase-1 expression in human intestinal epithelial cells. *Dig. Dis. Sci.* **2012**, *57*, 1792–1801. [CrossRef]

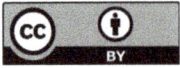 © 2019 by the authors. Licensee MDPI, Basel, Switzerland. This article is an open access article distributed under the terms and conditions of the Creative Commons Attribution (CC BY) license (http://creativecommons.org/licenses/by/4.0/).

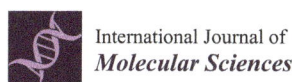

Review

Nutrition and Wound Healing: An Overview Focusing on the Beneficial Effects of Curcumin

Martina Barchitta [1], Andrea Maugeri [1], Giuliana Favara [1], Roberta Magnano San Lio [1], Giuseppe Evola [2], Antonella Agodi [1,*] and Guido Basile [3]

1. Department of Medical and Surgical Sciences and Advanced Technologies "GF Ingrassia", University of Catania, Via S. Sofia 87, 95123 Catania, Italy; martina.barchitta@unict.it (M.B.); andreamaugeri88@gmail.com (A.M.); giuliana.favara@gmail.com (G.F.); robimagnano@gmail.com (R.M.S.L.)
2. General and Emergency Surgery Department, Garibaldi Hospital, Piazza Santa Maria di Gesù, 95100 Catania, Italy; giuseppe_evola@hotmail.it
3. Department of General Surgery and Medical-Surgical Specialties, University of Catania, Via Plebiscito 628, 95124 Catania, Italy; gbasile@unict.it
* Correspondence: agodia@unict.it

Received: 25 January 2019; Accepted: 1 March 2019; Published: 5 March 2019

Abstract: Wound healing implicates several biological and molecular events, such as coagulation, inflammation, migration-proliferation, and remodeling. Here, we provide an overview of the effects of malnutrition and specific nutrients on this process, focusing on the beneficial effects of curcumin. We have summarized that protein loss may negatively affect the whole immune process, while adequate intake of carbohydrates is necessary for fibroblast migration during the proliferative phase. Beyond micronutrients, arginine and glutamine, vitamin A, B, C, and D, zinc, and iron are essential for inflammatory process and synthesis of collagen. Notably, anti-inflammatory and antioxidant properties of curcumin might reduce the expression of *tumor necrosis factor alpha* (*TNF-α*) and *interleukin-1* (*IL-1*) and restore the imbalance between reactive oxygen species (ROS) production and antioxidant activity. Since curcumin induces apoptosis of inflammatory cells during the early phase of wound healing, it could also accelerate the healing process by shortening the inflammatory phase. Moreover, curcumin might facilitate collagen synthesis, fibroblasts migration, and differentiation. Although curcumin could be considered as a wound healing agent, especially if topically administered, further research in wound patients is recommended to achieve appropriate nutritional approaches for wound management.

Keywords: wound; wound healing; diet; nutrition; micronutrients; macronutrients; curcumin; amino-acids; vitamins; minerals

---

1. Introduction

Wound healing implicates a well-orchestrated complex of biological and molecular events that involve cell migration, cell proliferation, and extracellular matrix deposition. Although these processes are similar to those driving embryogenesis, tissue and organ regeneration, and even pathological conditions [1,2], certain differences exist between adult wounds and these other systems. In acute wounds—cutaneous injuries that do not have an underpinning pathophysiological defect—the main evolutionary force may have been to achieve repair quickly and with the smallest amount of energy [2]. In contrast, evolutionary adaptations have probably not occurred in chronic wounds with pre-existing pathophysiological abnormalities, resulting in impaired healing [3]. Wound care places an enormous drain on healthcare resources worldwide. For instance, in the United States, it has been estimated that 3% individuals over 65 years will have a wound at any one time [4], with an estimated cost to the healthcare system of approximately US $25 billion each year [5]. In low-income countries, an even higher incidence, due to traumatic injuries and ulcers, is expected. Recently, the World Health Organization (WHO) has recognized the unmet need for an interdisciplinary approach facing this global challenge, which has been accordingly addressed by the Association for the Advancement of Wound Care (AAWC) Global Volunteers program [6].

Despite strides in technological innovations of a wide range of treatments against wounds, non-healing wounds continue to challenge physicians. Hence, further efforts are needed to improve our scientific understanding of the repair process and how that knowledge can be used to develop new approaches to treatment. Malnutrition is a common risk factor that might contribute to impaired wound healing [7–9]. In recent years, several lines of evidence have pointed out biochemical and molecular effects of several nutrients in the wound healing process, supporting the notion that a complementary nutritional approach might be useful in wound treatment, especially for chronic non-healing wounds [10]. Here, we provide an overview of biological and molecular events in wound healing and the effects of malnutrition and specific nutrients on this process (search strategy and selection criteria are shown in Figure 1). In line with the current Special Issue "Curcumin in Health and Disease", we have also focused on beneficial effects and related molecular mechanisms of curcumin—a natural phenol from the rhizome of *Curcuma longa*—which might enhance healing processes via antioxidant and anti-inflammatory properties [11]. In fact, curcumin was commonly used in traditional medicine for the treatment of biliary and hepatic disorders, cough, diabetic ulcers, rheumatism and sinusitis [11]. More recently, curcumin has been investigated extensively as an anti-cancer [12], anti-aging [13], and wound healing agent [11]. For instance, it has been demonstrated the beneficial effect of curcumin on the progression of endometriosis, a common disorder affecting women during reproductive age which shares some molecular events with wound healing (i.e., adhesion and proliferation, cellular invasion and angiogenesis) [14]. To date, most of the current knowledge on wound healing derives from in vitro and in vivo studies, while epidemiological investigations are scarce. To solve the question of whether curcumin is a suitable wound healing agent, we have summarized its biochemical and molecular effects during the different phases of wound healing, as well as evidence from epidemiological studies.

> **Search strategy and selection criteria**
>
> We searched PubMed by using the following terms: ("Wound healing" OR "Wounds") AND ("Nutrition" OR "Nutrients" OR "Curcumin"). We selected articles from inception to December 2018. Original articles and reviews were included with no restriction on language of publication.

Figure 1. Search strategy and selection criteria.

1.1. The Wound Healing Process and Impaired Healing

The type, size, and depth of wounds have significant repercussions on cellular and molecular events that occur after cutaneous injury. As reviewed by Falanga [15], it is useful to divide the wound healing process into four overlapping steps of coagulation, inflammation, migration-proliferation, and remodeling (Figure 2). While acute wounds show a linear progression of these overlapping events, the progression in chronic wounds does not occur in synchrony, with some areas being in different phases at the same time [15].

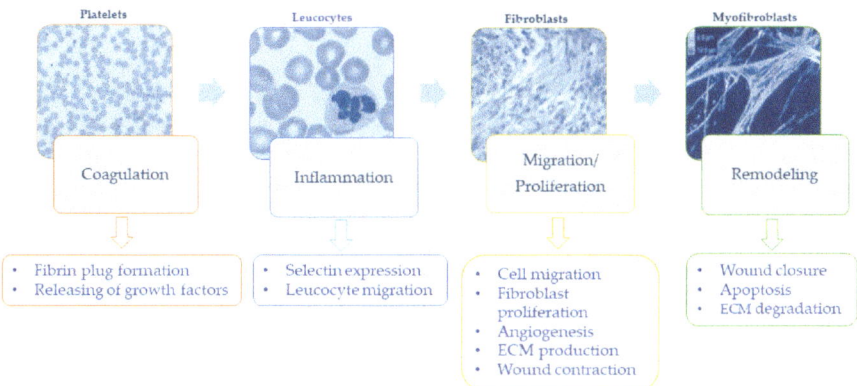

Figure 2. Phases and specific events of the wound healing process.

In the first phase after injury, the formation of a fibrin plug (i.e., an aggregate of platelets, fibrinogen, fibronectin, vitronectin, and thrombospondin) is necessary both for hemostasis and for covering and protecting the wound from bacteria [2,16]. Beyond that, fibrin plug also provides an extracellular matrix for cell migration [2] and releases growth factors (e.g., platelet-derived growth factor—PDGF—and transforming growth factor—TGF) involved in the recruitment of cells to the wound [1,2]. In the inflammatory phase, endothelial expression of selectins slows down leukocytes in the bloodstream, so as to enable them to move through endothelial gaps by binding to integrins into the extracellular area [1]. Neutrophils and macrophages recruited to the wound remove foreign particles and produce a wide range of growth factors and cytokines that promote fibroblast migration and proliferation [17]. Hypoxia—which occurs immediately after injury—is one of the main triggers of keratinocyte migration, angiogenesis, fibroblast proliferation, and the releasing of growth factors and cytokines (i.e., PDGF, vascular endothelial growth factor, and TGF) [18]. Later, fibroblasts and endothelial cells form the early granulation tissue that begins the processes of wound contraction, which in turn is an efficient driver of wound closure [2]. Extracellular matrix proteins are crucial in this phase because they provide substrates for cell migration and structures that restore the function and integrity of the tissue [18]. The formation of new blood vessels re-establishes tissue perfusion, allowing for the re-supply of oxygen and other nutrients [17]. Finally, once closure of wound has been achieved, remodeling of the resulting scar takes places over weeks or months, with a reduction of both cell content and blood flow, degradation of extracellular matrix, and further contraction and tensile strength [15].

While venous or arterial insufficiency, diabetes, and local-pressure are the most common pathophysiological causes of wounds and ulcers, several local and systemic factors can impair wound healing. The first ones consist of the presence of foreign bodies, tissue maceration, ischemia, and infection. The second ones include aging, malnutrition, diabetes, and renal diseases. In addition to these factors, a reduction in active growth factors may partially explain why certain wounds fail to heal. Chronic ulcers seem to have reduced levels of PDGF, TGF, and other growth factors than acute wounds [19]. Plausible explanations are that growth factors might be trapped by the extracellular matrix [20] or that they might be excessively degraded by proteases [21]. Moreover, in chronic wounds, fibroblasts show a decreased potential of proliferation accompanied by an increased number of senescent cells that might impair responsiveness to growth hormones [22].

1.2. Malnutrition, Macronutrients, and Chronic Wounds

According to the WHO, malnutrition refers to all forms of deficiency, excess, or imbalance in a person's intake of energy and/or nutrients [23]. In old people—who are at the highest risk of chronic wounds also due to coexisting diseases—malnutrition often consists of either protein-energy malnutrition or specific vitamin and mineral deficiencies [8]. Several age-related conditions increase the risk of developing nutritional deficiencies, such as clinical, physiological, and socio-economic difficulties that usually affect the elderly [8]. Particularly, in diabetic patients, higher glucose levels could interfere with the process of nutrient absorption, causing the depletion of several nutrients (i.e., magnesium, zinc, B12, B6, folic acid) [24]. While the response to an injury may increase the metabolic needs of the wound area, large amounts of protein can be continually lost through wound exudates [25]. Hence, protein and energy requirements of chronic wound patients may rise by 250% and 50%, respectively [26]. Since cells involved in wound healing require proteins for their formation and activity, protein loss may negatively affect the whole immune process. Proteins are also necessary for immune response, which in turn, if impaired, may delay the progression from the inflammatory to the proliferative phase. In the proliferative and remodeling phases, protein-energy deficiency may also decrease fibroblast activity, delaying angiogenesis and reducing collagen formation [8]. Moreover, protein-calorie deficiency is also associated with weight loss and decreased lean body mass [27]. Hence, implications of weight loss and decreased lean body mass should be recognized when considering the effect of protein-calorie deficiency on the healing process. In general, losing ≈10% lean mass is associated with impaired immunity and increased risk of infection. In case patients lose more than 10% lean body mass, wound healing competes with body demands to restore lean mass: The metabolism gives priority to healing in patients who lose up to 20%, while it delays healing to restore lean body mass in those who lose more than 30% [25,28].

Beyond proteins, both carbohydrates and fats address increased energy needs to support inflammatory response, cellular activity, angiogenesis, and collagen deposition in the proliferative phase of healing process [26]. Particularly, adequate intake of carbohydrates is necessary for fibroblast production and movement, and leukocyte activity [29]. Carbohydrates also stimulate secretion of hormones and growth factors, including insulin that is helpful in the anabolic processes of the proliferative phase. In contrast, hyperglycemia and its complications might reduce granulocyte function and promote wound formation [7]. Fats have structural functions in the lipid bilayer of cell membranes during tissue growth. They are also precursors of prostaglandins—which in turn are mediators of cellular inflammation and metabolism—and participate in several signaling pathways [30]. To date, the effect of supplementation of essential fatty acids on wound healing is controversial. While omega-3 supplementation might decrease wound tensile strength with a harmful effect on healing [31], its combination with omega-6 decreases the progression of pressure ulcers [32]. In line with this evidence, the co-supplementation of omega-3 and omega-6 might lead to benefits, especially during the inflammatory phase [33].

1.3. Micronutrients and Wound Healing

1.3.1. Amino-Acids

Micronutrients involved in the wound healing process have been extensively reviewed [7–9,33]. Among amino-acids, those that play an important role in wound healing, are arginine and glutamine. The first is a precursor of nitric oxide and proline, which in turn are essential for the inflammatory process [34] and synthesis of collagen [35,36]. Arginine also stimulates the production and secretion of growth hormone, as well as the activation of T cells [37,38]. In wound patients with adequate protein intake, the recommended dose of arginine supplementation is 4.5 g/day, while it is useless in the context of protein deficiency [39]. Glutamine plays several roles via its metabolic, enzymatic, antioxidant, and immune properties. In wounds, it protects against the risk of infectious and inflammatory complications by up-regulating the expression of heat shock proteins [40]. Glutamine is also a precursor of glutathione—an antioxidant and an essential cofactor of several enzymatic reactions—which is important for stabilizing cell membranes and for transporting amino acids across them [41]. In addition, glutamine seems involved in the inflammatory phase of wound healing by regulating leukocyte apoptosis, superoxide production, antigen processing, and phagocytosis [40,42]. As for arginine, benefits of glutamine supplementation are still controversial [43] and confounded by the combinations of supplements [44].

1.3.2. Vitamins

Vitamins are undoubtedly the most investigated micronutrients in the wound healing process. Vitamin A deficiency impairs B cell and T cell function and antibody production during the inflammatory phase. It also decreases epithelialization, collagen synthesis, and granulation tissue development in the proliferative and remodeling phases [45]. In addition, vitamin A seems to work as a hormone that modulates the activity of epithelial and endothelial cells, melanocytes, and fibroblasts by binding to retinoic acid receptors [46]. In general, vitamin A is topically administered for the care of dermatologic conditions due to its stimulating properties of fibroplasia and epithelialization [33]. In wound patients, it has been recommended to have a short-term supplementation of 10,000–25,000 IU/day to avoid toxicity [33]. Interestingly, vitamin A supplementation counteracts the delay in wound healing caused by corticosteroids for the treatment of inflammatory diseases [47] by down-regulating *TGF-β* and insulin-like growth factor-1 (*IGF-1*) [48]. B vitamins, which consist of thiamine, riboflavin, pyridoxine, folic acid, pantothenate, and cobalamins, are essential cofactors in enzyme reactions involved in leukocyte formation and in anabolic processes of wound healing. Among these, thiamine, riboflavin, pyridoxine and cobalamins are also required for the synthesis of collagen [25]. Hence, vitamin B deficiencies indirectly affect the wound healing process by impairing antibody production and white blood cell function, which in turn increase the risk of infectious complications [49]. Vitamin C seems to be involved in wound healing with several roles in cell migration and transformation, collagen synthesis, antioxidant response, and angiogenesis.

In the inflammatory phase, it participates in the recruitment of cells to the wound and their transformation into macrophages [29]. During collagen synthesis, vitamin C forms extra-bounds between collagen fibers that increase stability and strength of collagen matrix [8]. Vitamin C is essential to counteract the production of free radicals in damaged cells, while its deficiency might increase the fragility of new vessels [50]. The current recommendation of vitamin C supplementation ranges from 500 mg/day in non-complicated wounds to 2 g/day in severe wounds [33]. However, vitamin C supplementation seems to have a beneficial effect only in combination with zinc and arginine, and in pressure ulcer patients [51]. Vitamin D and its receptor (i.e., VDR)—which is ubiquitously expressed in several tissues—modulate structural integrity and transport across epithelial barriers [52]. In line with its roles, recent evidence of vitamin D deficiency among venous and pressure ulcer patients has suggested the potential involvement of vitamin D in the wound healing process [53,54]. However, further research is recommended to understand how vitamin D supplementation might be used in wound care. Although most vitamins show beneficial effects in wound healing, vitamin E might negatively affect collagen synthesis, antioxidant response, and the inflammatory phase [55]. Moreover, vitamin E appears to counteract the benefits of vitamin A supplementation in wound management [56].

1.3.3. Minerals

Several minerals are involved in the wound healing process due to their roles as enzyme structural factors, metalloenzymes, and antioxidants. Among these, zinc is essential for DNA replication in cells with high cell division rates, such as inflammatory and epithelial cells, and fibroblasts. In the inflammatory phase, zinc promotes immune response and counteracts susceptibility to infectious complications by activating lymphocytes and producing antibodies [30]. In the proliferative and remodeling phases, it is essential for collagen production, fibroblast proliferation, and epithelialization by stimulating the activity of involved enzymes [8]. Although zinc supplementation of 40–220 mg/day for 10–14 days [57] might be useful in zinc-deficient patients, its benefits in non-deficient patients are currently under debate [9]. Interestingly, topical administration of zinc to surgical wounds significantly improves the healing process [58]. In contrast, conditions that affect zinc metabolism and potential drug-nutrient interactions should be considered for the management of wound patients with zinc supplementation [58]. Less evidence exists on the beneficial effects of iron supplementation for promoting wound healing. As iron transports oxygen to the tissues, it is essential for tissue perfusion and collagen synthesis. Hence, iron deficiency results in tissue ischemia, impaired collagen production, and decreased wound strength in the proliferative phase [30].

1.4. Curcumin and Wound Healing

In 1910, Milobedzka and colleagues described for the first time the structure of curcumin (Figure 3), one of the three curcuminoids extracted from the powdered rhizome of turmeric plant (*Curcuma longa*) [59]. More recently, it has been demonstrated that curcumin might modulate physiological and molecular events involved in the inflammatory and proliferative phases of the wound healing process [60].

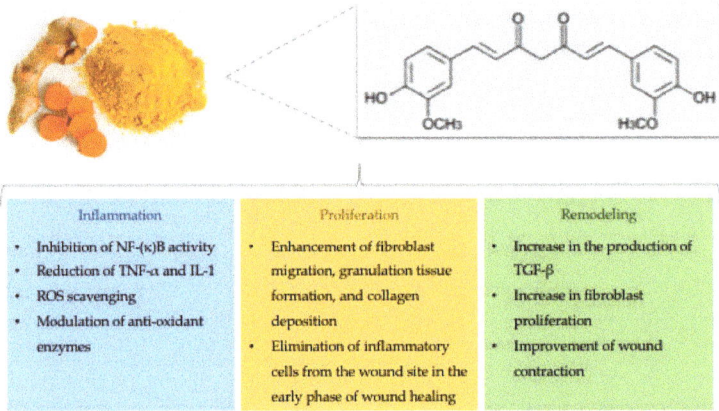

Figure 3. Structure and effects of curcumin on wound healing.

1.4.1. Effects on the Inflammatory Phase

With respect to the inflammatory phase, several studies have revealed the protective effect of curcumin that reduces the expression of pro-inflammatory cytokines, such as tumor necrosis factor alpha (*TNF-α*) and interleukin-1 (*IL-1*) [61]. Accordingly, curcumin recruits M2-like macrophages into white adipose tissues, thereby increasing the production of anti-inflammatory cytokines that are essential for the inflammatory response [62]. In addition, curcumin also inhibits nuclear factor κB (NF-κB) by suppressing the activity of kinases (i.e., AKT, PI3K, IKK) involved in several pathways. In general, NF-κB is physiologically inactivated by binding to its inhibitor IκB. During inflammation, the up-regulation of inflammatory mediators (i.e., cytokines and chemokines) activates NF-κB, which in turn translocates to the nucleus [63]. In wounded sites, curcumin might reduce inflammation caused by the activation of the NF-κB pathway [64]. The anti-inflammatory effects of curcumin are also involved in other signaling pathways, such as peroxisome proliferator-activated receptor-gamma (PPAR-γ) and myeloid differentiation protein 2-TLR 4 co-receptor (TLR4-MD2) [65–68]. Li and colleagues have reported that curcumin suppresses proliferation of vascular smooth muscle cells by increasing PPAR-γ activity to mitigate angiotensin II-induced inflammatory responses [67]. Additionally, it has been shown that curcumin reduces inflammation through competition with LPS for binding on MD2, thereby inhibiting the TLR4-MD2 signaling complex [68].

Since NF-κB has also several anti-oxidant targets, in 2004, Frey and Malik proposed a relationship between inflammation and oxidation during the wound healing process [69]. In wounds, ROS formation triggers the production and activity of various immune cells (i.e., T lymphocyte subsets, macrophages, dendritic cells, B lymphocytes, and natural killer cells). Moreover, prolonged high ROS concentrations are dangerous for cell structures leading to oxidative stress [70,71]. Particularly, hydrogen peroxide (H_2O_2) and superoxide (O_2^-) can be considered as potential markers for the amount of oxidative stress [72]. Although anti-oxidant enzymes (i.e., superoxide dismutase, glutathione peroxidase, and catalase) protect cells against toxic ROS levels [73], the imbalance between ROS concentrations and antioxidant activity could determine chronic diseases. Beyond its anti-inflammatory properties, curcumin also acts as an antioxidant by scavenging ROS, by restoring abnormal changes induced by external factors, and by suppressing transcription factors related to oxidation [74,75]. In vitro and in vivo studies have demonstrated the antioxidant activities of curcumin conferred by its electron-donating groups (i.e., the phenolic hydroxyl group) [76]. Moreover, it contributes to the production and activity of antioxidant enzymes [77,78] and their constituents, such as glutathione (GSH) [79]. In line with these findings, Phan and colleagues have revealed the protective role of curcumin against hydrogen peroxide in keratinocytes and fibroblasts [80].

1.4.2. Effects on the Proliferative and Remodeling Phases

As discussed below, curcumin also plays a critical role during the proliferative phase. Interestingly, Gopinath and colleagues have observed that curcumin ameliorates the above-mentioned process, resulting in an increase of hydroxyproline and collagen synthesis [74]. This is consistent with previous studies demonstrating that curcumin decreases the amount of membrane matrix metallo-proteinases (MMPs), which are usually higher in endometriotic mice and human ovarian endometriotic stromal cells. These pathological conditions, in fact, share some molecular events with wound healing, including adhesion and proliferation, cellular invasion, and angiogenesis. Particularly, curcumin could be involved in the process of endometriosis by decreasing the growth and number of endometriotic stromal cells [81]. With respect to wounds, Panchatcharam and colleagues have demonstrated that collagen fibers could mature earlier when wound rats are topically treated with curcumin [70]. Although curcumin does not seem to be involved in the migration of fibroblasts to the wound area in vitro [17], an in vivo study has suggested that curcumin mediates the infiltration of fibroblasts into wound sites, which in turn naturally differentiates into myofibroblasts during the formation of granulation tissue [82]. This controversy might be due to difficulties in creating an in vitro model of fibroblast migration in wounds. Treatment with curcumin also promotes the differentiation of fibroblasts into myofibroblasts [83–86] which marks the beginning of wound contraction [87]. A previous study has also demonstrated that curcumin reduces the epithelialization period of treated wounds if compared with the control group [70]. Finally, once closure of the wound has been achieved, apoptotic processes discard inflammatory cells from wound sites [88–90]. Since curcumin induces apoptosis during the early phase of wound healing, it could also accelerate the healing process by shortening the inflammatory phase [85].

2. Discussion

Our review summarizes current evidence about the main biochemical and molecular effects of nutrition, in terms of quality and quantity, on the wound healing process. In line with the Special Issue "Curcumin in Health and Disease", we have focused on the beneficial effects of curcumin, which exerts its anti-inflammatory and antioxidant properties during the different phases of the wound healing process [11]. Several lines of evidence from in vitro and in vivo studies have reported that curcumin might modulate physiological and molecular events during the inflammatory phase [60,61,65–68,85]. Moreover, it also exerts antioxidant effects by restoring the imbalance between ROS production and antioxidant activity [74–80]. In the proliferative phase, curcumin might facilitate collagen synthesis [70,74], fibroblasts migration [82], and differentiation [83–86]. In addition, curcumin appears to be beneficial for epithelialization [70] and for apoptotic processes that discard inflammatory cells from the wound site [88–90]. An in vivo study has suggested that curcumin mediates the infiltration of fibroblasts into wound sites, which in turn naturally differentiates into myofibroblasts during the formation of granulation tissue [82]. By contrast, curcumin does not seem to be involved in the migration of fibroblasts to the wound area in vitro [17].

This controversy might be due to difficulties in creating an in vitro model of fibroblast migration in wounds. In fact, fibroblast migration depends on several factors that cannot be entirely mimicked with in vitro models, such as cell-environment interactions and homeostatic mechanisms [17]. Recently, in wounds of diabetic rats, it has been demonstrated that topical curcumin treatment enhances angiogenesis, thereby ameliorating the healing process [91]. In line with these findings, curcumin could be considered an interesting phytochemical candidate for the treatment of non-healing wounds. Interestingly, its pleiotropic effect on several signaling pathways—by modulating cellular regulatory systems, such as NF-κB, AKT, growth factors, and Nrf2 transcription factor [92–95]—might be explained by its well-established role in epigenetic mechanisms, such as DNA methylation and histone modification [96]. An understanding of epigenetic regulation in the wound healing process is now becoming an attractive field of research [97], and more efforts should be made to uncover mechanisms underpinning beneficial effects of curcumin and other polyphenols [96,98]. As mentioned above, however, most of these findings come from in vitro or in vivo investigations, while evidence from epidemiological studies is scarce. Given its hydrophobicity and extensive first-pass metabolism [99,100], topical administration of curcumin has a greater effect on wound healing than oral administration [64,88,89]. Despite strides which have been made in the formulation of curcumin for topical application at the wound site [74,83–85,101], further research is recommended to improve curcumin delivery and to evaluate its effects in wound patients.

Beyond assessing the potential of curcumin as a wound healing agent, we have also indicated that nutritional assessment in patients at risk of chronic wounds could be the first step towards the prevention of non-healing wounds. In fact, these patients often exhibit protein-energy malnutrition or specific vitamin and mineral deficiencies [8]. The wound healing process, for its part, increases the needs of calories and proteins of the wound area, thereby increasing the requirements from chronic wound patients [26]. Given that protein-calorie deficiencies are further associated with weight loss and decreased lean body mass [27], their implications for wound patients should be also recognized. To meet the increased need of energy, especially during the proliferative phase, wounds also metabolize carbohydrates and fats [26], which in turn are necessary for fibroblast and leukocyte activities, secretion of hormones and growth factors, and structural functions [29,30]. Despite this evidence, the effect of macronutrient supplementation is currently controversial, raising the need for further research. For instance, it has been demonstrated that omega-6 supplementation decreases the progression of pressure ulcers [32], and its combination with omega-3 has beneficial effects on the inflammatory phase [33]. However, omega-3 supplementation alone has harmful effects on healing [31].

Beyond macronutrients, several micronutrients play a crucial role in the wound healing process, as extensively reviewed [7–9,33]. Arginine and glutamine exhibit several metabolic, enzymatic, antioxidant, and anti-inflammatory properties that are involved in the inflammatory phase [34,37,38,40,42] and in collagen synthesis [35,36]. However, the beneficial effect of the supplementation of glutamine and arginine, alone or in combination, is still controversial [43,44], probably due to differences in study design, patient characteristics, and type of supplementation. Most of the evidence comes from research on vitamins, with several lines of evidence supporting the benefits of vitamin A [33,47,48], vitamin B [49], vitamin C [8,29,50] and vitamin D [53,54] supplementation. However, to what extent they support wound healing process remains unclear until now. For instance, vitamin C seems to act only in combination with zinc and arginine [51], while vitamin E appears to counteract the benefits of vitamin A [56]. Among minerals, zinc is essential for the inflammatory, proliferative, and remodeling phases by promoting immune response, collagen production, fibroblast proliferation, and epithelialization [8]. Accordingly, topical zinc administration to surgical wounds significantly facilitates wound healing process [58]. These findings cumulatively suggest that nutritional approaches might be useful in the treatment of wounds, especially of chronic non-healing wounds [10]. However, benefits in non-deficient patients are currently under debate [9], and further research should take into account conditions that affect nutrient metabolism, such as diabetes and potential nutrient–nutrient interactions [58].

3. Conclusions

In conclusion, we support the notion that curcumin could be considered as a wound healing agent, especially if topically administered. However, most of the current knowledge is derived from in vitro and in vivo investigations, while studies in wound patients remain scarce or controversial. Moreover, since nutrition and nutrients in general might affect the wound healing process, nutritional assessment of patients at risk of non-healing wounds could be the first step towards prevention and treatment. However, further research is recommended to develop appropriate nutritional approaches for wound management.

Author Contributions: Conceptualization, A.M., M.B., A.A. and G.B.; methodology, A.M. and M.B.; writing—original draft preparation, A.M., G.F., R.M.S.L., G.E., and A.A.; writing—review and editing, all the authors.

Funding: This research was partially funded by the Department of Medical and Surgical Sciences and Advanced Technologies "GF Ingrassia", University of Catania, Catania, Italy.

Conflicts of Interest: The authors declare no conflict of interest.

Abbreviations

AAWC	Advancement of Wound Care
GSH	Glutathione
H_2O_2	Hydrogen Peroxide
IGF-1	Insulin-Like Growth Factor-1
IL-1	Interleukin-1
NF-κB	Nuclear Factor κB
O_2^-	Hydrogen Superoxide
PDGF	Platelet-Derived Growth Factor
PPAR-γ	Peroxisome Proliferator-Activated Receptor-Gamma
ROS	Reactive Oxygen Species
TGF	Transforming Growth Factor
TLR4-MD2	Myeloid Differentiation Protein 2-TLR 4 Co-Receptor
TNF-α	Tumor Necrosis Factor Alpha
VDR	Vitamin D Receptor
WHO	World Health Organization

References

1. Martin, P. Wound healing—Aiming for perfect skin regeneration. *Science* **1997**, *276*, 75–81. [CrossRef] [PubMed]
2. Singer, A.J.; Clark, R.A. Cutaneous wound healing. *N. Engl. J. Med.* **1999**, *341*, 738–746. [CrossRef] [PubMed]
3. Harding, K.G.; Morris, H.L.; Patel, G.K. Science, medicine and the future: Healing chronic wounds. *BMJ* **2002**, *324*, 160–163. [CrossRef] [PubMed]
4. Reiber, G.E. Diabetic foot care. Financial implications and practice guidelines. *Diabetes Care* **1992**, *15* (Suppl. 1), 29–31. [CrossRef]
5. Sen, C.K.; Gordillo, G.M.; Roy, S.; Kirsner, R.; Lambert, L.; Hunt, T.K.; Gottrup, F.; Gurtner, G.C.; Longaker, M.T. Human skin wounds: A major and snowballing threat to public health and the economy. *Wound Repair Regen.* **2009**, *17*, 763–771. [CrossRef] [PubMed]
6. Serena, T.E. A Global Perspective on Wound Care. *Adv. Wound Care (New Rochelle)* **2014**, *3*, 548–552. [CrossRef] [PubMed]
7. Quain, A.M.; Khardori, N.M. Nutrition in Wound Care Management: A Comprehensive Overview. *Wounds* **2015**, *27*, 327–335. [PubMed]

8. Harris, C.L.; Fraser, C. Malnutrition in the institutionalized elderly: The effects on wound healing. *Ostomy Wound Manag.* **2004**, *50*, 54–63.
9. Thompson, C.; Fuhrman, M.P. Nutrients and wound healing: Still searching for the magic bullet. *Nutr. Clin. Pract.* **2005**, *20*, 331–347. [CrossRef] [PubMed]
10. Enoch, S.; Grey, J.E.; Harding, K.G. ABC of wound healing. Non-surgical and drug treatments. *BMJ* **2006**, *332*, 900–903. [CrossRef] [PubMed]
11. Akbik, D.; Ghadiri, M.; Chrzanowski, W.; Rohanizadeh, R. Curcumin as a wound healing agent. *Life Sci.* **2014**, *116*, 1–7. [CrossRef] [PubMed]
12. Agrawal, D.K.; Mishra, P.K. Curcumin and its analogues: Potential anticancer agents. *Med. Res. Rev.* **2010**, *30*, 818–860. [CrossRef] [PubMed]
13. Lima, C.F.; Pereira-Wilson, C.; Rattan, S.I. Curcumin induces heme oxygenase-1 in normal human skin fibroblasts through redox signaling: Relevance for anti-aging intervention. *Mol. Nutr. Food Res.* **2011**, *55*, 430–442. [CrossRef] [PubMed]
14. Arablou, T.; Kolahdouz-Mohammadi, R. Curcumin and endometriosis: Review on potential roles and molecular mechanisms. *Biomed. Pharmacother.* **2018**, *97*, 91–97. [CrossRef] [PubMed]
15. Falanga, V. Wound healing and its impairment in the diabetic foot. *Lancet* **2005**, *366*, 1736–1743. [CrossRef]
16. Velnar, T.; Bailey, T.; Smrkolj, V. The wound healing process: An overview of the cellular and molecular mechanisms. *J. Int. Med. Res.* **2009**, *37*, 1528–1542. [CrossRef] [PubMed]
17. Topman, G.; Lin, F.H.; Gefen, A. The natural medications for wound healing—Curcumin, Aloe-Vera and Ginger—Do not induce a significant effect on the migration kinematics of cultured fibroblasts. *J. Biomech.* **2013**, *46*, 170–174. [CrossRef] [PubMed]
18. Falanga, V. The chronic wound: Impaired healing and solutions in the context of wound bed preparation. *Blood Cells Mol. Dis.* **2004**, *32*, 88–94. [CrossRef] [PubMed]
19. Santoro, M.M.; Gaudino, G. Cellular and molecular facets of keratinocyte reepithelization during wound healing. *Exp. Cell Res.* **2005**, *304*, 274–286. [CrossRef] [PubMed]
20. Iyer, V.; Pumiglia, K.; DiPersio, C.M. Alpha3beta1 integrin regulates MMP-9 mRNA stability in immortalized keratinocytes: A novel mechanism of integrin-mediated *MMP* gene expression. *J. Cell Sci.* **2005**, *118*, 1185–1195. [CrossRef] [PubMed]
21. Choma, D.P.; Pumiglia, K.; DiPersio, C.M. Integrin alpha3beta1 directs the stabilization of a polarized lamellipodium in epithelial cells through activation of Rac1. *J. Cell Sci.* **2004**, *117*, 3947–3959. [CrossRef] [PubMed]
22. Nahm, W.K.; Philpot, B.D.; Adams, M.M.; Badiavas, E.V.; Zhou, L.H.; Butmarc, J.; Bear, M.F.; Falanga, V. Significance of N-methyl-D-aspartate (NMDA) receptor-mediated signaling in human keratinocytes. *J. Cell. Physiol.* **2004**, *200*, 309–317. [CrossRef] [PubMed]
23. Malnutrition. Available online: https://www.who.int/en/news-room/fact-sheets/detail/malnutrition (accessed on 1 January 2019).
24. Katsarou, A.; Gudbjörnsdottir, S.; Rawshani, A.; Dabelea, D.; Bonifacio, E.; Anderson, B.J.; Jacobsen, L.M.; Schatz, D.A.; Lernmark, Å. Type 1 diabetes mellitus. *Nat. Rev. Dis. Primers* **2017**, *3*, 17016. [CrossRef] [PubMed]
25. Russell, L. The importance of patients' nutritional status in wound healing. *Br. J. Nurs.* **2001**, *10*, S42–S49. [CrossRef] [PubMed]
26. Breslow, R.A.; Hallfrisch, J.; Guy, D.G.; Crawley, B.; Goldberg, A.P. The importance of dietary protein in healing pressure ulcers. *J. Am. Geriatr. Soc.* **1993**, *41*, 357–362. [CrossRef] [PubMed]
27. Chen, C.C.; Schilling, L.S.; Lyder, C.H. A concept analysis of malnutrition in the elderly. *J. Adv. Nurs.* **2001**, *36*, 131–142. [CrossRef] [PubMed]
28. Evans, C. Malnutrition in the elderly: A multifactorial failure to thrive. *Perm. J.* **2005**, *9*, 38–41. [CrossRef] [PubMed]
29. Casey, G. Nutritional support in wound healing. *Nurs. Stand.* **2003**, *17*, 55–58. [CrossRef] [PubMed]
30. Todorovic, V. Food and wounds: Nutritional factors in wound formation and healing. *Br. J. Community Nurs.* **2002**, *7*, 43–54. [CrossRef]
31. Albina, J.E.; Gladden, P.; Walsh, W.R. Detrimental effects of an omega-3 fatty acid-enriched diet on wound healing. *JPEN J. Parenter. Enter. Nutr.* **1993**, *17*, 519–521. [CrossRef] [PubMed]

32. Theilla, M.; Schwartz, B.; Cohen, J.; Shapiro, H.; Anbar, R.; Singer, P. Impact of a nutritional formula enriched in fish oil and micronutrients on pressure ulcers in critical care patients. *Am. J. Crit. Care* **2012**, *21*, e102–e109. [CrossRef] [PubMed]
33. Molnar, J.A.; Underdown, M.J.; Clark, W.A. Nutrition and Chronic Wounds. *Adv. Wound Care (New Rochelle)* **2014**, *3*, 663–681. [CrossRef] [PubMed]
34. Debats, I.B.; Wolfs, T.G.; Gotoh, T.; Cleutjens, J.P.; Peutz-Kootstra, C.J.; van der Hulst, R.R. Role of arginine in superficial wound healing in man. *Nitric Oxide* **2009**, *21*, 175–183. [CrossRef] [PubMed]
35. Schäffer, M.R.; Tantry, U.; Thornton, F.J.; Barbul, A. Inhibition of nitric oxide synthesis in wounds: Pharmacology and effect on accumulation of collagen in wounds in mice. *Eur. J. Surg.* **1999**, *165*, 262–267. [CrossRef] [PubMed]
36. Kirk, S.J.; Hurson, M.; Regan, M.C.; Holt, D.R.; Wasserkrug, H.L.; Barbul, A. Arginine stimulates wound healing and immune function in elderly human beings. *Surgery* **1993**, *114*, 155–159; discussion 160. [PubMed]
37. Wu, G.; Bazer, F.W.; Davis, T.A.; Kim, S.W.; Li, P.; Marc Rhoads, J.; Carey Satterfield, M.; Smith, S.B.; Spencer, T.E.; Yin, Y. Arginine metabolism and nutrition in growth, health and disease. *Amino Acids* **2009**, *37*, 153–168. [CrossRef] [PubMed]
38. Barbul, A. Proline precursors to sustain Mammalian collagen synthesis. *J. Nutr.* **2008**, *138*, 2021S–2024S. [CrossRef] [PubMed]
39. Leigh, B.; Desneves, K.; Rafferty, J.; Pearce, L.; King, S.; Woodward, M.C.; Brown, D.; Martin, R.; Crowe, T.C. The effect of different doses of an arginine-containing supplement on the healing of pressure ulcers. *J. Wound Care* **2012**, *21*, 150–156. [CrossRef] [PubMed]
40. Wischmeyer, P.E. Glutamine and heat shock protein expression. *Nutrition* **2002**, *18*, 225–228. [CrossRef]
41. Newsholme, P. Why is L-glutamine metabolism important to cells of the immune system in health, postinjury, surgery or infection? *J. Nutr.* **2001**, *131*, 2515S–2522S; discussion 2523S–2514S. [CrossRef] [PubMed]
42. Ardawi, M.S. Glutamine and glucose metabolism in human peripheral lymphocytes. *Metabolism* **1988**, *37*, 99–103. [CrossRef]
43. Peng, X.; Yan, H.; You, Z.; Wang, P.; Wang, S. Clinical and protein metabolic efficacy of glutamine granules-supplemented enteral nutrition in severely burned patients. *Burns* **2005**, *31*, 342–346. [CrossRef] [PubMed]
44. Blass, S.C.; Goost, H.; Tolba, R.H.; Stoffel-Wagner, B.; Kabir, K.; Burger, C.; Stehle, P.; Ellinger, S. Time to wound closure in trauma patients with disorders in wound healing is shortened by supplements containing antioxidant micronutrients and glutamine: A PRCT. *Clin. Nutr.* **2012**, *31*, 469–475. [CrossRef] [PubMed]
45. Stadelmann, W.K.; Digenis, A.G.; Tobin, G.R. Impediments to wound healing. *Am. J. Surg.* **1998**, *176*, 39S–47S. [CrossRef]
46. Reichrath, J.; Lehmann, B.; Carlberg, C.; Varani, J.; Zouboulis, C.C. Vitamins as hormones. *Horm. Metab. Res.* **2007**, *39*, 71–84. [CrossRef] [PubMed]
47. Hunt, T.K.; Ehrlich, H.P.; Garcia, J.A.; Dunphy, J.E. Effect of vitamin A on reversing the inhibitory effect of cortisone on healing of open wounds in animals and man. *Ann. Surg.* **1969**, *170*, 633–641. [CrossRef] [PubMed]
48. Wicke, C.; Halliday, B.; Allen, D.; Roche, N.S.; Scheuenstuhl, H.; Spencer, M.M.; Roberts, A.B.; Hunt, T.K. Effects of steroids and retinoids on wound healing. *Arch. Surg.* **2000**, *135*, 1265–1270. [CrossRef] [PubMed]
49. Williams, J.Z.; Barbul, A. Nutrition and wound healing. *Crit. Care Nurs. Clin. N. Am.* **2012**, *24*, 179–200. [CrossRef] [PubMed]
50. Shepherd, A.A. Nutrition for optimum wound healing. *Nurs. Stand.* **2003**, *18*, 55–58. [PubMed]
51. Ellinger, S.; Stehle, P. Efficacy of vitamin supplementation in situations with wound healing disorders: Results from clinical intervention studies. *Curr. Opin. Clin. Nutr. Metab. Care* **2009**, *12*, 588–595. [CrossRef] [PubMed]
52. Zhang, Y.G.; Wu, S.; Sun, J. Vitamin D, Vitamin D Receptor, and Tissue Barriers. *Tissue Barriers* **2013**, *1*, e23118. [CrossRef] [PubMed]
53. Burkievcz, C.J.; Skare, T.L.; Malafaia, O.; Nassif, P.A.; Ribas, C.S.; Santos, L.R. Vitamin D deficiency in patients with chronic venous ulcers. *Rev. Col. Bras. Cir.* **2012**, *39*, 60–63. [CrossRef] [PubMed]
54. Kalava, U.R.; Cha, S.S.; Takahashi, P.Y. Association between vitamin D and pressure ulcers in older ambulatory adults: Results of a matched case-control study. *Clin. Interv. Aging* **2011**, *6*, 213–219. [CrossRef] [PubMed]

55. Mazzotta, M.Y. Nutrition and wound healing. *J. Am. Podiatr. Med. Assoc.* **1994**, *84*, 456–462. [CrossRef] [PubMed]
56. Trujillo, E.B. Effects of nutritional status on wound healing. *J. Vasc. Nurs.* **1993**, *11*, 12–18. [PubMed]
57. Fosmire, G.J. Zinc toxicity. *Am. J. Clin. Nutr.* **1990**, *51*, 225–227. [CrossRef] [PubMed]
58. Lansdown, A.B.; Mirastschijski, U.; Stubbs, N.; Scanlon, E.; Agren, M.S. Zinc in wound healing: Theoretical, experimental, and clinical aspects. *Wound Repair Regen.* **2007**, *15*, 2–16. [CrossRef] [PubMed]
59. Milobedzka, J.; Kostanecki, S.; Lampe, V. Zur Kenntnis des Curcumins. *Ber. Dtsch. Chem. Ges.* **1910**, *43*, 2163–2170. [CrossRef]
60. Bielefeld, K.A.; Amini-Nik, S.; Alman, B.A. Cutaneous wound healing: recruiting developmental pathways for regeneration. *Cell. Mol. Life Sci.* **2013**, *70*, 2059–2081. [CrossRef] [PubMed]
61. Wu, N.C.; Wang, J.J. Curcumin attenuates liver warm ischemia and reperfusion-induced combined restrictive and obstructive lung disease by reducing matrix metalloprotease 9 activity. *Transplant. Proc.* **2014**, *46*, 1135–1138. [CrossRef] [PubMed]
62. Song, Z.; Revelo, X.; Shao, W.; Tian, L.; Zeng, K.; Lei, H.; Sun, H.S.; Woo, M.; Winer, D.; Jin, T. Dietary Curcumin Intervention Targets Mouse White Adipose Tissue Inflammation and Brown Adipose Tissue *UCP1* Expression. *Obesity (Silver Spring)* **2018**, *26*, 547–558. [CrossRef] [PubMed]
63. Hunter, C.J.; De Plaen, I.G. Inflammatory signaling in NEC: Role of NF-κB, cytokines and other inflammatory mediators. *Pathophysiology* **2014**, *21*, 55–65. [CrossRef] [PubMed]
64. Merrell, J.G.; McLaughlin, S.W.; Tie, L.; Laurencin, C.T.; Chen, A.F.; Nair, L.S. Curcumin-loaded poly(epsilon-caprolactone) nanofibres: Diabetic wound dressing with anti-oxidant and anti-inflammatory properties. *Clin. Exp. Pharmacol. Physiol.* **2009**, *36*, 1149–1156. [CrossRef] [PubMed]
65. Wang, J.; Wang, H.; Zhu, R.; Liu, Q.; Fei, J.; Wang, S. Anti-inflammatory activity of curcumin-loaded solid lipid nanoparticles in IL-1β transgenic mice subjected to the lipopolysaccharide-induced sepsis. *Biomaterials* **2015**, *53*, 475–483. [CrossRef] [PubMed]
66. Antoine, F.; Girard, D. Curcumin increases gelatinase activity in human neutrophils by a p38 mitogen-activated protein kinase (MAPK)-independent mechanism. *J. Immunotoxicol.* **2015**, *12*, 188–193. [CrossRef] [PubMed]
67. Li, H.Y.; Yang, M.; Li, Z.; Meng, Z. Curcumin inhibits angiotensin II-induced inflammation and proliferation of rat vascular smooth muscle cells by elevating PPAR-γ activity and reducing oxidative stress. *Int. J. Mol. Med.* **2017**, *39*, 1307–1316. [CrossRef] [PubMed]
68. Zhang, Y.; Liu, Z.; Wu, J.; Bai, B.; Chen, H.; Xiao, Z.; Chen, L.; Zhao, Y.; Lum, H.; Wang, Y.; et al. New MD2 inhibitors derived from curcumin with improved anti-inflammatory activity. *Eur. J. Med. Chem.* **2018**, *148*, 291–305. [CrossRef] [PubMed]
69. Frey, R.S.; Malik, A.B. Oxidant signaling in lung cells. *Am. J. Physiol. Lung Cell. Mol. Physiol.* **2004**, *286*, L1–L3. [CrossRef] [PubMed]
70. Panchatcharam, M.; Miriyala, S.; Gayathri, V.S.; Suguna, L. Curcumin improves wound healing by modulating collagen and decreasing reactive oxygen species. *Mol. Cell. Biochem.* **2006**, *290*, 87–96. [CrossRef] [PubMed]
71. Roy, S.; Khanna, S.; Nallu, K.; Hunt, T.K.; Sen, C.K. Dermal wound healing is subject to redox control. *Mol. Ther.* **2006**, *13*, 211–220. [CrossRef] [PubMed]
72. Imlay, J.A. Pathways of oxidative damage. *Annu. Rev. Microbiol.* **2003**, *57*, 395–418. [CrossRef] [PubMed]
73. Matés, J.M.; Segura, J.A.; Alonso, F.J.; Márquez, J. Roles of dioxins and heavy metals in cancer and neurological diseases using ROS-mediated mechanisms. *Free Radic. Biol. Med.* **2010**, *49*, 1328–1341. [CrossRef] [PubMed]
74. Gopinath, D.; Ahmed, M.R.; Gomathi, K.; Chitra, K.; Sehgal, P.K.; Jayakumar, R. Dermal wound healing processes with curcumin incorporated collagen films. *Biomaterials* **2004**, *25*, 1911–1917. [CrossRef]
75. Tapia, E.; Sánchez-Lozada, L.G.; García-Niño, W.R.; García, E.; Cerecedo, A.; García-Arroyo, F.E.; Osorio, H.; Arellano, A.; Cristóbal-García, M.; Loredo, M.L.; et al. Curcumin prevents maleate-induced nephrotoxicity: Relation to hemodynamic alterations, oxidative stress, mitochondrial oxygen consumption and activity of respiratory complex I. *Free Radic. Res.* **2014**, *48*, 1342–1354. [CrossRef] [PubMed]
76. Zheng, Q.T.; Yang, Z.H.; Yu, L.Y.; Ren, Y.Y.; Huang, Q.X.; Liu, Q.; Ma, X.Y.; Chen, Z.K.; Wang, Z.B.; Zheng, X. Synthesis and antioxidant activity of curcumin analogs. *J. Asian Nat. Prod. Res.* **2017**, *19*, 489–503. [CrossRef] [PubMed]

77. Reddy, A.C.; Lokesh, B.R. Effect of dietary turmeric (Curcuma longa) on iron-induced lipid peroxidation in the rat liver. *Food Chem. Toxicol.* **1994**, *32*, 279–283. [CrossRef]
78. Subudhi, U.; Chainy, G.B. Expression of hepatic antioxidant genes in l-thyroxine-induced hyperthyroid rats: Regulation by vitamin E and curcumin. *Chem. Biol. Interact.* **2010**, *183*, 304–316. [CrossRef] [PubMed]
79. Dai, C.; Tang, S.; Li, D.; Zhao, K.; Xiao, X. Curcumin attenuates quinocetone-induced oxidative stress and genotoxicity in human hepatocyte L02 cells. *Toxicol. Mech. Methods* **2015**, *25*, 340–346. [CrossRef] [PubMed]
80. Phan, T.T.; See, P.; Lee, S.T.; Chan, S.Y. Protective effects of curcumin against oxidative damage on skin cells in vitro: Its implication for wound healing. *J. Trauma* **2001**, *51*, 927–931. [CrossRef] [PubMed]
81. Zhang, Y.; Cao, H.; Yu, Z.; Peng, H.Y.; Zhang, C.J. Curcumin inhibits endometriosis endometrial cells by reducing estradiol production. *Iran. J. Reprod. Med.* **2013**, *11*, 415–422. [PubMed]
82. Petroll, W.M.; Cavanagh, H.D.; Barry, P.; Andrews, P.; Jester, J.V. Quantitative analysis of stress fiber orientation during corneal wound contraction. *J. Cell Sci.* **1993**, *104 Pt 2*, 353–363.
83. Durgaprasad, S.; Reetesh, R.; Hareesh, K.; Rajput, R. Effect of topical curcumin preparation (BIOCURCUMAX) on burn wound healing in rats. *J. Pharm. Biomed. Sci. (JPBMS)* **2011**, *8*, 1–3.
84. Dai, M.; Zheng, X.; Xu, X.; Kong, X.; Li, X.; Guo, G.; Luo, F.; Zhao, X.; Wei, Y.Q.; Qian, Z. Chitosan-alginate sponge: Preparation and application in curcumin delivery for dermal wound healing in rat. *J. Biomed. Biotechnol.* **2009**, *2009*, 595126. [CrossRef] [PubMed]
85. Mohanty, C.; Das, M.; Sahoo, S.K. Sustained wound healing activity of curcumin loaded oleic acid based polymeric bandage in a rat model. *Mol. Pharm.* **2012**, *9*, 2801–2811. [CrossRef] [PubMed]
86. Jagetia, G.C.; Rajanikant, G.K. Acceleration of wound repair by curcumin in the excision wound of mice exposed to different doses of fractionated γ radiation. *Int. Wound J.* **2012**, *9*, 76–92. [CrossRef] [PubMed]
87. Welch, M.P.; Odland, G.F.; Clark, R.A. Temporal relationships of F-actin bundle formation, collagen and fibronectin matrix assembly, and fibronectin receptor expression to wound contraction. *J. Cell Biol.* **1990**, *110*, 133–145. [CrossRef] [PubMed]
88. Sidhu, G.S.; Singh, A.K.; Thaloor, D.; Banaudha, K.K.; Patnaik, G.K.; Srimal, R.C.; Maheshwari, R.K. Enhancement of wound healing by curcumin in animals. *Wound Repair Regen.* **1998**, *6*, 167–177. [CrossRef] [PubMed]
89. Sidhu, G.S.; Mani, H.; Gaddipati, J.P.; Singh, A.K.; Seth, P.; Banaudha, K.K.; Patnaik, G.K.; Maheshwari, R.K. Curcumin enhances wound healing in streptozotocin induced diabetic rats and genetically diabetic mice. *Wound Repair Regen.* **1999**, *7*, 362–374. [CrossRef] [PubMed]
90. Brown, D.L.; Kao, W.W.; Greenhalgh, D.G. Apoptosis down-regulates inflammation under the advancing epithelial wound edge: Delayed patterns in diabetes and improvement with topical growth factors. *Surgery* **1997**, *121*, 372–380. [CrossRef]
91. Kant, V.; Gopal, A.; Kumar, D.; Pathak, N.N.; Ram, M.; Jangir, B.L.; Tandan, S.K. Curcumin-induced angiogenesis hastens wound healing in diabetic rats. *J. Surg. Res.* **2015**, *193*, 978–988. [CrossRef] [PubMed]
92. Abe, Y.; Hashimoto, S.; Horie, T. Curcumin inhibition of inflammatory cytokine production by human peripheral blood monocytes and alveolar macrophages. *Pharmacol. Res.* **1999**, *39*, 41–47. [CrossRef] [PubMed]
93. Balogun, E.; Hoque, M.; Gong, P.; Killeen, E.; Green, C.J.; Foresti, R.; Alam, J.; Motterlini, R. Curcumin activates the haem oxygenase-1 gene via regulation of Nrf2 and the antioxidant-responsive element. *Biochem. J.* **2003**, *371*, 887–895. [CrossRef] [PubMed]
94. Huang, M.T.; Lysz, T.; Ferraro, T.; Abidi, T.F.; Laskin, J.D.; Conney, A.H. Inhibitory effects of curcumin on in vitro lipoxygenase and cyclooxygenase activities in mouse epidermis. *Cancer Res.* **1991**, *51*, 813–819. [PubMed]
95. Woo, J.H.; Kim, Y.H.; Choi, Y.J.; Kim, D.G.; Lee, K.S.; Bae, J.H.; Min, D.S.; Chang, J.S.; Jeong, Y.J.; Lee, Y.H.; et al. Molecular mechanisms of curcumin-induced cytotoxicity: Induction of apoptosis through generation of reactive oxygen species, down-regulation of *Bcl-XL* and *IAP*, the release of cytochrome c and inhibition of Akt. *Carcinogenesis* **2003**, *24*, 1199–1208. [CrossRef] [PubMed]
96. Maugeri, A.; Mazzone, M.G.; Giuliano, F.; Vinciguerra, M.; Basile, G.; Barchitta, M.; Agodi, A. Curcumin Modulates DNA Methyltransferase Functions in a Cellular Model of Diabetic Retinopathy. *Oxid. Med. Cell. Longev.* **2018**, *2018*, 5407482. [CrossRef] [PubMed]
97. Lewis, C.J.; Mardaryev, A.N.; Sharov, A.A.; Fessing, M.Y.; Botchkarev, V.A. The Epigenetic Regulation of Wound Healing. *Adv. Wound Care (New Rochelle)* **2014**, *3*, 468–475. [CrossRef] [PubMed]

98. Maugeri, A.; Barchitta, M.; Mazzone, M.G.; Giuliano, F.; Basile, G.; Agodi, A. Resveratrol modulates *SIRT1* and *DNMT* functions and restores *LINE-1* methylation levels in ARPE-19 cells under oxidative stress and inflammation. *Int. J. Mol. Sci.* **2018**, *19*, 2118. [CrossRef] [PubMed]
99. Ravindranath, V.; Chandrasekhara, N. Absorption and tissue distribution of curcumin in rats. *Toxicology* **1980**, *16*, 259–265. [CrossRef]
100. Asai, A.; Miyazawa, T. Occurrence of orally administered curcuminoid as glucuronide and glucuronide/sulfate conjugates in rat plasma. *Life Sci.* **2000**, *67*, 2785–2793. [CrossRef]
101. Hegge, A.B.; Andersen, T.; Melvik, J.E.; Bruzell, E.; Kristensen, S.; Tønnesen, H.H. Formulation and bacterial phototoxicity of curcumin loaded alginate foams for wound treatment applications: Studies on curcumin and curcuminoides XLII. *J. Pharm. Sci.* **2011**, *100*, 174–185. [CrossRef] [PubMed]

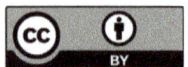

© 2019 by the authors. Licensee MDPI, Basel, Switzerland. This article is an open access article distributed under the terms and conditions of the Creative Commons Attribution (CC BY) license (http://creativecommons.org/licenses/by/4.0/).

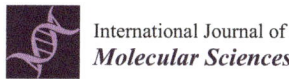

Review

Neuroprotective and Neurological/Cognitive Enhancement Effects of Curcumin after Brain Ischemia Injury with Alzheimer's Disease Phenotype

Ryszard Pluta [1,*], Marzena Ułamek-Kozioł [1,2] and Stanisław J. Czuczwar [3]

1 Laboratory of Ischemic and Neurodegenerative Brain Research, Mossakowski Medical Research Centre, Polish Academy of Sciences, 02-106 Warsaw, Poland; mulamek@imdik.pan.pl
2 First Department of Neurology, Institute of Psychiatry and Neurology, 02-957 Warsaw, Poland
3 Department of Pathophysiology, Medical University of Lublin, 20-090 Lublin, Poland; czuczwarsj@yahoo.com
* Correspondence: pluta@imdik.pan.pl; Tel.: +48-22-6086-540 or +48-22-6086-469; Fax: +48-22-6086-627 or +48-22-6685-532

Received: 16 November 2018; Accepted: 10 December 2018; Published: 12 December 2018

Abstract: In recent years, ongoing interest in ischemic brain injury research has provided data showing that ischemic episodes are involved in the development of Alzheimer's disease-like neuropathology. Brain ischemia is the second naturally occurring neuropathology, such as Alzheimer's disease, which causes the death of neurons in the CA1 region of the hippocampus. In addition, brain ischemia was considered the most effective predictor of the development of full-blown dementia of Alzheimer's disease phenotype with a debilitating effect on the patient. Recent knowledge on the activation of Alzheimer's disease-related genes and proteins—e.g., amyloid protein precursor and tau protein—as well as brain ischemia and Alzheimer's disease neuropathology indicate that similar processes contribute to neuronal death and disintegration of brain tissue in both disorders. Although brain ischemia is one of the main causes of death in the world, there is no effective therapy to improve the structural and functional outcomes of this disorder. In this review, we consider the promising role of the protective action of curcumin after ischemic brain injury. Studies of the pharmacological properties of curcumin after brain ischemia have shown that curcumin has several therapeutic properties that include anti-excitotoxic, anti-oxidant, anti-apoptotic, anti-hyperhomocysteinemia and anti-inflammatory effects, mitochondrial protection, as well as increasing neuronal lifespan and promoting neurogenesis. In addition, curcumin also exerts anti-amyloidogenic effects and affects the brain's tau protein. These results suggest that curcumin may be able to serve as a potential preventive and therapeutic agent in neurodegenerative brain disorders.

Keywords: brain ischemia; curcumin; Alzheimer's disease; neurodegeneration; amyloid; tau protein; autophagy; mitophagy; apoptosis; genes

1. Introduction

Brain ischemic injury in humans is the third cause of disability and the second cause of death, which may soon become the leading cause of full-blown dementia of Alzheimer's disease type [1–9]. Unexpected cerebral ischemia refers to a global and local cerebral episode that causes sudden neurological deficits [10]. Recent epidemiological data indicate that approximately 17 million people suffer from ischemic brain damage every year [6,11]. The number of patients after ischemic cerebral episode has now reached 33 million [6,11]. According to epidemiological predictions, this figure will increase to 77 million in 2030 [11]. In addition, people with cerebral ischemia are at high risk of cognitive impairment. Physical impairment after ischemic stroke tends to improve to a greater or lesser extent. However, for some unknown reasons, the impairment of cognitive functions gradually progresses. Currently used treatment of made ischemic stroke involves the use of thrombolysis, but thrombolysis has a limited window of therapeutic time and the potential risk of hemorrhagic transformation [10]. Now, post-ischemic stroke has a huge impact on global public healthcare and clinical practice.

Patients with ischemic stroke frequently have cognitive deficits with varying degrees of differentiation [4,12]. Animals after experimental cerebral ischemia also show cognitive deficits [13–16]. Recently, the key role of episodic cerebral ischemia in the development of dementia has appeared at the forefront of clinical and experimental research [17–28]. Studies in recent years suggest that ischemic brain damage may promote neurodegeneration of the Alzheimer's disease-type by damaging neuronal energy, generating reactive oxygen species [27,29], neuroinflammation [29–32], various parts of amyloid protein precursor accumulation [18,29,33], and tau protein dysfunction [34,35], which in turn damage neuronal cells, especially in the hippocampus and contribute to brain atrophy [33,36–39]. The vast majority of people who survived brain ischemia, experience progressive motor and cognitive deficits, which makes the development of new therapies to improve neurological outcomes even more urgent. Although many experimental studies have identified acute strategies to reduce the loss of nerve cell number during and after brain ischemia, only therapeutic hypothermia translates into use in a human clinic [40]. Therefore, due to the lack of translation of experimental neuroprotective agents for use in clinical conditions [41], we have focused our attention on improving functional outcomes after ischemia, instead of protecting neurons during ischemic damage. To this end, we should improve the function of persistent neurons after ischemia [14,16], and new therapies should be designed to reverse synaptic plasticity deficits to improve the functional outcome after brain ischemia, effectively extending the therapeutic window. This review presents current advances in the study of cerebral ischemia, focusing on ischemia-induced neurodegeneration of Alzheimer's disease-type. It should be emphasized that despite the fact that brain ischemia is one of the leading causes of death and disability in the world, there is no effective treatment to improve the structural and functional consequences of this disorder. Therefore, in this review, we will also look at the promising role of the protective action of curcumin on the function and survival of persistent neurons after ischemic brain damage. Finally, we present the latest evidence that provides new information on the role and mechanisms of curcumin in inhibiting ischemia-reperfusion brain injury and potential therapeutic strategies in the treatment of ischemic brain damage of Alzheimer's disease phenotype.

2. Similar Multifactorial Processes in the Post-Ischemic Brain and Alzheimer's Disease

Post-ischemic brain damage is undoubtedly one of the most common multifactorial forms of neurodegeneration, including a series of abnormal cell/molecular processes taking place at different times during recirculation and progressively various areas of the brain. It seems that ischemic episodes favor the development of Alzheimer's disease-like neurodegeneration through numerous mechanisms including neuronal loss, synaptic dysfunction, neuroinflammation, accumulation of various parts of the amyloid protein precursor, tau protein dysfunction and dysregulation of Alzheimer's disease-related genes, white matter lesions, and general brain atrophy. The progress in understanding the key processes of brain ischemia-induced changes of the Alzheimer's disease phenotype and genotype will help to develop the prevention and treatment strategies against neurodegeneration and dementia generated by ischemia.

2.1. Neurodegeneration after Brain Ischemia

In the hippocampus, necrotic and apoptotic neuronal cells were observed in the CA1 region 2–7 days after brain ischemia [29,33,42]. After two days of recirculation, the loss of neurons was superimposed with damaged nerve cells. In later times of observations up to six months, the number of neurons with pathological changes has been reduced and replaced by the loss of nerve cells. The above changes were mainly located in the hippocampus and third, fifth, and sixth layer of the cortex. The borderline zones of the brain cortex were also the site of serious neuropathological changes. Over six months after ischemic brain damage, apart from the local loss of neurons, various types of pathological neuronal changes have been observed. The first of these was the form of chronic neuronal degeneration, which was observed in the early periods following brain ischemia. Other changes were typical of early ischemic lesions but were observed in those areas of the brain that were not involved in early changes, such as the hippocampus region CA2, CA3, and CA4 [29,33,42]. The death of neurons in the CA1 region of the hippocampus, along with the decrease in the acetylcholine level in the cerebral cortex and striatum, is evident after cerebral ischemia, suggesting that the loss of neurons may result from the insufficiency of neuronal excitable transmission [43,44].

The synaptic integrity of the brain is essential for physiological activities, including memory and learning. Decreased levels of both synaptophysin and postsynaptic density protein 95 were found in the rat hippocampus after local cerebral ischemia [45,46]. Similarly, these rats presented ultrastructural synaptic changes in the CA1 region of the hippocampus. Other studies have shown that ischemic brain damage leads to an increase in both synaptic autophagy and asymmetric synapses that may be associated with the death of neurons in the CA1 region of the hippocampus after transient cerebral ischemia [47–49]. There is experimental evidence of an isolated and persistent abnormal synaptic function resulting from transient cerebral ischemia [50]. In the CA1 region of the hippocampus, depression of excitatory synaptic transmission after brain ischemia has been demonstrated [43]. Ischemia-induced increase in intracellular Ca^{2+} regulates the activity of calpain in neurons, and calpain target proteins are present in GABAergic and glutaminergic synapses. In brain ischemia, calpain cleaves pre- and postsynaptic proteins. The distribution of protein cleavage via calpain contributes to neuronal death in brain ischemia [51].

The damage of the white matter and the activation of glial cells are observed both in animals and in people after brain ischemia [29,32,36,37,42,52–54]. In models of rat brain ischemia, it seems that ischemia causes more serious changes in the subcortical white matter and corpus callosum [29,36,37,55]. These findings are consistent with glial activation in the corpus callosum following ischemia-reperfusion brain injury [56]. Brain ischemia favors the increase of blood–brain barrier permeability, which facilitates the penetration of inflammatory cells into the brain parenchyma and releases a large number of serine proteases, as well as β-amyloid peptides and tau protein from the blood into the brain tissue, which in turn leads to white matter lesions [18,32,57–66].

Evidence suggests that transient ischemic brain damage in rats causes extensive loss of neurons, in structures belonging to or not to selectively sensitive areas of the brain [29,42]. Ischemic changes in the brain represent a gradually progressive process that stretches for a long time during reperfusion after an ischemic episode [29]. They are characterized not only by early changes in the brain, but also by an active pathological process in the late stage following ischemic injury. Within one to two years after cerebral ischemia, the neuropathological process leads to generalized brain atrophy [29,42,67]. Brain gross examination, carried out from 9 to 24 months following ischemia-reperfusion episode, showed symptoms of brain hydrocephalus [42,67]. Dilatation of the subarachnoid space around the cerebral hemispheres was also observed [42]. Complete disappearance of the hippocampus with massive pyramidal neuron loss in its CA1 area and atrophy of the striatum was noted [42]. The brain cortex was narrow, which suggested an increased density of neurons. An additional feature of late atrophy of the brain was manifested as scattered changes of the white matter, taking the form of rarefaction and cavitations, manifesting as advanced spongiosis. This phenomenon can be explained by the huge loss of neurons along with the ischemic acute and chronic increased permeability of the blood–brain barrier [48], for example for neurotoxic amyloid and tau protein [57–59,61,63–66].

2.2. Amyloid Generation after Brain Ischemia

Amyloid deposits occur in both the brain parenchyma and the vascular walls of the brain after ischemic episodes in humans and animals [19,29,68–73]. Animals that survived up to seven days after ischemic brain injury showed intense brain immunoreactivity for the N-terminal of the amyloid protein precursor, the β-amyloid peptide, and for the C-terminal of the amyloid protein precursor. In animals that survived up to one year after ischemic brain injury, increased staining was reported only for the C-terminal of the amyloid protein precursor and the β-amyloid peptide [29–31,42]. Staining was observed intra- and extracellular [19,29]. Extracellular different parts of the amyloid protein precursor deposits ranged from scattered small dots to irregularly dispersed diffuse plaques [19,29,74–78]. In the hippocampus, entorhinal cortex, corpus callosum, around lateral ventricles and in the thalamus multifocal scattered amyloid plaques were observed. The time-dependent accumulation of the β-amyloid peptide in the hippocampus, especially in fields with the open blood–brain barrier, occurred after experimental brain ischemia [18,36,37,45,62,63,79,80]. It should be emphasized that β-amyloid peptide deposits observed after experimental cerebral ischemia did not stain with thioflavin S [19,81], while in humans some amyloid deposits were stained with thioflavin S [69]. Accumulation of amyloid in the vessel walls caused by ischemic brain damage with vasospasm may additionally cause ischemic changes and develop a self-propelling vicious cycle of ischemic episodes, ultimately leading to irreversible damage to the brain parenchyma [29,82].

2.3. Dysfunction of Tau Protein after Brain Ischemia

The microtubule-associated tau protein is hypophosphorylated in the ischemic brains of patients and in experimental cerebral ischemia and ultimately generates intraneuronal neurofibrillary tangles and/or neurofibrillary tangle-like tauopathy that are a key in the ongoing neuropathology of Alzheimer's disease [35,83]. Cyclin-dependent kinase 5 is involved in neurofibrillary tangle-like tauopathy, which is caused by ischemic hyperphosphorylation of tau protein [34]. Also, phosphorylation of tau protein in many places specific for Alzheimer's disease caused by experimental cerebral ischemia was observed [46]. Increased phosphorylation of tau protein with cyclin-dependent kinase 5 parallel activation, glycogen synthase kinase-3b and calcium/calmodulin dependent protein kinase II, as well as inhibition of protein phosphatase 2A have been reported after focal rat brain ischemia [84]. It can therefore be suggested that increased phosphorylation of tau protein and overproduction of β-amyloid peptide appear to be very sensitive to brain ischemic injury.

2.4. Dysregulation of Genes Associated with Alzheimer's Disease after Brain Ischemia

In the CA1 area of hippocampus, the expression of the amyloid protein precursor gene was lowered below the control value within two days after ischemic brain injury [85,86]. Seven and 30 days after cerebral ischemia, the expression of the amyloid protein precursor gene increased above the control value [85,86]. In the temporal cortex, the expression of the amyloid protein precursor gene has been lowered below the control value two days after ischemic brain injury [87]. However, on days 7 and 30 after brain ischemia, the expression of the amyloid protein precursor gene was increased above the control value [87]. Expression of the β-secretase gene increased above the control value after cerebral ischemia in the rat hippocampal CA1 area two to seven days after the injury [85,86]. However, 30 days after cerebral ischemia, expression of the β-secretase gene decreased below the control value [85,86]. Expression of the β-secretase gene was regulated upward in the temporal cortex two days after brain ischemia [87]. Seven and 30 days after temporal cortex ischemia, the expression of the β-secretase gene was significantly reduced [87]. In the hippocampal CA1 region, the expression of the presenilin 1 and 2 gene was above the control value two and seven days after brain ischemia [85,86]. However, 30 days after an ischemic injury, the gene expression of presenilin 1 and 2 decreased below the control value [85,86]. In the temporal cortex, presenilin 1 gene expression decreased below the control value, but presenilin 2 increased above control 2 days after ischemic brain injury [88]. Seven days after cerebral ischemia, gene expression of presenilin 1 was reduced, and presenilin 2 was significantly elevated [88]. Thirty days after the termination of cerebral ischemia, the expression of presenilin 1 gene increased above the control value and presenilin 2 decreased below the control [88].

There is only one study in the literature indicating the relationship between the ischemic CA1 area of the hippocampus and the expression of the tau protein gene following transient brain ischemia in rats with 2, 7, and 30 days survival [35,89]. In the CA1 area of the hippocampus, the expression of the tau protein gene increased approximately 3-fold with respect to control values on the second day following brain ischemia [89]. On the 7th and 30th day after brain ischemia, the expression of the tau protein gene oscillated in the range of control values [89]. Statistically significant changes in the expression of the tau protein gene after brain ischemia were between 2 and 7 and 2 and 30 days of survival [89].

It was found that the autophagy gene in the hippocampal CA1 region was not significantly modified 2, 7, and 30 days after ischemic brain injury [90]. However, the mitophagy gene was significantly elevated on day 2 and fell below baseline on days 7 and 30 [90]. Expression of the caspase 3 gene in the CA1 region of the hippocampus two days after brain ischemia increased by more than 300% compared to baseline. However, seven days after ischemic injury, its expression was close to its basic value. Thirty days after ischemic injury, the gene expression was lowered below baseline in the above area [90]. In the temporal cortex, gene expression of autophagy increased within 2–30 days after transient brain ischemia in rats [91]. However, the gene of mitophagy fell below the normal value within two days after brain ischemia. Seven and 30 days after cerebral ischemia, the expression of the mitophagy gene increased above control values. Expression of the apoptotic caspase 3 gene was reduced below normal values two days after brain ischemia. Seven and 30 days after ischemia, the expression of caspase 3 gene increased above control values [91].

2.5. Behavioral Changes after Brain Ischemia with Alzheimer's Disease Phenotype

After brain ischemia in animals, behavioral abnormalities were also observed in addition to neurodegenerative changes [13–16,92,93]. It should be emphasized that neurodegenerative changes after ischemia do not cause noticeable long-term neurological deficits in animals [92]. After the ischemic episode, a spontaneous return of the sensory-motor function in animals was observed [14,94,95]. After ischemic brain injury, excessive locomotor activity was noted [96,97], as in people with Alzheimer's disease. Longer brain ischemia causes longer locomotor hyperactivity [32,63,92,98]. An impairment of habituation was observed after ischemic brain injury, which results in longer exploration time [99,100]. Brain ischemia causes a reference and working memory deficits [14,101,102]. In addition, ischemic brain damage in animals gradually leads to deficits in spatial memory during post-ischemic survival [14,103,104]. Progression of cognitive impairment has been demonstrated at different times during recirculation [14,104,105]. In addition, evidence of recurrent ischemic brain injury in animals showed persistent locomotor hyperactivity, severe cognitive deficits, and reduced level of anxiety [106]. Vigilance and sensory-motor efficiency are damaged for one or two days, while deficits in learning and memory seem to be irreversible and indefinitely persistent [14,98]. The aforementioned behavioral changes were associated with the loss of neurons in the CA1 region of the hippocampus, cerebral cortex, caudate nucleus [29,63,106], amygdala and perirhinal cortex [13], and with significant brain atrophy [29–31,42,107].

3. Effect of Curcumin on Neurodegenerative Changes and Neurological/Cognitive Function after Brain Ischemia

3.1. Neuroprotective Effects

The administration of curcumin before reperfusion in the model of middle cerebral artery occlusion in rats reduced the size of cerebral infarction and cerebral edema (Table 1) [108]. Before reperfusion after middle cerebral artery occlusion, treatment with curcumin reduced neutrophil rolling and adhesion to the endothelium of the cerebrovascular system by 76% and 67%, respectively. Because neutrophils are the main source of oxidant damage during reperfusion, curcumin blocks the major contributing factor to reperfusion injury, preventing neutrophil attack and accumulation in ischemic sites after experimental brain ischemia [108]. Curcumin reduced reperfusion injury in ischemic stroke by preventing neutrophil adhesion to cerebrovascular microcirculation [108]. In the rat model of embolic stroke, the efficacy of curcumin after ischemia was demonstrated, in which curcumin reduced infarct volume, improved sensory motor function, and significantly reduced the stress associated with nitrosis [109]. Curcumin can protect against local ischemic brain damage with reperfusion and also stimulate neurogenesis by activating the Notch signaling pathway [110]. There was also a clear decrease in the apoptotic index after three days of reperfusion in groups receiving curcumin. Significantly more TUNEL-positive neuronal cells were found in the ischemic group compared to curcumin-treated ischemic groups [111]. In addition, Kalani et al., [112] have shown that embryonic stem cell exosomes loaded with curcumin reduced astrogliosis and improved neuronal survival after brain ischemia in mice. Embryonic stem cell exosomes loaded with curcumin restored the neurovascular unit after ischemic brain injury [112,113]. These results suggest that combining exosomal potentials from embryonic stem cells with curcumin may help restore the neurovascular unit after ischemic brain injury in mice. All acute therapies with curcumin reduced the activity of matrix metalloproteinase-9 and hemorrhagic transformation of ischemic stroke in diabetic rats [113]. In addition, curcumin has reduced cerebral edema in these animals. Administration of curcumin for two months significantly reduced the ischemia-induced death of neurons in the CA1 region of the hippocampus, as well as impaired glial activation [114]. Administration of curcumin in the above condition also reduced lipid peroxidation, mitochondrial dysfunction, and apoptotic indices. After intranasal administration of curcumin, locomotor activity, and reduction in grip strength were improved after middle cerebral artery occlusion [115].

Table 1. Summary of the protective action of curcumin on post-ischemic brain damage.

Kind of Ischemia	Animal	Treatment Time	Protective Action	References
Focal brain ischemia	Rat	Pre-treatment	Reduction of reperfusion injury by preventing neutrophil adhesion to the brain microcirculation	[108]
Incomplete brain ischemia	Rat	Pre-treatment	Inhibition of mitochondrial ROS generation, lipid peroxidation and neuro-protection by inhibiting apoptosis	[116]
Forebrain ischemia	Rat	Pre-treatment and post-ischemia	Reduction of apoptosis	[111]
Focal brain ischemia	Rat	Post-ischemia	Reduction in volume of infarct and brain edema	[117]
Focal embolic ischemia	Rat	Post-ischemia	Reduction in volume of infarct and improvement of sensory motor activity	[109]
Focal brain ischemia	Mouse	Post-ischemia	Reduced volume of infarct, brain edema, and blood–brain barrier permeability	[118,119]
Focal brain ischemia	Rat	Post-ischemia	Stimulation of neurogenesis and smaller neurobehavioral deficits	[110]
Forebrain ischemia	Gerbil	Post-ischemia	Reduction of neuronal death, glial activation, apoptotic indices and mitigation of changes in locomotor activity	[114]
Focal brain ischemia	Rat	Post-ischemia	Reduction of hemorrhagic transformation, brain edema and improvement of neurological function	[113]
Focal brain ischemia	Mouse	Post-ischemia curcumin-loaded mouse embryonic stem cell exosomes	Reduction of neurological score, infarct volume, edema, inflammation and astrogliosis and restoration of neurovascular system	[112]
Focal brain ischemia	Rat	Post-ischemia	Reduced neurological score, infarct area, apoptosis, caspase-3 mRNA expression and autophagy activity	[120,121]

3.2. Neurological/Cognitive Effects

Treatment with curcumin also improved neurological outcomes after focal cerebral ischemia [108]. Administration of curcumin after ischemia improved sensory-motor activity [109]. Rats with focal cerebral ischemia treated with curcumin showed significantly smaller neurobehavioral deficits than animals treated with vehicle after 3, 7, and 12 days of reperfusion [110]. After one and three days, a significant reduction in neurological score was noted in the curcumin-treated groups compared to the control ischemic group [111,112]. Improvement in neurological function was observed, as evidenced by gait results, modified Bederson's scores and grip strength, but the size of the infarct was similar to untreated animals with ischemia and diabetes [112,113]. Biochemical changes resulting from the administration of curcumin also correlated very well with the ability to relieve changes in locomotor activity after ischemia-reperfusion brain injury [114,115].

4. Possible Molecular Mechanisms Underlying the Protective Action of Curcumin after Ischemia-Reperfusion Brain Injury

Apoptosis is one of the main routes that lead to the process of neuronal cell death after brain ischemia [122]. Curcumin contributes to the protection of neurons, probably through anti-apoptotic mechanisms [123]. Curcumin increased the level of anti-apoptotic Bcl-2 protein in the mitochondria and reduced the subsequent translocation of cytochrome c to the cytosol, thereby weakening the activation of caspase [123]. It is suggested that the mitochondrial pathway is an important target for curcumin. Curcumin administration has been shown to completely inhibit ischemia-induced cytochrome c release [114]. Another mechanism by which curcumin prevents damage to the ischemic brain is to increase the expression of the silent information regulator 1, a key neuroprotective molecule that participates in protection against ischemia-reperfusion brain damage. In this respect, the activation of the silent information regulator 1 leads to deacetylation of p53 and attenuation of apoptosis in the brain after ischemia [124]. It has been documented that the number of mitochondria and their mass, mitochondrial biogenesis and mitochondrial uncoupling protein 2 are significantly reduced in rats with ischemic brain injury, and these changes are reversed by pre-treatment with curcumin. It was also shown that mitochondrial biogenesis was increased in the focal model of brain ischemia in rats after administration of curcumin [125]. The data suggest that curcumin can alleviate ischemia-reperfusion injury of the brain by preventing $ONOO^-$-induced damage to the blood–brain barrier, and this indicates that curcumin alleviates vasogenic edema of the brain by protecting the integrity of the blood–brain barrier [118].

It is suggested that in response to ischemia-reperfusion injury of the brain, numerous factors predisposing to stress from the endoplasmic reticulum are activated in neurons, including depletion of the endoplasmic reticulum of Ca^{2+}, proteins aggregation, reduced proteins degradation, and accumulation of lipid peroxidation products in the endoplasmic reticulum and structures of Golgi apparatus [126]. Endoplasmic reticulum stress can induce proapoptotic processes and lead to apoptosis [127,128]. The growth arrest- and DNA damage-inducible gene 153 and caspase 12 are among the main factors of apoptosis mediated by stress of the endoplasmic reticulum [129]. Growth arrest- and DNA damage-inducible gene 153 is a signaling molecule that is involved in the development of apoptosis via pathways, such as the effect on intracellular Ca^{2+} metabolism and a reduction in Bcl-2 [129–131]. Caspase-12 is released from the endoplasmic reticulum during stress of the endoplasmic reticulum, and then activates the caspase cascade and apoptosis. It has been observed that curcumin can reduce the stress of the endoplasmic reticulum by reducing the expression of growth arrest- and DNA damage-inducible gene 153 and caspase-12, thus exhibiting a protective effect against brain ischemia-reperfusion injury in animals [129].

In the early stages after ischemic damage to the brain, neuroinflammation accelerates the damage process and determines the degree of brain damage [32,132]. Oxidative stress and overproduction of reactive oxygen species is a permanent element and an important mechanism of brain damage after ischemia-reperfusion [133]. Available studies have shown that the administration of curcumin prevents ischemia-reperfusion injury due to its antioxidant activity [115,134–137]. Possible mechanisms for the protective effect of curcumin on oxidative stress include reduction of lipid peroxidation, increased protein synthesis, free radical scavenging, increased glutathione content, and maintenance of cell membrane integrity [115,137,138]. It was shown that the increase in peroxiredoxin 6 level by curcumin weakened ischemic oxidative damage by induction of factor specific protein 1 in post-ischemic rats [137]. Ischemic in vitro studies have shown that curcumin increases thioredoxin levels and protects neurons from death due to deprivation of oxygen and glucose [139]. In addition, curcumin protects the brain against ischemia-reperfusion injury by inhibiting neuroinflammatory cytokines, such as IL-6 and TNF-α [124].

It was found that the antioxidant and anti-inflammatory action of curcumin contributed to the reversal of cognitive deficits related to the neurotoxicity of the β-amyloid peptide [140]. In experimental models both in vivo and in vitro, it has been shown that curcumin reduces the level of soluble β-amyloid peptide and the density of β-amyloid peptide plaques in brain tissue [141,142]. It has been revealed that curcumin prevents aggregation of the β-amyloid peptide in vitro and promotes the clearance of aggregates of the β-amyloid peptide. In addition, it has been presented that curcumin inhibits the maturation of the amyloid protein precursor and inhibits the generation of β-amyloid peptide in vitro [142]. Curcumin—by reducing the level of soluble tau protein, increasing the heat shock protein associated with the removal of tau protein, even after the formation of tangles—indicates that synaptic and behavioral dysfunctions caused by the tau protein are reversible [143]. It has been shown that curcumin inhibits oligomerization of the β-amyloid peptide and phosphorylation of tau protein in brain parenchyma and reverses cognitive deficits in the Alzheimer's disease model [144]. Curcumin has been documented to stimulate neuronal stem cell proliferation and neuronal differentiation and reverses β-amyloid peptide-induced inhibition of hippocampal neurogenesis and memory deficits in the Alzheimer's disease model [144,145]. Curcumin reduced the level of amyloid deposits and inhibited tau protein aggregation in the transgenic model of Alzheimer's disease and reduced oxidative damage, neuroinflammatory, and neurological response, as well as cognitive deficit after infusion of amyloid into the brain [146]. Curcumin reduces the level and activity of beta-secretase, aggregation of beta-amyloid peptide and accumulation, and increases amyloid clearance [147]. Curcumin also induces amyloid uptake by macrophages and stimulates metal chelation [147]. A summary of protective action of curcumin after brain ischemia injury is presented in Table 1.

5. Conclusions

In the present review, we discussed the neuroprotective effects of curcumin after ischemia-reperfusion brain injury. Accumulating evidence has clearly shown the role of the neuroprotective and neurological/cognitive enhancement effects of curcumin after brain ischemia-reperfusion injury with the phenotype of Alzheimer's disease (Table 1). Based on the data presented, it appears that curcumin has its own effective therapeutic potential through anti-amyloid, anti-tau protein hyperphosphorylation, anti-hyperhomocysteinemia, anti-oxidant, anti-inflammatory, and anti-apoptotic effects (Table 1) [116,117,119,143], which clearly indicates that curcumin can be used as a neuroprotective substance not only in ischemic neurodegeneration [33,148] but also in a neurodegenerative disease similar to Alzheimer's disease as a response to brain ischemia associated with hyperhomocysteinemia [149,150]. The available data show that curcumin induces neuroprotection and neurogenesis and may be a new therapeutic agent for both regenerative medicine and for the treatment of neurodegenerative disorders such as neurodegeneration after brain ischemia with the phenotype of Alzheimer's disease. Therefore, curcumin may be a promising supplementary agent against brain ischemia-reperfusion injury in the future. Indeed, there is a rational scientific basis for the use of curcumin for the prophylaxis and treatment of ischemic neurodegeneration. Nevertheless, despite initial hard data, prospective studies are needed to further clarify how curcumin could exert protective action against ischemic brain damage and how it can be used therapeutically. In particular, evidence from clinical randomized controlled trials would be helpful.

Funding: This research received no external funding.

Acknowledgments: The authors acknowledge support by the Mossakowski Medical Research Centre, Polish Academy of Sciences, Warsaw, Poland (T3-RP) and by the Medical University of Lublin, Poland (DS 475/18-SJC).

Conflicts of Interest: The authors declare no conflict of interest.

References

1. Desmond, D.W.; Moroney, J.T.; Sano, M.; Stern, Y. Incidence of dementia after ischemic stroke: Results of a longitudinal study. *Stroke* **2002**, *33*, 2254–2260. [CrossRef] [PubMed]
2. Honig, L.S.; Tang, M.X.; Albert, S.; Costa, R.; Luchsinger, J.; Manly, J.; Stern, Y.; Mayeux, R. Stroke and the risk of Alzheimer disease. *Arch. Neurol.* **2003**, *60*, 1707–1712. [CrossRef] [PubMed]
3. Jellinger, K.A. The enigma of vascular cognitive disorder and vascular dementia. *Acta Neuropathol.* **2007**, *113*, 349–388. [CrossRef] [PubMed]
4. Pinkston, J.B.; Alekseeva, N.; Toledo, E.G. Stroke and dementia. *Neurol. Res.* **2009**, *31*, 824–831. [CrossRef] [PubMed]
5. Gemmell, E.; Bosomworth, H.; Allan, L.; Hall, R.; Khundakar, A.; Oakley, A.E.; Deramecourt, V.; Polvikoski, T.M.; O'Brien, J.T.; Kalaria, R.N. Hippocampal neuronal atrophy and cognitive function in delayed poststroke and aging-related dementias. *Stroke* **2012**, *43*, 808–814. [CrossRef] [PubMed]
6. Brainin, M.; Tuomilehto, J.; Heiss, W.D.; Bornstein, N.M.; Bath, P.M.; Teuschl, Y.; Richard, E.; Guekht, A.; Quinn, T.; Post Stroke Cognition Study Group. Post-stroke cognitive decline: An update and perspectives for clinical research. *Eur. J. Neurol.* **2015**, *22*, 229–238. [CrossRef] [PubMed]
7. Mok, V.C.T.; Lam, B.Y.K.; Wang, Z.; Liu, W.; Au, L.; Leung, E.Y.L.; Chen, S.; Yang, J.; Chu, W.C.W.; Lau, A.Y.L.; et al. Delayed-onset dementia after stroke or transient ischemic attack. *Alzheimers Dement.* **2016**, *12*, 1167–1176. [CrossRef]
8. Portegies, M.L.; Wolters, F.J.; Hofman, A.; Ikram, M.K.; Koudstaal, P.J.; Ikram, M.A. Prestroke vascular pathology and the risk of recurrent stroke and poststroke dementia. *Stroke* **2016**, *47*, 2119–2122. [CrossRef]
9. Kim, J.H.; Lee, Y. Dementia and death after stroke in older adults during a 10-year follow-up: Results from a competing risk model. *J. Nutr. Health Aging* **2018**, *22*, 297–301. [CrossRef]
10. Cassella, C.R.; Jagoda, A. Ischemic stroke: Advances in diagnosis and management. *Emerg. Med. Clin. N. Am.* **2017**, *35*, 911–930. [CrossRef]
11. Bejot, Y.; Daubail, B.; Giroud, M. Epidemiology of stroke and transient ischemic attacks: Current knowledge and perspectives. *Rev. Neurol.* **2016**, *172*, 59–68. [CrossRef] [PubMed]
12. Ruitenberg, A.; den Heijer, T.; Bakker, S.L.; van Swieten, J.C.; Koudstaal, P.J.; Hofman, A.; Breteler, M.M. Cerebral hypoperfusion and clinical onset of dementia: The Rotterdam Study. *Ann. Neurol.* **2005**, *57*, 789–794. [CrossRef] [PubMed]
13. Barra de la Tremblaye, P.; Plamondon, H. Impaired conditioned emotional response and object recognition are concomitant to neuronal damage in the amygdale and perirhinal cortex in middle-aged ischemic rats. *Behav. Brain Res.* **2011**, *219*, 227–233. [CrossRef] [PubMed]
14. Kiryk, A.; Pluta, R.; Figiel, I.; Mikosz, M.; Ułamek, M.; Niewiadomska, G.; Jabłoński, M.; Kaczmarek, L. Transient brain ischemia due to cardiac arrest causes irreversible long-lasting cognitive injury. *Behav. Brain Res.* **2011**, *219*, 1–7. [CrossRef] [PubMed]
15. Li, J.; Wang, Y.J.; Zhang, M.; Fang, C.Q.; Zhou, H.D. Cerebral ischemia aggravates cognitive impairment in a rat model of Alzheimer's disease. *Life Sci.* **2011**, *89*, 86–92. [CrossRef] [PubMed]
16. Cohan, C.H.; Neumann, J.T.; Dave, K.R.; Alekseyenko, A.; Binkert, M.; Stransky, K.; Lin, H.W.; Barnes, C.A.; Wright, C.B.; Perez-Pinzon, M.A. Effect of cardiac arrest on cognitive impairment and hippocampal plasticity in middle-aged rats. *PLoS ONE* **2015**, *10*, e0124918. [CrossRef] [PubMed]
17. Pluta, R. Resuscitation of the rabbit brain after acute complete ischemia lasting up to 1 h. Pathophysiological and pathomorphological observations. *Resuscitation* **1987**, *15*, 267–287. [CrossRef]
18. Pluta, R.; Lossinsky, A.S.; Wisniewski, H.M.; Mossakowski, M.J. Early blood-brain barrier changes in the rat following transient complete cerebral ischemia induced by cardiac arrest. *Brain Res.* **1994**, *633*, 41–52. [CrossRef]

19. Pluta, R.; Kida, E.; Lossinsky, A.S.; Golabek, A.A.; Mossakowski, M.J.; Wisniewski, H.M. Complete cerebral ischemia with shortterm survival in rats induced by cardiac arrest: I. Extracellular accumulation of Alzheimer's β-amyloid protein precursor in the brain. *Brain Res.* **1994**, *649*, 323–328. [CrossRef]
20. Pluta, R. From brain ischemia-reperfusion injury to possible sporadic Alzheimer's disease. *Curr. Neurovasc. Res.* **2004**, *1*, 441–453. [CrossRef]
21. Pluta, R. Is the ischemic blood-brain barrier insufficiency responsible for full-blown Alzheimer's disease? *Neurol. Res.* **2006**, *28*, 266–271. [CrossRef] [PubMed]
22. Pluta, R. Role of ischemic blood–brain barrier on amyloid plaques development in Alzheimer's disease brain. *Curr. Neurovasc. Res.* **2007**, *4*, 121–129. [CrossRef] [PubMed]
23. Pluta, R.; Kocki, J.; Maciejewski, R.; Ułamek-Kozioł, M.; Jabłoński, M.; Bogucka-Kocka, A.; Czuczwar, S.J. Ischemia signalling to Alzheimer-related genes. *Curr. Neurovasc. Res.* **2012**, *50*, 322–329. [CrossRef]
24. Akinyemi, R.O.; Mukaetova-Ladinska, E.B.; Attems, J.; Ihara, M.; Kalaria, R.N. Vascular risk factors and neurodegeneration in ageing related dementias: Alzheimer's disease and vascular dementia. *Curr. Alzheimer Res.* **2013**, *10*, 642–653. [CrossRef] [PubMed]
25. Kelleher, R.J.; Soiza, R.L. Evidence of endothelial dysfunction in the development of Alzheimer's disease: Is Alzheimer's a vascular disorder? *Am. J. Cardiovasc. Dis.* **2013**, *3*, 197–226. [PubMed]
26. Pluta, R.; Furmaga-Jabłońska, W.; Maciejewski, R.; Ułamek-Kozioł, M.; Jabłoński, M. Brain ischemia activates β- and γ secretase cleavage of amyloid precursor protein: Significance in sporadic Alzheimer's disease. *Mol. Neurobiol.* **2013**, *47*, 425–434. [CrossRef]
27. Pluta, R.; Jabłoński, M.; Ułamek-Kozioł, M.; Kocki, J.; Brzozowska, J.; Januszewski, S.; Furmaga-Jabłońska, W.; Bogucka-Kocka, A.; Maciejewski, R.; Czuczwar, S.J. Sporadic Alzheimer'sdisease begins as episodes of brain ischemia and ischemically dysregulated Alzheimer's disease genes. *Mol. Neurobiol.* **2013**, *48*, 500–515. [CrossRef] [PubMed]
28. Roh, J.H.; Lee, J.H. Recent updates on subcortical ischemic vascular dementia. *J. Stroke* **2014**, *16*, 18–26. [CrossRef]
29. Pluta, R.; Ułamek, M.; Jabłoński, M. Alzheimer's mechanisms in ischemic brain degeneration. *Anat. Rec.* **2009**, *292*, 1863–1881. [CrossRef]
30. Pluta, R. Glial expression of the β-amyloid peptide in cardiac arrest. *J. Neurol. Sci.* **2002**, *204*, 277–280. [CrossRef]
31. Pluta, R. Astroglial expression of the beta-amyloid in ischemia-reperfusion brain injury. *Ann. N. Y. Acad. Sci.* **2002**, *977*, 102–108. [CrossRef] [PubMed]
32. Sekeljic, V.; Bataveljic, D.; Stamenkovic, S.; Ułamek, M.; Jabłoński, M.; Radenovic, L.; Pluta, R.; Andjus, P.R. Cellular markers of neuroinflammation and neurogenesis after ischemic brain injury in the long-term survival rat model. *Brain Struct. Funct.* **2012**, *217*, 411–420. [CrossRef] [PubMed]
33. Pluta, R.; Ułamek-Kozioł, M.; Januszewski, S.; Czuczwar, S.J. From brain ischemia to Alzheimer-like neurodegeneration. *Neuropsychiatry* **2018**, *8*, 1708–1714. [CrossRef]
34. Wen, Y.; Yang, S.H.; Liu, R.; Perez, E.J.; Brun-Zinkernagel, A.M.; Koulen, P.; Simpkins, J.W. Cdk5 is involved in NFT-like tauopathy induced by transient cerebral ischemia in female rats. *Biochim. Biophys. Acta* **2007**, *1772*, 473–483. [CrossRef] [PubMed]
35. Pluta, R.; Ułamek-Kozioł, M.; Januszewski, S.; Czuczwar, S.J. Tau protein dysfunction after brain ischemia. *J. Alzheimers Dis.* **2018**, *66*, 429–437. [CrossRef] [PubMed]
36. Pluta, R.; Ułamek, M.; Januszewski, S. Microblood-brain barrier openings and cytotoxic fragments of amyloid precursor protein accumulation in white matter after ischemic brain injury in long-lived rats. *Acta Neurochir.* **2006**, *96*, 267–271.
37. Pluta, R.; Januszewski, S.; Ułamek, M. Ischemic blood–brain barrier and amyloid in white matter as etiological factors in leukoaraiosis. *Acta Neurochir.* **2008**, *102*, 353–356.
38. Urabe, T. Molecular mechanism and new protective strategy for ischemic white matter damages. *Rinsho Shinkeigaku* **2012**, *52*, 908–910. [CrossRef]
39. Bang, J.; Jeon, W.K.; Lee, I.S.; Han, J.S.; Kim, B.Y. Biphasic functional regulation in hippocampus of rat with chronic cerebral hypoperfusion induced by permanent occlusion of bilateral common carotid artery. *PLoS ONE* **2013**, *8*, e70093. [CrossRef]
40. Arrich, J.; Holzer, M.; Havel, C.; Müllner, M.; Herkner, H. Hypothermia for neuroprotection in adults after cardiopulmonary resuscitation. *Cochrane Database Syst. Rev.* **2012**, *9*, CD004128.

41. Herson, P.S.; Traystman, R.J. Animal models of stroke: Translational potential at present and in 2050. *Future Neurol.* **2014**, *9*, 541–551. [CrossRef] [PubMed]
42. Pluta, R. The role of apolipoprotein E in the deposition of β-amyloid peptide during ischemia–reperfusion brain injury. A model of early Alzheimer's disease. *Ann. N. Y. Acad. Sci.* **2000**, *903*, 324–334. [CrossRef] [PubMed]
43. Pluta, R.; Salińska, E.; Puka, M.; Staniej, A.; Nazarewicz, J.W. Early changes in extracellular amino acids and calcium concentrations in rabbit hippocampus following complete 15-min cerebral ischemia. *Resuscitation* **1988**, *16*, 193–210. [CrossRef]
44. Scheff, S.W.; Price, D.A.; Schmitt, F.A.; Scheff, M.A.; Mufson, E.J. Synaptic loss in the inferior temporal gyrus in mild cognitive impairment and Alzheimer's disease. *J. Alzheimers Dis.* **2011**, *24*, 547–557. [CrossRef] [PubMed]
45. Wang, X.; Xing, A.; Xu, C.; Cai, Q.; Liu, H.; Li, L. Cerebrovascular hypoperfusion induces spatial memory impairment, synaptic changes, and amyloid-beta oligomerization in rats. *J. Alzheimers Dis.* **2010**, *21*, 813–822. [CrossRef] [PubMed]
46. Zhao, Y.; Gu, J.H.; Dai, C.L.; Liu, Q.; Iqbal, K.; Liu, F.; Gong, C.X. Chronic cerebral hypoperfusion causes decrease of O-GlcNAcylation, hyperphosphorylation of tau and behavioral deficits in mice. *Front. Aging Neurosci.* **2014**, *6*, 10. [CrossRef]
47. Ni, J.W.; Matsumoto, K.; Li, H.B.; Murakami, Y.; Watanabe, H. Neuronal damage and decrease of central acetylcholine level following permanent occlusion of bilateral common carotid arteries in rat. *Brain Res.* **1995**, *673*, 290–296. [CrossRef]
48. Ruan, Y.W.; Han, X.J.; Shi, Z.S.; Lei, Z.G.; Xu, Z.C. Remodeling of synapses in the CA1 area of the hippocampus after transient global ischemia. *Neuroscience* **2012**, *218*, 268–277. [CrossRef]
49. Ułamek-Kozioł, M.; Furmaga-Jabłońska, W.; Januszewski, S.; Brzozowska, J.; Sciślewska, M.; Jabłoński, M.; Pluta, R. Neuronal autophagy: Self-eating or self-cannibalism in Alzheimer's disease. *Neurochem. Res.* **2013**, *38*, 1769–1773. [CrossRef]
50. Hofmeijer, J.; van Putten, M.J. Ischemic cerebral damage: An appraisal of synaptic failure. *Stroke* **2012**, *43*, 607–615. [CrossRef]
51. Curcio, M.; Salazar, I.L.; Mele, M.; Canzoniero, L.M.; Duarte, C.B. Calpains and neuronal damage in the ischemic brain: The swiss knife in synaptic injury. *Prog. Neurobiol.* **2016**, *143*, 1–35. [CrossRef] [PubMed]
52. Fernando, M.S.; Simpson, J.E.; Matthews, F.; Brayne, C.; Lewis, C.E.; Barber, R.; Kalaria, R.N.; Forster, G.; Esteves, F.; Wharton, S.B.; et al. White matter lesions in an unselected cohort of the elderly: Molecular pathology suggests origin from chronic hypoperfusion injury. *Stroke* **2006**, *37*, 1391–1398. [CrossRef] [PubMed]
53. Scherr, M.; Trinka, E.; Mc Coy, M.; Krenn, Y.; Staffen, W.; Kirschner, M.; Bergmann, H.J.; Mutzenbach, J.S. Cerebral hypoperfusion during carotid artery stenosis can lead to cognitive deficits that may be independent of white matter lesion load. *Curr. Neurovasc. Res.* **2012**, *9*, 193–199. [CrossRef] [PubMed]
54. Thiebaut de Schotten, M.; Tomaiuolo, F.; Aiello, M.; Merola, S.; Silvetti, M.; Lecce, F.; Bartolomeo, P.; Doricchi, F. Damage to white matter pathways in subacute and chronic spatial neglect: A group study and 2 single-case studies with complete virtual "in vivo" tractography dissection. *Cereb. Cortex* **2014**, *24*, 691–706. [CrossRef] [PubMed]
55. Wakita, H.; Tomimoto, H.; Akiguchi, I.; Kimura, J. Glial activation and white matter changes in the rat brain induced by chronic cerebral hypoperfusion: An immunohistochemical study. *Acta Neuropathol.* **1994**, *87*, 484–492. [CrossRef] [PubMed]
56. Yoshizaki, K.; Adachi, K.; Kataoka, S.; Watanabe, A.; Tabira, T.; Takahashi, K.; Wakita, H. Chronic cerebral hypoperfusion induced by right unilateral common carotid artery occlusion causes delayed white matter lesions and cognitive impairment in adult mice. *Exp. Neurol.* **2008**, *210*, 585–591. [CrossRef] [PubMed]
57. Pluta, R.; Barcikowska, M.; Januszewski, S.; Misicka, A.; Lipkowski, A.W. Evidence of blood–brain barrier permeability/leakage for circulating human Alzheimer's β-amyloid-(1–42)-peptide. *NeuroReport* **1996**, *7*, 1261–1265. [CrossRef]
58. Pluta, R.; Barcikowska, M.; Misicka, A.; Lipkowski, A.W.; Spisacka, S.; Januszewski, S. Ischemic rats as a model in the study of the neurobiological role of human β-amyloid peptide. Time-dependent disappearing diffuse amyloid plaques in brain. *NeuroReport* **1999**, *10*, 3615–3619. [CrossRef]

59. Pluta, R.; Misicka, A.; Barcikowska, M.; Spisacka, S.; Lipkowski, A.W.; Januszewski, S. Possible reverse transport of β-amyloid peptide across the blood-brain barrier. *Acta Neurochir.* **2000**, *76*, 73–77.
60. Anfuso, C.D.; Assero, G.; Lupo, G.; Nicota, A.; Cannavo, G.; Strosznajder, R.P.; Rapisarda, P.; Pluta, R.; Alberghia, M. Amyloid β(1-42) and its β(25-35) fragment induce activation and membrane translocation of cytosolic phospholipase A(2) in bovine retina capillary pericytes. *Biochim. Biophys. Acta* **2004**, *1686*, 125–138. [CrossRef]
61. Lee, P.H.; Bang, O.Y.; Hwang, E.M.; Lee, J.S.; Joo, U.S.; Mook-Jung, I.; Huh, K. Circulating β amyloid peptide is elevated in patients with acute ischemic stroke. *J. Neurol. Transm.* **2005**, *112*, 1371–1379. [CrossRef] [PubMed]
62. Pluta, R. Pathological opening of the blood–brain barrier to horseradish peroxidase and amyloid precursor protein following ischemia-reperfusion brain injury. *Chemotherapy* **2005**, *51*, 223–226. [CrossRef] [PubMed]
63. Pluta, R.; Januszewski, S.; Jabłoński, M.; Ułamek, M. Factors in creepy delayed neuronal death in hippocampus following brain ischemia-reperfusion injury with long-term survival. *Acta Neurochir.* **2010**, *106*, 37–41.
64. Mörtberg, E.; Zetterberg, H.; Nordmark, J.; Blennow, K.; Catry, C.; Decraemer, H.; Vanmechelen, E.; Rubertsson, S. Plasma tau protein in comatose patients after cardiac arrest treated with therapeutic hypothermia. *Acta Anaesthesiol. Scand.* **2011**, *55*, 1132–1138. [CrossRef] [PubMed]
65. Zetterberg, H.; Mörtberg, E.; Song, L.; Chang, L.; Provuncher, G.K.; Patel, P.P.; Ferrell, E.; Fournier, D.R.; Kan, C.W.; Campbell, T.G.; et al. Hypoxia due to cardiac arrest induces a time-dependent increase in serum amyloid β levels in humans. *PLoS ONE* **2011**, *6*, e28263. [CrossRef] [PubMed]
66. Randall, J.; Mörtberg, E.; Provuncher, G.K.; Fournier, D.R.; Duffy, D.C.; Rubertsson, S.; Blennow, K.; Zetterberg, H.; Wilson, D.H. Tau proteins in serum predict neurological outcome after hypoxic brain injury from cardiac arrest: Results of a pilot study. *Resuscitation* **2013**, *84*, 351–356. [CrossRef] [PubMed]
67. Jabłoński, M.; Maciejewski, R.; Januszewski, S.; Ułamek, M.; Pluta, R. One year follow up in ischemic brain injury and the role of Alzheimer factors. *Physiol. Res.* **2011**, *60*, 113–119.
68. Jendroska, K.; Poewe, W.; Daniel, S.E.; Pluess, J.; Iwerssen-Schmidt, H.; Paulsen, J.; Barthel, S.; Schelosky, L.; Cervos-Navarro, J.; DeArmond, S.J. Ischemic stress induces deposition of amyloid β immunoreactivity in human brain. *Acta Neuropathol.* **1995**, *90*, 461–466. [CrossRef]
69. Wisniewski, H.M.; Maślinska, D. β-Protein immunoreactivity in the human brain after cardiac arrest. *Curr. Neurovasc. Res.* **1996**, *34*, 65–71.
70. Jendroska, K.; Hoffmann, O.M.; Patt, S. Amyloid β peptide and precursor protein (APP) in mild and severe brain ischemia. *Ann. N. Y. Acad. Sci.* **1997**, *826*, 401–405. [CrossRef]
71. Qi, J.; Wu, H.; Yang, Y.; Wand, D.; Chen, Y.; Gu, Y.; Liu, T. Cerebral ischemia and Alzheimer's disease: The expression of amyloid-β and apolipoprotein E in human hippocampus. *J. Alzheimers Dis.* **2007**, *12*, 335–341. [CrossRef] [PubMed]
72. Maślińska, D.; Laure-Kamionowska, M.; Taraszewska, A.; Deręgowski, K.; Maśliński, S. Immunodistribution of amyloid β protein (Aβ) and advanced glycation end-product receptors (RAGE) in choroid plexus and ependyma of resuscitated patients. *Curr. Neurovasc. Res.* **2011**, *49*, 295–300.
73. Ułamek-Kozioł, M.; Pluta, R.; Bogucka-Kocka, A.; Januszewski, S.; Kocki, J.; Czuczwar, S.J. Brain ischemia with Alzheimer phenotype dysregulates Alzheimer's disease-related proteins. *Pharmacol. Rep.* **2016**, *68*, 582–591. [CrossRef] [PubMed]
74. Hall, E.D.; Oostveen, J.A.; Dunn, E.; Carter, D.B. Increased amyloid protein precursor and apolipoprotein E immunoreactivity in the selectively vulnerable hippocampus following transient forebrain ischemia in gerbils. *Exp. Neurol.* **1995**, *135*, 17–27. [CrossRef] [PubMed]
75. Ishimaru, H.; Ishikawa, K.; Haga, S.; Shoji, M.; Ohe, Y.; Haga, C.; Sasaki, A.; Takahashi, A.; Maruyama, Y. Accumulation of apolipoprotein E and β-amyloid-like protein in a trace of the hippocampal CA1 pyramidal cell layer after ischaemic delayed neuronal death. *NeuroReport* **1996**, *7*, 3063–3067. [CrossRef] [PubMed]
76. Yokota, M.; Saido, T.C.; Tani, E.; Yamaura, I.; Minami, N. Cytotoxic fragment of amyloid precursor protein accumulates in hippocampus after global forebrain ischemia. *J. Cereb. Blood Flow Metab.* **1996**, *16*, 1219–1223. [CrossRef] [PubMed]
77. Lin, B.; Schmidt-Kastner, R.; Busto, R.; Ginsberg, M.D. Progressive parenchymal deposition of β-amyloid precursor protein in rat brain following global cerebral ischemia. *Acta Neuropathol.* **1999**, *97*, 359–368. [CrossRef]

78. Sinigaglia-Coimbra, R.; Cavalheiro, E.A.; Coimbra, C.G. Postischemic hypertermia induces Alzheimer-like pathology in the rat brain. *Acta Neuropathol.* **2002**, *103*, 444–452.
79. Mossakowski, M.J.; Lossinsky, A.S.; Pluta, R.; Wiśniewski, H.M. Abnormalities of the blood brain barrier in global cerebral ischemia in rats due to experimental cardiac arrest. *Acta Neurochir.* **1994**, *60*, 274–276.
80. Pluta, R. Blood-brain barrier dysfunction and amyloid precursor protein accumulation in microvascular compartment following ischemia-reperfusion brain injury with 1-year survival. *Acta Neurochir.* **2003**, *86*, 117–122.
81. van Groen, T.; Puurunen, K.; Maki, H.M.; Sivenius, J.; Jolkkonen, J. Transformation of diffuse β-amyloid precursor protein and β-amyloid deposits to plaques in the thalamus after transient occlusion of the middle cerebral artery in rats. *Stroke* **2005**, *36*, 1551–1556. [CrossRef] [PubMed]
82. Wiśniewski, H.M.; Pluta, R.; Lossinsky, A.S.; Mossakowski, M.J. Ultrastructural studies of cerebral vascular spasm after cardiac arrest-related global cerebral ischemia in rats. *Acta Neuropathol.* **1995**, *90*, 432–440. [CrossRef] [PubMed]
83. Kato, T.; Hirano, A.; Katagiri, T.; Sasaki, H.; Yamada, S. Neurofibrillary tangle formation in the nucleus basalis of Meynert ipsilateral to a massive cerebral infarct. *Ann. Neurol.* **1988**, *23*, 620–623. [CrossRef] [PubMed]
84. Yao, Z.H.; Zhang, J.J.; Xie, X.F. Enriched environment prevents cognitive impairment and tau hyperphosphorylation after chronic cerebral hypoperfusion. *Curr. Neurovasc. Res.* **2012**, *9*, 176–184. [CrossRef] [PubMed]
85. Kocki, J.; Ułamek-Kozioł, M.; Bogucka-Kocka, A.; Januszewski, S.; Jabłoński, M.; Gil-Kulik, P.; Brzozowska, J.; Petniak, A.; Furmaga-Jabłońska, W.; Bogucki, J.; et al. Dysregulation of amyloid-β protein precursor, β-secretase, presenilin 1 and 2 genes in the rat selectively vulnerable CA1 subfield of hippocampus following transient global brain ischemia. *J. Alzheimers Dis.* **2015**, *47*, 1047–1056. [CrossRef] [PubMed]
86. Ułamek-Kozioł, M.; Pluta, R.; Januszewski, S.; Kocki, J.; Bogucka-Kocka, A.; Czuczwar, S.J. Expression of Alzheimer's disease risk genes in ischemic brain degeneration. *Pharmacol. Rep.* **2016**, *68*, 1345–1349. [CrossRef] [PubMed]
87. Pluta, R.; Kocki, J.; Ułamek-Kozioł, M.; Petniak, A.; Gil-Kulik, P.; Januszewski, S.; Bogucki, J.; Jabłoński, M.; Brzozowska, J.; Furmaga-Jabłońska, W.; et al. Discrepancy in expression of β-secretase and amyloid-β protein precursor in Alzheimer-related genes in the rat medial temporal lobe cortex following transient global brain ischemia. *J. Alzheimers Dis.* **2016**, *51*, 1023–1031. [CrossRef] [PubMed]
88. Pluta, R.; Kocki, J.; Ułamek-Kozioł, M.; Bogucka-Kocka, A.; Gil-Kulik, P.; Januszewski, S.; Jabłoński, M.; Petniak, A.; Brzozowska, J.; Bogucki, J.; et al. Alzheimer-associated presenilin 2 gene is dysregulated in rat medial temporal lobe cortex after complete brain ischemia due to cardiac arrest. *Pharmacol. Rep.* **2016**, *68*, 155–161. [CrossRef] [PubMed]
89. Pluta, R.; Bogucka-Kocka, A.; Ułamek-Kozioł, M.; Bogucki, J.; Januszewski, S.; Kocki, J.; Czuczwar, S.J. Ischemic tau protein gene induction as an additional key factor driving development of Alzheimer's phenotype changes in CA1 area of hippocampus in an ischemic model of Alzheimer's disease. *Pharmacol. Rep.* **2018**, *70*, 881–884. [CrossRef]
90. Ułamek-Kozioł, M.; Kocki, J.; Bogucka-Kocka, A.; Januszewski, S.; Bogucki, J.; Czuczwar, SJ.; Pluta, R. Autophagy, mitophagy and apoptotic gene changes in the hippocampal CA1 area in a rat ischemic model of Alzheimer's disease. *Pharmacol. Rep.* **2017**, *69*, 1289–1294. [CrossRef]
91. Ułamek-Kozioł, M.; Kocki, J.; Bogucka-Kocka, A.; Petniak, A.; Gil-Kulik, P.; Januszewski, S.; Bogucki, J.; Jabłoński, M.; Furmaga-Jabłońska, W.; Brzozowska, J.; et al. Dysregulation of autophagy, mitophagy and apoptotic genes in the medial temporal lobe cortex in an ischemic model of Alzheimer's disease. *J. Alzheimers Dis.* **2016**, *54*, 113–121. [CrossRef] [PubMed]
92. Block, F. Global ischemia and behavioural deficits. *Prog. Neurobiol.* **1999**, *58*, 279–295. [CrossRef]
93. Pluta, R.; Jolkkonen, J.; Cuzzocrea, S.; Pedata, F.; Cechetto, D.; PopaWagner, A. Cognitive impairment with vascular impairment and degeneration. *Curr. Neurovasc. Res.* **2011**, *8*, 342–350. [CrossRef] [PubMed]
94. Popa-Wagner, A. Alzheimer's disease pathological factors in ischemic aged brain. In *Ischemia-Reperfusion Pathways in Alzheimer's Disease*; Pluta, R., Ed.; Nova Science Publishers, Inc.: New York, NY, USA, 2007; pp. 51–84.

95. Yang, S.H.; Simpkins, J.W. Ischemia–reperfusion promotes tau and beta-amyloid pathology and a progressive cognitive impairment. In *Ischemia-Reperfusion Pathways in Alzheimer's Disease*; Pluta, R., Ed.; Nova Science Publishers, Inc.: New York, NY, USA, 2007; pp. 113–138.
96. Kuroiwa, T.; Bonnekoh, P.; Hossmann, K.A. Locomotor hyperactivity and hippocampal CA1 injury after transient forebrain ischemia in gerbils. *Neurosci. Lett.* **1991**, *122*, 141–144. [CrossRef]
97. Karasawa, Y.; Araki, H.; Otomo, S. Changes in locomotor activity and passive avoidance task performance induced by cerebral ischemia in mongolian gerbils. *Stroke* **1994**, *25*, 645–650. [CrossRef] [PubMed]
98. Langdon, K.D.; Granter-Button, S.; Corbett, D. Persistent behavioral impairments and neuroinflammation following global ischemia in the rat. *Eur. J. Neurosci.* **2008**, *28*, 2310–2318. [CrossRef] [PubMed]
99. Mileson, B.E.; Schwartz, R.D. The use of locomotor activity as a behavioral screen for neuronal damage following transient forebrain ischemia in gerbils. *Neurosci. Lett.* **1991**, *128*, 71–76. [CrossRef]
100. Colbourne, F.; Corbett, D. Delayed postischemic hypothermia: A six month survival study using behavioral and histological assessments of neuroprotection. *J. Neurosci.* **1995**, *15*, 7250–7260. [CrossRef]
101. Davis, H.P.; Tribuna, J.; Pulsinelli, W.A.; Volpe, B.T. Reference and working memory of rats following hippocampal damage induced by transient forebrain ischemia. *Physiol. Behav.* **1986**, *37*, 387–392. [CrossRef]
102. Kiyota, Y.; Miyamoto, M.; Nagaoka, A. Relationship between brain damage and memory impairment in rats exposed to transient forebrain ischemia. *Brain Res.* **1991**, *538*, 295–302. [CrossRef]
103. Block, F.; Schwarz, M. Global ischemic neuronal damage relates to behavioural deficits: A pharmacological approach. *Neuroscience* **1998**, *82*, 791–803. [CrossRef]
104. Karhunen, H.; Pitkanen, A.; Virtanen, T.; Gureviciene, I.; Pussinen, R.; Ylinen, A.; Sivenius, J.; Nissinen, J.; Jolkkonen, J. Long-term functional consequences of transient occlusion of the middle cerebral artery in rats: A 1-year follow-up of the development of epileptogenesis and memory impairment in relation to sensorimotor deficits. *Epilepsy Res.* **2003**, *54*, 1–10. [CrossRef]
105. Roof, R.L.; Schielke, G.P.; Ren, X.; Hall, E.D. A comparison of longterm functional outcome after 2 middle cerebral artery occlusion models in rats. *Stroke* **2001**, *32*, 2648–2657. [CrossRef] [PubMed]
106. Ishibashi, S.; Kuroiwa, T.; LiYuan, S.; Katsumata, N.; Li, S.; Endo, S.; Mizusawa, H. Long-term cognitive and neuropsychological symptoms after global cerebral ischemia in Mongolian gerbils. *Acta Neurochir.* **2006**, *96*, 299–302.
107. Hossmann, K.A.; Schmidt-Kastner, R.; Grosse Ophoff, B. Recovery of integrative central nervous function after one hour global cerebro-circulatory arrest in normothermic cat. *J. Neurol. Sci.* **1987**, *77*, 305–320. [CrossRef]
108. Funk, J.L.; Frye, J.B.; Davis-Gorman, G.; Spera, A.L.; Bernas, M.J.; Witte, M.H.; Weinand, M.E.; Timmermann, B.N.; McDonagh, P.F.; Ritter, L. Curcuminoids limit neutrophil-mediated reperfusion injury in experimental stroke by targeting the endothelium. *Microcirculation* **2013**, *20*, 544–554. [CrossRef]
109. Dohare, P.; Garg, P.; Jain, V.; Nath, C.; Ray, M. Dose dependence and therapeutic window for the neuroprotective effects of curcumin in thromboembolic model of rat. *Behav. Brain Res.* **2008**, *193*, 289–297. [CrossRef]
110. Liu, S.; Cao, Y.; Qu, M.; Zhang, Z.; Feng, L.; Ye, Z.; Xiao, M.; Hou, S.T.; Zheng, R.; Han, Z. Curcumin protects against stroke and increases levels of Notch intracellular domain. *Neurol. Res.* **2016**, *38*, 553–559. [CrossRef]
111. Altinay, S.; Cabalar, M.; Isler, C.; Yildirim, F.; Celik, D.S.; Zengi, O.; Tas, A.; Gulcubuk, A. Is chronic curcumin supplementation neuroprotective against ischemia for antioxidant activity, neurological deficit, or neuronal apoptosis in an experimental stroke model? *Turk Neurosurg.* **2017**, *27*, 537–545.
112. Kalani, A.; Chaturvedi, P.; Kamat, P.K.; Maldonado, C.; Bauer, P.; Joshua, I.G.; Tyagi, S.C.; Tyagi, N. Curcumin-loaded embryonic stem cell exosomes restored neurovascular unit following ischemia-reperfusion injury. *Int. J. Biochem. Cell Biol.* **2016**, *79*, 360–369. [CrossRef]
113. Kelly-Cobbs, A.I.; Prakash, R.; Li, W.; Pillai, B.; Hafez, S.; Coucha, M.; Johnson, M.H.; Ogbi, S.N.; Fagan, S.C.; Ergul, A. Targets of vascular protection in acute ischemic stroke differ in type 2 diabetes. *Am. J. Phys. Heart Circ. Phys.* **2013**, *304*, H806–H815. [CrossRef] [PubMed]
114. Wang, Q.; Sun, A.Y.; Simonyi, A.; Jensen, M.D.; Shelat, P.B.; Rottinghaus, G.E.; MacDonald, R.S.; Miller, D.K.; Lubahn, D.E.; Weisman, G.A.; et al. Neuroprotective mechanisms of curcumin against cerebral ischemia-induced neuronal apoptosis and behavioral deficits. *J. Neurosci. Res.* **2005**, *82*, 138–148. [CrossRef] [PubMed]

115. Ahmad, N.; Umar, S.; Ashafaq, M.; Akhtar, M.; Iqbal, Z.; Samim, M.; Ahmad, F.J. A comparative study of PNIPAM nanoparticles of curcumin, demethoxycurcumin, and bisdemethoxycurcumin and their effects on oxidative stress markers in experimental stroke. *Protoplasma* **2013**, *250*, 1327–1338. [CrossRef] [PubMed]
116. Mukherjee, A.; Sarkar, S.; Jana, S.; Swarnakar, S.; Das, N. Neuro-protective role of nanocapsulated curcumin against cerebral ischemia-reperfusion induced oxidative injury. *Brain Res.* **2019**, *1704*, 164–173. [CrossRef] [PubMed]
117. Thiyagarajan, M.; Sharma, S.S. Neuroprotective effect of curcumin in middle cerebral artery occlusion induced focal cerebral ischemia in rats. *Life Sci.* **2004**, *74*, 969–985. [CrossRef] [PubMed]
118. Jiang, J.; Wang, W.; Sun, Y.J.; Hu, M.; Li, F.; Zhu, D.Y. Neuroprotective effect of curcumin on focal cerebral ischemic rats by preventing blood–brain barrier damage. *Eur. J. Pharmacol.* **2007**, *561*, 54–62. [CrossRef] [PubMed]
119. Tyagi, N.; Qipshidze, N.; Munjal, C.; Vacek, J.C.; Metreveli, N.; Givvimani, S.; Tyagi, S.C. Tetrahydrocurcumin ameliorates homocysteinylated cytochrome-c mediated autophagy in hyperhomocysteinemia mice after cerebral ischemia. *J. Mol. Neurosci.* **2012**, *47*, 128–138. [CrossRef]
120. Huang, L.; Chen, C.; Zhang, X.; Li, X.; Chen, Z.; Yang, C.; Liang, X.; Zhu, G.; Xu, Z. Neuroprotective effect of curcumin against cerebral ischemia-reperfusion via mediating autophagy and inflammation. *J. Mol. Neurosci.* **2018**, *64*, 129–139. [CrossRef]
121. Zhang, Y.; Fang, M.; Sun, Y.; Zhang, T.; Shi, N.; Li, J.; Jin, L.; Liu, K.; Fu, J. Curcumin attenuates cerebral ischemia injury in Sprague-Dawley rats and PC12 cells by suppressing overactivated autophagy. *J. Photochem. Photobiol. B* **2018**, *184*, 1–6. [CrossRef]
122. Barreto, G.E.; Sun, X.; Xu, L.; Giffard, R.G. Astrocyte proliferation following stroke in the mouse depends on distance from the infarct. *PLoS ONE* **2011**, *6*, e27881. [CrossRef]
123. Zhao, J.; Yu, S.; Zheng, W.; Feng, G.; Luo, G.; Wang, L.; Zhao, Y. Curcumin improves outcomes and attenuates focal cerebral ischemic injury via anti-apoptotic mechanisms in rats. *Neurochem. Res.* **2010**, *35*, 374–379. [CrossRef]
124. Miao, Y.; Zhao, S.; Gao, Y.; Wang, R.; Wu, Q.; Wu, H.; Luo, T. Curcumin pretreatment attenuates inflammation and mitochondrial dysfunction in experimental stroke: The possible role of Sirt1 signaling. *Brain Res. Bull.* **2016**, *121*, 9–15. [CrossRef] [PubMed]
125. Liu, L.; Zhang, W.; Wang, L.; Li, Y.; Tan, B.; Lu, X.; Deng, Y.; Zhang, Y.; Guo, X.; Mu, J.; et al. Curcumin prevents cerebral ischemia reperfusion injury via increase of mitochondrial biogenesis. *Neurochem. Res.* **2014**, *39*, 1322–1331. [CrossRef] [PubMed]
126. DeGracia, D.J.; Montie, H.L. Cerebral ischemia and the unfolded protein response. *J. Neurochem.* **2004**, *91*, 1–8. [CrossRef] [PubMed]
127. Avila, M.F.; Cabezas, R.; Torrente, D.; Gonzalez, J.; Morales, L.; Alvarez, L.; Capani, F.; Barreto, G.E. Novel interactions of GRP78: UPR and estrogen responses in the brain. *Cell Biol. Int.* **2013**, *37*, 521–532. [CrossRef] [PubMed]
128. Martin-Jiménez, C.A.; García-Vega, Á.; Cabezas, R.; Aliev, G.; Echeverria, V.; González, J.; Barreto, G.E. Astrocytes and endoplasmic reticulum stress: A bridge between obesity and neurodegenerative diseases. *Prog. Neurobiol.* **2017**, *158*, 45–68. [CrossRef] [PubMed]
129. Zhu, H.; Fan, Y.; Sun, H.; Chen, L.; Man, X. Curcumin inhibits endoplasmic reticulum stress induced by cerebral ischemia reperfusion injury in rats. *Exp. Ther. Med.* **2017**, *14*, 4047–4052. [CrossRef]
130. Ferri, K.F.; Kroemer, G. Organelle-specific initiation of cell death pathways. *Nat. Cell Biol.* **2001**, *3*, E255. [CrossRef]
131. Li, G.; Mongillo, M.; Chin, K.-T.; Harding, H.; Ron, D.; Marks, A.R.; Tabas, I. Role of ERO1-α–mediated stimulation of inositol 1, 4, 5-triphosphate receptor activity in endoplasmic reticulum stress–induced apoptosis. *J. Cell Biol.* **2009**, *186*, 783–792. [CrossRef]
132. Berner, M.D.; Sura, M.E.; Alves, B.N.; Hunter, K.W., Jr. IFN-γ primes macrophages for enhanced TNF-α expression in response to stimulatory and non-stimulatory amounts of microparticulate β-glucan. *Immunol. Lett.* **2005**, *98*, 115–122. [CrossRef]
133. Raza, S.S.; Khan, M.M.; Ahmad, A.; Ashafaq, M.; Khuwaja, G.; Tabassum, R.; Javed, H.; Siddiqui, M.S.; Safhi, M.M.; Islam, F. Hesperidin ameliorates functional and histological outcome and reduces neuroinflammation in experimental stroke. *Brain Res.* **2011**, *1420*, 93–105. [CrossRef] [PubMed]

134. Jayaprakasha, G.; Rao, L.J.; Sakariah, K. Antioxidant activities of curcumin, demethoxycurcumin and bisdemethoxycurcumin. *Food Chem.* **2006**, *98*, 720–724. [CrossRef]
135. Sandur, S.K.; Pandey, M.K.; Sung, B.; Ahn, K.S.; Murakami, A.; Sethi, G.; Limtrakul, P.; Badmaev, V.; Aggarwal, B.B. Curcumin, demethoxycurcumin, bisdemethoxycurcumin, tetrahydrocurcumin and turmerones differentially regulate anti-inflammatory and antiproliferative responses through a ROS-independent mechanism. *Carcinogenesis* **2007**, *28*, 1765–1773. [CrossRef] [PubMed]
136. Sun, M.; Zhao, Y.; Gu, Y.; Xu, C. Inhibition of nNOS reduces ischemic cell death through down-regulating calpain and caspase-3 after experimental stroke. *Neurochem. Int.* **2009**, *54*, 339–346. [CrossRef] [PubMed]
137. Jia, G.; Tan, B.; Ma, J.; Zhang, L.; Jin, X.; Li, C. Prdx6 upregulation by curcumin attenuates ischemic oxidative damage via SP1 in rats after stroke. *Biomed. Res. Int.* **2017**, *2017*, 1–9. [CrossRef] [PubMed]
138. Avci, G.; Kadioglu, H.; Sehirli, A.O.; Bozkurt, S.; Guclu, O.; Arslan, E.; Muratli, S.K. Curcumin protects against ischemia/reperfusion injury in rat skeletal muscle. *J. Surg. Res.* **2012**, *172*, e39–e46. [CrossRef] [PubMed]
139. Wu, J.; Zhang, L.; Chen, Y.; Yu, S.; Zhao, Y.; Zhao, J. Curcumin pretreatment and post-treatment both improve the antioxidative ability of neurons with oxygen-glucose deprivation. *Neural Regen. Res.* **2015**, *10*, 481.
140. Frautschy, S.A.; Hu, W.; Kim, P.; Miller, S.A.; Chu, T.; Harris-White, M.E.; Cole, G.M. Phenolic anti-inflammatory antioxidant reversal of Abeta-induced cognitive deficits and neuropathology. *Neurobiol. Aging* **2001**, *22*, 993–1005. [CrossRef]
141. Dong, S.; Zeng, Q.; Mitchell, E.S.; Xiu, J.; Duan, Y.; Li, C.H.; Tiwari, J.K.; Hu, Y.; Cao, X.; Zhao, Z. Curcumin enhances neurogenesis and cognition in aged rats: Implications for transcriptional interactions related to growth and synaptic plasticity. *PLoS ONE* **2012**, *7*, e31211. [CrossRef]
142. Estabeyoglu, T.; Huebbe, P.; Ernst, I.M.A.; Chin, D.; Wagner, A.E.; Rimbach, G. Curcumin from molecule to biological function. *Angew. Rev. Int. Ed.* **2012**, *51*, 5308–5332. [CrossRef]
143. Ma, Q.L.; Zuo, X.; Yang, F.; Ubeda, O.J.; Gant, D.J.; Alaverdyan, M.; Teng, E.; Hu, S.; Chen, P.P.; Maiti, P.; et al. Curcumin suppresses soluble tau dimers and corrects molecular chaperone, synaptic, and behavioral deficits in aged human tau transgenic mice. *J. Biol. Chem.* **2013**, *288*, 4056–4065. [CrossRef]
144. Tiwari, S.K.; Agrawal, S.; Seth, B.; Yadav, A.; Nair, S.; Bhatnagar, P.; Karmakar, M.; Kumari, M.; Chauhan, L.K.S.; Patel, D.K.; et al. Curcumin-loaded nanoparticles potently induce adult neurogenesis and reverse cognitive deficits in Alzheimer's disease model via canonical Wnt/β-catenin pathway. *ACS Nano* **2014**, *8*, 76–103. [CrossRef] [PubMed]
145. Wang, Y.; Yin, H.; Wang, L.; Shuboy, A.; Lou, J.; Han, B.; Zhang, X.; Li, J. Curcumin as a potential treatment for Alzheimer's disease: A study of the effects of curcumin on hippocampal expression of glial fibrillary acidic protein. *Am. J. Chin. Med.* **2013**, *41*, 59–70. [CrossRef] [PubMed]
146. Ishrat, T.; Hoda, M.N.; Khan, M.B.; Yousuf, S.; Ahmad, M.; Khan, M.M.; Ahmad, A.; Islam, F. Amelioration of cognitive deficits and neurodegeneration by curcumin in rat model of sporadic dementia of Alzheimer's type (SDAT). *Eur. Neuropsychopharm.* **2009**, *19*, 636–647. [CrossRef]
147. Chen, M.; Du, Z.Y.; Zheng, X.; Li, D.L.; Zhou, R.P.; Zhang, K. Use of curcumin in diagnosis, prevention, and treatment of Alzheimer's disease. *Neural Regen. Res.* **2018**, *13*, 742–752. [PubMed]
148. Pluta, R.; Ułamek-Kozioł, M. The role of degenerative pathways in the development of irreversible consequences after brain ischemia. *Neural Regen. Res.* **2019**, in press.
149. Kovalska, M.; Tothova, B.; Kovalska, L.; Tatarkova, Z.; Kalenska, D.; Tomascova, A.; Adamkov, M.; Lehotsky, J. Association of induced hyperhomocysteinemia with Alzheimer's disease-like neurodegeneration in rat cortical neurons after global ischemia-reperfusion injury. *Neurochem. Res.* **2018**, *43*, 1766–1778. [CrossRef]
150. Tóthová, B.; Kovalská, M.; Kalenská, D.; Tomaščová, A.; Lehotský, J. Histone hyperacetylation as a response to global brain ischemia associated with hyperhomocysteinemia in rats. *Int. J. Mol. Sci.* **2018**, *19*, 3147. [CrossRef]

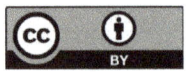

© 2018 by the authors. Licensee MDPI, Basel, Switzerland. This article is an open access article distributed under the terms and conditions of the Creative Commons Attribution (CC BY) license (http://creativecommons.org/licenses/by/4.0/).

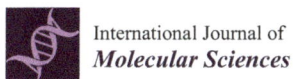

Review

Uncovering the Neuroprotective Mechanisms of Curcumin on Transthyretin Amyloidosis

Nelson Ferreira [1], Maria João Saraiva [2,3] and Maria Rosário Almeida [2,3,4,*]

1. Danish Research Institute of Translational Neuroscience, Nordic EMBL Partnership for Molecular Medicine, Department of Biomedicine, Aarhus University, 8000 Aarhus C, Denmark; nelson@biomed.au.dk
2. Molecular Neurobiology Group, IBMC-Instituto de Biologia Molecular e Celular, Universidade do Porto, 4200-135 Porto, Portugal; mjsaraiv@ibmc.up.pt
3. Instituto de Investigação e Inovação em Saúde (I3S), Universidade do Porto, 4200-135 Porto, Portugal
4. Molecular Biology Department, ICBAS-Instituto de Ciências Biomédicas Abel Salazar, Universidade do Porto, 4050-313 Porto, Portugal
* Correspondence: ralmeida@ibmc.up.pt; Tel.: +351 220 408 800

Received: 15 February 2019; Accepted: 7 March 2019; Published: 14 March 2019

Abstract: Transthyretin (TTR) amyloidoses (ATTR amyloidosis) are diseases associated with transthyretin (TTR) misfolding, aggregation and extracellular deposition in tissues as amyloid. Clinical manifestations of the disease are variable and include mainly polyneuropathy and/or cardiomyopathy. The reasons why TTR forms aggregates and amyloid are related with amino acid substitutions in the protein due to mutations, or with environmental alterations associated with aging, that make the protein more unstable and prone to aggregation. According to this model, several therapeutic approaches have been proposed for the diseases that range from stabilization of TTR, using chemical chaperones, to clearance of the aggregated protein deposited in tissues in the form of oligomers or small aggregates, by the action of disruptors or by activation of the immune system. Interestingly, different studies revealed that curcumin presents anti-amyloid properties, targeting multiple steps in the ATTR amyloidogenic cascade. The effects of curcumin on ATTR amyloidosis will be reviewed and discussed in the current work in order to contribute to knowledge of the molecular mechanisms involved in TTR amyloidosis and propose more efficient drugs for therapy.

Keywords: curcumin; transthyretin; amyloidosis; protein aggregation; protein misfolding; drug discovery

---

1. General Introduction

Transthyretin (TTR) is a plasma protein that functions mainly as a transporter for thyroid hormones, in particular thyroxine (T_4) and retinol (vitamin A) in complex with retinol binding protein (RBP) [1]. TTR is also known to interact with other protein ligands and small molecules, either natural or synthetic compounds. In plasma, TTR interacts with apolipoprotein AI (apo A-I) [2], with the receptor of advanced glycation end-products (RAGE) [3] and with metallothionein [4]. In the cerebrospinal fluid (CSF), TTR interacts with neuropeptide Y (NPY) [5] and with amyloid-β (Aβ) peptide, indicating a neuroprotective role for TTR in the central nervous system [6,7].

Concerning small ligands, TTR binds various types of compounds [8] besides T_4 and retinol. It binds pterins [9], halogenated polyphenols [10] and pharmacologic agents, such as some non-steroid anti-inflammatory drugs (NSAIDS) [11] and natural polyphenols of plant origin [12–15].

In humans and rodents, TTR is mainly synthetized by the liver and the choroid plexus of the brain [16,17] and is secreted to the plasma and cerebrospinal fluid, respectively [18]. In minor amounts, TTR is also synthesized in other tissues, such as the retinal pigmented epithelium, intestine, pancreas, and meninges [19,20].

At the molecular level, TTR is composed of four identical subunits of 127 amino acids forming a tetramer [21,22]. Each polypeptide chain is organized in eight segments with a β-chain structure and only a very small segment of alpha helix. The four monomers in the tetramer interact with each other through non-covalent bonds, establishing a strong interaction between two monomers, forming dimers that assemble as a tetramer originating a central hydrophobic channel limited by amino acids from both dimers. This channel has two similar binding sites for thyroxine molecules [23]. The binding sites can also accommodate other small TTR ligands that might occur in plasma as a result of metabolism, diet origin, or even compounds administered for therapeutic purposes. For an extensive review of TTR-ligand complex X-ray crystal structures, see a review by Pallaninathan et al. [24].

The predominance of the β-chain structure in the polypeptide chains of the TTR tetramer, and its organization as β-sheets contribute to the intrinsic amyloid potential of the protein, leading to aggregation, fibril formation, and deposition under specific conditions, originating transthyretin amyloidosis (ATTR amyloidosis).

2. ATTR Amyloidosis

ATTR amyloidosis is a systemic amyloidosis of hereditary or non-hereditary origin. The hereditary forms of the disease are due to mutations in the *TTR* gene that originate variants with a single amino acid substitution [25,26] (Available online: amyloidosismutations.com). In the non-hereditary forms, the main component of the amyloid fibrils is the wild type protein. In both cases, for different reasons, namely amino acid alterations and/or environmental conditions, TTR becomes less stable and dissociates into monomers that are partially unfolded and present a high tendency to aggregate and form fibrils that deposit in the extracellular space. More than 120 TTR variants have been described until now, related with different hereditary forms of ATTR (ATTRv). Though these are mainly systemic forms of the disease, the most affected tissues or organs where amyloid gets deposited are the peripheral nerves, gastro intestinal system, kidney, heart, carpal tunnel, eye, and in less cases the meninges [27]. The non-hereditary form of the disease is mainly associated with cardiomyopathy of aged people, over 80 years old, and the deposits are composed of wild type protein (ATTR wt) [28]. The most frequent TTR variant is TTR V30M that causes ATTRV30M amyloidosis (formerly designated familial amyloid polyneuropathy (FAP)) [29]. The disease occurs in several foci in the world, the biggest ones located in Portugal, Sweden, Japan, Brazil, Italy, France, and USA [30]. Concerning the hereditary forms of the disease, TTR V122I is also a very frequent variant, in particular, in the Black American population, being this variant related with a predominant involvement of the heart [31,32], now designated as ATTR amyloidosis with cardiomyopathy [33].

The clinical expression of the disease is highly heterogeneous in ATTR amyloidosis. In particular the age of onset of the disease is variable for different variants and even for patients with the same TTR variant, namely TTR V30M, in which the onset can vary from the 2nd to the 6th decade of life [34,35]. Early onset cases are mainly characterized by predominant loss of small-diameter nerve fibers, severe autonomic dysfunction, and cardiac conduction alterations, resulting in peripheral neuropathy leading to loss of sensation, to pain and heat, lower and upper members muscle atrophy, gastro-intestinal disturbances, and cardiomyopathy. In contrast, late onset TTR V30M patients show loss of both small and large fibers, less severe polyneuropathy, mild autonomic dysfunction and frequent cardiomegaly [36]. Among different TTR variants, there is also high variability of predominance of polyneuropathy or cardiomyopathy as main clinical manifestations in ATTRv amyloidosis (reviewed in Reference [26,37]).

3. Inhibitors of TTR Aggregation: Pharmacologic and Natural Inhibitors of TTR Amyloidosis

Since plasma TTR is mainly synthesized by the liver, liver transplant has been one of the first therapeutic approaches proposed and found effective for the disease [38]. However, as expected, liver transplant is an invasive therapy, not suitable for all patients and with several limitations and risks [39]. In addition, recently, it was found that after liver transplant, some patients develop TTR cardiomyopathy due to deposition of wild-type TTR in their heart [40–42]. This supports the need for alternative therapeutic approaches that aim to stabilize TTR using small molecules that, by binding to TTR, stabilize it and inhibit its aggregation and deposition [43]. The first evidence of TTR stabilization through binding of small compounds came from the fact that when TTR is bound to T_4 it is less prone to aggregation. In addition, T_4 binding sites in TTR are mostly unoccupied due to the high TTR/T_4 ratio in plasma, allowing TTR stabilization by binding of small compounds to TTR with high affinity [44].

Several nonsteroidal anti-inflammatory drugs (NSAIDs), have been known for a long time to compete with T_4 for the binding to TTR, such as salicylates, diclofenac, flufenamic acid and diflunisal [45]. Among these, diflunisal was one of the most promising compounds due to its affinity and specificity to bind TTR. In addition, several diflunisal derivatives have been synthetized to improve its affinity and selectivity to bind TTR in plasma [46,47]. Diflunisal is still one of the compounds in use for ATTR amyloidosis therapy in countries where Tafamidis has not yet been approved [48,49]. Tafamidis, diclorofenol benzoxazole carboxylic acid, is a more recent and widely-used drug that binds to TTR and stabilizes it [50,51]. Tafamidis is highly safe and tolerable and has been found efficient in slowing disease progression and preserving quality of life of TTR V30M patients [52]. Meanwhile, other strategies for ATTR amyloidosis therapy have also been pursued, namely targeting different steps in the cascade of amyloid formation, fibril disruption, and clearance [53]. An example of such strategies is to use compounds that bind to TTR and block its polymerization or disrupt the amyloid fibrils formed, such as molecular tweezers (CLR01) and doxycycline, respectively [54,55].

4. Natural Inhibitors—Polyphenols

In the search for compounds of therapeutic interest, presenting very low toxicity and structural similarities to other TTR ligands, several polyphenols of plant origin have been studied as inhibitors of TTR amyloidogenesis. Some polyphenols were previously reported as inhibiting protein aggregation and amyloid formation in neurodegenerative diseases, such as Alzheimer's and Parkinson's disease [56]. One of the most studied polyphenols is resveratrol. In vitro studies using the AC16 cardiomyocyte cell line demonstrate that resveratrol is able to stabilize the native TTR tetramer, preventing the formation of cytotoxic species and promoting aggregation of monomeric into non-toxic species [12]. Furthermore, administration of resveratrol to Alzheimer's disease (AD) mice revealed an increase in TTR levels in plasma that does not result from higher expression of the protein, but, instead, might be related with increased TTR stability and longer half-life in circulation [57]. However, resveratrol seems to have not only these direct effects on TTR but also other properties namely those involving protection against oxidation, which is difficult to discern.

Other polyphenols, like nordihydroguaiaretic acid (NDGA), rosmarinic acid, caffeic acid and epigallocatechin gallate (EGCG), have also been investigated in vitro for their interaction with TTR [58–62]. Contrary to most polyphenols, EGCG did not compete with T_4 for binding to TTR, revealing that it binds at a different binding site in the molecule [62]. Indeed, the crystallographic structure of the complex of TTR with EGCG revealed that it binds at different regions at the surface of the molecule and not at the T_4 binding sites [63]. In a subsequent structure–activity study, the galloyl moiety has been highlighted as a key structural feature of EGCG by greatly enhancing its anti-amyloid chaperone activity of TTR [61].

When administered to a model mice expressing human TTR V30M, EGCG inhibited TTR deposition in the gastrointestinal tract and in the dorsal root ganglia (DRG), the main sites of aggregated TTR deposition in this animal model for the disease [64]. In addition, when administered to old mice, EGCG treatment resulted in a decrease of TTR deposits in tissues, indicating a disruptive effect on aggregated TTR deposits. A small pilot study with EGCG administration to human carriers of amyloidogenic TTR mutations including TTR V30M revealed a reduction of myocardial mass in the case of cardiomyopathy, indicating an inhibitory effect of EGCG on TTR amyloid fibril formation [65,66]. The reported studies show improvement in the cardiac function without increase of the patient's survival. The low toxicity and high tolerability to EGCG, confirmed in these studies, encourage continuation of treatment with EGCG [67].

Among the polyphenols studied in vitro, curcumin revealed a particular behavior suggesting different mechanism of inhibition of ATTR amyloidosis [58].

5. In Vitro Studies with Curcumin

5.1. Curcumin Binds to TTR and Increases Its Resistance to Dissociation

A decade ago, Pullakhandam and colleagues first reported curcumin interaction with TTR [68]. Using Scatchard analysis of fluorescence quenching, the authors showed that curcumin binds to wild-type TTR with a molar ratio of 1.2:1 and K_d of 2.3×10^{-6} M [68]. In addition, curcumin was found to dose-dependently displace 1-anilino-8-naphalene sulfonate (ANS) at pH 7.2 from TTR's central ligand-binding channel, to which various ligands are known to bind [68].

Shortly after, we further detailed the interaction between curcumin and TTR by unequivocally showing that curcumin competed with radiolabeled T_4 ($[^{125}I]T_4$) for its binding to wild-type and V30M mutant TTR, both in vitro and in whole human plasma [58]. These observations were later corroborated by the crystal structures of TTR complexes with curcumin and also its degradation product, ferulic acid, [15], and other curcumin-like compounds [69], showing that curcumin interacts with Ser 117 and Lys15 and with Val 121 and Thr123 through a water molecule [15]. By filling the largely unoccupied T_4 binding pockets at the weaker dimer–dimer interface, curcumin increases TTR tetramer resistance to dissociation in non-native monomers as shown by isoelectric focusing (IEF) studies in semi-denaturing conditions (4 M urea) [58]. This, together with selective binding of curcumin to TTR over other plasma proteins, resulted in a 25% increase of the tetramer/total TTR ratio in plasma from controls and TTR V30M heterozygote carriers [58].

5.2. Curcumin Redirects TTR Aggregation into "Off-Pathway" Oligomers and Disaggregates Pre-Formed TTR Amyloid Fibrils

Despite its inability to prevent the acid induced aggregation of TTR wild-type [68], we have shown that curcumin robustly inhibits aggregation of the highly amyloidogenic Y78F variant under physiological conditions (phosphate buffered saline, pH 7.4, 37 °C) [58]. This supports the hypothesis that protonation and isomerization of the phenolic and enolic hydroxyl groups of curcumin at low pH might impair interaction with TTR [68]. Under transmission electron microscopy (TEM) and dynamic light scattering (DLS), curcumin redirected the TTR Y78F amyloid formation pathway into a monodispersed, highly stable population of "off-pathway" oligomers with approximately 80 nm in hydrodynamic diameter (dH) [58]. In addition, we found that Schwann cells exposed to TTR Y78F aggregates incubated with curcumin presented significantly reduced endoplasmic reticulum (ER) stress and were protected from entering into the apoptotic signaling pathway [70], highlighting that curcumin-induced oligomers are less toxic than untreated "on-pathway" aggregate intermediates. Moreover, dot–blot analysis of conditioned medium from Rat Schwannoma (RN22) cells expressing TTR L55P incubated with curcumin revealed almost complete inhibition of TTR aggregation (90%). This variant is associated with an aggressive form of ATTR amyloidosis, further supporting the protective role of curcumin on the early stages of TTR aggregation, either by inhibiting tetramer dissociation and/or redirecting pathological misfolding and aggregation into more innocuous counterparts [58]. Similar observations were later reported relative to different aggregation-prone proteins associated with neurodegeneration, including Aβ [71], tau [72] and α-synuclein [73].

Beyond sharing many structural similarities with classical amyloid-binding dyes, such as Thioflavin-S, Congo red, and crysamine-G, curcumin showed specific labeling of amyloid deposits [74–76]. Although the precise atomic-detailed characteristics underlying the ability of curcumin to break down β-sheet rich aggregates remain unclear, solid-state NMR studies have highlighted the structural importance of the aromatic carbons adjacent to the methoxy and/or hydroxy groups of curcumin in its binding with Aβ fibrils [77].

Overall, multiple lines of evidence favor the hypothesis that the non-specific modulatory role of curcumin on amyloid formation and toxicity in vitro depends on aggregate-related conformational structure rather than protein primary sequence.

6. In Vivo Studies with Curcumin

6.1. Curcumin Reduces TTR Load and Degrades Amyloid Deposits in Tissues

In recent years, an increasing amount of evidence supporting the anti-amyloidogenic role of curcumin in different proteins prone to misfolding have paved the way to preclinical trials in transgenic animal models [78].

With regard to ATTR amyloidosis, we have shown that chronically feeding young transgenic mice for human TTR V30M with curcumin (2% w/w) results in micromolar steady-state levels of curcumin in plasma (21.4 ± 3.6 μM) [79]. Selective competition of curcumin with T_4 (42%) for the binding to TTR in plasma significantly reduced tetramer dissociation into non-native monomeric intermediaries under semi-dissociating conditions [79]. Beyond stabilizing TTR native fold, curcumin supplementation alleviated TTR load and associated biomarkers in the gastrointestinal tract, the primary target organ in this mouse model [79]. Dietary intake of curcumin was well-tolerated and non-toxic to animals and the treatment did not interfere with TTR plasma levels in vivo [79].

In a later study, we evaluated the effect of curcumin in aged mice expressing the TTR V30M variant on an *Hsf-1* heterozygous background (hTTR V30M/Hsf), in which deposition of aggregated TTR coexists with birefringent congophilic material in tissues. We found that curcumin intake not only reduced non-fibrillar extracellular TTR burden in both gastrointestinal tract and dorsal root ganglia, but also remodeled pre-existing congophilic amyloid material in tissues [70].

Our findings are in close alignment with recent observations made by others showing that curcumin promotes remodeling of existing amyloid deposits and counteracts the formation of new amyloid deposits, or even reduce the amount of remaining deposits [72,76,78,80].

6.2. Other Neuroprotective Mechanisms of Curcumin

Although we hypothesize that curcumin alleviates TTR extracellular burden most likely due to its ability to directly interact and modify multiple partners of the TTR amyloid cascade, as summarized in Figure 1, we speculate whether the pleiotropic therapeutic actions of curcumin [78] might synergistically potentiate its efficacy in vivo.

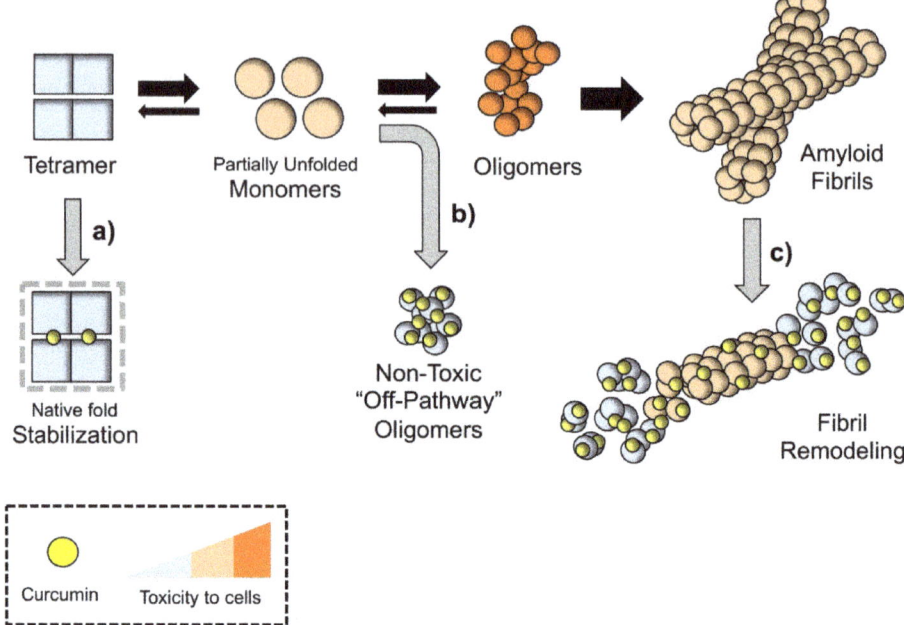

Figure 1. Proposed mechanism for TTR aggregation pathway modulation by curcumin. Rate-limiting tetramer dissociation of TTR into partially unfolded monomers precedes the formation of toxic oligomeric intermediates that evolve into β-sheets enriched mature fibrils. Curcumin modulates TTR cascade by directly interacting with different binding partners: (**a**) Curcumin interaction with TTR at the T_4 binding pockets stabilizes the tetrameric fold and blocks its dissociation into unfolded monomeric species [15,58,68]; (**b**) Curcumin interaction with partially misfolded non-native monomers redirects TTR aggregation into "off-pathway" unstructured oligomers innocuous to cells [58,68]; (**c**) Curcumin breaks down and remodels β-sheet rich TTR fibrils in smaller amorphous aggregates in in vitro [58] and in vivo [70].

Recently, increasing relevance has been attributed to endothelial abnormalities associated with ATTRv amyloidosis and in particular ATTR V30M [81,82]. It has been suggested that TTR variants may affect endothelial cells function even before amyloid fibril formation. Thus, microangiopathy could play an important role in an initial lesion leading to organ damage [83]. Interestingly, curcumin appears to improve endothelial cell function and, though its mechanisms of action are not completely known, it seems that by lowering the expression of pro-inflammatory molecules, and by reducing levels of reactive oxygen species, such as Nox-2 in endothelial cells, curcumin not only decreases trans-endothelial monocyte migration, but also maintains adequate NO levels for the proper function of cells [84].

Accumulating evidence has linked autophagy impairment to neurodegeneration and neuronal cell death [85,86]. Given that stimulation of autophagy can potentially enhance degradation of aggregation prone-proteins, development of autophagy-inducing therapies, in which toxic misfolded proteins are used as autophagy substrates, might be a valuable pharmacological approach for neurodegenerative diseases, including ATTR amyloidosis [85,86].

In preclinical studies performed with TTR V30M transgenic mice, curcumin has been shown to effectively reverse accumulation of p62, a key cargo receptor involved in selective autophagy, re-establishing the autophagic flux and mitigating apoptosis [87]. Nevertheless, since curcumin can mediate crosstalk between different signaling pathways [88,89] it remains unclear to which extent restoration of the autophagic flux in vivo occurs because: (i) curcumin promotes autophagy or (ii) its anti-amyloid activity prevents TTR "on-pathway" aggregation reaching a critical threshold beyond which the autophagic machinery would be overwhelmed and irreversibly damaged.

In recent years, macrophage-mediated clearance of amyloid by a variety of phagocytic and digestive mechanisms has been receiving increasing attention in the literature [90]. Several small-molecules, including derivatives of curcumin, have been found to promote phagocytosis of Aβ by macrophages [91–93]. Similarly, we have shown that pre-treatment of macrophages isolated from aged FAP mice with physiologically achievable doses of curcumin, improves phagocytic uptake and degradation of extracellular TTR aggregates, supporting that curcumin restores the inefficient macrophage TTR clearance characteristic of pathological conditions [70].

7. Final Remarks

Several lines of evidence suggest that curcumin has neuroprotective properties in many protein-misfolding disorders, including Alzheimer's and Parkinson's diseases and ATTR amyloidosis [78]. Curcumin is a biologically well-tolerated polyphenol, with a long established safety history [94]. According to JECFA (The Joint United Nations and World Health Organization Expert Committee on Food Additives) and EFSA (European Food Safety Authority) guidelines, the recommended allowable daily intake (ADI) amount of curcumin is 0–3 mg/kg body weight [94]. Nonetheless, some minor undesired side effects have been reported in a single dose escalation study where healthy subjects were given increasing doses from 0.5 to 12 g of curcumin [95].

Despite its well-documented therapeutic efficacy, the poor absorption and rapid metabolism of curcumin, has hindered its progress as a prospective pharmacological agent. To increase its bioavailability, a wide array of novel formulations have been developed, including nanoparticles, liposomes, micelles, and phospholipid complexes, which increase the bioavailability of curcumin by providing longer circulation, enhanced permeability, and resistance to metabolic degradation and excretion [78].

Presently, numerous disease-modifying targeted therapies for TTR amyloidosis are being tested in human clinical trials, including TTR stabilizers (diflunisal, tafamidis), fibril disruptors (doxycycline/TUDCA) and the most recent gene therapies to block TTR expression (small interference RNAs (siRNAs) and antisense oligonucleotides therapy (ASOs)) [26,37,96,97]. Although development of these strategies greatly improved the perspectives in ATTR amyloidosis, the complex nature of the disease, in which several pathways are known to contribute to the pathology, prompts to seek multi-stage interventions that not only block TTR synthesis and/or misfolding, but also suppress inflammation and oxidative damage and enhance cellular protein degradation systems. Taken together, the pleiotropic activities of curcumin provide multiple ways to tackle TTR pathophysiology, either through direct interaction of curcumin with TTR, or indirect effects affecting signaling pathways associated with TTR amyloid fibril formation and clearance. Accordingly, the works here reviewed, and summarized in Figure 2, demonstrate interaction of curcumin with TTR through binding at the thyroxine binding sites, resulting in TTR tetramer stabilization and consequent modulation of the TTR misfolding cascade inhibiting aggregation and /or inducing formation of non-toxic aggregates. This leads to restoring the autophagy flux and improving phagocytic uptake and clearance of extracellular TTR. Curcumin also appears to directly induce disaggregation of TTR pre-formed fibrils and to promote clearance of TTR aggregates through endocytose by fibroblasts and macrophages. Concomitant with these effects, curcumin presents several non-specific effects counteracting common pathogenic events in amyloidosis, such as oxidative stress, inflammation, apoptosis and extracellular matrix dysregulation within a range of dosing with proven safety.

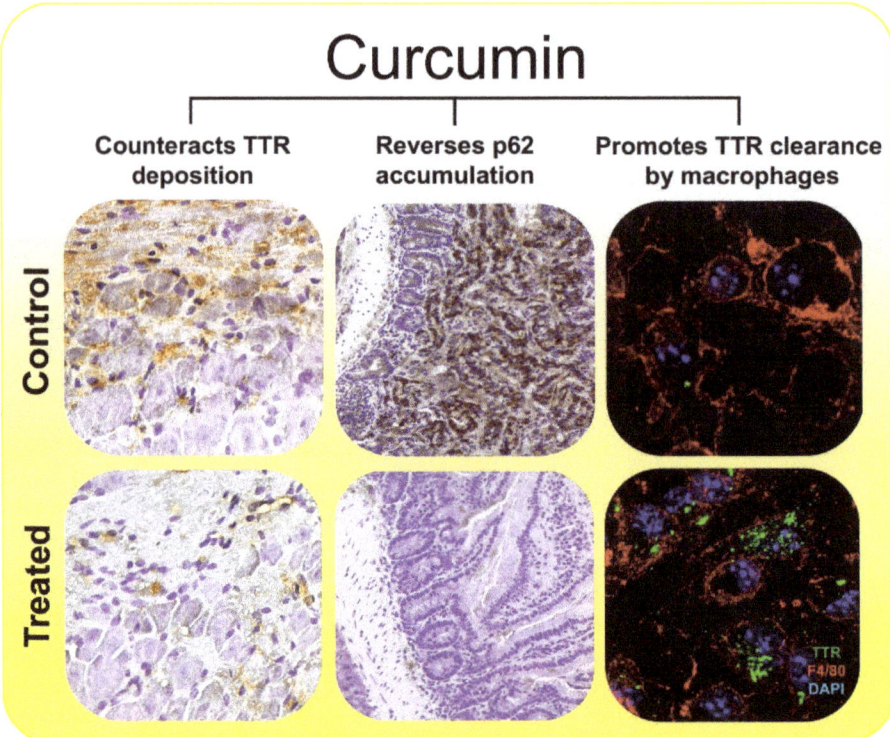

Figure 2. The pleiotropic effects of curcumin on the molecular pathways associated with ATTR amyloidosis. Curcumin exerts neuroprotective effects on ATTR amyloidosis by modulating TTR abnormal aggregation and counteracting TTR tissue deposition (left panels, 20× magnification) immunohistochemistry (IHC) analysis of TTR in dorsal root ganglia (DRG) from mice expressing human TTR V30M (hTTRV30M mice) treated with curcumin and age-matched controls [70]), re-establishing the autophagic flux by reversing p62 accumulation (center panels, 20× magnification), IHC analysis of p62, in duodenum samples from hTTRV30M mice treated with curcumin and age-matched controls [87]) and improving the phagocytic uptake and degradation of extracellular TTR aggregates by macrophages (right panels, 63× magnification), double immunofluorescence labeling for TTR, in green, and F4/80, in red, of primary macrophages from hTTRV30M mice that were pre-incubated in presence of curcumin or its absence (control), before addition of TTR aggregates to cell culture medium [70]). Nevertheless, other well-known neuroprotective properties of curcumin, such as its anti-inflammatory, anti-apoptotic, and anti-oxidative activities [78,94], might potentiate its in vivo effects.

In conclusion, in this context, curcumin remains a promising scaffold for the development of potent multi-stage disease-modifying drugs for the treatment of TTR amyloidosis.

Funding: This research was funded by the European Regional Development Fund (FEDER) through the Norte Portugal Regional Operational Programme (NORTE 2020), under the PORTUGAL 2020 Partnership Agreement, grant number Norte-01-0145-FEDER-000008—Porto Neurosciences and Neurologic Disease Research Initiative at I3S. Nelson Ferreira was a recipient of a Postdoctoral Fellowship R171-2014-591 from Lundbeck foundation and by Lundbeck Foundation grant R248-2016-2518 for Danish Research Institute of Translational Neuroscience—DANDRITE, Nordic-EMBL Partnership for Molecular Medicine, Aarhus University, Denmark.

Acknowledgments: The authors thank Cristina Teixeira (MSc) (from Molecular Neurobiology Group, IBMC and I3S, University of Porto, Portugal) for the immunohistochemistry pictures of p62 in duodenum included in Figure 2.

Conflicts of Interest: The authors declare no conflicts of interest.

References

1. Raz, A.; Goodman, D.S. The interaction of thyroxine with human plasma prealbumin and with the prealbumin-retinol-binding protein complex. *J. Biol. Chem.* **1969**, *244*, 3230–3237.
2. Sousa, M.M.; Berglund, L.; Saraiva, M.J. Transthyretin in high density lipoproteins: Association with apolipoprotein A-I. *J. Lipid Res.* **2000**, *41*, 58–65.
3. Sousa, M.M.; Yan, S.D.; Stern, D.; Saraiva, M.J. Interaction of the receptor for advanced glycation end products (RAGE) with transthyretin triggers nuclear transcription factor kB (NF-kB) activation. *Lab. Investig.* **2000**, *80*, 1101–1110. [CrossRef]
4. Gonçalves, I.; Quintela, T.; Baltazar, G.; Almeida, M.R.; Saraiva, M.J.M.; Santos, C.R. Transthyretin interacts with metallothionein 2. *Biochemistry* **2008**, *47*, 2244–2251. [CrossRef]
5. Nunes, A.F.; Saraiva, M.J.; Sousa, M.M. Transthyretin knockouts are a new mouse model for increased neuropeptide Y. *FASEB J.* **2006**, *20*, 166–168. [CrossRef]
6. Costa, R.; Gonçalves, A.; Saraiva, M.J.; Cardoso, I. Transthyretin binding to A-Beta peptide–impact on A-Beta fibrillogenesis and toxicity. *FEBS Lett.* **2008**, *582*, 936–942. [CrossRef]
7. Liz, M.A.; Mar, F.M.; Franquinho, F.; Sousa, M.M. Aboard transthyretin: From transport to cleavage. *IUBMB Life* **2010**, *62*, 429–435. [CrossRef]
8. Almeida, M.R.; Gales, L.; Damas, A.M.; Cardoso, I.; Saraiva, M.J. Small transthyretin (TTR) ligands as possible therapeutic agents in TTR amyloidoses. *Curr. Drug Targets CNS Neurol. Disord.* **2005**, *4*, 587–596. [CrossRef]
9. Ernström, U.; Pettersson, T.; Jörnvall, H. A yellow component associated with human transthyretin has properties like a pterin derivative, 7,8-dihydropterin-6-carboxaldehyde. *FEBS Lett.* **1995**, *360*, 177–182. [CrossRef]
10. Lans, M.C.; Klasson-Wehler, E.; Willemsen, M.; Meussen, E.; Safe, S.; Brouwer, A. Structure-dependent, competitive interaction of hydroxy-polychlorobiphenyls, -dibenzo-p-dioxins and -dibenzofurans with human transthyretin. *Chem. Biol. Interact.* **1993**, *88*, 7–21. [CrossRef]
11. Baures, P.W.; Oza, V.B.; Peterson, S.A.; Kelly, J.W. Synthesis and evaluation of inhibitors of transthyretin amyloid formation based on the non-steroidal anti-inflammatory drug, flufenamic acid. *Bioorg. Med. Chem.* **1999**, *7*, 1339–1347. [CrossRef]
12. Bourgault, S.; Choi, S.; Buxbaum, J.N.; Kelly, J.W.; Price, J.L.; Reixach, N. Erratum to "Mechanisms of transthyretin cardiomyocyte toxicity inhibition by resveratrol analogs" [Biochem. Biophys. Res. Commun. 410 (2011) 707–713]. *Biochem. Biophys. Res. Commun.* **2011**, *412*, 196. [CrossRef]
13. Trivella, D.B.B.; dos Reis, C.V.; Lima, L.M.T.R.; Foguel, D.; Polikarpov, I. Flavonoid interactions with human transthyretin: Combined structural and thermodynamic analysis. *J. Struct. Biol.* **2012**, *180*, 143–153. [CrossRef] [PubMed]
14. Yokoyama, T.; Kosaka, Y.; Mizuguchi, M. Inhibitory activities of propolis and its promising component, caffeic acid phenethyl ester, against amyloidogenesis of human transthyretin. *J. Med. Chem.* **2014**, *57*, 8928–8935. [CrossRef]
15. Ciccone, L.; Tepshi, L.; Nencetti, S.; Stura, E.A. Transthyretin complexes with curcumin and bromo-estradiol: Evaluation of solubilizing multicomponent mixtures. *New Biotechnol.* **2015**, *32*, 54–64. [CrossRef] [PubMed]
16. Aleshire, S.L.; Bradley, C.A.; Richardson, L.D.; Parl, F.F. Localization of human prealbumin in choroid plexus epithelium. *J. Histochem. Cytochem.* **2017**, *31*, 608–612. [CrossRef]
17. Dickson, P.W.; Howlett, G.J.; Schreiber, G. Rat transthyretin (prealbumin). Molecular cloning, nucleotide sequence, and gene expression in liver and brain. *J. Biol. Chem.* **1985**, *260*, 8214–8219. [PubMed]
18. Richardson, S.J. Cell and molecular biology of transthyretin and thyroid hormones. *Int. Rev. Cytol.* **2007**, *258*, 137–193. [PubMed]
19. Cavallaro, T.; Martone, R.L.; Dwork, A.J.; Schon, E.A.; Herbert, J. The retinal pigment epithelium is the unique site of transthyretin synthesis in the rat eye. *Investig. Ophthalmol. Vis. Sci.* **1990**, *31*, 497–501.
20. Richardson, S.J. Evolutionary changes to transthyretin: Evolution of transthyretin biosynthesis. *FEBS J.* **2009**, *276*, 5342–5356. [CrossRef] [PubMed]
21. Blake, C.C.; Geisow, M.J.; Oatley, S.J.; Rérat, B.; Rérat, C. Structure of prealbumin: Secondary, tertiary and quaternary interactions determined by Fourier refinement at 1.8 A. *J. Mol. Biol.* **1978**, *121*, 339–356. [CrossRef]

22. Hamilton, J.A.; Steinrauf, L.K.; Braden, B.C.; Liepnieks, J.; Benson, M.D.; Holmgren, G.; Sandgren, O.; Steen, L. The X-ray crystal structure refinements of normal human transthyretin and the amyloidogenic Val-30->Met variant to 1.7-A resolution. *J. Biol. Chem.* **1993**, *268*, 2416–2424. [PubMed]
23. Wojtczak, A. Crystal structure of rat transthyretin at 2.5 A resolution: First report on a unique tetrameric structure. *Acta Biochim. Pol.* **1997**, *44*, 505–517.
24. Palaninathan, S.K. Nearly 200 X-ray crystal structures of transthyretin: What do they tell us about this protein and the design of drugs for TTR amyloidoses? *Curr. Med. Chem.* **2012**, *19*, 2324–2342. [CrossRef] [PubMed]
25. Benson, M.D.; Kincaid, J.C. The molecular biology and clinical features of amyloid neuropathy. *Muscle Nerve* **2007**, *36*, 411–423. [CrossRef]
26. Sekijima, Y. Transthyretin (ATTR) amyloidosis: Clinical spectrum, molecular pathogenesis and disease-modifying treatments. *J. Neurol. Neurosurg. Psychiatry* **2015**, *86*, 1036–1043. [CrossRef]
27. Sousa, M.M.; Saraiva, M.J. Neurodegeneration in familial amyloid polyneuropathy: From pathology to molecular signaling. *Prog. Neurobiol.* **2003**, *71*, 385–400. [CrossRef]
28. Patel, K.S.; Hawkins, P.N. Cardiac amyloidosis: Where are we today? *J. Intern. Med.* **2015**, *278*, 126–144. [CrossRef]
29. Saraiva, M.J.; Birken, S.; Costa, P.P.; Goodman, D.S. Amyloid fibril protein in familial amyloidotic polyneuropathy, Portuguese type. Definition of molecular abnormality in transthyretin (prealbumin). *J. Clin. Investig.* **1984**, *74*, 104–119. [CrossRef]
30. Planté-Bordeneuve, V.; Kerschen, P. Transthyretin familial amyloid polyneuropathy. *Handb. Clin. Neurol.* **2013**, *115*, 643–658.
31. Jacobson, D.R.; Gorevic, P.D.; Buxbaum, J.N. A homozygous transthyretin variant associated with senile systemic amyloidosis: Evidence for a late-onset disease of genetic etiology. *Am. J. Hum. Genet.* **1990**, *47*, 127–136.
32. Saraiva, M.J.; Sherman, W.; Marboe, C.; Figueira, A.; Costa, P.; de Freitas, A.F.; Gawinowicz, M.A. Cardiac amyloidosis: Report of a patient heterozygous for the transthyretin isoleucine 122 variant. *Scand. J. Immunol.* **1990**, *32*, 341–346. [CrossRef]
33. Gertz, M.A.; Benson, M.D.; Dyck, P.J.; Grogan, M.; Coelho, T.; Cruz, M.; Berk, J.L.; Plante-Bordeneuve, V.; Schmidt, H.H.-J.; Merlini, G. Diagnosis, Prognosis, and Therapy of Transthyretin Amyloidosis. *J. Am. Coll. Cardiol.* **2015**, *66*, 2451–2466. [CrossRef]
34. Conceiçao, I.; Gonzalez-Duarte, A.; Obici, L.; Schmidt, H.H.-J.; Simoneau, D.; Ong, M.-L.; Amass, L. "Red-flag" symptom clusters in transthyretin familial amyloid polyneuropathy. *J. Peripher. Nerv. Syst.* **2016**, *21*, 5–9. [CrossRef]
35. Ando, Y.; Coelho, T.; Berk, J.L.; Cruz, M.W.; Ericzon, B.-G.; Ikeda, S.-I.; Lewis, W.D.; Obici, L.; Plante-Bordeneuve, V.; Rapezzi, C.; et al. Guideline of transthyretin-related hereditary amyloidosis for clinicians. *Orphanet J. Rare Dis.* **2013**, *8*, 31. [CrossRef]
36. Koike, H.; Misu, K.; Sugiura, M.; Iijima, M.; Mori, K.; Yamamoto, M.; Hattori, N.; Mukai, E.; Ando, Y.; Ikeda, S.; et al. Pathology of early- vs. late-onset TTR Met30 familial amyloid polyneuropathy. *Neurology* **2004**, *63*, 129–138. [CrossRef]
37. Plante-Bordeneuve, V. Transthyretin familial amyloid polyneuropathy: An update. *J. Neurol.* **2018**, *265*, 976–983. [CrossRef]
38. Holmgren, G.; Ericzon, B.G.; Groth, C.G.; Steen, L.; Suhr, O.; Andersen, O.; Wallin, B.G.; Seymour, A.; Richardson, S.; Hawkins, P.N. Clinical improvement and amyloid regression after liver transplantation in hereditary transthyretin amyloidosis. *Lancet* **1993**, *341*, 1113–1116. [CrossRef]
39. Carvalho, A.; Rocha, A.; Lobato, L. Liver transplantation in transthyretin amyloidosis: Issues and challenges. *Liver Transpl.* **2015**, *21*, 282–292. [CrossRef]
40. Liepnieks, J.J.; Zhang, L.Q.; Benson, M.D. Progression of transthyretin amyloid neuropathy after liver transplantation. *Neurology* **2010**, *75*, 324–327. [CrossRef]
41. Okamoto, S.; Zhao, Y.; Lindqvist, P.; Backman, C.; Ericzon, B.-G.; Wijayatunga, P.; Henein, M.Y.; Suhr, O.B. Development of cardiomyopathy after liver transplantation in Swedish hereditary transthyretin amyloidosis (ATTR) patients. *Amyloid* **2011**, *18*, 200–205. [CrossRef]

42. Ericzon, B.-G.; Wilczek, H.E.; Larsson, M.; Wijayatunga, P.; Stangou, A.; Pena, J.R.; Furtado, E.; Barroso, E.; Daniel, J.; Samuel, D.; et al. Liver Transplantation for Hereditary Transthyretin Amyloidosis: After 20 Years Still the Best Therapeutic Alternative? *Transplantation* **2015**, *99*, 1847–1854. [CrossRef]
43. Miroy, G.J.; Lai, Z.; Lashuel, H.A.; Peterson, S.A.; Strang, C.; Kelly, J.W. Inhibiting transthyretin amyloid fibril formation via protein stabilization. *Proc. Natl. Acad. Sci. USA* **1996**, *93*, 15051–15056. [CrossRef]
44. Johnson, S.M.; Wiseman, R.L.; Sekijima, Y.; Green, N.S.; Adamski-Werner, S.L.; Kelly, J.W. Native state kinetic stabilization as a strategy to ameliorate protein misfolding diseases: A focus on the transthyretin amyloidoses. *Acc. Chem. Res.* **2005**, *38*, 911–921. [CrossRef]
45. Munro, S.L.; Lim, C.F.; Hall, J.G.; Barlow, J.W.; Craik, D.J.; Topliss, D.J.; Stockigt, J.R. Drug competition for thyroxine binding to transthyretin (prealbumin): Comparison with effects on thyroxine-binding globulin. *J. Clin. Endocrinol. Metab.* **1989**, *68*, 1141–1147. [CrossRef]
46. Adamski-Werner, S.L.; Palaninathan, S.K.; Sacchettini, J.C.; Kelly, J.W. Diflunisal analogues stabilize the native state of transthyretin. Potent inhibition of amyloidogenesis. *J. Med. Chem.* **2004**, *47*, 355–374. [CrossRef]
47. Miller, S.R.; Sekijima, Y.; Kelly, J.W. Native state stabilization by NSAIDs inhibits transthyretin amyloidogenesis from the most common familial disease variants. *Lab. Investig.* **2004**, *84*, 545–552. [CrossRef]
48. Tojo, K.; Sekijima, Y.; Kelly, J.W.; Ikeda, S.-I. Diflunisal stabilizes familial amyloid polyneuropathy-associated transthyretin variant tetramers in serum against dissociation required for amyloidogenesis. *Neurosci. Res.* **2006**, *56*, 441–449. [CrossRef]
49. Sekijima, Y.; Dendle, M.A.; Kelly, J.W. Orally administered diflunisal stabilizes transthyretin against dissociation required for amyloidogenesis. *Amyloid* **2006**, *13*, 236–249. [CrossRef]
50. Johnson, S.M.; Connelly, S.; Wilson, I.A.; Kelly, J.W. Biochemical and structural evaluation of highly selective 2-arylbenzoxazole-based transthyretin amyloidogenesis inhibitors. *J. Med. Chem.* **2008**, *51*, 260–270. [CrossRef]
51. Johnson, S.M.; Connelly, S.; Fearns, C.; Powers, E.T.; Kelly, J.W. The transthyretin amyloidoses: From delineating the molecular mechanism of aggregation linked to pathology to a regulatory-agency-approved drug. *J. Mol. Biol.* **2012**, *421*, 185–203. [CrossRef] [PubMed]
52. Coelho, T.; Maia, L.F.; da Silva, A.M.; Cruz, M.W.; Plante-Bordeneuve, V.; Suhr, O.B.; Conceiçao, I.; Schmidt, H.H.-J.; Trigo, P.; Kelly, J.W.; et al. Long-term effects of tafamidis for the treatment of transthyretin familial amyloid polyneuropathy. *J. Neurol.* **2013**, *260*, 2802–2814. [CrossRef]
53. Adams, D.; Cauquil, C.; Labeyrie, C.; Beaudonnet, G.; Algalarrondo, V.; Théaudin, M. TTR kinetic stabilizers and TTR gene silencing: A new era in therapy for familial amyloidotic polyneuropathies. *Expert Opin. Pharmacother.* **2016**, *17*, 791–802. [CrossRef] [PubMed]
54. Ferreira, N.; Pereira-Henriques, A.; Attar, A.; Klärner, F.-G.; Schrader, T.; Bitan, G.; Gales, L.; Saraiva, M.J.; Almeida, M.R. Molecular tweezers targeting transthyretin amyloidosis. *Neurotherapeutics* **2014**, *11*, 450–461. [CrossRef] [PubMed]
55. Galant, N.J.; Westermark, P.; Higaki, J.N.; Chakrabartty, A. Transthyretin amyloidosis: An under-recognized neuropathy and cardiomyopathy. *Clin. Sci.* **2017**, *131*, 395–409. [CrossRef] [PubMed]
56. Ngoungoure, V.L.N.; Schluesener, J.; Moundipa, P.F.; Schluesener, H. Natural polyphenols binding to amyloid: A broad class of compounds to treat different human amyloid diseases. *Mol. Nutr. Food Res.* **2014**, *59*, 8–20. [CrossRef] [PubMed]
57. Santos, L.M.; Rodrigues, D. Resveratrol Administration Increases Transthyretin Protein Levels, Ameliorating AD Features: The Importance of Transthyretin Tetrameric Stability. *Mol. Med.* **2016**, *22*, 1. [CrossRef] [PubMed]
58. Ferreira, N.; Saraiva, M.J.; Almeida, M.R. Natural polyphenols inhibit different steps of the process of transthyretin (TTR) amyloid fibril formation. *FEBS Lett.* **2011**, *585*, 2424–2430. [CrossRef]
59. Florio, P.; Folli, C.; Cianci, M.; Del Rio, D.; Zanotti, G.; Berni, R. Transthyretin Binding Heterogeneity and Anti-amyloidogenic Activity of Natural Polyphenols and Their Metabolites. *J. Biol. Chem.* **2015**, *290*, 29769–29780. [CrossRef]
60. Ortore, G.; Orlandini, E.; Braca, A.; Ciccone, L.; Rossello, A.; Martinelli, A.; Nencetti, S. Targeting Different Transthyretin Binding Sites with Unusual Natural Compounds. *ChemMedChem* **2016**, *11*, 1865–1874. [CrossRef]

61. Ferreira, N.; Pereira-Henriques, A.; Almeida, M.R. Transthyretin chemical chaperoning by flavonoids: Structure-activity insights towards the design of potent amyloidosis inhibitors. *Biochem. Biophys. Rep.* **2015**, *3*, 123–133. [CrossRef]
62. Ferreira, N.; Cardoso, I.; Domingues, M.R.; Vitorino, R.; Bastos, M.; Bai, G.; Saraiva, M.J.; Almeida, M.R. Binding of epigallocatechin-3-gallate to transthyretin modulates its amyloidogenicity. *FEBS Lett.* **2009**, *583*, 3569–3576. [CrossRef]
63. Miyata, M.; Sato, T.; Kugimiya, M.; Sho, M.; Nakamura, T.; Ikemizu, S.; Chirifu, M.; Mizuguchi, M.; Nabeshima, Y.; Suwa, Y.; et al. The crystal structure of the green tea polyphenol (−)-epigallocatechin gallate-transthyretin complex reveals a novel binding site distinct from the thyroxine binding site. *Biochemistry* **2010**, *49*, 6104–6114. [CrossRef]
64. Ferreira, N.; Saraiva, M.J.; Almeida, M.R. Epigallocatechin-3-gallate as a potential therapeutic drug for TTR-related amyloidosis: "in vivo" evidence from FAP mice models. *PLoS ONE* **2012**, *7*, e29933. [CrossRef]
65. Kristen, A.V.; Lehrke, S.; Buss, S.; Mereles, D.; Steen, H.; Ehlermann, P.; Hardt, S.; Giannitsis, E.; Schreiner, R.; Haberkorn, U.; et al. Green tea halts progression of cardiac transthyretin amyloidosis: An observational report. *Clin. Res. Cardiol.* **2012**, *101*, 805–813. [CrossRef]
66. Aus dem Siepen, F.; Bauer, R.; Aurich, M.; Buss, S.J.; Steen, H.; Altland, K.; Katus, H.A.; Kristen, A.V. Green tea extract as a treatment for patients with wild-type transthyretin amyloidosis: An observational study. *Drug Des. Dev. Ther.* **2015**, *9*, 6319–6325. [CrossRef]
67. Cappelli, F.; Martone, R.; Taborchi, G.; Morini, S.; Bartolini, S.; Angelotti, P.; Farsetti, S.; Di Mario, C.; Perfetto, F. Epigallocatechin-3-gallate tolerability and impact on survival in a cohort of patients with transthyretin-related cardiac amyloidosis. A single-center retrospective study. *Intern. Emerg. Med.* **2018**, *13*, 873–880. [CrossRef]
68. Pullakhandam, R.; Srinivas, P.N.B.S.; Nair, M.K.; Reddy, G.B. Binding and stabilization of transthyretin by curcumin. *Arch. Biochem. Biophys.* **2009**, *485*, 115–119. [CrossRef]
69. Polsinelli, I.; Nencetti, S.; Shepard, W.; Ciccone, L.; Orlandini, E.; Stura, E.A. A new crystal form of human transthyretin obtained with a curcumin derived ligand. *J. Struct. Biol.* **2016**, *194*, 8–17. [CrossRef]
70. Ferreira, N.; Gonçalves, N.P.; Saraiva, M.J.; Almeida, M.R. Curcumin: A multi-target disease-modifying agent for late-stage transthyretin amyloidosis. *Sci. Rep.* **2016**, *6*, 503. [CrossRef]
71. Thapa, A.; Jett, S.D.; Chi, E.Y. Curcumin Attenuates Amyloid-β Aggregate Toxicity and Modulates Amyloid-β Aggregation Pathway. *ACS Chem. Neurosci.* **2015**, *7*, 56–68. [CrossRef] [PubMed]
72. Rane, J.S.; Bhaumik, P.; Panda, D. Curcumin Inhibits Tau Aggregation and Disintegrates Preformed Tau Filaments in vitro. *J. Alzheimer's Dis.* **2017**, *60*, 999–1014. [CrossRef] [PubMed]
73. Singh, P.K.; Kotia, V.; Ghosh, D.; Mohite, G.M.; Kumar, A.; Maji, S.K. Curcumin modulates α-synuclein aggregation and toxicity. *ACS Chem. Neurosci.* **2013**, *4*, 393–407. [CrossRef] [PubMed]
74. Yang, F.; Lim, G.P.; Begum, A.N.; Ubeda, O.J.; Simmons, M.R.; Ambegaokar, S.S.; Chen, P.P.; Kayed, R.; Glabe, C.G.; Frautschy, S.A.; et al. Curcumin inhibits formation of amyloid beta oligomers and fibrils, binds plaques, and reduces amyloid in vivo. *J. Biol. Chem.* **2005**, *280*, 5892–5901. [CrossRef] [PubMed]
75. Garcia-Alloza, M.; Borrelli, L.A.; Rozkalne, A.; Hyman, B.T.; Bacskai, B.J. Curcumin labels amyloid pathology in vivo, disrupts existing plaques, and partially restores distorted neurites in an Alzheimer mouse model. *J. Neurochem.* **2007**, *102*, 1095–1104. [CrossRef] [PubMed]
76. Maiti, P.; Hall, T.C.; Paladugu, L.; Kolli, N.; Learman, C.; Rossignol, J.; Dunbar, G.L. A comparative study of dietary curcumin, nanocurcumin, and other classical amyloid-binding dyes for labeling and imaging of amyloid plaques in brain tissue of 5×-familial Alzheimer's disease mice. *Histochem. Cell Biol.* **2016**, *146*, 609–625. [CrossRef] [PubMed]
77. Masuda, Y.; Fukuchi, M.; Yatagawa, T.; Tada, M.; Takeda, K.; Irie, K.; Akagi, K.-I.; Monobe, Y.; Imazawa, T.; Takegoshi, K. Solid-state NMR analysis of interaction sites of curcumin and 42-residue amyloid β-protein fibrils. *Bioorg. Med. Chem.* **2011**, *19*, 5967–5974. [CrossRef] [PubMed]
78. Maiti, P.; Dunbar, G.L. Use of Curcumin, a Natural Polyphenol for Targeting Molecular Pathways in Treating Age-Related Neurodegenerative Diseases. *Int. J. Mol. Sci.* **2018**, *19*, 1637. [CrossRef] [PubMed]
79. Ferreira, N.; Santos, S.A.O.; Domingues, M.R.M.; Saraiva, M.J.; Almeida, M.R. Dietary curcumin counteracts extracellular transthyretin deposition: Insights on the mechanism of amyloid inhibition. *Biochim. Biophys. Acta* **2013**, *1832*, 39–45. [CrossRef]

80. Chongtham, A.; Agrawal, N. Curcumin modulates cell death and is protective in Huntington's disease model. *Sci. Rep.* **2016**, *6*, 18736. [CrossRef]
81. Nunes, R.J.; de Oliveira, P.; Lages, A.; Becker, J.D.; Marcelino, P.; Barroso, E.; Perdigoto, R.; Kelly, J.W.; Quintas, A.; Santos, S.C.R. Transthyretin proteins regulate angiogenesis by conferring different molecular identities to endothelial cells. *J. Biol. Chem.* **2013**, *288*, 31752–31760. [CrossRef] [PubMed]
82. Koike, H.; Ikeda, S.; Takahashi, M.; Kawagashira, Y.; Iijima, M.; Misumi, Y.; Ando, Y.; Ikeda, S.-I.; Katsuno, M.; Sobue, G. Schwann cell and endothelial cell damage in transthyretin familial amyloid polyneuropathy. *Neurology* **2016**, *87*, 2220–2229. [CrossRef] [PubMed]
83. Koike, H.; Katsuno, M. Ultrastructure in Transthyretin Amyloidosis: From Pathophysiology to Therapeutic Insights. *Biomedicines* **2019**, *7*, 11. [CrossRef]
84. Karimian, M.S.; Pirro, M.; Johnston, T.P.; Majeed, M.; Sahebkar, A. Curcumin and Endothelial Function: Evidence and Mechanisms of Protective Effects. *Curr. Pharm. Des.* **2017**, *23*, 2462–2473. [CrossRef] [PubMed]
85. Rahman, M.A.; Rhim, H. Therapeutic implication of autophagy in neurodegenerative diseases. *BMB Rep.* **2017**, *50*, 345–354. [CrossRef] [PubMed]
86. Fujikake, N.; Shin, M.; Shimizu, S. Association Between Autophagy and Neurodegenerative Diseases. *Front. Neurosci.* **2018**, *12*, 255. [CrossRef]
87. Teixeira, C.A.; Almeida, M.D.R.; Saraiva, M.J. Impairment of autophagy by TTR V30M aggregates: In vivo reversal by TUDCA and curcumin. *Clin. Sci.* **2016**, *130*, 1665–1675. [CrossRef]
88. Rainey, N.; Motte, L.; Aggarwal, B.B.; Petit, P.X. Curcumin hormesis mediates a cross-talk between autophagy and cell death. *Cell Death Dis.* **2015**, *6*, e2003. [CrossRef]
89. Moustapha, A.; Pérétout, P.A.; Rainey, N.E.; Sureau, F.; Geze, M.; Petit, J.-M.; Dewailly, E.; Slomianny, C.; Petit, P.X. Curcumin induces crosstalk between autophagy and apoptosis mediated by calcium release from the endoplasmic reticulum, lysosomal destabilization and mitochondrial events. *Cell Death Discov.* **2015**, *1*, 15017. [CrossRef]
90. Lai, A.Y.; McLaurin, J. Clearance of amyloid-β peptides by microglia and macrophages: The issue of what, when and where. *Future Neurol.* **2012**, *7*, 165–176. [CrossRef]
91. Zhang, L.; Fiala, M.; Cashman, J.; Sayre, J.; Espinosa, A.; Mahanian, M.; Zaghi, J.; Badmaev, V.; Graves, M.C.; Bernard, G.; et al. Curcuminoids enhance amyloid-β uptake by macrophages of Alzheimer's disease patients. *J. Alzheimer's Dis.* **2006**, *10*, 1–7. [CrossRef]
92. Masoumi, A.; Goldenson, B.; Ghirmai, S.; Avagyan, H.; Zaghi, J.; Abel, K.; Zheng, X.; Espinosa-Jeffrey, A.; Mahanian, M.; Liu, P.T.; et al. 1α,25-dihydroxyvitamin D3 Interacts with Curcuminoids to Stimulate Amyloid-β Clearance by Macrophages of Alzheimer's Disease Patients. *J. Alzheimer's Dis.* **2009**, *17*, 703–717. [CrossRef] [PubMed]
93. Fiala, M.; Mahanian, M.; Rosenthal, M.; Mizwicki, M.T.; Tse, E.; Cho, T.; Sayre, J.; Weitzman, R.; Porter, V. MGAT3 mRNA: A Biomarker for Prognosis and Therapy of Alzheimer's Disease by Vitamin D and Curcuminoids. *J. Alzheimer's Dis.* **2011**, *25*, 135–144. [CrossRef] [PubMed]
94. Hewlings, S.J.; Kalman, D.S. Curcumin: A Review of Its' Effects on Human Health. *Foods* **2017**, *6*, 92. [CrossRef] [PubMed]
95. Lao, C.D.; Ruffin, M.T.; Normolle, D.; Heath, D.D.; Murray, S.I.; Bailey, J.M.; Boggs, M.E.; Crowell, J.; Rock, C.L.; Brenner, D.E. Dose escalation of a curcuminoid formulation. *BMC Complement. Altern. Med.* **2006**, *6*, 10. [CrossRef]
96. Adams, D.; Gonzalez-Duarte, A.; O'Riordan, W.D.; Yang, C.-C.; Ueda, M.; Kristen, A.V.; Tournev, I.; Schmidt, H.H.; Coelho, T.; Berk, J.L.; et al. Patisiran, an RNAi Therapeutic, for Hereditary Transthyretin Amyloidosis. *N. Engl. J. Med.* **2018**, *379*, 11–21. [CrossRef] [PubMed]
97. Benson, M.D.; Waddington-Cruz, M.; Berk, J.L.; Polydefkis, M.; Dyck, P.J.; Wang, A.K.; Plante-Bordeneuve, V.; Barroso, F.A.; Merlini, G.; Obici, L.; et al. Inotersen Treatment for Patients with Hereditary Transthyretin Amyloidosis. *N. Engl. J. Med.* **2018**, *379*, 22–31. [CrossRef]

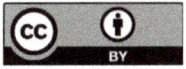 © 2019 by the authors. Licensee MDPI, Basel, Switzerland. This article is an open access article distributed under the terms and conditions of the Creative Commons Attribution (CC BY) license (http://creativecommons.org/licenses/by/4.0/).

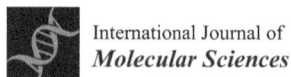

Article

Antimicrobial Potential of Single Metabolites of Curcuma longa Assessed in the Total Extract by Thin-Layer Chromatography-Based Bioautography and Image Analysis

Lidia Czernicka [1], Agnieszka Grzegorczyk [2], Zbigniew Marzec [1], Beata Antosiewicz [3], Anna Malm [2] and Wirginia Kukula-Koch [4],*

1. Chair and Department of Food and Nutrition, Medical University of Lublin, 4a Chodźki Str., 20-093 Lublin, Poland; lidiaczernicka@umlub.pl (L.C.); zbigniew.marzec@umlub.pl (Z.M.)
2. Department of Pharmaceutical Microbiology with Laboratory for Microbiological Diagnostics, Faculty of Pharmacy with Medical Analytics Division, Medical University of Lublin, 1 Chodźki, Lublin 20-093, Poland; agnieszka.grzegorczyk@umlub.pl (A.G.); anna.malm@umlub.pl (A.M.)
3. Department of Cosmetology, University of Information Technology and Management in Rzeszow, 35-225 Rzeszów, Poland; bantosiewicz@wsiz.rzeszow.pl
4. Chair and Department of Pharmacognosy with Medicinal Plants Unit, Medical University of Lublin, 20-093 Lublin, Poland
* Correspondence: virginia.kukula@gmail.com; Tel.: +48-81-4487087

Received: 16 January 2019; Accepted: 11 February 2019; Published: 19 February 2019

Abstract: *Curcuma longa* from Zingiberaceae belongs to the major spices consumed around the world, known from its cholagogue, anti-inflammatory, and antimicrobial properties. Lack of data on the activity of single components of turmeric extract encouraged the authors to apply TLC (thin-layer chromatography) based bioautography studies to reveal its antimicrobial constituents and construct a universal platform for the bioactivity assessment of crude extracts, with help of a freeware ImageJ software. This optimized chromatographic bioassay performed on diethyl ether and methanol extracts of *Curcuma longa* was successfully applied on the total extract and revealed the antimicrobial potential of single components against a variety of Gram-positive strains, with no need for their isolation from the mixture. The obtained results were further confronted with a classic microdilution antimicrobial assay on the isolates, purified from the crude extracts by centrifugal partition chromatography in the following solvent system: heptane-chloroform-methanol-water (5:6:3:2) ($v/v/v/v$).

Keywords: *Curcuma longa*; turmeric tuber; Zingiberaceae; TLC bioautography; antimicrobial agents; ImageJ; TLC-MS; hydrostatic counter-current chromatography; centrifugal partition chromatography

1. Introduction

In recent years, the development of bacterial resistance against antibiotics available in the pharmaceutical market constitutes a serious pharmacological issue. There are many cases of hospital infections, bacterial diseases originating from tropical countries, or infections caused by mutant bacteria, which are difficult to treat [1]. Since the beginning of the 80 s, there have been numerous attempts to discover new potent antimicrobial agents and develop novel antibiotics that can overcome severe problems associated with bacterial resistance. Even though the costs of conducted studies are high, as in any field of research, the results still do not bring much novelty to the field. Moreover, significant adverse or side effects caused by the currently administered drugs to the macroorganism constitute another important issue that needs a special focus. For these reasons, phytotherapy has become a popular field of study for both patients searching for new and more effective therapeutical strategies and for researchers searching for ideas in the process of new drug design, as nature has already given a variety of chemical structures to modern pharmacology.

Turmeric (*Curcuma longa* L.) is one of the most widely recognized medicinal plants. It is a tropical, perennial spice that belongs to the Zingiberaceae family and is widely cultivated in Malaysia, India, and Indonesia for its flavoring, coloring, and medicinal applications [2], together with its low toxicity (doses of 12 g/day are reported to be safe to humans [3]). The first information about its medicinal uses come from Ayurveda, Siddha, and Unani medicine systems and concerns its antibacterial, wound healing, anti-inflammatory, digestive, and anticancer properties [4].

Turmeric extracts contain both precious sesquiterpenes (α-zingiberene, β-sesquiphellandrene, and *ar*-turmerone as the leading constituents of terpene fraction) and polyphenols (curcuminoids). Among the latter group, curcumin, demethoxycurcumin, and bisdemethoxycurcumin can be distinguished as the leading compounds [2]. These ferulic acid derivatives are responsible for the major pharmacological effects of turmeric. Their strong antioxidant potential affects the inhibition of tumor growth and promotes antisclerotic or neuroprotective activity of the plant [5]. Interestingly, the majority of scientific publications describe the activity of crude extracts or focus on the properties of curcumin—the major phenolic metabolite of the plant. Because of some difficulties in the isolation of curcuminoids caused by a marked structural similarity between one another, much less is known about the potential of the remaining constituents of this plant.

Several publications have reported the antimicrobial activity of turmeric extract against oral bacteria [6,7] or compared its potential by considering the extraction conditions used [8–10]. A large majority of the papers, however, describe the antibacterial potential of the crude turmeric extract or crude turmeric oil [11–14].

The aim of this study was to evaluate the antimicrobial potential of single constituents of methanol and diethyl ether extracts of *C. longa* L., without any need for their isolation from the crude extract. This task was performed by the application of TLC bioautography with image analysis on the selected strains of Gram-positive bacteria, and the result was expressed as the antimicrobial potential according to the values of minimum inhibitory quantity (MIQ) of the compounds. The subsequent identification of potent components was performed using a TLC-MS interface in a direct MS analysis of an indicated spot, which clearly determined the structure of the analyzed compounds. The accuracy of this methodology was assessed by the authors on the isolated single metabolites in the microdilution test in order to compare the results with those from image analyses. The latter task was performed through the application of centrifugal partition chromatography (CPC) on the crude extract.

This study was performed to show a new approach—the performance of a rapid screening protocol that enables the identification of natural antimicrobial metabolites present in the mixtures and can be applied in the studies of other plant extracts.

2. Results and Discussion

Antimicrobial potential of the members of the Zingiberaceae family has been extensively studied in recent years. Turmeric, one of the most known species of this family, is perceived as an efficient antimicrobial herb with low toxicity, which can be supplemented or eaten as a spice [15]. The authors in their works underline a marked potential of both—essential oil and alcoholic extracts obtained from different species of *Curcuma* grown worldwide. Although there are many reports on the activity of the total extracts, only a few papers have focused on the potential of single metabolites present in turmeric tuber [16–18]. None of them have actually answered the question on which metabolites plays a crucial role in the process of bacterial growth inhibition.

The present work shows the efficiency of chromatographic separation coupled with image processing software in the estimation of antimicrobial activity of turmeric metabolites, tested against a large selection of Gram-positive bacteria.

2.1. LC-ESI-Q-TOF-MS Analysis of the Extracts' Qualitative and Quantitative Composition

Qualitative and quantitative composition of the obtained extracts was studied by a mass spectrometer coupled with liquid chromatography, which provided high accuracy mass measurements with low error of measurement values. Several compounds were identified by the authors in both extracts on the basis of the fragmentation patterns and the available scientific literature. For the purpose of this study, the below-described inhibitors of bacterial growth were quantified.

The optimized methodology allowed high sensitivity of the measurement and precise determination of molecular formulas, without any doubt concerning the number of defined elements in the metabolites' structures. The positive ionization mode was found to be preferable for the determination of both phenolic compounds and terpenes present in the turmeric. The applied fragmentation voltage of 150 V and the CID energies of 10 and 20 V allowed sufficient sensitivity and good fragmentation of molecular ions.

Table 1 shows the list of identified components of the evaluated turmeric extracts together with the recognition of other major peaks present in the analyzed sample with the total ion chromatogram and their spectral data. All identified compounds were found in both MeOH and diethyl ether extracts. The extracted ion chromatograms of the described components are present in the Supplementary file.

Table 1. LC-ESI-Q-TOF-MS accurate mass measurements of phenolics and terpenes identified in the MeOH and diethyl ether extracts of *Curcuma longa* tubers.

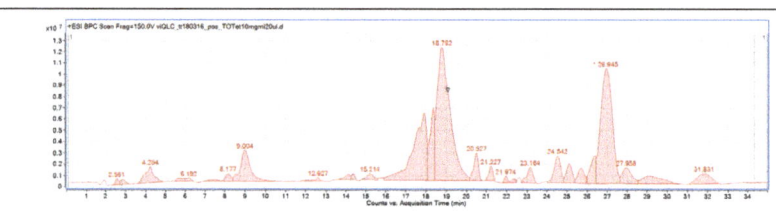

			The total ion chromatogram of diethyl ether extract from turmeric tuber				
No.	Compound	Molecular Formula	Experimental Mass [M+H]$^+$	Calculated Mass [M+H]$^+$	Mass Error (ppm)	DBE	MS/MS Fragments
1	CU	$C_{21}H_{20}O_6$	369.1336	369.1333	−0.91	12	177, 145
2	DMCU	$C_{20}H_{18}O_5$	339.1233	339.1227	−1.77	12	177, 147
3	BDMCU	$C_{19}H_{16}O_4$	309.1122	309.1121	−0.21	12	147, 119
4	TUR	$C_{15}H_{20}O$	217.1586	217.1587	0.42	12	119, 91
5	Dihydro-BDMCU	$C_{19}H_{18}O_4$	311.1286	311.1278	−2.63	11	225, 147
6	Dihydro-CU	$C_{21}H_{22}O_6$	371.1468	371.1489	5.71	11	245, 177, 147
7	Dihydro-DMCU	$C_{20}H_{20}O_5$	341.1377	341.1384	1.91	11	177, 147
8	Tetrahydro-BDMCU	$C_{19}H_{20}O_4$	313.1286	313.1434	3.0	10	-

(DBE—double bond equivalent values; CU—curcumin; DMCU—dimethoxycurcumin; BDMCU—bisdemethoxycurcumin).

The first four identified components are the compounds later confirmed to be responsible for the antimicrobial activity. They constitute 22.1 ± 0.4% (CU), 9.14 ± 0.2% (DMCU), 11.33 ± 0.2% (BDMCU), and 3.48 ± 0.06% (TUR) of the MeOH extract and 19.2 ± 0.2% (CU), 7.21 ± 0.4% (DMCU), 8.95 ± 0.3% (BDMCU), and 4.58 ± 0.1% (TUR) of the diethyl ether extract of turmeric tubers, measured in four separate injections of the extracts. As presented above, the influence of the extractant used on the final composition of the extracts was not significant.

Our studies on the composition of the extracts are in accordance with the previously published papers. Other authors describe a similar ratio of these three pigments with curcumin as the leading component, however, the total concentration of those differ depending on the place of origin. According to the studies of Peret-Almeida and co-workers (2008) the quantity of curcumin reached 50%, DMCU—29% and BDMCU—12% in the extract. According to the studies of Jayaprakasha and colleagues, the ferulic acid derivatives varied in four varieties of the plant and stayed within the range of 1.06–5.65%, DMCU: 0.83–3.36% and BDMCU: 0.42–2.16% in the tubers [19,20].

Detailed LC-MS analysis of the extract' composition revealed the presence of other phenolic compounds, which were tentatively identified by the authors based on the scientific literature and fragmentation patterns [21]. The derivatives of the investigated three pigments are characterized by a different quantity of unsaturated bonds. Even if present in the extracts, their concentration was scarce (Table 1).

2.2. TLC Bioautography Tests and Identification of Active Metabolites by TLC-LC-ESI-TOF-MS

From the optimization studies, two mobile phases were selected for the analyses of extracts: MeOH: DCM (0.5: 9.5 v/v) for the more polar MeOH extract, and n-hexane: DCM (1:9 v/v) for the diethyl ether extract. The evaluated conditions provided effective separation of both polar and nonpolar compounds present in the extracts.

As mentioned in the Materials and Methods section, seven strains of Gram-positive bacteria were used for the determination of antimicrobial properties of turmeric. All the strains grew well on the MHA agar, and after re-incubation with TTC, they provided evenly colored plates with colorless zones of inhibition. The preliminary studies revealed that the most efficient bacterial inoculum concentration was 1.5×10^6 CFU; it assured an even colorization of the plate with no zones of color lightening. An absolute condition for conducting the tests was the need to dry out the mobile phase from the TLC plates before applying the bacteria strain and to keep them closed inside the Petri dishes prior to covering with the medium.

In the next step of the experiment, on the uncoated but developed TLC plates, all zones corresponding to the zones of inhibition were analyzed by a mass spectrometer. In the optimized TLC development conditions for the identification of single components present on the uncoated TLC plates were afforded by a TLC-MS interface, thus providing high accuracy mass measurements of metabolites and their fragmentation patterns; this allowed data- and literature-based identification [15,21]. Among the metabolites which were found to be active in the applied concentrations of the total extracts, three curcuminoids—curcumin (CU), demethoxycurcumin (DMCU), and bisdemethoxycurcumin (BDMCU)—in both extracts and turmerone (TUR) in the nonpolar extract were identified. Table S1 (in the Supplementary file) presents the identity of these metabolites, the total chromatograms of the analyzed spots, and the MS spectra of major peaks. All the below-presented data were obtained in the positive ionization mode.

The behavior of the identified metabolites was different, depending on the strain tested. Table 2. shows the bacterial strains sensitive to the identified compounds. The obtained values come from a careful analysis of all developed TLC plates. The spots of the lowest extract concentration, with an unambiguous red color clearance were selected for the determination of MIQ value. To obtain the final result, the concentration of the spotted total extract was divided by the actual content of each curcuminoid and *ar*-turmerone in the extract to deliver the values presented in Table 2, which constitute an estimated quantification.

Differences in the action of individual compounds result from the varied sensitivity of each microorganism and each strain of a given species. Typically, *S. epidermidis* or *B. subtilis* are more sensitive than *S. aureus*. In addition, the *S. aureus* ATCC 43300 strain is a methicillin resistant strain, and therefore may be less susceptible to tested drugs.

ar-Turmerone did not inhibit all tested bacteria. It was found to be active against *S. aureus* ATCC 43300, *S. epidermidis* ATCC 12228, and *B. subtilis* ATCC 6633, with the lowest MIQ value for the first strain.

As previously mentioned, the studies on the antimicrobial potential of turmeric metabolites are scarce. The activity of ar-turmerone described in this paper is, however, in accordance with the publication of Peret-Almeida and colleagues [19], who confirmed the antimicrobial activity of turmeric oil with the main metabolite identified as ar-turmerone, against *Bacillus subtilis* (the diameters around the discs increased by 131%) [15].

Table 2. Evaluation of the antimicrobial activity of four identified compounds against all tested Gram-positive bacteria strains, in relation to the isolated curcumin studied in a microdilution assay. The MIQ values are given in μg.

Strains of Bacteria	MIQ (μg)			
	CU	DMCU	BDMCU	TUR
Staphylococcus aureus ATCC 25923	4.42	0.91	0.57	-
Staphylococcus aureus ATCC 6538	0.55	0.23	0.28	-
Staphylococcus aureus ATCC 43300	8.84	1.83	0.57	0.23
Staphylococcus epidermidis ATCC 12228	0.55	0.23	0.14	1.80
Bacillus subtilis ATCC 6633	4.42	0.46	0.28	1.83
Bacillus cereus ATCC 10876	<0.28	<0.11	<0.14	-

Interestingly, all curcuminoids inhibited the growth of bacteria. Considering their concentration in the total extract, as described above, BDMCU, as a less abundant component in the extract, showed the strongest inhibition of the growth of bacteria. Its lowest MIQ values were noted for *S. aureus* ATCC 43300 (MIQ = 0.28 μg) and *B. cereus* ATCC 10876 (MIQ ≤ 0.14 μg)), whereas its weakest activity was observed for two strains: *S. aureus* ATCC 25923 and *S. aureus* ATCC 43300. In the only study on single curcuminoids antimicrobial activity which is known to the authors, BDMCU was also found the most active among the tested three curcuminoids, with a particular antimicrobial potential against *Bacillus subtilis* at a concentration of 10 μg/μL [15].

The other curcumin derivative—DMCU—even if present in the smallest quantity, was found to show stronger inhibitory properties from curcumin itself. *Bacillus cereus* ATCC 10876 was the most susceptible to DMCU (MIQ = <0.11 μg) among all four studied compounds.

Interestingly, similar tendency in the pharmacological activity strength of the herein described phenolics was also observed in the works related to the anticancer activity assessment [22].

2.3. Purification of Single Curcuminoids by CPC Chromatography

The applied separation conditions enabled a successful purification of curcuminoids: bisdemethoxycurcumin was present in fractions no. 8–12, demethoxycurcumin in fractions no. 16–18, and curcumin in fractions no. 22–26. The identification of the ferulic acid derivatives and their purity was performed by LC-MS spectrometry on the basis of their fragmentation pattern, the retention time, and the scientific literature, as shown in the Supplementary Material (Figures S2 and S3). The purity of all compounds exceeded 95.5%, and for curcumin, the purity was calculated as 98.2%. From the injected total extract, the authors obtained as much as 178 mg of curcumin, which was used to perform a microdilution antimicrobial assay. The data on the purity of isolated curcumin are presented in the Supplementary file (Figure S1).

A standard microdilution antimicrobial assay was performed on the sample of pure curcumin to assess the accuracy of the TLC bioautography technique.

2.4. Antibacterial Potential of Turmeric Metabolites in Relation to the Commonly-Used Antibiotic Vancomycin

As shown in the Tables 2 and 3, the MIQ values obtained for curcumin differ, depending on the method used. This result seems to be valid as the quantity of microorganisms in both tests differs significantly. The concept of microdilution assay is to study a sample dipped in the medium containing a certain concentration of bacteria. As a consequence, the tested sample can interact with all bacterial cells inside the well. In the TLC bioautography tests, the effect of tested compounds on the microorganisms is limited to the place where the spot is located; thus, every metabolite affects a much smaller quantity of the microorganisms than in the microdilution assay.

Table 3. Determination of curcumin antibacterial activity in relation to vancomycin, by a standard microdilution assay, measured in µg.

Strains of Bacteria	MIQ (µg)	
	CU	Vancomycin
Staphylococcus aureus ATCC 25923	25	0.098
Staphylococcus aureus ATCC 6538	6.25	0.049
Staphylococcus aureus ATCC 43300	50	0.049
Staphylococcus epidermidis ATCC 12228	6.25	0.098
Bacillus subtilis ATCC 6633	25	0.024
Bacillus cereus ATCC 10876	25	0.098

To relate the bioautographic results presented in Table 2 to those obtained by the standard microdilution assay, we found it necessary to analyze the behavior of the reference compound vancomycin on a TLC plate under the same analytical conditions as those used for the extracts.

For this purpose, chromatograms with different concentrations of vancomycin were prepared. During the chromatogram processing of images, the concentration of the antibacterial activity of the compounds was reflected in their peak areas. The higher the concentration, the larger the absolute value of its peak area.

The set of peak areas of vancomycin obtained from an ImageJ image processing was used for the preparation of calibration curves for each bacterial strain evaluated in the study.

The calibration curve equations are presented in Table 4. All of them showed high linearity (R^2 values were higher than 0.95) and could be successfully used for the determination of vancomycin equivalents, which characterize the tested natural products. Table 4 shows the calculations of vancomycin equivalents for curcumin, as the major constituent of the extracts, determined in both antimicrobial assays.

Table 4. Determination of vancomycin equivalents for curcumin determined in the bioautographic and microdilution tests.

Strains of Bacteria	Calibration Curve Equation (Vancomycin)	Vancomycin Equivalents (TLC Bioutography)		Vancomycin Equivalents (Microdilution Assay)
		CU (µg ± SD)	RSD (%)	CU [µg]
Staphylococcus aureus ATCC 25923	y = 9731ln(x) − 12434	206 ± 12	5.8	255
Staphylococcus aureus ATCC 6538	y = 17492ln(x) − 7990.8	142 ± 10	6.9	127
Staphylococcus aureus ATCC 43300	y = 1381.9ln(x) + 5925.8	1310 ± 69	5.3	1020
Staphylococcus epidermidis ATCC 12228	y = 1340.3ln(x) + 128.79	49 ± 4	8.7	64
Bacillus subtilis ATCC 6633	y = 13889ln(x) + 22510	1328 ± 56	4.2	1041
Bacillus cereus ATCC 10876	y = 629.12ln(x) + 10915	202 ± 13	6.5	255

The above-presented data show that the findings of TLC-based bioautographic test were identical to the results of antimicrobial studies performed in a traditional way by using the microdilution method and were performed by the authors of the manuscript [23]. With a relatively low error, the antimicrobial potential of curcumin could be assessed without any need for their purification from the total extract.

The herein presented approach is universal and may be applied to the analyses of other complex matrices such as plant extracts, where the process of isolation is time-, money- and solvent-consuming.

Image processing by the freeware software ImageJ program is an interesting alternative for biological screening studies, as it is easy to operate and offers a wide range of image modifications. Initial screening of biological properties by imaging software may provide important information on the pharmacological potential of the ingredients of various mixtures, without any need for their isolation; this favors the green chemistry approach and reduces the efforts of researchers.

3. Materials and Methods

3.1. General

Silica gel 60 F254 neutral TLC plates were purchased from Merck (Darmstadt, Germany) for TLC bioautography assays. Hamilton micropipette 705 (Hamilton, Bonaduz, Switzerland) was used for the extracts' application onto the TLC plates. TLC chromatograms were photographed with a Canon Power Shot G5 camera digital camera with standard 18-35 lens. The pictures were processed using an ImageJ 1.48v image processing program (Wayne Rasband, National Institutes of Health, Maryland, USA).

An accelerated solvent extraction apparatus (ASE, Model ASE 100, Dionex, CA, USA) was used for the extraction of plant material. A centrifugal partition chromatograph SCPC-250-L system by Armen (Saint Ave, France) equipped with a 250 mL column, a quaternary pump, a fraction collector (LS-5600) and a UV detector (Flesh06S DAD 600) provided the isolation of curcuminoids.

An LC-ESI-Q-TOF-MS qualitative and quantitative analysis of extracts and isolates was performed using an Agilent G3250AA LC/MSD TOF system containing a photodiode array detector (G1315D), an HP 1200 chromatograph and a Q-TOF-MS spectrometer (Agilent Technologies, Santa Clara, CA, USA) with an ESI ionization source. The apparatus contained a column thermostate, a degasser (G1322A), an autosampler (G1329B) and the binary pump (G1312C). The analysis was performed on an HPLC column: Zorbax RP 18 (150 mm × 2.1 mm, dp = 3.5 μm) with a fast gradient elution method.

The identification of active components directly from a TLC plate was performed using an LC-ESI-TOF spectrometer Agilent Technologies (Santa Clara, CA, USA) equipped with an HPLC system G3250AA LC composed of a binary pump, an autosampler, a thermostated column, a photodiode-array (PDA) detector and a degasser, and a mass spectrometer: 6210 MSD TOF with ESI dual-spray source. The system with a TLC-MS interface (Camag, Muttenz, Switzerland) contained a Zorbax RP-18 Rapid Resolution column (50 × 2.1 mm, 5 μm diameter).

3.2. Chemicals and Reagents

The chemicals used in the study: methanol, ethanol, dichloromethane, diethyl ether, n-hexane, ammonia, sulphuric acid, heptane, chloroform, and vanillin were produced by Avantor Performance Materials (Gliwice, Poland), whereas water and acetonitrile of spectroscopic grade were obtained from Merck (Darmstadt, Germany). Vancomycin was purchased from Sigma Aldrich (St. Louis, CA, USA) as well as 2,3,5-triphenyltetrazolium chloride (TTC), which is the dye used in this work to observe, stain colonies of microorganisms on solid culture media such as Mueller-Hinton Agar (MHA) on TLC plates.

3.3. Plant Extract Preparation

Fresh turmeric rhizomes were purchased from Tex Plants & More Philipp Foerster, Annaberg-Buchholz, Germany; they were immediately frozen after the delivery and then thawed in the required quantity shortly before the extraction. For the preparation of extracts, the tubers were cut into small pieces and placed in a 30 mL stainless steel extraction cell with a cellulose filter at the bottom end (methanol extracts) or in a mortar (diethyl ether extracts). Two types of extractants were used to enrich the final extract either in more or less polar constituents to obtain a more comprehensive picture in the antimicrobial tests. The extraction with methanol was conducted under the following conditions in an ASE apparatus: temperature, 70 °C; purge volume, 70%; purge time, 100 s; analysis time, 10 min; number of cycles, 3; this extraction was done after an initial purification from unipolar components with n-hexane under the same conditions, but with 1 cycle [22]. The extraction with diethyl ether was performed by pounding crushed turmeric rhizomes in a mortar with solvent, followed by drying of the sample over silica gel. Methanol extracts were evaporated on a rotary evaporator at the temperature of 45 °C and re-dissolved in methanol to obtain following concentrations: 2, 1, 0.5, 0.25, 0.125, and 0.0625 mg/mL. Diethyl ether extracts were left under the fume hood until they became dry. Methanol was used to obtain similar concentrations as those for the other extracts.

3.4. Thin-Layer Chromatography (TLC) Conditions

TLC chromatograms were performed using aluminum TLC plates (silica gel 60 F254, Merck, Darmstadt, Germany).

An initial evaluation of the chromatographic conditions and the composition of a solvent system was performed using a 1% solution of vanillin, which provided a successful visualization of the extracts' constituents. The 1% vanillin-sulfuric acid reagent was prepared by dissolving 2 mL of sulfuric acid in a 1% methanolic solution of vanillin (w/v). After spraying, the TLC plates were heated at 110 °C for optimal color development.

Every plate used in the TLC bioautography studies was sized 7 × 6 cm and contained six concentrations of each extract, namely 2, 1, 0.5, 0.25, 0.125, and 0.0625 mg/mL, spotted quantitatively by a Hamilton syringe with the following volumes, respectively: 20, 10, 5, 2.5, 1.25, and 0.675 µL. The applied volume resembled 40, 20, 10, 5, 2.5, and 1.25 µg of extract within the spot. Thus, 16 TLC plates were prepared for both extracts for each tested bacterial strain.

After the color development, the TLC plates were dried inside sterile Petri dishes in a laminar flow hood to minimize microbial contamination from the air. The active compounds were then visualized under UV light at 254 nm and 366 nm and marked on each TLC plate with a pencil. After drying they were subjected to further microbiological analysis. Each TLC plate was prepared in triplicate. Each time, three TLC plates were coated with a bacterial broth. Additionally, six TLC plates for each extract were prepared for the identification and quantitative studies.

3.5. Organisms and Media

Several Gram-positive bacterial strains applied onto the developed TLC plates for the estimation of active metabolites of both extracts: *Staphylococcus aureus* ATCC 25923, *Staphylococcus aureus* ATCC 6538, *Staphylococcus aureus* ATCC 43300, *Staphylococcus epidermidis* ATCC 12228, *Bacillus subtilis* ATCC 6633, *Bacillus cereus* ATCC 10876, and *Micrococcus luteus* ATCC 10240. The above microorganisms were obtained from American Type Culture Collection, which are used as microbiological standards in the study of the activity of various substances and compounds against microbes.

3.6. Bioautographic Methods

The developed TLC plates were covered (sprayed) manually by MHA containing the bacterial inoculum of 1.5×10^6 CFU (colony forming units)/mL. These bioautograms were placed in sterile Petri dishes and were incubated at 35 °C for 24 h under aerobic and humid conditions. After the completion of incubation, TTC was used to visualize zones of inhibition of bacterial growth. These salts were sprayed onto the bioautograms and were reincubated at 35 °C for 24 h. Transparent zones of bacterial growth inhibition indicated the antibacterial activity of the samples.

Additionally, vancomycin—an antibiotic with a wide spectrum of antibacterial activity against Gram-positive bacteria—was used to define the sensitivity of the assay. Several concentrations of the antibiotic were prepared as follows: 128, 32, 8, 2, 0.5, and 0.2 µg/mL (for *Staphylococcus aureus* ATCC 6538), and 64, 16, 4, 1, 0.25, and 0.1 µg/mL (for *S. aureus* ATCC 25923, *Bacillus subtilis* ATCC 6633, *Micrococcus luteus* ATCC 10240, *S. aureus* ATCC 43300, and *Bacillus cereus* ATCC 10876), and the solutions were spotted on the TLC plates in the following volumes: 20, 10, 5, 2.5, 1.25, and 0.675 µL, respectively. The test concentrations of this antibiotic were selected on the basis of previous studies, where this compound was studied in the microdilution tests, [24,25], and on the basis of the values of peak areas of active components of the extracts for the calibration curves to stay within a similar range.

Determination of the MIQ Values

MIQ values are the lowest concentration of a chemical compound that inhibits the visible growth of a microorganism after incubation [26]. In the present bioautography assay, the MIC values were determined from a series of dilution of samples, similar to a classical microdilution assay. The inhibition zones were observed as yellowish or clear areas against a red background on the plates. The lowest quantity of a compound that inhibited the growth of bacterial strain was considered as the MIQ value. On the basis of the obtained peak areas and known concentrations of active components in the total extract, the MIQ values were calculated for each active compound and each strain. Furthermore, to express the antimicrobial potential of metabolites relative to known reference standards, their antimicrobial potential was expressed in vancomycin equivalents, in respect to the prepared calibration curve equations for each bacterial strain.

To confirm the accuracy of TLC bioautography-based methodology the antimicrobial potential was also assessed for one of the active antimicrobial metabolites—curcumin, which was isolated by the authors by using centrifugal partition chromatography (see Table 4) and tested by the microdilution method according to the previously described methodology [27].

3.7. Image Processing

ImageJ—an image processing program—was used for the measurement of the area of inhibition zones to define the antimicrobial potential of single metabolites in the total extract (to determine their MIQ values and vancomycin equivalents) [28].

After 24 hours of incubation of TLC plates with the bacterial strain, the developed TLC plates were photographed by Canon Power Shot G5 camera. The obtained photos in the JPG format were processed by free, open source image processing software—ImageJ program 1.48 v—to quantitatively determine the MIQ values of all active constituents.

First, all documented photos were modified according to the procedure described by Olech et al. [20]. The images were converted into 8-bit type pictures, as initially they contained white or yellowish spots of active components against a red background, which would interfere with proper area quantitation. After this transformation, the spots were read as white against a dark gray background. Later the median filter was set at 5 pixels and the FFT Bandpass filter for large structures—was moved down to 40 pixels. To prepare an outline of the track, a "rectangular selection tool" parameter was selected, and the profile lines were then generated with the "plot lines" option. Thus, videoscan images were converted into chromatograms. Then, a "straight line selection tool" was applied to draw the baseline and the "wand tool" was used to determine the peak areas. The peaks of active metabolites were recorded as negative signals to the track's baseline (see Figure 1.).

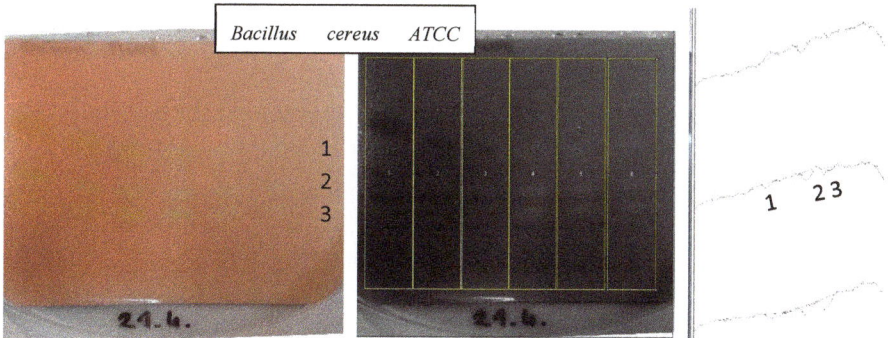

Figure 1. Determination of peak areas of active metabolites visualized by TLC bioautography. The example shows the TLC plate with MeOH extract of turmeric, covered with *B. cereus* ATCC 10876 strain, which was developed on NP silica gel TLC plates by using MeOH: DCM (0.5:99.5 v/v) as the mobile phase. The picture on the right shows the obtained densitometric data from the program.

3.8. Quantitative and Qualitative Analysis of the Samples by Mass Spectrometry

All obtained extracts and purified compounds were analyzed by the LC-ESI-Q-TOF-MS spectrometer from Agilent Technologies (see Section 2.1) in both positive and negative ionization modes. The analyses were performed on a Zorbax RP 18 (150 × 2.1 mm, d_p = 3.5 µm) chromatographic column using the following gradient of acetonitrile with 0.1% formic acid (FA) (solvent B) and 0.1% aqueous FA (solvent A): t = 0 min: 30% B, t = 20 min: 45% B, t = 20.1 min: 70% B, and t = 30 min: 60% B. The injection volume was 10 µL per sample, the flow rate: 0.2 mL/min and the post run was set at 5 min. Other operation parameters are listed below: drying gas flow: 12 L/min, nebulizer voltage: 35 psi, fragmentor voltage: 150 V, skimmer voltage: 65 V, capillary and vaporizer temperatures: 350 °C each, capillary voltage: 3.5 kV, the wavelength range of PDA detector: 190–500 nm. All spectra were recorded in both ionization modes in the mass range of 40–1000 m/z. The MS/MS spectra were automatically recorded for two the most intensive *m/z* signals in two CID energies: 10 and 20 V, which were later excluded for the following 0.3 min from fragmentation. The identification of metabolites was based on the retention times, fragmentation patterns, and scientific literature.

Additionally, a TLC-LC-ESI-TOF-MS (see Section 2.1) analysis was conducted on the developed TLC plates without derivatization (one TLC for each extract at different concentrations) to identify the spots responsible for the antimicrobial activity in the tested extracts and to check their purity. For the sake of quantitative estimations, the peak areas of the eventually occurring impurities were later subtracted from the total peak area of each active spot. That is why, the chromatograms were obtained in triplicate.

For this purpose, a simple gradient method was applied on a short chromatographic column. The spots of interest not covered with medium and/or bacteria, were collected by a TLC-MS interface (Camag, Muttenz, Switzerland) and the identification of each spot was performed by analyzing their MS spectra. The impurities were not visible in the chromatograms thanks to the mounting of a short chromatographic column (see Section 2.1) before the detectors. The following conditions of LC-MS operation were applied: gas temperature—350 °C, gas flow—10 L/min, *m/z* range—100–1500, nebulizer pressure—30 psi, capillary voltage—3500 V, fragmentor voltage—150 V, skimmer—65 V. The applied gradient of solvents (A—0.1% formic acid, and B—0.1% of formic acid in acetonitrile) was composed of the following steps: 0 min—35% B, 2 min—95% B, 3 min—95% B, 3.1 min—35% B. The run length was set at 10 min, the flow rate at 0.2 mL/ min, and the injection time at 3 sec.

3.9. Application of CPC Chromatography in the Isolation of Active Components of Turmeric Extract

To assess the accuracy of TLC-based bioautographic antimicrobial tests, the authors used previously reported separation conditions [22] to obtain pure curcumin and study its antimicrobial potential in a standard microdilution antimicrobial assay. These results were compared with those theoretically calculated using the imaging program.

Curcumin purification was performed using a centrifugal partition chromatograph SCPC-250-L from Armen (Saint-Ave, France), according to the method previously published by the authors [15]. The biphasic solvent system used in the separation process contained a mixture of heptane-chloroform-methanol-water (5:6:3:2) ($v/v/v/v$) and was prepared according to the calculations of partition coefficient values of all major peaks present in the chromatograms of the total extract. The following experimental conditions were applied: rotation speed: 1200 rpm, UV detection: 425 nm and 290 nm, flow rate: 6 mL/min, injection volume: 6 mL, mode of operation: ascending. The purification of active metabolites from turmeric was performed using 1.0 g of dried turmeric methanol extract dissolved in 3 mL of upper and 3 mL of lower phases. The mobile phase was the lighter, upper layer of the solvent system and the stationary phase was the heavier, lower layer. The fractions containing pure curcuminoids were combined together, evaporated to dryness on a rotary evaporator at 45 °C, analyzed for their purity by LC-ESI-Q-TOF-MS, and subjected to the antimicrobial assay.

Supplementary Materials: The following are available online at http://www.mdpi.com/1422-0067/20/4/898/s1: Figure S1 Purity of curcumin isolated by the centrifugal partition chromatography, Figure S2 EIC chromatograms of identified compounds present in the studied extracts of turmeric, Figure S3. Fragmentation patterns of curcuminoids isolated by centrifugal partition chromatography recorded in the CID collision energy of 20 V, Table S1. The identification of active zones on the TLC chromatograms by a TLC-MS interface coupled with a mass spectrometer.

Author Contributions: W.K.-K., A.G., L.C., A.M., and Z.M. conceived and designed the experiments; L.C., A.G., and W.K.-K. performed the experiments; L.C., A.G., W.K.-K., and B.A. analyzed the data; W.K.-K., A.M., Z.M., and B.A. contributed materials and equipment; L.C., A.G., and W.K.-K. wrote the manuscript in consultation with all co-authors. All authors accepted the final version of the manuscript.

Acknowledgments: The study was supported by the Sonata project no 2015/17/D/NZ7/00822 from the National Science Center, Poland.

Conflicts of Interest: The authors declare no conflict of interest. The founding sponsors had no role in the design of the study; in the collection, analyses, or interpretation of data; in the writing of the manuscript, or in the decision to publish the results.

References

1. Gupta, P.D.; Birdi, T.J. Development of botanicals to combat antibiotic resistance. *J. Ayurveda Integr. Med.* **2017**, *8*, 266–275. [CrossRef] [PubMed]
2. Chattopadhyay, I.; Biswas, K.; Bandyopadhyay, U.; Banerjee, R.K. Turmeric and curcumin: Biological actions and medicinal applications. *Curr. Sci.* **2004**, *87*, 44–53.
3. Anand, P.; Kunnumakkara, A.B.; Newman, R.A.; Aggarwal, B.B. Bioavailability of curcumin: Problems and promises. *Mol. Pharm.* **2007**, *4*, 807–818. [CrossRef] [PubMed]
4. Amalraja, A.; Pius, A.; Gopi, S.; Gopi, S. Biological activities of curcuminoids, other biomolecules from turmeric and their derivatives—A review. *J. Tradit. Complement Med.* **2017**, *7*, 205–233. [CrossRef] [PubMed]
5. Ruby, A.J.; Kuttan, G.; Babu, K.G.; Rajasekharan, K.N.; Kuttan, R. Anti-tumour and antioxidant activity of natural curcuminoids. *Cancer Lett.* **1995**, *94*, 79–83. [CrossRef]
6. Suvarna, R.; Bhat, S.S.; Hegde, K.H. Antibacterial Activity of Turmeric against Enterococcus faecalis An In vitro Study. *Int. J. Curr. Microbiol. App. Sci.* **2014**, *3*, 498–504.
7. Mohammed, N.A.; Habil, N.Y. Evaluation of antimicrobial activity of Curcumin against two oral bacteria. *Autom. Control Intell. Syst.* **2015**, *3*, 18–21.
8. Moghadamtousi, S.Z.; Kadir, H.A.; Hassandarvish, P.; Tajik, H.; Abubakar, S.; Zandi, K. A Review on Antibacterial, Antiviral, and Antifungal Activity of Curcumin. *BioMed Res. Int.* **2014**, *2014*, 186864. [CrossRef]
9. Guptaa, A.; Mahajana, S.; Sharmab, R. Evaluation of antimicrobial activity of *Curcuma longa* rhizome extract against *Staphylococcus aureus*. *Biotechnol. Rep.* **2015**, *6*, 51–55. [CrossRef]

10. Naz, S.; Jabeen, S.; Ilyas, S.; Manzoor, F.; Pak, J. Antibacterial activity of *Curcuma longa* varieties against different strains of bacteria. *Pakistan J. of Bot.* **2010**, *42*, 455–462.
11. Gul, P.; Bakht, J. Antimicrobial activity of turmeric extract and its potential use in food industry. *J. Food Sci. Technol.* **2015**, *52*, 2272–2279. [CrossRef]
12. Negi, P.S.; Jayaprakasha, G.K.; Rao, L.J.M.; Sakariah, K.K. Antibacterial Activity of Turmeric Oil: A Byproduct from Curcumin Manufacture. *J. Agric. Food Chem.* **1999**, *47*, 4297–4300. [CrossRef] [PubMed]
13. Apisariyakul, A.; Vanittanakom, N.; Buddhasukh, D. Antifungal activity of turmeric oil extracted from *Curcuma longa* (Zingiberaceae). *J. Ethnopharmacol.* **1995**, *49*, 163–169. [CrossRef]
14. Singh, R.; Chandra, R.; Bose, M.; Luthra, P.M. Antibacterial activity of *Curcuma longa* rhizome extract on pathogenic bacteria. *Curr. Sci.* **2002**, *83*, 737–740.
15. Dosoky, N.S.; Setzer, W.N. Chemical Composition and Biological Activities of Essential Oils of *Curcuma* Species. *Nutrients* **2018**, *10*, 1196. [CrossRef] [PubMed]
16. Vaughn, A.R.; Haas, K.N.; Burney, W.; Andersen, E.; Clark, A.K.; Crawford, R.; Sivamani, R.K. Potential Role of Curcumin Against Biofilm-Producing Organisms on the Skin: A Review. *Phytother. Res.* **2017**, *31*, 1807–1816. [CrossRef] [PubMed]
17. Neelakantan, P.; Subbarao, C.; Sharma, S.; Subbarao, C.V.; Garcia-Godoy, F.; Gutmann, J.L. Effectiveness of curcumin against Enterococcus faecalis biofilm. *Acta Odontol. Scand.* **2013**, *71*, 1453–1457. [CrossRef]
18. Seo, M.J.; Park, J.E.; Jang, M.S. Optimization of sponge cake added with turmeric (Curcuma longa L.) powder using mixture design. *Food Sci. Biotechnol* **2010**, *19*, 617–625. [CrossRef]
19. Péret-Almeida, L.; Naghetini, C.C.; de Aguiar Nunan, E.; Junqueira, R.G.; Glória, M.B.A. In vitro antimicrobial activity of the ground rhizome, curcuminoid pigments and essential oil of *Curcuma longa* L. *Ciêne. Agrotec* **2008**, *32*, 875–881.
20. Jayaprakasha, G.K.; Jagan Mohan Rao, L.; Sakariah, K.K. Improved HPLC Method for the Determination of Curcumin, Demethoxycurcumin, and Bisdemethoxycurcumin. *J. Agric. Food Chem.* **2002**, *50*, 3668–3672. [CrossRef]
21. Jiang, H.; Timmermann, B.N.; Gang, D.R. Use of liquid chromatography-electrospray ionization tandem mass spectrometry to identify diarylheptanoids in turmeric (*Curcuma longa* L.) rhizome. *J. Chromatogr. A* **2006**, *7*, 21–31. [CrossRef] [PubMed]
22. Kukuła-Koch, W.; Grabarska, A.; Łuszczki, J.; Czernicka, L.; Nowosadzka, E.; Gumbarewicz, E.; Jarząb, A.; Audo, G.; Upadhyay, S.; Głowniak, K.; et al. Superior anticancer activity is demonstrated by total extract of *Curcuma longa* L. as opposed to individual curcuminoids separated by centrifugal partition chromatography. *Phytother. Res.* **2018**, *32*, 933–942. [CrossRef] [PubMed]
23. Paneth, A.; Frączek, T.; Grzegorczyk, A.; Janowska, D.; Malm, A.; Paneth, P. A search for dual action HIV-1 reverse transcriptase, bacterial RNA polymerase inhibitors. *Molecules* **2017**, *22*, 1808. [CrossRef] [PubMed]
24. Isnard, C.; Dhalluin, A.; Malandain, D.; Bruey, Q.; Auzou, M.; Michon, J.; Giard, J.C.; Guérin, F.; Cattoir, V. In vitro activity of novel anti-MRSA cephalosporins and comparator antimicrobial agents against staphylococci involved in prosthetic joint infections. *J. Glob. Antimicrob. Resist.* **2018**, *13*, 221–225. [CrossRef] [PubMed]
25. Sá, S.; Chaul, L.T.; Alves, V.F.; Fiuza, T.S.; Tresvenzol, L.M.F.; Vaz, B.G.; Ferri, P.H.; Borges, L.L.; Paula, J.R. Phytochemistry and antimicrobial activity of *Campomanesia adamantium*. *Braz. J. Pharmacogn.* **2018**, *28*, 303–311. [CrossRef]
26. Andrews, J.M. Determination of minimum inhibitory concentrations. *J. Antimicrob. Chemother.* **2001**, *48*, 5–16. [CrossRef] [PubMed]
27. Skalicka-Woźniak, K.; Grzegorczyk, A.; Świątek, Ł.; Walasek, M.; Widelski, J.; Rajtar, B.; Polz-Dacewicz, M.; Malm, A.; Elansary, H.O. Biological activity and safety profile of the essential oil from fruits of *Heracleum mantegazzianum* Sommier & Levier (Apiaceae). *Food Chem. Toxicol.* **2017**, *109*, 820–826.
28. Olech, M.; Komsta, Ł.; Nowak, R.; Cieśla, Ł.; Waksmundzka-Hajnos, M. Investigation of antiradical activity of plant material by thin-layer chromatography with image processing. *Food Chem.* **2012**, *132*, 549–553. [CrossRef]

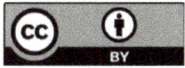

© 2019 by the authors. Licensee MDPI, Basel, Switzerland. This article is an open access article distributed under the terms and conditions of the Creative Commons Attribution (CC BY) license (http://creativecommons.org/licenses/by/4.0/).

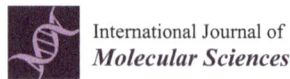

Article

Curcumin-Loaded Mesoporous Silica Nanoparticles Markedly Enhanced Cytotoxicity in Hepatocellular Carcinoma Cells

Zwe-Ling Kong *, Hsiang-Ping Kuo, Athira Johnson, Li-Cyuan Wu and Ke Liang B. Chang

Department of Food Science, National Taiwan Ocean University, Keelung 20224, Taiwan; williamkuococo@hotmail.com (H.-P.K.); athirajohnson07@gmail.com (A.J.); ninec9@hotmail.com (L.-C.W.); klchang@mail.ntou.edu.tw (K.L.B.C.)
* Correspondence: kongzl@mail.ntou.edu.tw; Tel.: +886-2-2462-2192; Fax: +886-2-2463-4203

Received: 3 May 2019; Accepted: 13 June 2019; Published: 14 June 2019

Abstract: Curcumin, a natural polyphenol extracted from a perennial herb *Curcuma longa* has been verified for many physiological activities such as anti-oxidant, anti-inflammatory, and anti-tumor properties. The direct use of curcumin cytotoxicity studies are limited due to its unstable chemical structure, low bioavailability, easy oxidation, and degradation by ultraviolet (UV) light etc. Trying to overcome this problem, silica-encapsulated curcumin nanoparticles (SCNP) and chitosan with silica co-encapsulated curcumin nanoparticles (CSCNP) were prepared by silicification and biosilicification methods, respectively, and encapsulated curcumin within it. We investigated the antitumor properties of SCNP and CSCNP on different tumor cell lines. Scanning electron microscopy (SEM) analysis revealed that both SCNP and CSCNP were almost spherical in shape and the average particle size of CSCNP was 75.0 ± 14.62 nm, and SCNP was 61.7 ± 23.04 nm. The results show that CSCNP has more anti-oxidant activity as compared to curcumin and SCNP. The higher cytotoxicity towards different cancerous cell lines was also observed in CSCNP treated tumor cells. It was noted that the SCNP and CSCNP has a high percentage of IC_{50} values in Hep G2 cells. The encapsulation of curcumin improved instability, antioxidant activity, and antitumor activity. Our results demonstrated that nanoencapsulation of curcumin with silica and chitosan not only increase curcumin stability but also enhance its cytotoxic activity on hepatocellular carcinoma cells. On the basis of these primary studies, the curcumin-loaded nanoparticles appear to be promising as an innovative therapeutic material for the treatment of tumors.

Keywords: curcumin; silica; chitosan; nanoparticles; anti-tumor; antioxidant activity

1. Introduction

Cancer is the second leading cause of mortality in the world and approximately 1,665,540 people in the United States suffered from cancer by 2014 [1]. A tumor (neoplasm) is an uncontrolled growth of cells and becomes less responsive to normal growth control. Invasion and metastasis are the major features of a tumor and is categorized into benign and malignant tumors. Benign tumors are non-cancerous and they will not spread to other areas. Malignant tumors are cancerous and can spread to other tissues (metastasis) via the bloodstream and lymph nodes [2]. Tumors may occur in any part of the body including the skin, lungs, bone, intestines, and breast etc. Uncontrolled proliferation, induction of angiogenesis, active invasion, metastasis, immortality, and evasion of growth suppressors are the major traits of cancerous cells [3]. Apoptosis is an ordered cell death mechanism involving many complex pathways. It is a key mechanism to eliminate damaged cells and control cell proliferation. The processes of apoptosis involve the shrinkage of cells, chromatin condensation, membrane blebbing, and deoxyribonucleic acid (DNA) fragmentation [4,5]. The resistance of tumor cells occurs due to the defective apoptosis signaling pathway by mutation [4]. During initiation, the oncogene is activated and the processes of oncogenesis leads to the formation of cancerous cells. In most cases, tumors are associated with *p53* gene mutation and it became known as the first tumor suppressor gene linked to apoptosis [6]. The primary trial of each chemotherapeutic drug is based on its potential cytotoxicity towards the cancer cell lines. A decrease in cell numbers over time is an important requirement for an in vitro cytotoxicity assessment [7]. Currently, the antitumor drug designs are based on their selective targeting towards tumor cells. This will be achieved by caspase activation, phosphatidylserine exposure, and poly (ADP-ribose) polymerase (PARP) cleavage [8]. The conventional treatments such as radiation and chemotherapy have not been widely recommended because of their side effects.

The emergence of nanotechnology has changed the conventional concepts and ideas of the pharmaceutical fields. Mesoporous silica nanoparticles (MSNs) were first introduced by Mobil corporation scientists in 1992. They have a unique mesoporous structure with high chemical stability, low toxicity, high drug loading capacity, controlled release, biocompatibility, high surface area, target delivery, large pore volume, and surface functionality [9]. The passive target of nanoparticles in cancer therapies is achieved because of the enhanced permeability and retention (EPR) effect of the cancerous cells. The impaired lymphatic system and defective vascular architecture allow the nanoparticles to enter into the cancerous cells. The MSNs are internalized into the cells via phagocytosis and pinocytosis [10]. Polypeptides and polysaccharides are responsible for the formation of biosilica via the repeated phase-separation mediated templating mechanism and the aggregation-based mechanism. Chitosan is a cationic polysaccharide having a terminal amino group has been proven to facilitate silicification through catalyzing the hydrolysis/condensation of the silica source and the subsequent aggregation of silica [11]. A recent study shown a targeted delivery of calcium leucovorin galactosylated chitosan-functionalized mesoporous silica nanoparticle to treat colon cancer. The surface of the MSNs contains a large number silanol groups, which allow easy functionalization, controlled drug release, and drug loading [12]. Chitosan is obtained from the deacetylation of chitin. It is composed of β-(1,4)-linked glucosamine units (2-amino-2-deoxy-β-d-glucopyranose) and N-acetylglucosamine units (2-acetamido-2-deoxy-β-d-glucopyranose) in different ratios [13]. The amino group on chitosan provide controlled release, permeation enhancement, mucoadhesion, in situ gelation etc. [14]. p^H responsive delivery of curcumin from chitosan mesoporous silica nanoparticles were reported by Nasab et al., 2018 [15]. Cytotoxicity assays revealed IC_{50} after 72 h treatment with free curcumin and curcumin-loaded nanoparticles on U87MG glioblastoma cancer cell line were 15.20 and 5.21 µg/mL ($p < 0.05$). respectively [15].

Curcumin (1, 7-bis (4-hydroxy-3-methoxyphenyl)-1, 6-heptadiene-3, 5-dione) is a yellow colored polyphenol obtained from turmeric (*Curcuma longa*) that has been known for thousands of years for its pharmacological activities [16]. It has a wide spectrum of therapeutic activities including anti-inflammatory, antioxidant, antitumor, antiviral, antimicrobial, and analgesic effects etc. It is insoluble in water but soluble in ethanol and acetone. The anti-inflammatory property of curcumin is carried out by blocking the IκK-mediated phosphorylation and degradation of IκBα. As a consequence, the nuclear factor (NF)-κB will bind to the IκBα and does not induce transcription [17]. The growth, invasion, and metastasis of the cancerous cells can be prevented by curcumin via interfering with their proliferation process [18]. Curcumin scavenges superoxide, nitric oxide, and hydrogen peroxide radicals and reduces the inflammation by lowering the histamine levels and produce an inflammatory response to cytokines [19]. Curcumin also induces apoptosis through the inhibition of cyclooxygenase (COX)–2 and affects various growth factor receptors and molecules involved in tumor growth, angiogenesis, and metastasis [20]. It was understood that curcumin causes cell cycle arrest at the G0/G1 phase and S and G2/M phases in leukemic cells and breast cancer cells respectively [21]. Apart from this, curcumin moderates transcription factors downregulates cytokines and inhibits the activity of c- Jun N-terminal kinase, protein tyrosine kinases and protein serine/threonine kinases of a wide variety of tumor cells and cancer stem cells [22]. The mode of action of curcumin is different in each type of cells. A recent study showed that miR-21/PTEN/Akt signaling pathway is the key mechanism of the anti-cancer effects of curcumin on breast cancer cells [23]. Reduction in vascular endothelial growth factor (VEGF) expression and PI3K/AKT signaling were noticed in hepatocellular carcinoma model [24]. Curcumin inhibited zeste homolog 2 (EZH2) in lung cancer cells both transcriptionally and post-transcriptionally, thereby decreasing the expression of NOTCH1 [25]. The process of nanoencapsulation enhances the site-specific activity and optimizes the therapeutic efficacy of curcumin [26]. Recent study showed that the curcumin-loaded nanoliposomes (Cur-NLs) protected the tetrachloromethane- (CCl$_4^-$) induced liver injury in mice. Cur-NLs attenuated the hepatic necrosis and decreased the malonaldehyde (MDA) level [27]. Another study demonstrated the inhibition of the growth and *hTERT* gene expression in human breast cancer cells by nano-encapsulated metformin-curcumin in poly (lactic-co-glycolic acid)/polyethylene glycol (PLGA/PEG) [28]. 5-flurouracil and curcumin loaded N,O-carboxymethyl chitosan nanoparticles 4 showed a sustained release and enhanced anti-cancer effects both in vitro and in vivo [29]. Song et al., 2018 [30] reported the high uptake efficiency, toxicity, and sustained release in human Caucasian breast adenocarcinoma cells (MDA-MB-231). It supported the dose-depended delivery of curcumin on cancer cells [30]. Higher toxicity of PEGylated curcumin nanoparticles (IC$_{50}$ = 4.2 µM) than the free curcumin at all doses were observed in CT-26 cells with an 8-fold decrease in the half-maximal inhibitory concentration (IC$_{50}$) values of the free Cur (IC$_{50}$ = 33.4 µM) after 24 h [31]. There is a significant difference between curcumin and nanocucumin effects on growth depression of on human breast adenocarcinoma cell line (MDA-MB231) ($p < 0.01$). The IC$_{50}$ curcumin after 24 h, 48 h and 72 was 79.58 µg/mL and 53.18 µg/mL and 30.78 µg/mL whereas this value for nanocurcumin was 37.75 µg/mL and 23.25 µg/h and 12.99 µg/mL, respectively ($p < 0.01$) [32]. A decreased proliferation of esophageal squamous cell carcinoma (KYSE-30) cells was observed after treatment with nanocurcumin (71.09%) without affecting the normal cells. In addition to this, it down-regulated the expression of cyclin D1 [33]. In vitro models of the toxicity studies have diverse application in the selection of cancerous cells and tumor microenvironments. The cancer cells grow easily and facilitate the direct comparison between the results under in vitro conditions [34]. The direct use of curcumin is limited due to its low water solubility, poor chemical stability, and low oral bioavailability [35]. Along with this, research based on the cytotoxicity of curcumin in various cancer cells are still rare. The present study examined the cytotoxic effect of curcumin- loaded mesoporous silica nanoparticles (MSNs) on different tumor cell lines together with an examination of curcumin parameters after storage.

2. Results

2.1. Characterization of Silica-Encapsulated Curcumin Nanoparticles (SCNP) and Chitosan with Silica Co-Encapsulated Curcumin Nanoparticles (CSCNP)

Silica-encapsulated curcumin nanoparticles (SCNP) and chitosan with silica co-encapsulated curcumin nanoparticles (CSCNP) were prepared by silicification and biosilicification methods respectively. The nanoparticles were characterized by scanning electron microscopy (SEM) and the dynamic light scattering (DLS) method. From SEM images, CSCNP were relatively spherical in shape with uniform size distributions as compared to SCNP (Figure 1). The average size of CSCNP was 75.0 ± 14.62 nm and SCNP was 61.7 ± 23. 04 nm. The sizes of nanoparticles were also confirmed by DLS analysis. The average particle sizes of SCNP and CSCNP were 111.0 ± 2.95 nm and 112.8 ± 3.00 nm, respectively (Table 1). The difference in the particle sizes between SEM and DLS was due to the dryness of the particle during SEM sample preparation. Nanoparticle-based drug carrier system increase the bioavailability of the drug in the targeted site. Literature showed that a particle between the size of 100 to 1000 nm can enter into the cancer cells instead of normal cells because of the EPR effect [36].

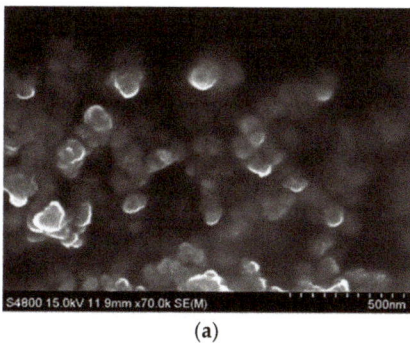 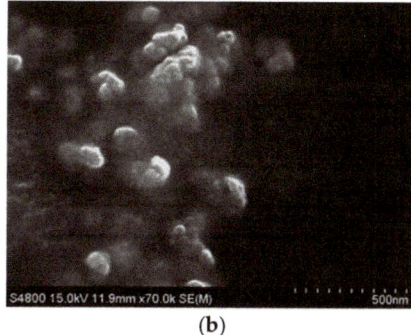

Figure 1. Scanning electron microscope (SEM) images of (**a**) CSCNP and (**b**) SCNP. SCNP: silica-encapsulated curcumin nanoparticles; CSCNP: chitosan with silica co-encapsulated curcumin nanoparticles.

Table 1. Particle sizes analyzed by SEM and DLS.

	CSCNP	SCNP
SEM	75.0 ± 14.62	61.8 ± 23.04
DLS	112.88 ± 3.00	111.05 ± 2.95

Data were shown by mean ± SD of 3 independent experiments ($n = 3$) with 3 technical replicates. SEM: scanning electron microscopy; DLS: dynamic light scattering; SCNP: silica-encapsulated curcumin nanoparticles; CSCNP: chitosan and silica co-encapsulated curcumin nanoparticles.

2.2. Antioxidant Activities of SCNP and CSCNP

The imbalance between the production of reactive oxygen species (ROS) and antioxidants generates oxidative stress within the cells. Under stress conditions, the cell structure is damaged and cell functions are altered. [37]. The antioxidant activities of SCNP and CSCNP were evaluated by 2, 2-diphenyl-1-picrylhydrazyl (DPPH) radical scavenging activity (Figure 2a) and ferrous ion chelating activity (Figure 2b). The DPPH radical scavenging activity increased with increasing concentrations of curcumin and nanoparticles. As compared to pure curcumin and SCNP, the CSCNP showed slightly better activity towards the DPPH radical scavenging and the half maximal effective concentration (EC_{50}) of curcumin, CSCNP and SCNP were 59 µg/mL, 32 µg/mL and 44 µg/mL, respectively (Figure 2a). Interestingly, curcumin has no ferrous ion chelating activity but both SCNP and CSCNP exhibited better activity at higher concentration (Figure 2b). Noting that curcumin itself does not have the property to chelate ferrous ion and CSCNP has better activity than SCNP indicated the involvement of chitosan in chelating ferrous ions. A previous study reported that the stimulation of ROS production is also a pro-apoptotic action of curcumin to induce cell death [38]. These results suggest that curcumin nanoparticles might also influence the ROS levels through free radicals scavenging or ferrous iron chelation. The increased antioxidant of nanoencapsulated curcumin (scavenging capacity, $SC_{50} = 13.9$ µg/mL) than free curcumin ($SC_{50} = 16.7$ µg/mL) by DPPH radical scavenging activity were reported by Huang et al., 2016 with the differences statistically significant at $p < 0.05$ [39].

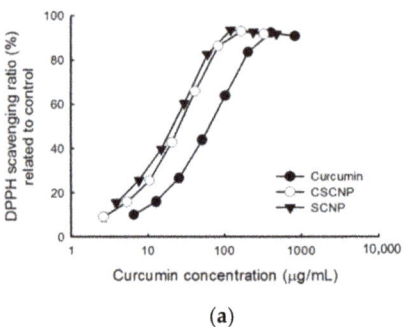
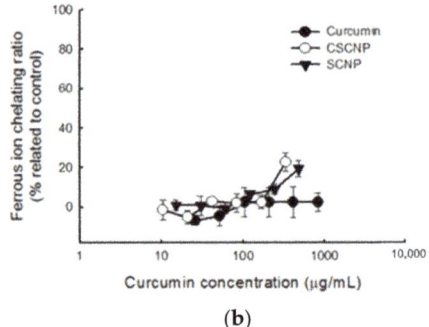

(a) (b)

Figure 2. Antioxidant activities of curcumin, SCNP, and CSCNP. (**a**) DPPH scavenging activity and (**b**) ferrous ion chelating activity of curcumin, SCNP and CSCNP. Data were shown by mean ± standard deviation (SD) of 3 independent experiments ($n = 3$) with 3 technical replicates. DPPH: 2, 2-diphenyl-1-picrylhydrazyl; SCNP: silica-encapsulated curcumin nanoparticles; CSCNP: chitosan with silica co-encapsulated curcumin nanoparticles.

2.3. Cytotoxicity of SCNP and CSCNP

Tumor cells are characterized by the uncontrolled proliferation of cells [40]. Regulations of the differentiation of cells are needed to control tumor growth. The non-toxicity of curcumin on normal cells where described elsewhere [41,42]. The cytotoxicy of curcumin (Figure 3a), SCNP (Figure 3c) and CSCNP (Figure 3b) were examined by performing the 3-(4,5-dimethylthiazol-2-yl)-2,5-diphenyltetrazolium bromide (MTT) assay against seven types of tumor cell lines. Figure 3a indicated that curcumin has significant toxicity towards the cancerous cells and the cell viabilities of each cell were decreased with the increase in concentrations. The similar results were also observed in SCNP and CSCNP treated cells. It was noticed that human cervical squamous carcinoma cell line HeLa was more sensitive to curcumin, SCNP and CSCNP. The human breast carcinoma cell line MCF-7 and the human gastric adenocarcinoma cell line MKN-28 were more tolerant towards curcumin and nanoparticles. The comparison of the IC_{50} value of each sample was listed in Table 2. IC_{50} values of CSCNP were lower than that of the curcumin and SCNP. It was also noted that the most significant difference between the percentage of IC_{50} values of curcumin and nanoparticles was observed in Hep G2 cells. About 49% (CSCNP) and 54% (SCNP) in IC_{50} value in Hep G2 cells indicated that both CSCNP and SCNP were more toxic to HepG2 cells than free curcumin. Consequently, further analyses were carried out using Hep G2 cells. A previous study reported the increased bioavailability of curcumin after encapsulation and both free and nanoencapsulated curcumin suppress COX-2 and VEGF expression and thereby reduced the proliferation of hepatocellular carcinoma cells [43]. It was also noted that curcumin cause toxicity via disturbing the cell homeostasis and affect cell function including intracellular free Ca^{2+} concentration and mitochondrial membrane potential in HepG2 cells [44].

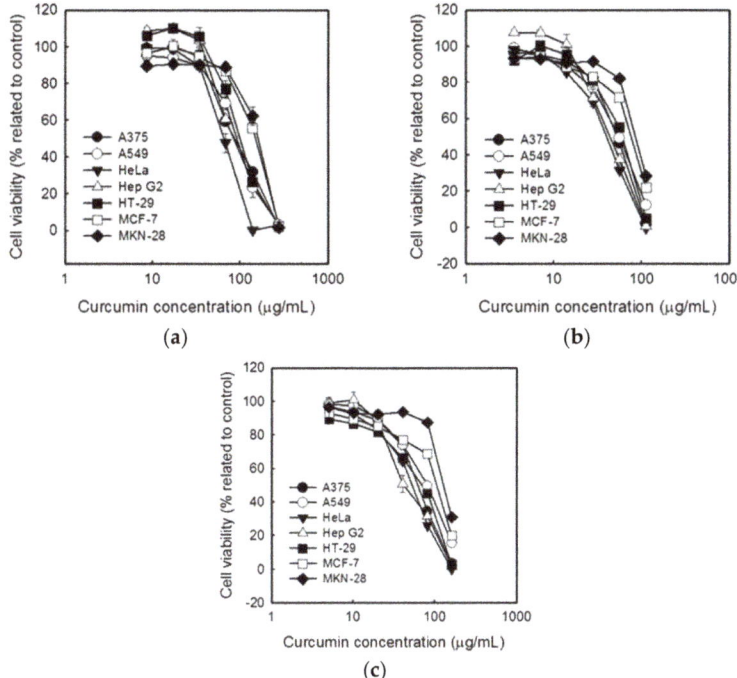

Figure 3. Effects of (**a**) curcumin, (**b**) CSCNP, and (**c**) SCNP on cancer cell viability. The cell number for 7 kinds of cells were adjusted to 2×10^5 cells/mL and treated with different concentrations of samples for 48 h. The cell viability was analyzed by MTT assay. Data were shown by mean ± SD of 3 independent experiments ($n = 3$) with 3 technical replicates. SCNP: silica-encapsulated curcumin nanoparticles; CSCNP: chitosan with silica co-encapsulated curcumin nanoparticles.

Table 2. Comparisons of IC_{50} (μg/mL) of curcumin, SCNP, and CSCNP toward seven cancer cell lines.

Cell line	Curcumin	CSCNP	Difference [a]	SCNP	Difference [b]
A375	93 ± 3	53 ± 1	43%	65 ± 1	30%
A549	98 ± 0	56 ± 4	43%	81 ± 2	17%
HeLa	68 ± 4	42 ± 0	38%	56 ± 1	18%
Hep G2	90 ± 2	46 ± 3	49%	41 ± 10	54%
HT-29	106 ± 2	62 ± 0	42%	72 ± 3	32%
MCF-7	153 ± 7	80 ± 0	48%	112 ± 1	27%
MKN-28	166 ± 9	89 ± 1	46%	135 ± 1	19%

Differences were shown as the percentage decrease in IC_{50} after nanoencapsulation. SCNP: silica-encapsulated curcumin nanoparticles; CSCNP: chitosan with silica co-encapsulated curcumin nanoparticles. Difference [a] and difference [b] were calculated by the following formulas: Difference [a] = 100 − (CSCNP IC_{50}/Curcumin IC_{50}) × 100; Difference [b] = 100 − (SCNP IC50/Curcumin IC_{50}) × 100.

2.4. Cytotoxicity of SCNP and CSCNP against Hep G2 Cells

Cytotoxicity of curcumin, SCNP, and CSCNP against Hep G2 cells were evaluated by 1-(4,5-Dimethylthiazol-2-yl)-3,5-diphenylformazan (MTT) assay. From Figure 4a, it was understood that the cell viability of Hep G2 cells dropped gradually after the cells were treated with curcumin and nanoparticles. As compared to curcumin and SCNP, the CSCNP showed more reduction in cell viability of cancerous cells at lower concentrations. The cell viability was also analyzed in a time-dependent manner (Figure 4b). The cell viability of Hep G2 cells was significantly reduced with

CSCNP treatment when compared to other groups at different time intervals. From Figure 4, it was understood that CSCNP was more efficient in cytotoxicity of Hep G2 than curcumin and SCNP.

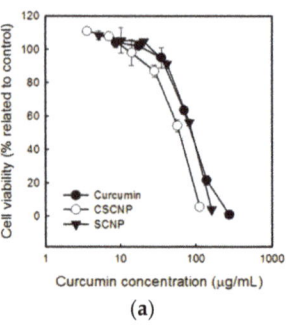 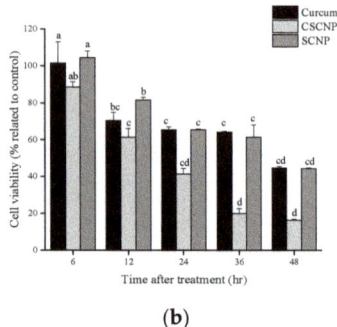

(a) (b)

Figure 4. MTT assay of Hep G2 cells after different curcumin or nanoparticle dosages and time durations. The cells were treated with samples for (**a**) 48 h at different dosages and (**b**) 100 µg/mL at different time intervals. The initial cell number was adjusted to 2×10^5 cells/mL. Data were shown by mean ± SD of 3 independent experiments ($n = 3$) with 3 technical replicates. SCNP: silica-encapsulated curcumin nanoparticles; CSCNP: chitosan with silica co-encapsulated curcumin nanoparticles.

2.5. Lactate Dehydrogenase (LDH) Leakage Assay

A higher concentration of lactate dehydrogenase LDH is present in tumor cells. The cytotoxicity of drugs was determined by evaluating the amount of LDH released from the damaged tumor cells [45]. DNA fragmentation is also associated with apoptosis during cancer therapy [46]. An LDH leakage assay was performed to analyze the cytotoxicity of curcumin and curcumin nanoparticles against Hep G2 cells. Figure 5a shows that all samples increased the percentage of LDH leakage at a concentration between approximately 70~80 µg/mL. The cytotoxicity of each sample increased with longer duration. A significant increase was observed in CSCNP treated cells at a lower curcumin concentration. In addition, more than 50% of LDH leakage was observed in CSCNP treated groups. This result supports the MTT assay and apparently CSCNP was more cytotoxic against Hep G2 cells.

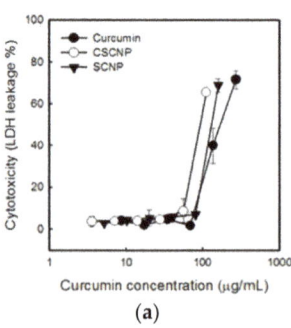 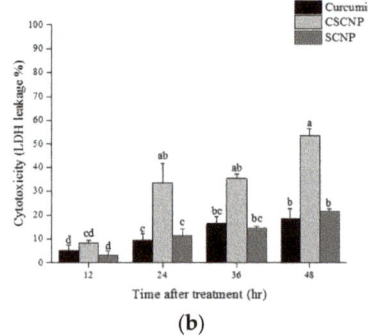

(a) (b)

Figure 5. Lactate dehydrogenase (LDH) leakage of Hep G2 after different curcumin, or nanoparticle dosages and time durations. The cells were treated with samples for (**a**) 48 h at different dosage and (**b**) 100 µg/mL at different times. The initial cell number was adjusted to 2×10^5 cells/mL. Data were shown by mean ± SD of three independent experiments ($n = 3$) with three technical replicates. LDH: lactate dehydrogenase; SCNP: silica-encapsulated curcumin nanoparticles; CSCNP: chitosan with silica co-encapsulated curcumin nanoparticles.

2.6. Storage Test

Curcumin is unstable due to its specific chemical and physical properties. The cell viability test (MTT assay) and anti-oxidation test were used to determine the stabilities of the particles. It was found that the effects of curcumin and nanoparticles on cell cytotoxicity were decreased with increasing storage time. Curcumin show a dramatic increase in the IC_{50} of the cell survival rate after 80 days of storage, while the CSCNP and SCNP only showed a slight increase. After the 80 days' storage, the efficiency defined in Table 3 of the curcumin was 28.9%, but both CSCNP and SCNP showed more than 80% of efficiency.

Table 3. Comparisons of the cell viability IC_{50} of curcumin, SCNP, and CSCNP in Hep G2 cells while stored in water for 80 days (μg/mL).

Sample Name	Storage at 0 Day	Storage after 80 Days	Efficiency [a] (%)
Curcumin	72	251	28.9
CSCNP	111	127	87.4
SCNP	140	166	84.3

[a] Formula = 1/(Storage after 80 days IC_{50}/Storage at 0 day IC_{50}) × 100. SCNP: silica-encapsulated curcumin nanoparticles; CSCNP: chitosan with silica co-encapsulated curcumin nanoparticles.

The oxidation resistance of samples after irradiated with an ultraviolet (UV) lamp was also determined. In the anti-oxidation test, the samples were simultaneously irradiated with an ultraviolet light tube (UV-C, 30 W) in an aseptic workstation (over 10 h), and followed by a DPPH radicals scavenging test. It was found that the UV-irradiated curcumin significantly reduced its antioxidant capacity (Figure 6) as compared to SCNP and CSCNP. The efficiency of both SCNP and CSCNP were higher than curcumin. The decrease in the ability of curcumin to scavenge DPPH free radicals is mainly due to the decomposition of curcumin by UV light. However, both SCNP and CSCNP showed more than 100% efficiency (Table 4)

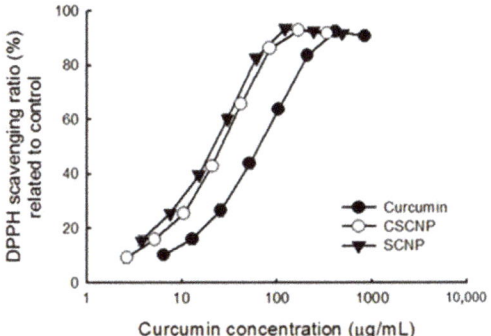

Figure 6. DPPH scavenging ability of curcumin, SCNP, and CSCNP after irradiated with an ultraviolet (UV-C) 30W lamp overnight (about 10 h). Data were shown by mean ± SD of 3 independent experiments (n = 3) with 3 technical replicates. DPPH: 2, 2-diphenyl-1-picrylhydrazyl; SCNP: silica-encapsulated curcumin nanoparticles; CSCNP: chitosan with silica co-encapsulated curcumin nanoparticles.

Table 4. Comparisons of DPPH scavenging EC$_{50}$ of curcumin, SCNP, and CSCNP while with and without UV irradiation (µg/mL).

Sample Name	Irradiated at 0 Hour	Irradiated at Overnight	Efficiency [a]
Curcumin	59	68	86.8%
CSCNP	32	28	114.3%
SCNP	44	23	191.3%

[a] Formula = 1/(Irradiated overnight EC$_{50}$/Irradiated 0-h EC$_{50}$) × 100. EC$_{50}$: half maximal effective concentration SCNP: silica-encapsulated curcumin nanoparticles; CSCNP: chitosan and silica co-encapsulated curcumin nanoparticles.

3. Discussion

Curcuma longa (turmeric) belongs to the family Zingiberaceae and has been well-known for its effect on treating inflammatory and other diseases. Curcumin (diferuloylmethane) is a less toxic polyphenol derived from *Curcuma longa* with chemical formula of (1, 7-bis (4-hydroxy-3-methoxyphenyl) -1,6-heptadiene-3,5-dione) [47]. Curcumin acts as a potent scavenger for a variety of reactive oxygen species (ROS), inhibits lipid peroxidation, and reduces oxidative cell injury etc. [48]. Previous studies showed that curcumin down-regulates cyclooxygenase-2, inhibits nuclear factor kappa B (NF-κB) expression and reduce tumor necrosis factor (TNF)-α expression. The anti-cancer effect of curcumin is achieved by the inhibition of cell cycle progression and the induction of apoptosis. It blocks the inhibition of protein tyrosine kinase and c-myc messenger ribonucleic acid (mRNA) expression. Curcumin damages the DNA and impairs the ubiquitin-proteasome system through the mitochondrial pathway and thereby promote apoptosis. Curcumin causes a rapid decrease in mitochondrial membrane potential and release of cytochrome c to activate caspase 9 and caspase 3 for apoptotic cell death [49]. MTT assay in A549 cells showed that the curcumin (CM)-loaded nanoparticles exhibited better cytotoxicity with higher number of apoptotic bodies than free CM at * $p < 0.05$. This was due to the increased intracellular uptake of nanoparticles by cells [50].

The direct use of curcumin is limited due to low water solubility, low bioavailability, chemical instability, rapid metabolization within the gastrointestinal tract (GIT), intense color, and strong flavor [35]. In order to overcome this problem, nanotechnology-based encapsulation methods are employed. Inorganic particles incorporated biomolecules exhibit improved properties of the drug. Mesoporous silica nanoparticles (MSN) have characteristics of tunable porosity and size, biocompatibility, and high surface area. The modification of MSN can control cellular uptake, drug release, and endosomal escape [51]. Chitosan is a biopolymer obtained by the deacetylation of chitin. It was shown that chitosan is able to control drug release, enhance efficiency, improves drug solubility and stability, and reduces toxicity [52]. Silica-encapsulated curcumin nanoparticles (SCNP) and chitosan with silica co-encapsulated curcumin nanoparticles (CSCNP) were prepared by silicification and biosilicification methods, respectively. Chitosan-mediated formation of biomimetic silica nanoparticles involving the hydrolysis/condensation and aggregation of silica source by the terminal amine groups of chitosan [11]. From SEM analysis, the average size of CSCNP and SCNP were 75.0 ± 14.62 nm and 61.7 ± 23. 04 nm, respectively. It was also observed that the particles were in a spherical shape (Figure 1). The particle size was confirmed by DLS analysis and the average particle sizes of SCNP and CSCNP were bigger than that analyzed with SEM (Table 1). The size variation was due to the different analysis methods. For SEM, the particles were analyzed in a dry form whereas in DLS analysis the samples were dissolved in water. The particle size was reduced in SEM due to the particle shrinkage because of the loss of moisture content. A previous study reported that the biocompatibility of silica can be improved in the presence of chitosan [53]. The small size, leaky vasculature, and EPR effect enable nanoparticle to accumulate in the body and then internalized into the cells via endocytosis [54].

DPPH radical scavenging and ferrous ion chelating activity were performed to evaluate the antioxidant activities of SCNP and CSCNP. Antioxidants reduce cell damage by decreasing the formation of reactive oxygen species (ROS) [55]. Free radical-mediated lipid peroxidation, DNA damage, and production of ROS are the key mechanisms exerted by curcumin to reduce tumor cell growth [56]. Studies showed that the ER stress, intracellular Ca^{2+}, and ROS production were increased after treatment with curcumin [57]. 2,2-diphenyl-1-picrylhydrazyl (DPPH) is a stable free radical with deep violet color. If the free radicals have been scavenged, the color will be changed to yellow. The hydrogen atom from the antioxidant reduces the odd electron of the nitrogen atom in DPPH [58]. It was understood that curcumin, SCNP, and CSCNP have DPPH radical scavenging activity and CSCNP showed slightly better activity than others (Figure 2b). The formation of free radicals by gain or loss of electrons is achieved by the transition metal ion Fe^{2+} and the reduction of ROS production by the chelation of metal ions with chelating agents [59]. Only SCNP and CSNP showed ferrous ion chelating activity at higher concentration. The better antioxidant activity of CSCNP may due to the participation of hydroxyl groups (-OH) and amino groups (NH_2) from chitosan. The donation of hydrogen or the lone pairs of electrons enables the chitosan to chelate metal ions or scavenge free radicals [60]. The increased antioxidant activity of curcumin when loaded to nanoparticles were shown by DPPH scavenging activity in the confidence interval of 99% ($p < 0.01$) [61]. The combined antioxidant activity of curcumin and chitosan were shown by Fan et al., 2017. The DPPH scavenging activity was 249 13.2 % for curcumin loaded chitosan (CS) and 43.8 % was for curcumin loaded chitosan-chlorogenic acid (CS-CA) at 10 μg/mL. It was reported that mechanism for antioxidant activities of CS is mainly due to the hydrogen-donating ability [62].

An MTT assay was carried out to analyze the cytotoxicity of curcumin, SCNP, and CSCNP towards the tumor cell lines such as human melanoma cell line A375, human lung carcinoma cell line A549, human cervical squamous carcinoma cell line HeLa, human hepatoma cell line Hep G2, human colon carcinoma cell line HT-29, human breast carcinoma cell line MCF-7, and human gastric adenocarcinoma cell line MKN-28. The MTT assay is a very useful method to determine the toxicity of chemotherapeutics to the tumor cells. The number of living cells is proportional to the amount formazan (dark blue) produced from MTT (yellow) by mitochondrial dehydrogenase enzymes in living cells. IC_{50} is a concentration of the tested drug able to cause the death of 50% of the cells. More cytotoxicity of the substance is denoted by a lower IC_{50} value [63]. The literature showed that the effect of curcumin varied from cell to cell and the cellular uptake of curcumin in cancer cells was higher than the normal cells [41]. Another important aspect is based on the level of glutathione. Studies showed that the low level of glutathione in cancer cells makes them more sensitive towards curcumin [42]. It was also noted that the high expression of NF-κB in cancerous could reduce after being treated with curcumin [41]. The good biocompatibility and biodegradation of both chitosan and silica were described elsewhere [64,65]. MSN has tunable pore size with good chemical and thermal stability but exerts certain toxicity at high doses. So, the addition of biopolymer chitosan will reduce the toxic nature of silica. In addition, the presence of amine groups make them pH-sensitive [66]. The presence of the acidic environment of tumor cells facilitates the swelling of chitosan and enables the easy release of the drug [66,67]. The cytotoxicity of each sample is shown in Figure 3, and it was noted that the curcumin, SCNP, and CSCNP showed significant cytotoxicity towards all tumor cell lines and the toxicities increased with the increasing the concentrations of samples. Studies showed that the curcumin induced different mechanisms of action in each cancer cells. Literature revealed that the curcumin-induced G2/M arrest, inhibiting the assembly dynamics of microtubules, and suppressed the expression of *zeste homolog 2* (*EZH2*) gene in breast cancer cell line MCF-7 [68]. Wu et al., pointed out that curcumin induces apoptosis in human non-small cell lung cancer NCI-H460 cells through the endoplasmic reticulum (ER) stress and caspase cascade and mitochondrial-dependent pathways [57]. HeLa cells were more sensitive to the samples, whereas MCF-7 and MKN-28 were more tolerant to the samples. The IC_{50} values of CSCNP were lower than that of the curcumin and SCNP. The highest difference in the percentage of IC_{50} value was observed in Hep G2 cells (Table 2). Therefore, further analysis was conducted based on Hep G2 cells. Previous studies also show that both silica and curcumin nanoparticles have the ability to produce cytotoxicity towards Hep G2 cells [69,70]. A previous study reported the significant reduction of cancer cells by curcumin nanoparticle as compared to free curcumin. It suggested the internalization and localization of drug-loaded nanoparticles into the cancer cells [71]. Hepatocellular carcinoma is known the cancer that causes the third most deaths worldwide [72]. HepG2 cells are used as a model for liver cancer because of the wild apoptotic p53 gene, high expression of COX-2, phenotypically more hepatocytic than others, and expresses many differentiated essential hepatic functions [73]. The cytotoxicity of curcumin, SCNP, and CSCNP were particularly evaluated in Hep G2 cells using MTT assay in both dose-dependent and time-dependent manners. The viability of Hep G2 cells was gradually dropped after curcumin, SCNP, and CSCNP treatment. CSCNP showed higher cytotoxicity towards Hep G2 cells at a lower concentration (Figure 4a). After 48 h, the cytotoxicity caused by CSCNP was significantly higher than both curcumin and SCNP. Less than 20% of cell viability was observed in CSCNP treated cells (Figure 4b). The dose-dependent relationship of curcumin with the cell viability of Hep G2 cells were reported by Wang et al., in 2011 [44]. They suggested that curcumin altered the cell morphology and promoted apoptosis by triggering pro-apoptotic factors [44]. Recent literature showed that the selenium nanoparticle-coated curcumin induced intracellular ROS production, activated p53, and induced AKT signal pathway [72]. The nanoparticles enter into the cells via endocytosis and the size, shape, stiffness, and surface properties of the nanoparticles will influence the uptake [74]. The nanoparticles are retained in the blood for an appropriate time. Because they are not small enough to be excreted by the kidney and not large enough to be recognized by the reticuloendothelial system (RES). Due to the enhanced permeation and retention effect (EPR), nanoparticle will enter into the tumor cells through leaky vasculature and retained due to reduced lymphatic drainage [75]. As a result, the leaky vascular nature of cancerous cells allows the uptake of more nanoparticles rather than normal cells. Studies reported that curcumin arrests cell growth at G2/M phase and induces apoptosis in the human hepatoma cell line HepG2. The compartmental lipophilic properties of curcumin allow them to localized in the cell membrane. Fluorescent microscopic images of free curcumin and curcumin nanoemulsions on HepG2 cells have shown that the intensity of curcumin faded significantly with time, while the nanoemulsion showed a high intensity after 24 h. This confirmed the gradual release of curcumin from nanoemulsion [76]. LDH is a stable cytoplasmic enzyme that is released from the cells when the plasma membrane is damaged. The LDH release from the cells during apoptosis or necrosis is quantified by measuring the NADH production during the conversion of lactate to pyruvate. This NADH is responsible for the reduction of a tetrazolium salt into formazan [77]. In our study, the LDH leakage in Hep G2 cells was estimated both in dose-dependent and time-dependent manners. The LDH leakage was increased at concentrations between approximately 70~80 µg/mL, indicated that higher concentration of samples can act as an apoptotic inducer. In the case of CSCNP, the LDH leakage was increased with longer duration, which was significantly higher than both curcumin and SCNP. From the results, it was apparent that the curcumin and curcumin nanoparticles promote the apoptosis in cancer cells and it was confirmed by MTT and LDH leakage assays (Figure 5). These results agreed with a previous study in which the cell viability decreased with higher concentrations of the silica nanoparticles on cancerous cells through inducing cell membrane damage [53]. In cancer cells, the formation of lactate occurred due to the conversion of aerobic conditions to anaerobic conditions (Warburg effect). Literature indicated that LDH plays a crucial role in Warburg effect [78]. LDH convert pyruvate to lactate under anaerobic condition and identified as a biomarker of glycolytic activity. Tumor invasion, initiation, metastasis, and recurrence are associated with LDH and lactate production [79].

During apoptosis, the condensation of cytoplasm and plasma membrane blebbing lead to the breakdown of nuclear DNA. The chromosomal DNA was cleaved into multiples of ~200bp oligonucleosomal size fragments during apoptosis [80]. The DNA fragmentation was assessed by electrophoresis. Figure S1 indicated that curcumin and curcumin nanoparticles promote apoptosis of Hep G2 cells by stimulating the DNA fragmentation and CSCNP caused more amount of DNA fragmentation than curcumin and SCNP. The expression of death receptor 5 (DR5) is an indicator of cell apoptosis. DR5 and/or DR4 promote cell death via TNF-related apoptosis-inducing ligand (TRAIL). Dominant-negative mutation in DR4 or DR5 that inhibits the apoptosis pathway is one of the characteristics of cancerous cells [81]. Because of the presence of a large number of a decoy receptors, TRAIL-mediated apoptosis does not cause toxicity to normal cells. Previous studies showed that curcumin promotes the upregulations of DR5 accompanying ROS generation and makes cells more sensitive to the cytotoxic activity of TRAIL [82]. Figure S2 showed that the DR5 expression in curcumin-treated cells were higher than that of nanoparticles. The lower expression of DR5 in Hep G2 cells may be due to the fact that nanoparticles do not interfere with the DR5 involved pathway. Further studies such as DR5 downstream event analysis or changes of sensitivity of the receptor and caspase assay (DNA fragmentation) are needed to confirm the activity of nanoencapsulated curcumin on cancer cells.

Recent literature showed that the chemical instability, low bioavailability, and poor water dispersibility of curcumin have been improved by encapsulation [83]. The stability and efficiency of curcumin and nanoparticles were determined via MTT assay and an anti-oxidation test. After 80 days of storage, the IC_{50} values of curcumin increased significantly but nanoparticles showed only a slight difference on day 0. The efficiencies of both SCNP and CSCNP were higher than 80% indicated the stability of the particles was still acceptable after 80 days. After irradiation with UV light, the antioxidant activity of curcumin was reduced. The decrease in the ability to scavenge DPPH free radicals is mainly due to the decomposition of curcumin by UV light. The DPPH scavenging EC_{50} efficiencies of SCNP and CSCNP were significantly higher than that of curcumin. It is concluded that nanoencapsulation improves the instability of curcumin and helps to stimulate its anti-oxidant and antitumor properties via promoting cell membrane leakage and DNA damage.

Curcumin is generally recognized as a safe material by the Food and Drug Administration (FDA) and are nontoxic, non-mutagenic, and non-genotoxic in nature [84]. The pathways involved in the anti-tumor activity of curcumin may originate from cyclin-dependent, (b) p53-dependent and (c) p53-independent pathways [85]. Literature indicated that the effect of curcumin in cancer cells and normal cells are different. A low level of glutathione and a high level of NF-κB in cancer cells make them more sensitive towards curcumin [86]. The neovasculature of the tumor cell is characterized by impaired vessel and widespread blood vessel. Consequently, the leaky vascular nature of tumor cell provides the easy entry for the nanoparticles to move across cell membrane [87]. It was observed that both SCNP and CSCNP induced potential cytotoxicity to several cancer cell line particularly, to Hep G2 cells (demonstrated in Table 2). The cytotoxicity of nanoparticles was significantly higher than the pure curcumin. Our results demonstrated that nanoencapsulation of curcumin with silica and chitosan not only increase curcumin stability but also enhance cytotoxic activity and LDH leakage on hepatocellular carcinoma cells. This study provided initial data regarding potential cytotoxic activity of SCNP and CSCNP in different cancer cell lines and can be considered as a novel drug delivery system for increasing the bioavailability of curcumin,

4. Materials and Methods

4.1. Materials

Human melanoma cell line A375, human lung carcinoma cell lineA549, human cervical squamous carcinoma cell line HeLa, human hepatoma cell line Hep G2, human colon carcinoma cell line HT-29, human breast carcinoma cell line MCF-7, and human gastric adenocarcinoma cell line MKN-28 were purchased from the American Type Culture Collection (ATCC) and Dr. Murakami's Research Laboratory, Kyushu University, Japan. Dulbecco's modified Eagle's medium (DMEM) and trypsin- ethylenediaminetetraacetic acid (EDTA) were obtained from Invitrogen, California, USA. Fetal bovine serum (FBS) was purchased from HyClone (Logan, UT, USA). Aquaresin Turmeric was purchased from KALSCE®, Michigan, USA. Sodium silicate solution was obtained from Wako Pure Chemical, Osaka, Japan. Chitosan was obtained from LYTONE Enterprise. Inc., Taipei, Taiwan. 2,2-diphenyl-1-picrylhydrazyl (DPPH) and 3-(4,5-dimethylthiazol-2-yl)-2,5-diphenyltetrazolium bromide (MTT) were purchased from Sigma Aldrich, Missouri, USA. Lactate dehydrogenase (LDH) leakage kit was acquired from Promega, Wisconsin,

USA. PE-conjugated anti-human DR5 was purchased from ebioscience, San Diego, CA, USA. Ferrous chloride and ferrozine (3-(2-pyridyl)-5,6-diphenyl-1,2,4-triazine-4′,4″-disulfonic acid sodium salt) were purchased from Sigma, St. Louis, MO, USA.

4.2. Methods

4.2.1. Cell Culture

All cells (except human gastric adenocarcinoma cell line MKN-28) were cultured in Dulbecco's modified Eagle's medium (DMEM) supplemented with 10% FBS at 37 °C in a 5% CO_2 incubator. Roswell Park Memorial Institute (RPMI) 1640 Medium was used for human gastric adenocarcinoma cell line MKN-28.

4.2.2. Preparation of Nano-Encapsulated Curcumin

Chitosan samples were purchased from a commercial supplier were analyzed for the degree of deacetylation (DD) and molecular weight (Mw) according to previous reports [88]. The DD of chitosan samples were 90% with an Mw of 20kDa; 0.82% (*w/w*) sodium silicate solution was prepared by dissolving in 100 mL, 0.05 M sodium acetate buffer and stirred for 3 min [89]. Later, silica encapsulated curcumin nanoparticles (SCNP) were prepared by adding 10 mL curcumin solution to the above solution under strong agitation condition. The nanoencapsulated curcumin obtained was centrifuged (26,100× *g*) and freeze-dried. Chitosan with silica co-encapsulated curcumin nanoparticles (CSCNP) were obtained by stirring the mixture of sodium citrate solution, the chitosan solution, and curcumin solution (10:1:1) for three days. After centrifugation (26,100× *g*), the supernatants were discarded, dialyzed (one day), and freeze-dried [53].

4.2.3. Characterization of Nano-Encapsulated Curcumin

The particle size was measured by using dynamic light scattering (DLS) method using Malvern 4700c submicron particle analyzer (Malvern Instruments, Malvern, Worcestershire, UK). 0.1 g of nanoencapsulated curcumin particles were dispersed in 50 mL deionized water and sonicated for 30 min before the analysis. Hitachi S-4800 scanning electron microscope (SEM) was used to observe the size and morphology of the nanoparticles. Lyophilized nanoparticles were transferred to carbon discs and coated with a gold layer at an accelerating voltage of 20 kV.

4.2.4. 2,2-diphenyl-1-picrylhydrazyl (DPPH) Radical Scavenging Activity

100 µL of samples were added to 100 µL of freshly prepared 1 mM DPPH solution and stirred for 30 min at room temperature. The absorbance was measured at 517 nm. The concentration at which scavenged 50% (EC50) was determined by linear interpolation [90].

$$\% \text{ DPPH inhibition} = [1 - (A517_{sample}/A517_{blank})] \times 100 \quad (1)$$

4.2.5. Determination of the Ability to Chelate Ferrous Ions

0.5 mL of Methanol and 0.025 mL of 2 mM Iron (II) chloride were added to 0.5 mL of different concentrations of the samples. After 30 s, 0.05 mL of 5 mM ferrozine was added. After 10 min, the absorbance was measured at 562 nm using a spectrophotometer [91].

$$\text{Chelating ratio \%} = [1 - (\text{sample A562} - \text{background value A562}) / (\text{control group A562} - \text{background value A562})] \times 100 \quad (2)$$

4.2.6. Cell Viability Assay

2×10^5 cells/mL (100 µL/well) were seeded into 96-well plate containing medium supplemented with 2% FBS and incubated in 5% CO_2 incubator for overnight. Cells were treated with 20 µL of different concentrations of samples and incubated for 12–48 h. Later, the medium was aspirated from the wells and 120 µL of fresh medium was added. After 1 hour, 100 µL of the MTT solution (0.5 mg/mL) was added to the cells and incubated for 4 h. The absorbance was measured at 570 nm. The concentration at which cell growth was inhibited by 50% (the 50% inhibitory concentration (IC_{50}) was determined by linear interpolation [(50% − low percentage)/(high percentage − low percentage)] × (high concentration − low concentration) + low concentration] [92].

$$\text{Relative viability (\%)} = [A \text{ sample}]/[A \text{ control}] \times 100 \tag{3}$$

where [A]sample and [A]control denote the absorbance of the sample and control, respectively [53].

4.2.7. Lactate Dehydrogenase Leakage Assay

The CytoTox96 nonradioactive assay kit (LDH assay) was used to perform the LDH assay. Hep G2 cells were seeded in 96-well plates, exposed to samples, and incubated for 48 h. After incubation, the 96-well plates were centrifuged at 430× g for 5 min and the cell medium was transferred to another new 96-well plates (50 µL/well). After the addition of LDH substrate (50 µL/well), the plates were kept under a dark atmosphere for 30 min. 1N hydrochloric acid (HCl) (25 µL/well) was then added to each sample to terminate the reaction. The absorbance was measured at 490 nm. Control experiments were performed with 0.1% (*w/v*) Triton X-100 set as 100% cytotoxicity.

LDH release was calculated by the following equation:

$$\text{LDH (\%)} = ([A]\text{sample} - [A]\text{medium})/([A]100\% - [A]\text{medium}) \times 100 \tag{4}$$

where [A]sample, [A]medium, [A] 100% denote the absorbance of the sample, medium control, and Triton X-100 control, respectively. All experiments were run in triplicate [53].

4.2.8. DNA Fragmentation

Hep G2 cells were seeded into 10 cm dishes at a density of 2×10^5 cells/mL (10 mL/dish) in medium supplemented with 2% FBS and incubated overnight. Different concentrations of nanoparticles were added to dishes (2 mL/dish) under the dark condition and incubated for 12–48 hours. After treatment, the cells were centrifuged at 250× g. Cells were lysed in a buffer containing 10 mM Tris (pH 7.4), 150 mM NaCl, 5 mM EDTA and 0.5% Triton X-100 for 10 min on ice. Lysates were vortexed and centrifuged at 14,000× g for 10 min. Fragmented DNA in the supernatant was extracted with an equal volume of neutral phenol: chloroform: isoamyl alcohol mixture (25:24:1) and analyzed electrophoretically on 2% agarose gels. Later, stained with ethidium bromide, and imaged with a FluoroImager (Pharmacia Biotech, D & R, Israel) [82].

4.2.9. Analysis of Cell Surface Death Receptor 5 (DR5)

The cell number was adjusted to 2×10^5. After the incubation with samples for one day, the cells were detached with 0.5 mM EDTA and washed three times with phosphate-buffered saline (PBS) wash buffer supplemented with 0.5% bovine serum albumin (BSA). Cells were resuspended in 200 µL of PBS, stained with the PE-conjugated anti-human DR5 (ebioscience, San Diego, CA) antibody (1 µg/mL) and incubated for 30 min at 4 °C. The unreacted antibody was removed by washing the cells twice with the same PBS buffer. Cell surface expression of the DR5 receptor was determined by flow cytometry (FACscan, BD Biosciences, Franklin Lake, NJ, USA). Fluorescent intensity of the cells is directly proportional to the density of receptor [82].

4.2.10. Storage Test

Curcumin was dissolved in dimethyl sulfoxide (DMSO, Sigma-Aldrich Company, St. Louis, MO, USA) and nano-encapsulated curcumin was dissolved in distilled-deionized water.

The final volume was adjusted to 10 mL and the concentration of DMSO was 0.1%. The samples were stored in a moisture proof cabinet and protected from light for 80 days. The cell viability and DPPH radical scavenging activity were analyzed according to Sections 4.2.4 and 4.2.6, respectively.

4.3. Statistical Analysis

Data were expressed as means ± SD and analyzed using Student's *t*-test of Sigma Plot 9.

Supplementary Materials: Supplementary materials can be found at http://www.mdpi.com/1422-0067/20/12/2918/s1.

Author Contributions: Conceptualization, supervision, Z.-L.K., and K.L.B.C.; formal analysis, L.-C.W.; writing—original draft preparation, A.J., L.-C.W., and H.-P.K.; writing—review and editing, Z.-L.K., A.J. and H.-P.K.

Funding: This work was financially supported by the Centre of Excellence for the Oceans, National Taiwan Ocean University, from the Featured Areas Research Centre Program within the framework of Higher Education Sprout Project by the Ministry of Education (MOE), Taiwan. This work also received a grant from the Ministry of Science and Technology (MOST 106-2320-B-019-006), Taiwan.

Acknowledgments: The authors have no any further acknowledgments.

Conflicts of Interest: The authors declare no conflict of interest.

Abbreviations

SCNP	silica encapsulated curcumin nanoparticles
CSCNP	chitosan with silica co-encapsulated curcumin nanoparticles
MSNs	mesoporous silica nanoparticles
EPR	enhanced permeability and retention effect
ROS	reactive oxygen species
DR5	death receptor 5
DISC	death-inducing signaling complex

References

1. Hassanpour, S.H.; Dehghani, M. Review of cancer from perspective of molecular. *J. Cancer Res. Pract.* **2017**, *4*, 127–129. [CrossRef]
2. Carr, I.; Orr, F.W. Invasion and metastasis. *Can. Med. Assoc. J.* **1983**, *128*, 1164–1167.
3. Hanahan, D.; Weinberg, R.A. Hallmarks of cancer: The next generation. *Cell* **2011**, *144*, 646–674. [CrossRef] [PubMed]
4. Debatin, K.M. Apoptosis pathways in cancer and cancer therapy. *Cancer Immunol. Immunother.* **2004**, *53*, 153–159. [CrossRef]
5. Lowe, S.W.; Lin, A.W. Apoptosis in cancer. *Carcinogenesis* **2000**, *21*, 485–495. [CrossRef] [PubMed]
6. Wallace-Brodeur, R.R.; Lowe, S.W. Clinical implications of p53 mutations. *Cell. Mol. Life Sci.* **1999**, *55*, 64–75. [CrossRef] [PubMed]
7. Eastman, A. Improving anticancer drug development begins with cell culture: Misinformation perpetrated by the misuse of cytotoxicity assays. *Oncotarget* **2016**, *8*, 8854–8866. [CrossRef] [PubMed]
8. Letai, A. Apoptosis and Cancer. *Annu. Rev. Cancer Biol.* **2017**, *1*, 275–294. [CrossRef]
9. Bharti, C.; Nagaich, U.; Pal, A.K.; Gulati, N. Mesoporous silica nanoparticles in target drug delivery system: A review. *Int. J. Pharm. Investig.* **2015**, *5*, 124–133. [CrossRef] [PubMed]
10. Zhou, Y.; Quan, G.; Wu, Q.; Zhang, X.; Niu, B.; Wu, B.; Huang, Y.; Pan, X.; Wu, C. Mesoporous silica nanoparticles for drug and gene delivery. *Acta Pharm. Sin. B* **2018**, *8*, 165–177. [CrossRef]
11. Luan, P.-P.; Jiang, Y.-J.; Zhang, S.-P.; Gao, J.; Zu, Z.-J.; Ma, G.-H.; Zhang, Y.-F. Chitosan-mediated formation of biomimetic silica nanoparticles: An effective method for manganese peroxidase immobilization and stabilization. *J. Biosci. Bioeng.* **2014**, *118*, 575–582. [CrossRef] [PubMed]
12. Liu, W.; Wang, F.; Zhu, Y.; Li, X.; Liu, X.; Pang, J.; Pan, W. Galactosylated chitosan-functionalized mesoporous silica nanoparticle loading by calcium leucovorin for colon cancer cell-targeted drug delivery. *Molecules* **2018**, *12*, 3082. [CrossRef]

13. De Queiroz Antonino, R.S.C.M.; Lia Fook, B.R.P.; de Oliveira Lima, V.A.; de Farias Rached, R.Í.; Lima, E.P.N.; da Silva Lima, R.J.; Peniche Covas, C.A.; Lia Fook, M.V. Preparation and Characterization of Chitosan Obtained from Shells of Shrimp (Litopenaeus vannamei Boone). *Mar. Drugs* **2017**, *15*, 141. [CrossRef] [PubMed]
14. Bernkop-Schnürch, A.; Dünnhaupt, S. Chitosan-based drug delivery systems. *Eur. J. Pharm. Biopharm.* **2012**, *81*, 463–469. [CrossRef] [PubMed]
15. Ahmadi Nasab, N.; Hassani Kumleh, H.; Beygzadeh, M.; Teimourian, S.; Kazemzad, M. Delivery of curcumin by a pH-responsive chitosan mesoporous silica nanoparticles for cancer treatment. *Artif. Cells Nanomed. Biotechnol.* **2018**, *1*, 75–81. [CrossRef] [PubMed]
16. Hewlings, S.J.; Kalman, D.S. Curcumin: A Review of Its' Effects on Human Health. *Foods* **2017**, *6*, 92. [CrossRef]
17. Wilken, R.; Veena, M.S.; Wang, M.B.; Srivatsan, E.S. Curcumin: A review of anti-cancer properties and therapeutic activity in head and neck squamous cell carcinoma. *Mol. Cancer* **2011**, *10*, 12. [CrossRef] [PubMed]
18. Deng, Y.I.; Verron, E.; Rohanizadeh, R. Molecular mechanisms of anti-metastatic activity of curcumin. *Anticancer Res.* **2016**, *36*, 5639–5647. [CrossRef]
19. Alok, A.; Singh, I.D.; Singh, S.; Kishore, M.; Jha, P.C. Curcumin—Pharmacological Actions And its Role in Oral Submucous Fibrosis: A Review. *J. Clin. Diagn. Res.* **2015**, *9*, ZE1–ZE3. [CrossRef]
20. Goel, A.; Boland, C.R.; Chauhan, D.P. Specific inhibition of cyclooxygenase-2 (COX-2) expression by dietary curcumin in HT-29 human colon cancer cells. *Cancer Lett.* **2001**, *172*, 111–118. [CrossRef]
21. Tuorkey, M.J. Curcumin a potent cancer preventive agent: Mechanisms of cancer cell killing. *Interv. Med. Appl. Sci.* **2014**, *6*, 139–146. [CrossRef] [PubMed]
22. Reeves, A.; Vinogradov, S.V.; Morrissey, P.; Chernin, M.; Ahmed, M.M. Curcumin-encapsulating Nanogels as an Effective Anticancer Formulation for Intracellular Uptake. *Mol. Cell. Pharmacol.* **2015**, *7*, 25–40. [CrossRef] [PubMed]
23. Wang, X.; Hang, Y.; Liu, J.; Hou, Y.; Wang, N.; Wang, M. Anticancer effect of curcumin inhibits cell growth through miR-21/PTEN/Akt pathway in breast cancer cell. *Oncol. Lett.* **2017**, *13*, 4825–4831. [CrossRef] [PubMed]
24. Pan, Z.; Zhuang, J.; Ji, C.; Cai, Z.; Liao, W.; Huang, Z. Curcumin inhibits hepatocellular carcinoma growth by targeting VEGF expression. *Oncol. Lett.* **2018**, *15*, 4821–4826. [CrossRef] [PubMed]
25. Wu, G.Q.; Chai, K.Q.; Zhu, X.M.; Jiang, H.; Wang, X.; Xue, Q.; Zheng, A.H.; Zhou, H.Y.; Chen, Y.; Chen, X.C.; et al. Anti-cancer effects of curcumin on lung cancer through the inhibition of EZH2 and NOTCH1. *Oncotarget* **2016**, *7*, 26535–26550. [CrossRef]
26. Hussain, Z.; Thu, H.E.; Ng, S.F.; Khan, S.; Katas, H. Nanoencapsulation, an efficient and promising approach to maximize wound healing efficacy of curcumin: A review of new trends and state-of-the-art. *Colloids Surf B Biointerfaces* **2017**, *150*, 223–241. [CrossRef] [PubMed]
27. Li, J.; Niu, R.; Dong, L.; Gao, L.; Zhang, J.; Zheng, Y.; Shi, M.; Liu, Z.; Li, K. Nanoencapsulation of curcumin and its protective effects against CCl_4-induced hepatotoxicity in mice. *J. Nanomater.* **2019**, *2019*. [CrossRef]
28. Farajzadeh, R.; Pilehvar-Soltanahmadi, Y.; Dadashpour, M.; Javidfar, S.; Lotfi-Attari, J.; Sadeghzadeh, H.; Shafiei-Irannejad, V.; Zarghami, N. Nano-encapsulated metformin-curcumin in PLGA/PEG inhibits synergistically growth and hTERT gene expression in human breast cancer cells. *Artif. Cells Nanomed. Biotechnol.* **2018**, *46*, 917–925. [CrossRef]
29. Anitha, A.; Sreeranganathan, M.; Chennazhi, K.P.; Lakshmanan, V.K.; Jayakumar, R. In vitro combinatorial anticancer effects of 5-fluorouracil and curcumin loaded N,O-carboxymethyl chitosan nanoparticles toward colon cancer and in vivo pharmacokinetic studies. *Eur. J. Pharm. Biopharm.* **2014**, *88*, 238–251. [CrossRef] [PubMed]
30. Song, W.; Su, X.; Gregory, D.A.; Li, W.; Cai, Z.; Zhao, W. Magnetic alginate/chitosan nanoparticles for targeted delivery of curcumin into human breast cancer cells. *Nanomaterials* **2018**, *11*, 907. [CrossRef]
31. Zhang, J.; Li, S.; An, F.-F.; Liu, J.; Jin, S.; Zhang, J.-C.; Wang, P.-C.; Zhang, X.; Lee, C.-S.; Liang, S.-J. Self-carried curcumin nanoparticles for in vitro and in vivo cancer therapy with real-time monitoring of drug release. *Nanoscale* **2015**, *7*, 13503–13510. [CrossRef]

32. Khosropanah, M.H.; Dinarvand, A.; Nezhadhosseini, A.; Haghighi, A.; Hashemi, S.; Nirouzad, F.; Khatamsaz, S.; Entezari, M.; Hashemi, M.; Dehghani, H. Analysis of the antiproliferative effects of curcumin and nanocurcumin in MDA-MB231 as a breast cancer cell line. *Iran. J. Pharm. Res.* **2016**, *15*, 231–239.
33. Hosseini, S.; Chamani, J.; Rahimi, H.; Azmoodeh, N.; Ghasemi, F.; Abadi, P.H. An in vitro study on curcumin delivery by nano-micelles for esophageal squamous cell carcinoma (KYSE-30). *Rep. Biochem. Mol. Biol.* **2018**, *6*, 137–143.
34. Katt, M.E.; Placone, A.L.; Wong, A.D.; Xu, Z.S.; Searson, P.C. In vitro tumor models: Advantages, disadvantages, variables, and selecting the right platform. *Front. Bioeng. Biotechnol.* **2016**, *4*, 12. [CrossRef]
35. Zhang, Z.; Zhang, R.; Zou, L.; Chen, L.; Ahmed, Y.; Bishri, W.A.; Balamash, K.; McClements, D.J. Encapsulation of curcumin in polysaccharide-based hydrogel beads: Impact of bead type on lipid digestion and curcumin bioaccessibility. *Food Hydrocoll.* **2016**, *58*, 160–170. [CrossRef]
36. Xin, Y.; Yin, M.; Zhao, L.; Meng, F.; Luo, L. Recent progress on nanoparticle-based drug delivery systems for cancer therapy. *Cancer Biol. Med.* **2017**, *14*, 228–241. [CrossRef]
37. Reuter, S.; Gupta, S.C.; Chaturvedi, M.M.; Aggarwal, B.B. Oxidative stress, inflammation, and cancer: How are they linked? *Free Radic. Biol. Med.* **2010**, *49*, 1603–1616. [CrossRef]
38. Sánchez, Y.; Simón, G.P.; Calviño, E.; de Blas, E.; Aller, P. Curcumin stimulates reactive oxygen species production and potentiates apoptosis induction by the antitumor drugs arsenic trioxide and lonidamine in human myeloid leukemia cell lines. *J. Pharmacol. Exp. Ther.* **2010**, *335*, 114–123. [CrossRef]
39. Huang, X.; Huang, X.; Gong, Y.; Xiao, H.; Mc Clements, D.J.; Hu, K. Enhancement of curcumin water dispersibility and antioxidant activity using core-shell protein-polysaccharide nanoparticles. *Food Res. Int.* **2016**, *87*, 1–9. [CrossRef]
40. Feitelson, M.A.; Arzumanyan, A.; Kulathinal, R.J.; Blain, S.W.; Holcombe, R.F.; Mahajna, J.; Marino, M.; Martinez-Chantar, M.L.; Nawroth, R.; Sanchez-Garcia, I.; et al. Sustained proliferation in cancer: Mechanisms and novel therapeutic targets. *Semin. Cancer Biol.* **2015**, *35*, S25–S54. [CrossRef]
41. Ravindran, J.; Prasad, S.; Aggarwal, B.B. Curcumin and cancer cells: How many ways can curry kill tumor cells selectively? *AAPS J.* **2009**, *11*, 495–510. [CrossRef]
42. Syng-Ai, C.; Kumari, A.L.; Khar, A. Effect of curcumin on normal and tumor cells: Role of glutathione and bcl-2. *Mol. Cancer Ther.* **2004**, *3*, 1101–1108.
43. Duan, J.; Zhang, Y.; Han, S.; Chen, Y.; Li, B.; Liao, M.; Chen, W.; Deng, X.; Zhao, J.; Huang, B. Synthesis and in vitro/in vivo anti-cancer evaluation of curcumin-loaded chitosan/poly(butyl cyanoacrylate) nanoparticles. *Int. J. Pharm.* **2010**, *1*, 211–220. [CrossRef]
44. Wang, M.; Ruan, Y.; Chen, Q.; Li, S.; Wang, Q.; Cai, J. Curcumin induced HepG2 cell apoptosis-associated mitochondrial membrane potential and intracellular free Ca (2+) concentration. *Eur. J. Pharmacol.* **2011**, *650*, 41–47. [CrossRef]
45. Jurisic, V.; Bumbasirevic, V. In vitro assays for cell death determination. *Arch. Oncol.* **2008**, *16*, 49–54. [CrossRef]
46. Khodarev, N.N.; Sokolova, I.A.; Vaughan, A.T.M. Review Mechanisms of induction of apoptotic DNA fragmentation. *Int. J. Radiat.* **1998**, *73*, 455–467. [CrossRef]
47. Zorofchian Moghadamtousi, S.; Kadir, H.A.; Hassandarvish, P.; Tajik, H.; Abubakar, S.; Zandi, K. A Review on Antibacterial, Antiviral, and Antifungal Activity of Curcumin. *BioMed. Res. Int.* **2014**, *2014*, 12. [CrossRef]
48. Maheshwari, R.K.; Singh, A.K.; Gaddipati, J.; Srimal, R.C. Multiple biological activities of curcumin: A short review. *Life Sci.* **2006**, *78*, 2081–2087. [CrossRef]
49. Chattopadhyay, I.; Biswas, K.; Bandyopadhyay, U.; Banerjee, R.K. Turmeric and Curcumin: Biological actions and medicinal applications. *Curr. Sci.* **2003**, *87*, 44–53.
50. Yin, H.; Zhang, H.; Liu, B. Superior anticancer efficacy of curcumin-loaded nanoparticles against lung cancer. *Acta Biochim. Biophys. Sin.* **2013**, *8*, 634–640. [CrossRef]
51. Watermann, A.; Brieger, J. Mesoporous Silica Nanoparticles as Drug Delivery Vehicles in Cancer. *Nanomaterials* **2017**, *7*, 189. [CrossRef]
52. Wang, J.J.; Zeng, Z.W.; Xiao, R.Z.; Xie, T.; Zhou, G.L.; Zhan, X.R.; Wang, S.L. Recent advances of chitosan nanoparticles as drug carriers. *Int. J. Nanomed.* **2011**, *6*, 765–774. [CrossRef]
53. Chang, J.-S.; Chang, K.L.B.; Hwang, D.-F.; Kong, Z.-L. In vitro cytotoxicitiy of silica nanoparticles at high concentrations strongly depends on the metabolic activity type of the cell line. *Environ. Sci. Technol.* **2007**, *41*, 2064–2068. [CrossRef]

54. Bahrami, B.; Hojjat-Farsangi, M.; Mohammadi, H.; Anvari, E.; Ghalamfarsa, G.; Yousefi, M.; Jadidi-Niaragh, F. Nanoparticles and targeted drug delivery in cancer therapy. *Immunol. Lett.* **2017**, *190*, 64–83. [CrossRef]
55. Nimse, S.B.; Pal, D. Free radicals, natural antioxidants, and their reaction mechanisms. *RSC Adv.* **2015**, *5*, 27986–28006. [CrossRef]
56. Khan, M.A.; Gahlot, S.; Majumdar, S. Oxidative stress induced by curcumin promotes the death of cutaneous T-cell lymphoma (HuT-78) by disrupting the function of several olecular targets. *Mol. Cancer Ther.* **2012**, *11*, 1873–1883. [CrossRef]
57. Wu, S.H.; Hang, L.W.; Yang, J.S.; Chen, H.Y.; Lin, H.Y.; Chiang, J.H.; Lu, C.C.; Yang, J.L.; Lai, T.Y.; Ko, Y.C.; et al. Curcumin Induces Apoptosis in Human Non-small Cell Lung Cancer NCI-H460 Cells through ER Stress and Caspase Cascade-and Mitochondria-dependent Pathways. *Anticancer Res.* **2010**, *30*, 2125–2133.
58. Kedare, S.B.; Singh, R.P. Genesis and development of DPPH method of antioxidant assay. *J. Food Sci. Technol.* **2011**, *48*, 412–422. [CrossRef]
59. Sudan, R.; Bhagat, M.; Gupta, S.; Singh, J.; Koul, A. Iron (FeII) Chelation, Ferric Reducing Antioxidant Power, and Immune Modulating Potential of Arisaema jacquemontii (Himalayan Cobra Lily). *J. BioMed. Res. Int.* **2014**, *2014*, 179865. [CrossRef]
60. Rajalakshmi, A.; Krithiga, N.; Jayachitra, A. Antioxidant activity of the chitosan extracted from shrimp exoskeleton. *Middle East J. Sci. Res.* **2013**, *16*, 1446–1451. [CrossRef]
61. Pathak, L.; Kanwal, A.; Agrawal, Y. Curcumin loaded self assembled lipid-biopolymer nanoparticles for functional food applications. *J. Food Sci. Technol.* **2015**, *10*, 6143–6156. [CrossRef]
62. Fan, Y.; Yi, J.; Zhang, Y.; Yokoyama, W. Improved chemical stability and antiproliferative activities of curcumin-loaded nanoparticles with a chitosan chlorogenic acid conjugate. *J. Agric. Food Chem.* **2017**, *49*, 10812–10819. [CrossRef]
63. Florento, L.; Matias, R.; Tuaño, E.; Santiago, K.; Dela Cruz, F.; Tuazon, A. Comparison of Cytotoxic Activity of Anticancer Drugs against Various Human Tumor Cell Lines Using In Vitro Cell-Based Approach. *Int. J. Biomed. Sci.* **2012**, *8*, 76–80.
64. Kean, T.; Thanou, M. Biodegradation, biodistribution and toxicity of chitosan. *Adv. Drug Deliv. Rev.* **2010**, *62*, 3–11. [CrossRef]
65. Mai, W.X.; Meng, H. Mesoporous silica nanoparticles: A multifunctional nano therapeutic system. *Integr. Biol.* **2013**, *5*, 19–28. [CrossRef]
66. Liu, W.T. Facile and simple preparation of pH-sensitive chitosan-mesoporous silica nanoparticles for future breast cancer treatment. *Express Polym. Lett.* **2015**, *9*, 1068–1075. [CrossRef]
67. Kato, Y.; Ozawa, S.; Miyamoto, C.; Maehata, Y.; Suzuki, A.; Maeda, T.; Baba, Y. Acidic extracellular microenvironment and cancer. *Cancer Cell Int.* **2013**, *13*, 89. [CrossRef]
68. Liu, D.; Chen, Z. The effect of curcumin on breast cancer cells. *J. Breast Cancer* **2013**, *16*, 133–137. [CrossRef]
69. Loutfy, S.A.; El-Din, H.M.A.; Elberry, M.H.; Allam, N.G.; Hasanin, M.T.M.; Abdellah, A.M. Synthesis, characterization and cytotoxic evaluation of chitosan nanoparticles: In vitro liver cancer model. *ANSN* **2016**, *7*, 1–9. [CrossRef]
70. Lu, X.; Qian, J.; Zhou, H.; Gan, Q.; Tang, W.; Lu, J.; Yuan, Y.; Liu, C. In vitro cytotoxicity and induction of apoptosis by silica nanoparticles in human HepG2 hepatoma cells. *Int. J. Nanomed.* **2011**, *6*, 1889–1901. [CrossRef]
71. Punfa, W.; Yodkeeree, S.; Pitchakarn, P.; Ampasavate, C.; Limtrakul, P. Enhancement of cellular uptake and cytotoxicity of curcumin-loaded PLGA nanoparticles by conjugation with anti-P-glycoprotein in drug resistance cancer cells. *Acta Pharmacol. Sin.* **2012**, *6*, 823–831. [CrossRef]
72. Guo, M.; Li, Y.; Lin, Z.; Zhao, M.; Xiao, M.; Wang, C.; Xu, T.; Xia, Y.; Zhu, B. Surface decoration of selenium nanoparticles with curcumin induced HepG2 cell apoptosis through ROS mediated p53 and AKT signaling pathways. *RSC Adv.* **2017**, *7*, 52456–52464. [CrossRef]
73. Abdallah, F.M.; Helmy, M.W.; Katary, M.A.; Ghoneim, A.I. Synergistic antiproliferative effects of curcumin and celecoxib in hepatocellular carcinoma HepG2 cells. *Naunyn Schmiedebergs Arch. Pharmacol.* **2018**, *391*, 1399–1410. [CrossRef]
74. Zhao, J.; Stenzel, M.H. Entry of nanoparticles into cells: The importance of nanoparticle properties. *Polym. Chem.* **2018**, *9*, 259–272. [CrossRef]
75. Nakamura, Y.; Mochida, A.; Choyke, P.L.; Kobayashi, H. Nanodrug delivery: Is the enhanced permeability and retention effect sufficient for curing cancer? *Bioconjug. Chem.* **2016**, *27*, 2225–2238. [CrossRef]

76. Ucisik, M.H.; Küpcü, S.; Schuster, B.; Sleytr, U.B. Characterization of curcuemulsomes: Nanoformulation for enhanced solubility anddelivery of curcumin. *J. Nanobiotechnol.* **2013**, *1*, 1–13. [CrossRef]
77. Kumar, P.; Nagarajan, A.; Uchil, P.D. Analysis of Cell Viability by the Lactate Dehydrogenase Assay. *Cold Spring Harb. Protoc.* **2018**, *2018*. [CrossRef]
78. Jurisic, V.; Radenkovic, S.; Konjevic, G. The actual role of LDH as tumor marker, biochemical and clinical aspects. *Adv. Exp. Med. Biol.* **2015**, *867*, 115–124. [CrossRef]
79. Miao, P.; Sheng, S.; Sun, X.; Liu, J.; Huang, G. Lactate dehydrogenase a in cancer: A promising target for diagnosis and therapy. *IUBMB Life* **2013**, *65*, 904–910. [CrossRef]
80. Loannou, Y.A.; Chen, F.W. Quantitation of DNA Fragmentation in Apoptosis. *Nucleic Acids Res.* **1996**, *24*, 992–993. [CrossRef]
81. Di, X.; Zhang, G.; Zhang, Y.; Takeda, K.; Rosado, L.A.R.; Zhang, B. Accumulation of autophagosomes in breast cancer cells induces TRAIL resistance through downregulation of surface expression of death receptors 4 and 5. *Oncotarget* **2013**, *4*, 1349–1364. [CrossRef]
82. Jung, E.M.; Lim, J.H.; Lee, T.J.; Park, J.W.; Choi, K.S.; Kwon, T.K. Curcumin sensitizes tumor necrosis factor-related apoptosis-inducing ligand (TRAIL)-induced apoptosis through reactive oxygen species-mediated upregulation of death receptor 5 (DR5). *Carcinogenesis* **2005**, *26*, 1905–1913. [CrossRef]
83. Kharat, M.; Du, Z.; Zhang, G.; McClements, D.J. Physical and chemical stability of curcumin in aqueous solutions and emulsions: Impact of pH, temperature, and molecular environment. *J. Agric. Food Chem.* **2016**, *65*, 1525–1532. [CrossRef]
84. Liu, Z.; Huang, P.; Law, S.; Tian, H.; Leung, W.; Xu, C. Preventive effect of curcumin against chemotherapy-induced side-effects. *Front. Pharmacol.* **2018**, *9*, 1374. [CrossRef]
85. Sa, G.; Das, T. Anti cancer effects of curcumin: Cycle of life and death. *Cell Div.* **2008**, *3*, 14. [CrossRef]
86. Allegra, A.; Innao, V.; Russo, S.; Gerace, D.; Alonci, A.; Musolino, C. Anticancer activity of curcumin and its analogues: Preclinical and clinical studies. *Cancer Investig.* **2017**, *35*, 1–22. [CrossRef]
87. Ngoune, R.; Peters, A.; von Elverfeldt, D.; Winkler, K.; Pütz, G. Accumulating nanoparticles by EPR: A route of no return. *J. Control. Release* **2016**, *238*, 58–70. [CrossRef]
88. Chang, K.L.B.; Tai, M.-C.; Cheng, F.-H. Kinetics and products of the degradation of chitosan by hydrogen peroxide. *J. Agric. Food Chem.* **2001**, *49*, 4845–4851. [CrossRef]
89. Chang, J.-S.; Kong, Z.-L.; Hwang, D.-F.; Chang, K.L.B. Chitosan-catalyzed aggregation during the biomimetic synthesis of silica nanoparticles. *Chem. Mater.* **2006**, *18*, 1714. [CrossRef]
90. Blois, M.S. Antioxidant Determinations by the Use of a Stable Free Radical. *Nature* **1958**, *181*, 1199–1200. [CrossRef]
91. Boyer, R.F.; McCleary, C.J. Superoxide ion as a primary reductant in ascorbate-mediated ferretin iron release. *Free Radic. Biol. Med.* **1987**, *3*, 389–395. [CrossRef]
92. Li, L.; Braiteh, F.S.; Kurzrock, R. Liposome-encapsulated curcumin. *Cancer* **2005**, *104*, 1322–1331. [CrossRef]

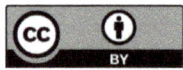

© 2019 by the authors. Licensee MDPI, Basel, Switzerland. This article is an open access article distributed under the terms and conditions of the Creative Commons Attribution (CC BY) license (http://creativecommons.org/licenses/by/4.0/).

MDPI\
St. Alban-Anlage 66\
4052 Basel\
Switzerland\
Tel. +41 61 683 77 34\
Fax +41 61 302 89 18\
www.mdpi.com

International Journal of Molecular Sciences Editorial Office\
E-mail: ijms@mdpi.com\
www.mdpi.com/journal/ijms

www.ingramcontent.com/pod-product-compliance
Lightning Source LLC
LaVergne TN
LVHW071940080526
838202LV00064B/6644